Orthopedic Rehabilitation

Orthopedic Rehabilitation

Edited by

Vernon L. Nickel, M.D.

Professor of Surgery/Orthopedics and Rehabilitation
University of California at San Diego
Director of Rehabilitation
Sharp Rehabilitation Center
San Diego, California

Churchill Livingstone
New York, Edinburgh, London, and Melbourne
1982

© Churchill Livingstone Inc. 1982

Distributed in the United Kingdom by Churchill Livingstone,
Robert Stevenson House, 1–3 Baxter's Place, Leith Walk,
Edinburgh EH1 3AF and associated companies, branches
and representatives throughout the world.

First published 1982
Printed in U.S.A.

ISBN 0-443-08060-7
9 8 7 6 5 4 3 2 1

Library of Congress Cataloging in Publication Data
Main entry under title:

Orthopedic rehabilitation.

   Bibliography: p.
   Includes index.
   1. Physically handicapped—Rehabilitation.
I. Nickel, Vernon L.
RD797.077   617'.3   82-1256
ISBN 0-443-08060-7   AACR2

Manufactured in the United States of America

List of Contributors

Sidney J. Blair, M.D.
Chief, Section of Hand Surgery, Loyola University, Stritch School of Medicine, Maywood, Illinois

Henry H. Bohlman, M.D.
Associate Professor, Department of Orthopedic Surgery, Case Western University Medical School; Chief, Spinal Cord Injury Service, Veterans Administration Medical Center, Cleveland, Ohio

John H. Bowker, M.D.
Professor, Department of Orthopaedic Surgery; Head, Section of Rehabilitation, University of Arkansas College of Medicine; Medical Director, Arkansas Rehabilitation Institute, Little Rock, Arkansas

Richard M. Braun, M.D.
Associate Clinical Professor of Orthopedic Surgery, The University of California at San Diego, San Diego, California; Assistant Clinical Professor and Consultant in Upper Extremity Surgery, Rancho Los Amigos Hospital, The University of Southern California, Los Angeles, California

Ruth Cox Brunings, M.S.W.
Director of Social Work, Rancho Los Amigos Hospital, Downey, California

Wilton H. Bunch, M.D., Ph.D.
Professor and Chairman, Department of Orthopedics and Rehabilitation, Loyola University Medical Center, Maywood, Illinois

Ernest M. Burgess, M.D.
Clinical Professor of Orthopaedic Surgery, University of Washington School of Medicine; Director, Prosthetics Research Study Center, Seattle, Washington

Douglas Cairns, Ph.D.
Head Clinical Psychologist, Rancho Los Amigos Hospital, Downey, California

J. Pierce Conaty, M.D.
Clinical Professor of Orthopaedic Surgery, University of Southern California, Los Angeles, California; Chief, Arthritis Service (Surgical), Rancho Los Amigos Hospital, Downey, California

Gordon L. Engler, M.D.
Director of Scoliosis and Spinal Deformities, New York University Medical Center, New York, New York

William F. Enneking, M.D.
Distinguished Service Professor and Eugene L. Jewett Professor of Orthopaedic Surgery, Department of Orthopaedics, College of Medicine, University of Florida, Gainesville, Florida

E. Burke Evans, M.D.
Professor of Surgery and Chief of Orthopaedic Surgery, University of Texas Medical Branch, Galveston, Texas

Shirley M. Forsgren
Administrator, Prosthetics Research Study, Seattle, Washington

William P. Fortune, M.D.
Professor of Orthopaedic Surgery and Medicine, Department of Orthopaedic Surgery, George Washington University Medical Center, Washington, D.C.

Gary K. Frykman, M.D., F.A.C.S.
Associate Professor of Orthopedic Surgery; Medical Director, Hand Rehabilitation Center, Loma Linda University, Loma Linda, California

Douglas E. Garland, M.D.
Chief, Adult Head Trauma and Problem Fractures Services, Rancho Los Amigos Hospital, Downey, California; Associate Clinical Professor of Orthopedics, University of Southern California, Los Angeles, California

Alice L. Garrett, M.D.
Valley Cottage, New York

Donald R. Gunn, M.B., Ch.B., M.Ch.Orth., F.R.C.S., Ed., D.Sc.Hon.
Clinical Professor of Orthopaedics, University of Washington, Seattle, Washington

Linda Mills Hennig, M.A., R.N.
Director of Nursing, Dallas Rehabilitation Institute, Dallas, Texas

M. Mark Hoffer, M.D.
Chief, Children's Orthopedics, Rancho Los Amigos Hospital, Downey, California; Clinical Professor of Orthopedics and Pediatrics, University of Southern California, Los Angeles, California

Robert W. Hussey, M.D.
Chief, Spinal Cord Injury Service (128), Veterans Administration Medical Center; Associate Professor of Orthopedic Surgery, Medical College of Virginia, Richmond, Virginia

Christopher Jordan, M.D.
Chief, Stroke Service, Rancho Los Amigos Hospital, Downey, California

Robert D. Keagy, M.D.
Associate Professor of Clinical Orthopaedic Surgery, Northwestern University Medical School; Lecturer, Department of Orthopaedic Surgery, The Abraham Lincoln School of Medicine, University of Illinois; Member, Strauss Surgical Group Associates, S.C., Chicago, Illinois

Martin Koffman, M.D.
Consultant in Cerebral Palsy, Rancho Los Amigos Hospital, Downey, California; Clinical Instructor in Orthopedics, University of Southern California, Los Angeles, California; Assistant Clinical Professor of Orthopedics, Loma Linda University, Loma Linda, California

Judy Leonard, O.T.R.
Jenison, Michigan

Randall J. Lewis, M.D.
Orthopaedic Surgeon, Washington, D.C.

Marilyn J. Lister, B.S.
Editor, *Physical Therapy,* American Physical Therapy Association, Washington, D.C.

Mary W. McKenzie, B.S., L.O.T.R., F.A.O.T.A.
Instructor, Louisiana State University Medical Center, School of Allied Health Professions, New Orleans, Louisiana

Donald R. McNeal, Ph.D.
Co-Director, Rancho Los Amigos Rehabilitation Engineering Center, Downey, California

Vert Mooney, M.D.
Professor and Chairman, Division of Orthopaedic Surgery, University of Texas Southwestern Medical School, Dallas, Texas

Robert J. Neviaser, M.D.
Professor of Orthopedic Surgery and Director, Hand and Upper Extremity Service, The George Washington University Medical Center, Washington, D.C.

Vernon L. Nickel, M.D.
Professor of Surgery/Orthopedics and Rehabilitation, University of California at San Diego; Director of Rehabilitation, Sharp Rehabilitation Center, San Diego, California

Donald H. Parks, M.D., F.R.C.S.(C), F.A.C.S.
Acting Chief of Staff, Shriners Burns Institute; Associate Professor of Surgery, Division of Plastic Surgery, University of Texas Medical Branch, Galveston, Texas

Maurice D. Schnell, M.D.
Mercy Hospital, Davenport, Iowa

Sheldon R. Simon, M.D.
Director, Gait Analysis Laboratory, Boston Children's Hospital; Assistant Professor of Orthopedics, Harvard University Medical School; Director, Acute Rehabilitation Unit, Brigham and Women's Hospital, Boston, Massachusetts

Michael J. Smith, M.D.
Orthopedic Surgeon; Director, Sports Medicine Clinic, All Children's Hospital, St. Petersburg, Florida

Dempsey S. Springfield, M.D.
Assistant Professor, Department of Orthopaedics, College of Medicine, University of Florida, Gainesville, Florida

Marcus J. Stewart, M.D.
Professor of Orthopaedics, University of Tennessee Center for the Health Sciences; Chief of Orthopaedics, United States Veterans Hospital, Memphis, Tennessee

Alfred B. Swanson, M.D., F.A.C.S.
Chief, Orthopaedic and Hand Surgery Training Program, Blodgett and Butterworth Hospitals; Chief, Orthopaedic Research, Blodgett Memorial Hospital, Grand Rapids, Michigan; Clinical Professor of Surgery, Michigan State University, Lansing, Michigan

Genevieve deGroot Swanson, M.D.
Plastic Surgeon, Blodgett Memorial Hospital, Grand Rapids, Michigan; Assistant Clinical Professor of Surgery, Michigan State University, Lansing, Michigan

Carolyn L. Vash, Ph.D.
Vice President, Institute for Information Studies, Falls Church, Virginia

F. William Wagner, Jr., M.D.
Clinical Professor of Orthopedic Surgery, University of Southern California School of Medicine; Chief, Foot Clinic, Los Angeles County–University of Southern California Medical Center, Los Angeles, California; Chief of the Ortho-Diabetes Services, Rancho Los Amigos Hospital, Downey, California

Robert L. Waters, M.D.
Chief, Surgical Services, Rancho Los Amigos Hospital, Downey, California

Honora K. Wilson, M.S.W.
Clinical Social Worker (private practice); Social Work Consultant, Rancho Los Amigos Hospital, Downey, California

Barbara Ziemba, O.T.R.
Blodgett Memorial Hospital, Grand Rapids, Michigan

Rehabilitation: A Definition

Rehabilitation is a therapeutic program designed to minimize the consequences of a permanent or protracted disability. It stands in sharp contrast to standard medical care, which concentrates on curing the patient's pathology and assumes that function will recover spontaneously. Failure to cure is considered an unfortunate consequence of an imperfect system, an event to be tabulated as a statistical reminder of improvement needed. The patient is left alone to cope with the residuals.

The basic difference between curative and rehabilitative medicine lies in the direction of effort. The focus of curative medicine is on reversing the primary disease process; every procedure is directed that way. Rehabilitation concentrates on restoring function; emphasis is placed on preventing contractures, developing muscle strength, stimulating latent control, training the patient to use residual function in an effective manner, providing assistive devices, and guiding patient and family in accommodating to an altered way of life.

Rehabilitation is a therapeutic program that works most effectively when integrated with the curative process. Then attention to pathology and attention to function are exercised simultaneously, and the debilitating consequences of uninterrupted bed rest are avoided. The therapeutic continuum gradually shifts from an emphasis on control of pathology to one of restoration of function.

By necessity, rehabilitation is a multidisciplinary program and often a multispecialty one as well. There must be an appropriate blend of physical therapy, occupational therapy, communication therapy, medical social work, psychology, vocational counselling, prosthetics, orthotics, and recreational therapy as well as rehabilitation-focused nursing, medicine, and reconstructive surgery.

Thus for a person with a catastrophic disability normal function is not possible, but effective performance and reentry into active society may be achieved if all the measures influencing a patient's capacity to function are provided.

Jacquelin Perry, M.D.
1981

Contents

Introduction

Rehabilitation as an idea applicable to human disability began with the care and treatment of conditions considered to belong to the sphere of the early orthopedic surgeon. The term rehabilitation first appeared in a paper entitled "Problems in Rehabilitation of the Victims of War," which Dr. E. McIver Law read before the Florida Midland Medical Society at St. Petersburg, Florida on October 12, 1921.[6] The author was presenting a detailed account of the care of amputees following World War I. Long before the word rehabilitation was used, however, the specialty of orthopedics provided this type of care for the physically disabled.

The specialty of orthopedics received its name from a man deeply concerned with the plight of persons deformed by birth or circumstances—Nicholas Andry, Professor of Medicine and later Dean of the Faculty of Medicine of the University of Paris, then probably the most prestigious medical school in the world. In 1741 Andry coined the word orthopaedia, from the Greek *orthos* (straight) and *pais* (child).[1] His work concentrated primarily on the problems of children, because poor crippled children then were virtual outcasts of society. They were often left to die. The diseases they suffered included such congenital abnormalities as clubfoot and dislocated hips as well as residuals of poliomyelitis or infections and consequences of trauma.

For many years physicians who treated chronic crippling conditions were called "strap and buckle doctors," and they concerned themselves chiefly with problems of the lower extremity. But by the end of the 19th century Sir Hugh Owens Thomas of Liverpool was able to bring lower-extremity care to a very high level. His nephew, Sir Robert Jones, strongly supported and carried on this work.[5]

Jones was a leading advocate of the evolving concept that orthopedists should also be surgeons.[8] The experience of Jones and other pioneering orthopedic surgeons with the use of the Thomas splint in conditions such as tuberculosis of the knee led to a widespread practice of splinting fractures, particularly in the British armed forces. The success of the orthopedists in treating fractures during World War I made it clear that orthopedic surgeons were best qualified to assume responsibility for fracture care.[7] This factor, along with the increasing involvement of the orthopedist in surgical services, quickened the evolution of orthopedic surgery as a specialty. Further experiences in World War II gave additional impetus to the specialty's development, and by 1950 orthopedists were unquestionably the leaders in caring for fractures. They shifted their attention to acute problems. Except for the treatment of polio, clubfoot, and dislocated hips, the care of chronic crippling disorders was progressively relegated to other physicians or health care workers or not done at all.

As orthopedic surgeons became more and more immersed in acute trauma and posttraumatic conditions, certain orthopedic surgeons, notably Goldthwait,[4] became concerned that the surgical aspects of orthopedics were superseding nonoperative care. Goldthwait insisted that surgical procedures should take a subordinate position in the orthopedist's practice and that surgery could be delegated to other well-trained surgeons. This notion did not prevail. However, Goldthwait's reservations about the excessive emphasis on surgical procedures were probably well founded.

In England Sir Robert Jones, and later Reginald Watson-Jones, continued to stress the importance of rehabilitation in the care of all persons with musculoskeletal disabilities—adults as well as children and patients with congenital as well as acquired conditions.[3] Watson-Jones also recognized the urgent need of adults disabled by industrial injuries for orthopedic rehabilitation. He argued for both nonoperative therapy and a more than superficial involvement of allied health professionals in chronic care,[10] and he spent the remaining years of his career reminding society of its unfulfilled obligation to the adult cripple.[11]

Unfortunately, these attempts to develop adult rehabilitation units in England were not successful. Indeed, history reveals very few actual successes until after World War II. The one exception was the Hospital for Crippled Adults, which was established by Willis Campbell in Memphis, Tennessee with the financial support of regional Rotary clubs. Campbell's example showed what could be done when society concerned itself with the needs of the crippled adult. Regrettably, few followed his lead until 1952, when the Rancho Los Amigos Hospital in Downey, California was founded to care for patients with respiratory paralysis.

Two occurrences helped bring about this change in attitude. The first, of course, was the need of the soldiers who returned disabled from World War II. The second was the example of Franklin D. Roosevelt. Despite his severe physical deficits, Roosevelt achieved at heroic levels of endeavor. And because of his international prominence, he had tremendous impact on social thinking about the handicapped. People began entertaining the possibility of allowing disabled persons to become contributors to society instead of a drain on its resources.

As Americans have become more aware of the strain on the nation's resources imposed by caring for the physically handicapped, a sharp activation of interest in rehabilitation is taking place. With increased knowledge has also come more extensive legislative support, sparked by active lobbying by disabled people themselves, who are no longer willing to sit ignored or forgotten. Landmark legislation passed in 1945 and 1973, culminating in Public Law 95-602 in 1978, made facilities of medical organizations available to disabled adults. At one time hospitalization insurance plans excluded most reconstructive surgery from coverage; a sizable proportion still exclude rehabilitation if it is called by that name. All these factors—positive and negative—have directed notice to the adult with a musculoskeletal disability and reawakened the interest of many orthopedic surgeons in these patients' various problems.

This book deals with subjects that I believe rightly belong in the domain of any orthopedic surgeon who supervises rehabilitation and treatment of chronic disabling conditions. It is my conviction that subspecialization is the key to excellence in treating the various disease entities discussed throughout these pages. This concept will be reviewed extensively in regard both to disease entities (for example, spinal cord injury) and to the expertise of allied health professionals, such as physical therapists, in relation to these entities.

Because the economic cost to society of physical disability is enormous, and because the number of physically disabled persons increases every year, better rehabilitation following the time-tested mode of planned medical care—namely, clinical treatment, education, and research—promises great rewards, both in the salvage of human beings as far as their quality of life is concerned and in their contribution to society as a whole. It is most helpful for rehabilitation professionals to bear in mind the three major assets or work-related resources possessed by every human being. In her chapter on vocational rehabilitation Carolyn Vash separates these areas into brain, brawn, and personality. Each person differs from every other as to the capacity he or she has in each area. A physically disabled person might be deficient in brawn, as would be a poliomyelitis patient, but brain and personality remain unaffected and can often compensate sufficiently to allow for significant accomplishments. Someone who sustains deficits both in brain and brawn (as in cases of head injury) with extensive residuals has to learn to rely more heavily on personality traits to achieve more effective functioning. Another helpful way of viewing patients with chronic musculoskeletal disability is to compare them with an astronaut. Both require an environmental support system that will heighten sensorimotor function and lessen dependence, thereby increasing the ability to perform productively. The improved quality of life that results enables a worthwhile contribution to society to be made.

A highly successful model of orthopedic rehabilitation, and one widely understood by orthopedic surgeons, is that of sports medicine. This field provides a useful illustration of how rehabilitation practice can permeate the treatment of—and help alleviate—a specific kind of problem. The current practice for physicians who specialize in or who have a strong interest in orthopedic sports medicine is to emphasize the need for an intensive rehabilitation program at the onset of treatment and then continue that program aggressively for as long as it is indicated. The concept gained strength during World War II. Later De Lorme et al.[2] established the pattern of rigorous exercises after knee injuries. Since then, their ideas have significantly influenced the thinking of orthopedic surgeons who treat other conditions, with markedly improved results. Research activity in sports medicine has produced advances in arthroscopy and arthroscopic surgery. Such forceful, scientifically based orthopedic rehabilitation is urgently required for a large variety of other musculoskeletal disabilities.

Orthopedic Rehabilitation is dedicated to the premise that the best quality of rehabilitative care must be applied on the broadest possible scale. This desired goal is attainable within both the current framework of medical knowledge and the general political and social climate. The individual authors contributing to this work have been selected to represent a wide spectrum of specialties recognized for their indispensable role in the rehabilitation process. Each section of *Orthopedic Rehabilitation* stresses the categorical disease-oriented approach to the rehabilitation effort, aided by the extensive participation of allied health professionals who are skilled in their own disciplines and have additional specialized knowledge of particular disease states. As Dr. Alfred E. Shands wrote in 1961, rehabilitation "is not a chance happening, but the result of a careful plan which includes the active cooperation of many members of a reconstruction team. This team of workers should consist of the physician, the psychologist, the physical therapist, the occupational therapist, the social worker, the vocational teacher, the director of vocational guidance, the vocational placement worker, and sometimes other consultants in special fields."[9] These words are still true today.

In conclusion, I want to express my deepest gratitude to the orthopedic surgeons, other medical specialists, and allied health professionals who have contributed their valuable knowledge, expertise, and time to the writing of this book. They were both patient and conscientious. In particular, I would like to thank Natalie Neviaser, who typed the manuscripts and assisted with much of the paperwork, and Avis Berman, who coordinated the editing of this book.

Vernon L. Nickel, M.D.

REFERENCES

1. Andry, N.: *L'orthopédie ou l'art de Prevenir and de Corriger dan les Enfants, les Difformites du Corps.* La Venve Alix, Paris, 1741.
2. De Lorme, T. L., Shaw, R. S., and Austen, W. G.: Musculo-skeletal functions in the amputated perfused human being limb. Surg. Forum 15:450–452, 1964.
3. Girdlestone, G. R.: The Robert Jones tradition. J. Bone Joint Surg. 30B:187–195, 1948.
4. Goldthwait, J. E.: The backgrounds and foregrounds of orthopaedics. J. Bone Joint Surg. 15:279–301, 1933.
5. Jones, R.: The problem of the cripple. Practitioner 112:1–12, 1924.
6. Law, E. M.: Problems in rehabilitation of victims of war. J. Flor. Med. Assoc. 8:152–156, 1922.

7. Nickel, V. L.: Sir Robert Jones Lecture: Orthopedic rehabilitation—Challenges and opportunities. Bull. Hosp. Joint Dis. 29(1):153–161, 1969.

8. Paterson, D.: Who cares? Bull. Am. Acad. Orthop. Surg. 29:18–22, 1981.

9. Shands, A. R.: A few remarks on physical medicine, rehabilitation and orthopedic surgery. South. Med. J. 54:420–425, 1961.

10. Watson-Jones, R.: Dame Agnes Hunt. J. Bone Joint Surg. 30B:709–713, 1948.

11. Watson-Jones, R.: Death and growth of bone. J. Bone Joint Surg. 30B:736–737, 1948. (abstract)

Orthopedic Rehabilitation

General Principles of Orthopedic Rehabilitation

Vernon L. Nickel, M.D.

Two principles are fundamental to the planning of a rehabilitation program. First, the sequelae of the original insult, whether it be trauma or disease, must be minimized as much as possible. Second, all preventable complications should be averted. If they happen, they should be dealt with aggressively. When these basic rules are strongly enforced, the application of good rehabilitation techniques is most likely to obtain the maximal effect in the shortest time at the lowest cost.

A good illustration of the first concept involves the treatment of the patient with spinal cord injury. The spine must be reduced and maintained in a stable position at the earliest possible moment to allow for optimal recovery and forestall additional neurological loss. Some devastating complications that can and should be prevented are bladder infections, pressure sores, contractural deformities, and muscle atrophy from disuse. These medical problems, combined with the severe psychosocial deficits that many patients will develop under the circumstances, can impede or halt the rehabilitation process.

ORGANIZATION OF THE REHABILITATION SERVICE

The concept of a categorical approach to chronic disease was applied with great success in the treatment of respiratory poliomyelitis.[11,12] It is the author's firm conviction that this approach is far more effective in the rehabilitation setting than is grouping patients together regardless of diagnosis. This trend, which began after World War II, is referred to as comprehensive rehabilitation. Whenever the size of the service and the availability of personnel permit, patients should be grouped according to disease category. Grouping by the physician's medical specialty, which is customary in acute-care hospitals, does not apply to rehabilitation. The organization of this book is based on that belief.

A vital component in the organization of any rehabilitation service is the need for high-quality medical care and discipline. The demand for excellence can and must be satisfied in the chronic as well as acute-care hospital setting. The centers for respiratory poliomyelitis established in the early 1950s by the National Foundation for Infantile Paralysis,[1] in which the disease was managed as a category and serviced by physicians of different specialties, are superb instances of an area in which standards of excellence were sought and achieved. At present, a growing number of spinal cord injury centers are following their example.[6]

Direction

A major impediment to the effective organization of a rehabilitation service is the confusion that exists regarding the proper procedure for directing such a service. Physicians in the acute-care setting are accustomed to prescribing medications and precise therapeutic programs for their patients. They expect nurses and other health professionals to follow those directions exactly. In the rehabilitation environment, that model of care is not workable. It may, in fact, be a barrier to the development of a good program. The rehabilitation patient has direct contact with the physician and a variety of health professionals, each of whom is expert in dealing with the patient's problems. What these professionals need is general direction and supervision similar to the activities of the coach of a professional football team, who coordinates and acts as a catalyst for the team yet leaves the details of execution to subordinate specialists.

The term "prescription" is a misnomer for the directions given to allied health professionals by physicians, since it is impossible to detail all the procedures to be followed. These are designed by the experienced therapist, who is accustomed to exercise professional judgment in such matters. This is a controversial notion to accept for those who have worked in an environment where lip service was paid to such "prescriptions." The prescription cannot and should not be attempted. Unfortunately, it is still true that physicians write fairly detailed directions (commonly called "prescriptions") in the rehabilitation setting. Allied health professionals usually ignore these directions, chiefly because they may be impractical and often impossible to carry out. It is much more pertinent for the physician to give general directions and leave the details to other trained health professionals.

Those who persist in clinging to the unreasonable notion that detailed prescriptions can be written and should be followed must consider that these prescriptions, currently imposed on physical and occupational therapists, would also have to be given to speech therapists, social workers, and clinical pathologists. This is clearly unfeasible.

However, this does not mean that medications need not be ordered with precision. In this respect, the nurse on the rehabilitation service should be encouraged to exercise more independent judgment than is usually the case in the acute medical-surgical ward.

Physicians and administrators who are somewhat insecure about the idea of extensive delegation of responsibility might contemplate the design of the coronary care unit, in which nurses specializing in heart problems have excelled. If we have learned to delegate responsibility to specifically trained nurses when life itself is at risk, then we should surely be willing to give authority to competent health professionals in chronic disease situations of less immediate threat to life and limb.

By letting others have a share in making decisions, physicians can then use their time more efficiently and direct the care for a large number of patients.[2] This does not mean that the physician abdicates responsibility. The ability of the rehabilitation team to turn to strong leadership and have prompt, ready access to expert medical guidance is central to the concept of delegation.

TIMING

When should an active rehabilitation program begin? This is difficult to determine, but the general rule is the earlier the better. Fundamental to the concept of appropriate timing for an active rehabilitation program is the recognition that rehabilitation is not a separate process occurring when an inpatient or outpatient is transferred from an acute-care hospital, a physician's office, or from home to a rehabilitation center. Astute physicians and their colleagues in the allied health professions understand that the conventional progress of healing to an eventual cure is not likely to happen, and that the patient will require a formal, organized program of rehabilitation. As soon as this is recognized, planning and treatment should be aimed at lessening the consequences of major and permanent loss of function. The loss will not only be physical. The patient may well sustain mental and emotional problems.

The extent and complexity of a rehabilitation program will depend on many factors. For example, in one patient with backache, a large ruptured disc produces severe symptoms and disability. It is removed surgically, the patient recovers, and returns to his usual occupation in a relatively short time. In contrast, another patient exhibits a similar problem, but in this case there are significant neurological sequelae. The patient has considerable permanent loss of function, with the added problems of depression and a lack of confidence. The first person needs little or no rehabilitation, whereas the second would benefit greatly from a well-structured, intensive rehabilitation program staffed by allied health professionals specially instructed in rehabilitating patients with spinal complaints. Without access to such an effective program, the second patient might suffer marked impairment in ambulating (which could have been corrected by proper bracing), chronic renal disability from continued catheterization, and other preventable problems such as loss of motivation or the breaking up of family relationships.

Another example is the elderly person with Parkinson's disease who falls, fractures a hip, and undergoes total hip replacement. This patient is much more likely to resume ambulation in a rehabilitation setting than in the usual medical-surgical ward. A younger person with a fractured hip and no neurological problems would not require transfer to a rehabilitation setting under normal conditions. A stroke victim should be considered a rehabilitation candidate as soon as his medical condition stabilizes and he has the potential to resume some form of activity. A patient with spinal cord injury and severe neurological loss will always require an intensive rehabilitation program.

The rehabilitation effort is costly and the process is lengthy, because the problems involved are not straightforward or simple. They require many different kinds of professional personnel to deal with them. The expense is fully justified, however, because every dollar spent in rehabilitating patients with chronic conditions results in manifold dollar savings when these patients eventually return to society.[10]

More awareness of the relatedness of rehabilitation to the spectrum of acute care is needed among orthopedists, neurologists, and other physicians, in order for them to recognize more quickly the kind of patient who requires rehabilitation. The physician who has seen the patient from the beginning of the initial injury or illness is the appropriate one to continue treatment when it is clear that a rehabilitation program is needed. This physician has paid careful attention to preserving the patient's life and immediate physical well-being, and has also been alert to the barriers that commonly impede or detract from a rehabilitation program. When the doctor has a positive attitude toward preventing complications and points out the potential remaining to the patient, he or she is making a realistic assessment both of the disability and the potential for rehabilitation. The allied health specialists also contribute to this assessment, and their involvement is essential in planning the program.

THE SCOPE OF REHABILITATION

The scope of rehabilitation has not been clearly demarcated and is undergoing rapid change. Previously hospitalization was intrinsic to rehabilitation, but the current emphasis is increasingly on outpatient care. The team effort that has worked so well in hospitals can function equally as well in an outpatient setting as long as the organizational structure is suitable.

For many years, too, rehabilitation was chiefly focused on children. Orthopedists devoted themselves to such conditions as poliomyelitis, clubfoot, dislocated hips, and cerebral palsy. When it was customary for these children to spend long periods of time in hospitals, the Shriners' hospitals for crippled children provided excellent care for them.[19] Today, because of improved surgical procedures, extended periods of hospitalization are seldom indicated. We now try to see that children spend a short time away from their homes. Modern rehabilitation, of course, extends to adults crippled by a whole range of disorders.

The modern approach to rehabilitation was greatly stimulated by World War II because of the presence of the war-wounded amputee. Rehabilitation was largely on an outpatient basis, except for surgical procedures; amputation clinics became an example to emulate as a model of the categorical approach to a disease process. Amputation centers at that time were concentrated in Veterans Administration hospitals.[8] The outstanding level reached during the 1950s is underscored by the fact that the post of clinic chief of the amputation rehabilitation service was considered a high honor and an important professional achievement. It is unfortunate that the interest and the activity on behalf of amputees have dissipated and that the quality of amputee care has deteriorated accordingly.

Poliomyelitis is probably the disease that has been treated with the most success from the rehabilitation standpoint. For a few years before the use of vaccines, it is fair to state that almost every case of poliomyelitis received adequate care. This changed to some degree with the advent of respiratory poliomyelitis because of the complex nature of the problem, but after the organization of special centers in this area, excellent rehabilitative care was given to these patients.[3]

This is not true for many other disease categories. Only a small percentage of patients with stroke receive complete care. Similarly, many patients with head injuries are not given the medical treatment they require. Until recently, patients with spinal cord injury were scattered in many different areas of a region, and the cost of care was prohibitive. As centers for spinal care spread across the United States, outcomes are improving and costs are dropping.[15]

GOALS AND LIMITATIONS

Two facets of any treatment plan that must be kept in mind are assistance in making the best return or preservation of residual physical abilities, and the greater enhancement of that potential function by proper apparatus, training in substitute skills, and surgical procedures. Any reasonable means should be used to increase function beyond that which the patient could achieve alone. Operations, strengthening, training, fitting with correct appliances, and auxiliary devices all aid the rehabilitation team in attaining these goals.

The process of defining goals requires a high level of expertise, as well as the combined experience of the entire rehabilitation team. Once the initial effort is made and the goal-setting process is constantly under review, realistic predictions and limitations can be established. Poor goal setting, for example, would be the expectation that an elderly above-knee amputee with marked cardiovascular impairment will ambulate with an above-knee prosthesis. Continuing an extended period of training to reach the goal of ambulation must be avoided. In addition to the economic cost, the patient, family, and staff will suffer inevitable disappointment and frustration in the effort to attain an unachievable goal. Progressively accurate goal setting, with the patient's residual assets kept in mind, is based on the professional team's level of expertise, the rehabilitation environment, optimal medical care (which includes surgical procedures), and well-designed aids such as prosthetic and/or orthotic devices.

Goals can gradually be extended with the application of rehabilitation engineering to the severely disabled patient. For instance, the high quadriplegic who is unable to propel his or her own wheelchair will be able to consider vocational independence as a rational goal once he or she has a properly fitted wheelchair with adequate seating to control pressure and electrical controls that permit the driving of a van tailored to the patient's needs.

In viewing the total problems of drastically handicapped persons, physicians are subject to many preconceived notions and prejudices. Physicians generally spend most of their time treating conditions in their offices or a hospital for acute care. Reluctance to treat the chronically handicapped may arise from lack of personal experience in such care and from the disturbing realization that complete recovery is unlikely.[14] The potentially dangerous psychological impediment that must be overcome is that all health professionals have been trained to *cure*. They experience a sense of failure with anything less than a cure. Because many younger orthopedic surgeons have trained only in acute-care settings, this "cure syndrome" is ever present.

Another psychological hurdle is that our society, including people in the biomedical sciences, considers walking to be the ultimate goal of recovery. Ambulation, however, is frequently overemphasized. Although walking obviously is tremendously important, for many patients with chronic crippling disorders it may not be as essential as having effective use of the hands. It is far more important that the disabled individual be able to take care of personal needs and function socially and vocationally than walk. Patients, relatives, friends, and staff members need to be educated in rational expectations by professionals who themselves have a clear understanding of what constitutes an appreciable functional ability.

TRIAGE

Dorland's Illustrated Medical Dictionary defines triage as "the sorting out and classification of casualties of war or other disasters to determine the priority of need and proper place of treatment." The term as applied to medical care was reputedly first used at the Battle of Waterloo, when Napoleon's surgeon ordered his medical aides to concentrate their efforts and supplies on the wounded soldiers who would benefit most from them, rather than treating those who were beyond help or others less severely injured and not in immediate need of care.

Triage is vital to a successful rehabilitation program. It must be invoked with firmness when selecting patients with chronic disabling conditions for rehabilitation. Priority of treatment should be weighted toward persons who can make significant gains from the therapy. The steadily increasing numbers of patients who request rehabilitative care make it imperative that leaders of rehabilitation teams exercise some discrimination in selecting candidates for their programs to ensure that the greatest good is accomplished for the greatest number of people.

The total social and medical resources needed to rehabilitate everyone who could conceivably benefit are enormous. Even if such unlimited resources became available, it would be most inappropriate to devote them to the ongoing care of patients with little potential for functional gains. Costly treatment must be promptly curtailed after it appears that gains are minimal or nonexistent, even when the patients' families apply strong pressure to extend therapy. To preserve a physical system or body part that no longer has any functional meaning is not good medicine, and it is not good rehabilitation. It is, in fact, bad rehabilitation. Just preserving the body is not rehabilitation; life must be worthwhile for the individual.

The decision process of triage is determined by the availability of resources. These consist of the physical plant, the social and economic support for the patient, and the accessibility and expertise of various physicians and allied health professionals. It requires equating the therapeutic potential of maximal effort with the cost, time, and personnel involved in it. Therapeutic potential can be defined as the achieving of a reasonably good functional level upon the patient's return to society. This would encompass a person's physical condition, emotional and psychological attitudes, social situation, and vocational possibilities.

Measuring the value of any rehabilitation effort is not simple. One method is based on economics, represented by what disabled persons contribute to society or by the reduction in the cost of care when they gain independence. But further experience is urgently needed to estimate rehabilitation outcomes more accurately, because many handicapped people with no earning capacity have made important contributions to the arts, sciences, and family management. It is even less easy to evaluate the joy a happy person can bring to those around him. An unforgettable example is the woman I met who suffered frightful paralysis secondary to poliomyelitis. She required permanent use of respiratory equipment and had lost the function of her arms and legs. This patient went home to a strongly supportive family that despite her condition assisted her relatives and her community. She had a forceful personality and an active brain. With these assets left to her, she managed her household efficiently.

PREVENTABLE BARRIERS TO SUCCESSFUL REHABILITATION

A patient's rehabilitation is often seriously and sometimes disastrously impeded by complications. Such conditions as pressure sores, bladder infections, contractural deformities, unnecessary muscle atrophy, skeletal deformities, noxious spasticity, psychological regression, and social deterioration will increase the expense and extent of a rehabilitation program. These complications are singularly offensive to knowledgeable rehabilitationists, because they know that with few exceptions they could and should be prevented. Prevention is relatively simple and much less costly than treatment. In addition, major complications may not be completely correctable; the residuals that persist add to the patient's already serious loss of function. Typical, avoidable complications are discussed briefly here and in further detail in subsequent chapters.

Pressure Sores

One of the best examples of a preventable condition is the pressure sore,[4] which, until recently, was believed to be an inevitable sequel to a condition such as spinal cord injury. Even if a large pressure sore has healed, often with major surgical intervention required, a patient will still be much more susceptible to the reoccurrence of sores.

Pressure sores are caused by unrelieved pressure over an excessive period of time, making the body tissue necrotic. It is not neurological loss that alters the physiology of the skin and subcutaneous tissue. Factors such as hydration, spasm, protein depletion, rough bedding, moisture, and lack of cleanliness contribute to a patient's propensity for developing pressure sores. The optimal solution to the problem is to relieve pressure and avoid as many contributing variables as possible in patients with the likelihood of getting them.[17]

There are three clinical stages of a pressure sore. In the first, the skin is persistently red. This resolves quickly with the relief of pressure. The first stage offers the best opportunity to prevent later stages and their serious consequences. In the second stage, the skin shows bluish discoloration or blistering. These signs mean that some cutaneous necrosis has already occurred. With aggressive treatment, the sore may heal, although a longer period of time will be required for it. In the third and final stage, the skin becomes white (ischemic blanching) or black (actual necrosis), which represents the death of all layers of the skin in varying degrees in the subcutaneous and other underlying tissues. This stage always results in large ulcerations, and reaching it makes the patient increasingly vulnerable to new sores. Accordingly, it behooves the entire staff—and especially the nurse—to exert great diligence in seeing that no lesion progresses beyond the first stage.

Bladder Infections

The inability to urinate at will is a common problem for patients with a neuromusculoskeletal disorder. The condition of most of these patients has improved with the advent of intermittent catherization. This technique highlights the grave complication of bladder infection and the need for efficient therapy as a preventive or, if necessary, as a curative measure. The consequences of the indiscriminate and unchallenged use of an indwelling catheter for prolonged periods can usually be obviated early in the treatment program.[5]

Contractural Deformities

Recent research on the development of contractural deformities lends credence to the idea of a vigorous program of prevention.[4] The rehabilitation nurse, working with the physical and occupational therapists on a program of positioning and ranging, can in most instances eliminate this disturbing complication.

The nursing profession is to be commended for pursuing a thorough program of teaching and therapeutic intervention to avoid creating settings conducive to contractural deformities. It is well established that daily range of motion exercises are a good preventive measure.[11] In addition, the practical step of turning a patient to the prone position (face down) at intervals is most effective in discouraging contractures of the hips and knees. In this maneuver, the feet are placed over the edge of the bed against the footboard and the shoulders are elevated.[17] Unfortunately, it remains true that the correction of contractural deformities comprises the majority of surgical procedures seen in most rehabilitation units.

Atrophied Muscles

Patients who have already sustained a loss of functional muscle strength from disease or trauma often suffer additional wasting and weakness as a result of muscle disease. The earliest possible active exercise program following the acute episode is the best way to maintain maximal muscle strength.[14]

Poor Nutrition

The recovery of patients from major trauma may be considerably hindered by inadequate nourishment. The same deficiency may be true for patients with long-standing chronic diseases. Detailed assessments of a patient's specific dietary requirements and careful supervision by the dietitian are clearly indicated during the rehabilitation program.[9]

Noxious Spasticity

Whenever noxious spasticity interferes with a patient's function, prompt action should be taken to reduce the spasticity. There are few instances in which it cannot be controlled by medication, nerve injection, tenotomy, or tendon transfer. Medication, however, should be used sparingly because of frequently attendant and adverse side effects.[14]

Social and Psychological Problems

Skilled professionals who are familiar with the host of social adjustments necessary in cases of severe, chronic disability are as essential to the rehabilitation effort as those who deal with the physical disability itself. The term "social pressure sore"[7] points up dramatically the implication of such problems and the aspects of prevention that must be considered.

Historically, an attitude of helplessness and hopelessness has prevailed in the treatment and rehabilitation of patients with most of the chronic crippling disorders. The psychologist with a specialty in clinical psychology and expertise in dealing with various disease entities is of invaluable help to the rehabilitation program. It is vitally important to stress that the patient must focus on the possibilities and abilities remaining to him—not on what he has lost.[18]

PROGNOSES

It is difficult to assign a prognosis for a patient with a serious multi-organ chronic disorder. Not only are there primary physical deficits being evaluated—they are compounded by social, psychological, and vocational factors. Physicians who have had minimal contact with rehabilitation services are prone to be more gloomy in their prognoses than is warranted. Unless the prognosis is transparently obvious, or until they pile up more experiences in the rehabilitation setting, physicians should avoid being specific. The team conference, a group discussion characterized by frequent interchange of ideas among professionals from various backgrounds, is an extremely useful way to arrive at a prognosis. It fosters the establishment of reasonable goals and constantly emphasizes what the patient can still do and learn to do.

SURGICAL INTERVENTION IN REHABILITATION

Many professionals in rehabilitation settings have had little or no contact with surgeons, and a bias against surgical procedures clearly exists. One reason for their prejudice is that the rehabilitation hospital has been used inappropriately as a dumping ground for patients with failed surgical procedures. This practice is obviously not rehabilitation in the best sense. Furthermore, in many cases, the busy surgeon tends to focus attention on the merits of the surgical procedure and may not be sufficiently interested in or knowledgeable about the patient's total problem or sphere of activities. For instance, a quadriplegic patient who has been operated on for a hand problem may develop pressure sores and bladder infections during the acute-care phases of the hospitalization because these complications were not properly observed.

Another reason for the bias against surgery is that some physicians who are not successful in pursuing a surgical career may opt for a less demanding area of patient care and enter the rehabilitation field. These persons may nurture and retain a subconscious or open anti-surgical bias.

Surgical procedures in the rehabilitation setting should be recognized as having the potential for major complications, just as in acute medicine, and should be performed by physicians who have some specific perspective on the patient and the problems he faces as a whole, plus an extensive general understanding of the rehabilitation process. Surgery is advocated when the risk involved is exceeded by reasonable gains in the patient's potential to function. An example of wise surgical thinking is the decision to do a simple operation to correct a contractural deformity, supplanting a costly, time-consuming period of stretching the deformity, which will often yield a poor end result. The same preference—that is, the choice of surgery—is also valid for noxious spasticity, closure of pressure sores, stabilization of joints, and tendon transfers. Because this is a text on orthopedic rehabilitation, the theme of effective surgical intervention pervades it throughout.

SUMMARY

Initially orthopedists confined themselves to the practice of treating musculoskeletal disorders, or what is now called orthopedic rehabilitation. During the last few decades, however, they have primarily treated acute diseases and trauma in acute-care settings. I believe that orthopedic surgeons must once again devote themselves to caring for patients with chronic crippling conditions and accept responsibility for leadership in this regard.[16]

Several reasons make the return to this original obligation compelling. Acute ailments are better cared for and not neglected. More orthopedic surgeons are trained and available to rehabilitation. Lastly, our population contains an increasing number of elderly men and women. They will inevitably develop a variety of neuromusculoskeletal complaints, but their mortality rate will not be as high as it would have been decades ago. Accordingly, the number of people who will require rehabilitation is on the rise.

When orthopedic surgeons assume the role of rehabilitation team leader with the same intellectual and professional dedication that they have applied to acute care, the results are extremely promising. They can direct a large program that will consume a comparatively small portion of their total professional time. This would require simply an adjustment in attitude, since the actual techniques used differ very little from those employed in treating acute illnesses. The well-trained orthopedic surgeon is fully qualified to direct the rehabilitation of patients with chronic crippling conditions. The rewards are as great and the challenges as inspiring as those to be found in any other part of his or her professional life.[13]

REFERENCES

1. Affeldt, J. E.: Concept of patient care in a respiratory and rehabilitation center. In *Poliomyelitis: Papers and Discussions Presented at the Fourth International Poliomyelitis Conference*, pp. 618–623. J. B. Lippincott, Philadelphia, 1958.
2. Affeldt, J. E., Nickel, V. L., Perry, J., and Kriete, B. C.: Intensive rehabilitation. Recent experience in a chronic disease hospital. Calif. Med. 91:193–196, 1959.
3. Affeldt, J. E., West, H. F., Landauer, K. S., Wendland, L. V., and Arata, N. N.: Functional and vocational recovery in severe poliomyelitis. Clin. Orthop. 12:16–21, 1958.
4. Edberg, E.: Physical therapy for thoracic and lumbar paraplegia. In Pierce, D. S., and Nickel, V. L., Eds.: *The Total Care of Spinal Cord Injuries*, pp. 225–236. Little, Brown, Boston, 1977.
5. Guttmann, L., and Frankel, H.: The value of intermittent catheterization in the early management of traumatic paraplegia and tetraplegia. Paraplegia 7:38–41, 1969.
6. Inman, V. T.: Specialization and the physiatrist. Arch. Phys. Med. 45:765–770, 1966.
7. Kahn, E.: Social bracing in rehabilitation. J. Am. Phys. Ther. Assoc. 47:692–699, 1967.
8. Klopsteg, P. E., and Wilson, P. D.: *Human Limbs and Their Substitutes*. Hafner Publishing, New York, 1968.
9. Mitchell, H. S.: *Nutrition in Health and Disease*, 16th ed, pp. 278–283, 334–346. J. B. Lippincott, Philadelphia, 1976.
10. Nickel, V. L.: Rehabilitating the injured worker. In *Proceedings of the 1965 Conference on Occupational Health*, pp. 29–32. California Medical Association, 1965.
11. Nickel, V. L.: Sir Robert Jones Lecture: Orthopedic rehabilitation—Challenges and opportunities. Bull. Hosp. Joint Dis. 29(1):1–21, 1968.
12. Nickel, V. L.: Orthopedic rehabilitation—Challenges and opportunities. Clin. Orthop. 63:153–161, 1969.
13. Paterson, D.: Who cares? Bull. Am. Acad. Orthop. Surg. 29(2):18–22, 1981.
14. Perry, J. Orthopedic rehabilitation. In Goldsmith, H. S., Ed.: *Practice of Surgery*, pp. 1–12. Harper & Row, Hagerstown, Md., 1972.
15. Pierce, D. S., and Nickel, V. L., Eds.: *The Total Care of Spinal Cord Injuries*. Little, Brown, Boston, 1977.
16. Shands, A. R.: A few remarks on physical medicine, rehabilitation and orthopedic surgery. South. Med. J. 54:420–425, 1961.
17. Thomas, E. L.: Nursing care of the patient with spinal cord injury. In Pierce, D. S., and Nickel, V. L., Eds.: *The Total Care of Spinal Cord Injuries*, pp. 249–294. Little, Brown, Boston, 1977.
18. Vash, C.: *The Psychology of Disability*. Springer, New York, 1981.
19. Wilson, P. D.: Whither orthopedics? Bull. Hosp. Joint Dis. 24:1–21, 1963.

2

The Rationale and Rewards of Team Care

Vernon L. Nickel, M.D.

Most physicians, including orthopedic surgeons, have not concerned themselves as much with the care of chronic disabilities as they could and should have. For many years, the chief reason for this neglect has been the press of work in acute-care hospitals. Now that acute ailments generally are better looked after and enough specialists are available, it is time that these specialists devote themselves to chronic crippling conditions with the same attention. One factor compounding the problem of care for chronic diseases is a fortuitous one—the mortality of patients with such conditions is being progressively lowered. More and more patients are surviving their acute episodes, which means there is a growing population of persons requiring rehabilitation.

I believe that at least 25 percent of all patients with chronic diseases could be significantly aided by the rehabilitation process. Unfortunately for these patients, there is only a limited acceptance of coverage of rehabilitation by third-party payers, such as Blue Cross, Medicare, and Medicaid. And in contrast to the excellent example of the crippled children's services in correcting orthopedic conditions and rehabilitating children, the orthopedic profession has not assumed that degree of responsibility for rehabilitation of disabled adults. This deficiency was attested to and deplored by the profession's greatest leader, Sir Robert Jones.[1,5,6]

Because the techniques and skills the physician needs for treating chronic and acute disorders are so similar, someone trained in acute-care orthopedics is also well-qualified to lead a rehabilitation team for chronic neuromusculoskeletal disorders. The rehabilitation team leader should not be chosen because of belonging to a particular specialty, but rather because he or she has a great interest in the particular disease category. For that matter, physicians who are not orthopedists could be well-qualified to direct programs of neuromuscular rehabilitation.[13]

Physical medicine developed largely to fill a void that other expanding specialties created through their neglect. In some areas, the physiatrists are still the only group that concerns itself with the rehabilitation process. The skills of the many disciplines needed in the rehabilitation process cannot be fully encompassed or learned by one person.[3,14]

Occasionally, an allied health professional is chosen to direct the rehabilitation effort. This usually proves unsatisfactory, because a person who is sick demands a doctor. Although certain aspects of rehabilitation may not require close direction by a physician, for delegation can be extensive, the overall program should be coordinated and led by a physician.

In the sections that follow, I argue for the need to discard the myth of the physician as an omnipotent being who can successfully deal with all aspects of the rehabilitation process. My method is to emphasize the skills of each health professional required for a competent rehabilitation service and note the improvement in patient care that will result when all members are permitted to work to their full potential.* Delegation of authority and teamwork have been traditional and expected in the operating room and the intensive care unit but they are not of long standing in rehabilitation. Unfortunately, isolation and bickering among specialties have erected severe hurdles that have hampered progress severely.

NURSING

The nurse is the key person on the rehabilitation team, by virtue of her skills and interest in the rehabilitation process. The nursing profession has been one of the first to give status and recognition to its members who have specialized in the field of rehabilitative nursing.

The nurse's background and experience uniquely qualify her to step into roles for which she may not have specific training, to do what needs to be done under the existing circumstances, and then to step back when the specialists arrive to take over. At no time during this process does she lose professional dignity or status.[2,8]

In contrast to the acute-care setting, the nurse's pattern of operation changes somewhat when she enters the rehabilitation environment. Rather than performing every task for patients, the rehabilitation nurse must encourage and direct patients to expand maximum effort in their own care. She must never hover over them. Rather, she must instill self-confidence and assist in their relearning program. Patients are required to feed and dress themselves even though it is not the easiest path for the patients or the professionals caring for them.

---

* The history and contributions of specific allied health professionals in rehabilitation are discussed at length in Chapters 3–12.

Patients on rehabilitation services have many demands on their time and are kept busy. Their schedules may require that routine nursing care be done early or late in the day, on weekends, or even omitted. Priority must be given to the tasks that will speed up the patients's return to the outside community.

In a rehabilitation setting, nursing assumes responsibility for many activities that are not a part of acute care. At a rehabilitation facility, nurses do positioning, turning, and range of motion, and they constantly work to prevent pressure sores and contractural deformities. They are well aware of how these complications can devastate a patient's rehabilitation.

The nurse recognizes the intense competition for her patient's time by the various rehabilitation services, and she apportions it among the other professional services. It is not merely a question of freeing the physician from this chore, but rather she is best suited to supervise the patient's day most effectively. Her broad professional interests, skills, and 24-hour-a-day presence with the patient eminently qualify her to assume this responsibility.[16]

The nurse is rapidly assuming charge of arranging and maintaining continuity of care.[16] She is best qualified to plan and extend care into the patient's home environment, and she certainly is most effective in coordinating this effort.

ENGINEERING AND KINESIOLOGY

Rehabilitation engineers bring the scientific and technical knowledge of their profession to the clinical environment of chronic disability. Engineers are recruited from two main sources: the traditional specialties of electrical and mechanical engineering and the newer field of bioengineering. Engineers applying advanced technology to the problems of rehabilitation can well be compared to engineers who participate in space programs. The difficulties a physically disabled person has are similar in concept to those encountered by men in space. In each case, the engineer must manipulate the environment with the tools of science and technology in order to improve the quality of life for someone at a physical disadvantage. Rehabilitation engineers work to refine diagnostic as well as therapeutic measures. Their contribution to improved diagnostic tests is best represented by spinal cord monitoring; their progress in upgrading therapeutic methods is exemplified by functional electrical stimulation.

An important example of engineering research in the service of the disabled is that of kinesiology. Kinesiology does for individuals with motor dysfunction what cardiological assessment has done for heart disease. Kinesiology has made it possible for therapists and surgeons to measure limb function with reproducible precision, with excellent results for amputations, total joint replacement, and gait in cerebral palsy. Surgical decisions regarding muscle transplants in cerebral palsy and stroke have already been markedly improved. It is now possible to evaluate several aspects of phasic muscle activity, including gait velocity, stride length, and force and timing.

The kinesiology laboratory has also provided a rich opportunity for the physician, the therapist, and the engineer to work together in a scientific milieu that encourages pooling of knowledge and wholehearted professional cooperation.

PHYSICAL THERAPY

Traditionally the physical therapist has a comfortable and rewarding professional relationship with the orthopedic surgeon; this is even more true in the rehabilitation setting. In orthopedic rehabilitation, physical therapists help prevent and help correct deformities, strengthen and train weakened muscles, administer a variety of special techniques to improve function, and are highly skilled in the employment of special equipment and training patients in its use. Their duties do not include using such modalities as massage, ultrasound, ultraviolet or infrared radiation, diathermy, diapulse, or whirlpool baths. *These have no place whatsoever in rehabilitation.*

In the early years of this century, physical therapists were instrumental in cooperating with orthopedic surgeon in developing accurate muscle grading techniques. Their work contributed greatly to the care of thousands of poliomyelitis patients. Today we have a similar need for methods to grade spasticity,[11] and physical therapy is expected to be prominent in solving this problem.

OCCUPATIONAL THERAPY

The profession of occupational therapy has assumed important new dimensions in recent years. Although occupational therapists were once considered only for diversional or recreational activities,[2,9] they now are concentrating their efforts on improving upper extremity function, teaching patients how to carry out activities of daily living, and performing vocational testing. Never again can occupational therapists be asked to fritter away their valuable professional resources on anything less than functional training.

Many orthopedic surgeons have little or no knowledge of what a professional occupational therapist is and can do. Certainly these trained therapists are ideal partners for the surgeon in pioneering better hand surgery, better upper extremity function, and better neurological testing and training. They are invaluable assistants to the orthopedic surgeon and deserve the highest level of support.[19]

ORTHOTICS AND PROSTHETICS

After World War II, the field of prosthetics became the prototype in medicine for enlisting technology on behalf of serving the disabled. The introduction of plastics, the prefabrication of component parts for prostheses, and the strong emphasis on high standards of education for those wishing to become prosthetists greatly improved the care given to amputees as well as the status of the field itself. Today, the duties of prosthetists are not confined to fabricating and fitting devices. They also confer with the surgeon about the possibilities for immediate fitting and work with the physician, the occupational and physical therapists, and the social worker in orchestrating the patient's return to a stable life in the community.

The role of the orthotist is changing, much as the prosthetist's function did after World War II. Research, training, and clinical applications of knowledge promise rapid progress in orthotics.[4,15] The orthotist is a vital adjunct to the rehabilitation team, providing the know-how and professional training needed to fit patients with assistive devices. New and better braces and assistive devices make possible many activities that were impossible for patients not so long ago. The orthopedic surgeon is vitally interested in the progress being made in orthotics, especially as it relates to a rehabilitation program. Cooperation is essential between these two facets of medical care, for their combined efforts often convert a dependent person into a productive, independent one.

SOCIAL WORK

Patients with chronic diseases often suffer devastating social crippling in addition to their other disabilities. When a person's wage-earning capacity is diminished and this disability is heaped upon his impaired capability to care for himself, the blow to his morale can easily cause a patient to withdraw and isolate himself from his surroundings. Obviously, constructive social planning is necessary in a good rehabilitation program to prevent such behavior; thus the social worker is an integral part of the rehabilitation team.[7]

Orthopedic surgeons should encourage and expand the social workers' activities on the rehabilitation team. Their professional contribution to patients' physical well-being and mental restoration is substantial and demands cooperation from all members of the team.

CLINICAL PSYCHOLOGY

The clinical psychologist not only helps the patient adjust to disability, but he also helps other members of the professional rehabilitation team to understand the severe psychological problems of patients with chronic crippling disabilities.[17]

Clinical psychologists are well trained in experimental designs and the scientific method. They provide leadership for others who might not have as firm a background in validating information. The clinical psychologist has been far more successful in rehabilitation than the psychiatrist who, except in isolated instances, has not participated effectively on the rehabilitation team. The psychiatrists have had the tendency to consider patients with long-term disability as mentally ill. Psychologists, however, have seen them as normal people who have been disrupted or disturbed.

VOCATIONAL COUNSELING

Society has long recognized the tremendous financial and social benefits gained by returning a patient with a chronic physical disability to gainful employment.[12,18] Historically, more than any other specialty, orthopedics has led this effort, best exemplified by the success in caring for people with residuals of poliomyelitis and returning a large number of them to the work force.[10] From beginning to end, the efforts of the medical and allied health workers are pointed toward developing the disabled person's physical, intellectual, and emotional resources to their maximum potential for functioning as a productive member of society.

Although poliomyelitis is no longer a problem in the United States, we need to maintain the aggressive attitude that it spawned and apply it to employable adults with other chronic physical disorders. The vocational counselor—trained to lead patients through the frustrating steps to becoming an independent wage earner—is the person educated to do just that. The total rehabilitation process itself culminates in vocational preparation. All states now have very active and well-funded programs to create conditions conducive to help many patients sustaining disabilities of varying severity. These programs are led by vocational counselors.

REFERENCES

1. Girdlestone, G. R.: The Robert Jones tradition. J. Bone Joint Surg. 30B:187–195, 1948.
2. Goldthwait, J. E.: The backgrounds and foregrounds of orthopaedics. J. Bone Joint Surg. 15B:279–301, 1933.
3. Inman, V. T.: Specialization and the physiatrist. Arch. Phys. Med. Rehabil. 45:765–770, 1966.
4. Jones, R.: Treatment of fractures of the thigh. Br. Med. J. 1:1086–1087, 1914.
5. Jones, R.: The problem of the cripple. Practitioner 112:1–12, 1924.
6. Jones, R.: An address on the domain of orthopedic surgery. Br. Med. J. 1:295–297, 1931.
7. Kahn, E.: Social bracing in rehabilitation. J. Am. Phys. Ther. Assoc. 47(6):692–699, 1967.
8. Knoche, F. J., and Knoche, L. S.: *Orthopedic Nursing*. F. A. Davis, Philadelphia, 1951.
9. Nickel, V. L.: The therapist and the profession. In *Proceedings of the American Occupational Therapy Association Conference*, pp. 1–40. American Occupational Therapy Association, Washington, D.C., 1960.
10. Nickel, V. L.: Sir Robert Jones Lecture: Orthopedic rehabilitation—challenges and opportunities. Bull. Hosp. Joint Dis. 29:1–21, 1968.
11. Riebel, J. D., and Nashold, B. S., Jr.: Electronic method of measuring and recording resistance to passive muscle stretch. J. Am. Phys. Ther. Assoc. 42:21–27, 1962.
12. Rusk, H. A.: The advantage of disadvantage. Bull. Hosp. Joint Dis. 16:1–6, 1955.
13. Sarmiento, A., and McCullough, N. C.: The orthopaedist and rehabilitation. Clin. Orthop. 41:111–115, 1965.
14. Shands, A. R.: A few remarks on physical medicine, rehabilitation and orthopedic surgery. South. Med. J. 54:420–425, 1961.
15. Snelson, R., and Conry, J.: Recent advances in functional arm bracing correlated with orthopedic surgery for the severely paralyzed upper extremity. Orthop. Prosthet. Appl. J. 12:41–49, 1958.
16. Stanton, J.: Rehabilitation nursing related to stroke. Clin. Orthop. 63:39–53, 1969.
17. Wendland, L. V.: Psychologists at work. Am. Psych. Assoc. Bull. 22:1, 1964.
18. Wright, B. A.: *Physical Disability: A Psychological Approach*. Harper, New York, 1960.
19. Yerxa, E. J.: Authentic occupational therapy. Am. J. Occup. Ther. 21:1–9, 1967.

3

The Rehabilitation Nurse

Linda Mills Hennig, M.A., R.N.

Rehabilitation belongs to no one profession. It is dependent on the contributions of many professionals and on the active participation and comprehension of the patient. Not only are there areas of collaborative effort among the health care providers, plus a sharing of many roles and functions, but professional boundaries are not always well defined. Each discipline, however, makes a singular contribution and has definite areas of responsibility. Nursing is a pivotal factor in the recovery and progress of the patient undergoing rehabilitation. Without knowledgeable nursing intervention, the rehabilitation program can fail. The physician and therapists provide intermittent services; unless these services are sustained and *augmented* by continuous nursing contact and nursing therapy, the patient's progress is diminished.

This chapter addresses the role and some of the primary responsibilities of professional nurses in caring for persons with chronic diseases and those undergoing orthopedic procedures. It will also discuss the emergence of rehabilitation nursing, the preparation and qualifications of the nurse for rehabilitation, and the specific technological expertise required by the nurse.

EMERGENCE OF REHABILITATION NURSING

Opinions differ in regarding rehabilitation nursing as a specialty area or as a component of general nursing practice.[4,8,11] This author believes, given the advances in physical rehabilitation and nursing over the past 25 years, that rehabilitation nursing has emerged as a specialty. Yet the basic concepts and skills of rehabilitation nursing are fundamental and applicable to most of nursing practice.

Rehabilitation is not just a tertiary phase of medical or health care. Its philosophy and approaches should be initiated at the onset of disease or injury. The efforts by nurses and other health care professionals to maintain function, prevent further dysfunction, and deal with the psychological reactions during the initial phase of care will greatly enhance the results of long-term care and rehabilitation. In fact, if rehabilitation is integrated into acute care, long-term care can often be averted. Conversely, failure to integrate rehabilitation into acute care can markedly reduce the patient's potential for rehabilitation. The nurse is the primary person in the acute-care setting to initiate rehabilitative care.

Even though much rehabilitation can be accomplished within the acute-care hospital, treatment of patients with selected conditions is often beyond the scope of available services. Specialty centers for rehabilitation exist for the comprehensive management of these patients. Societal attitudes, legislative actions, and recognition by health professionals that rehabilitation can have positive results for the disabled individual have resulted in the establishment of more rehabilitation facilities. The proliferation of rehabilitation services has created a demand for knowledgeable and highly skilled professional nurses. Rehabilitation nursing as a specialty has evolved from this demand as well as a recognition within the nursing profession of the need for rehabilitation expertise in a variety of settings, including acute-care hospitals, rehabilitation centers, nursing homes, and patients' own residences.

IMPACT OF ORTHOPEDIC SURGERY ON REHABILITATION NURSING

Orthopedic surgery adds a dynamic dimension to the rehabilitation process. An artificial joint replacement will mean increased functional ability, improved motion, and decreased pain. Tendon transfers offer a new source of power for selected movements abolished by paralysis. Spinal fusion leads to stabilization and early mobilization, often resulting in more rapid rehabilitation. Numerous other procedures and advances in orthopedic surgery have had a direct impact on both orthopedic and rehabilitation nursing.

For the nurse in the general rehabilitation setting, advances in orthopedic surgery have necessitated the acquisition of knowledge about selected procedures and special equipment. These changes have also increased the numbers of patients requiring immediate postoperative care. For the nurse on the general orthopedic or surgical unit, orthopedic rehabilitation has necessitated a sharpening of rehabilitation skills and techniques. It has also given these nurses exposure to more persons with chronic diseases and disabling conditions, such as stroke, arthritis, and spinal cord injury. One result has been a sharing of knowledge and a recognition of commonalities between these two specialties. In essence, rehabilitation and orthopedic nursing go hand in hand, and may be viewed graphically as two partially overlapping circles. Indeed, one author has written, ''Although all rehabilitation is not necessarily concerned with orthopedics, it may be said that all orthopedics is concerned with rehabilitation.''[5]

THE PROFESSIONAL NURSE'S ROLE AND CONTRIBUTION TO REHABILITATION

The goal of rehabilitation is to attempt to restore maximum physical, psychological, social, economic, and vocational capacities to the person with a disabling condition. Rehabilitation also strives to help patients realize latent potentialities within themselves and to achieve some degree of self-actualization. As the *Guidelines for the Practice of Nursing on the Rehabilitation Team,* issued by the American Nurses' Association, state:[6]

> The rehabilitation program should help the patient to know himself as he is, and as he wishes to become; to communicate with his fellow team members; to assess himself; to learn and apply new techniques, substitutive processes, and perhaps even a new vocation in order to achieve the fullest possible life.

Nursing is concerned with maintenance of the patient's abilities, prevention of further disabilities or complications, restoration of bodily functions, and improving capacities for meeting self-care requirements. Self care may be defined as "the practice of activities that individuals personally initiate and perform on their own behalf in maintaining life, health, and well being."[7] Self-care requirements may be universal (such as food and elimination), or they can be demands secondary to the deviation in the patient's state of health. One role of the rehabilitation nurse is to assist patients in engaging in therapeutic self care and compensate for their deficiencies in performing these actions. Nursing also addresses itself to "facilitating a state of positive health for individuals and groups, attending to holistic man, and the interrelationships and feedback among his systems and subsystems, including the environment in which he interacts."[9]

Performing treatments and administering medications ordered by the physician are dependent functions of nursing. Independent functions include assessment of the patient's state of health on initial contact and throughout the period of care; interpretation of data derived from the assessment to arrive at a nursing diagnosis; development of goals for nursing care and a plan of action to achieve them; writing nursing orders; implementation of the plan; evaluation of the quality of the care given and the results of care; and initiation of health teaching. The nursing process (assessment, planning, implementation, evaluation) is ongoing, and its goals and actions are altered when necessary. The nursing regimen is consistent with, and complementary to, the prescribed medical regimen.

Assessment of the patient by the nurse includes, but is not limited to, the following broad categories:

> The patient's understanding of health problems
> Expectations of hospitalization or treatment
> General appearance and behavior
> Current health practices
> Communication abilities and limitations
> Nutritional status
> Rest and sleep pattern
> Elimination pattern
> Cardiopulmonary status
> Skin integrity and condition

   Gross motor and sensory evaluation
   Abilities, knowledge, motivation, and attitude to meet self-care requirements
   Present medications and understanding of actions
   Available resources—family, friends, financial status

The professional nurse has autonomy for decision-making within the realm of nursing practice. It is crucial for physicians to recognize and support this autonomy and nurses must exercise it and be accountable for the results. The role of autonomy in nursing practice is illustrated in the following examples.

Pressure sores are a monumental problem in persons with chronic conditions, especially those with sensory loss and immobilization of body parts. Maintaining the integrity of the skin and preventing problems is largely a nursing responsibility. It requires a thorough assessment of the patient's skin condition, the recognition of potential or real factors that contribute to skin breakdown, a comprehensive program of skin care, and constant re-evaluations of skin status. The nurse should select any special beds, mattresses, or positioning and skin care aids needed for management. These aids are adjuncts to deliberate actions, such as turning, repositioning, and skin inspection.

There is some overlap of responsibility between nurses and therapists in the area of skin protection. Equipment, such as wheelchairs, cushions, splints, and braces have a direct effect on the skin. The team works together with the patient to evaluate skin tolerance when using this equipment. Therapists must also be cognizant of tissue trauma when performing treatments and report potential problems to the nurse. The physician often orders or limits selected positions because of a surgical procedure or skeletal instability, but the nurse then works independently within those restrictions. Therapists may also recommend certain positions based on their evaluations and treatment plans, and the nurse follows through with these recommendations. The overall positioning program, however, is designed and implemented by the nurse.

Maintaining satisfactory elimination for the patient is within the nurse's realm. The nurse ensures that the patient has a regular pattern of bowel elimination by developing a suitable program on initial contact, based on an assessment of the patient's past history and present health status. The plan is implemented by explanations about the diet designed to aid the program, fluid regulation, abdominal exercises, regular toileting, and use of authorized medications, such as stool softeners, bulking agents, and suppositories. The nurse modifies the program when necessary. Disorders of the gastrointestinal tract would necessitate evaluation and management by the physician.

Health education is another important function of independent nursing. It may deal with any aspect of the patient's life, but it mainly concerns actions he is unable to perform or new knowledge required in light of his altered health status. For example, health education encompasses teaching patients and their families about the disease process or condition, the effects of immobilization, medications required, the skin maintenance program, the elimination program, methods of self-care, and adjustments to the disability.

The professional nurse has the responsibility for coordinating the 24-hour program for the patient. This means not only organizing and supervising nursing care delivery, but coordinating all of the other services to the patient. The nurse often needs to reschedule a patient's appointments or recommend restructuring the daily program if, in her evaluation, the patient's energy level, need for rest, or overall condition warrants it. As the patient acquires greater functional abilities, self-care capacities, and knowledge, nursing assistance is withdrawn. Although physical aid may be decreased, such nursing actions as guiding, teaching, and providing a therapeutic environment are all continued as needed.

SPECIAL ATTRIBUTES AND KNOWLEDGE OF THE REHABILITATION NURSE

The rehabilitation nurse has a sound foundation in anatomy and physiology, particularly of the neurological and musculoskeletal subsystems, and understands the processes of normal growth and development, including aging, and the normal behavioral reactions to injury and loss. The proper use of specialized equipment commonly used in rehabilitation and orthopedics must also be understood. Underlying all of this is an understanding of biomechanics and kinesiology. The nurse must have the ability to use manual skills, such as positioning, transferring, and ambulating, plus techniques to aid patients in carrying out the daily activities of living.

The nurse must comprehend the therapies of the other members of the rehabilitation team and be able to apply their techniques to the nursing area. Informed supervision of the patient performing a newly learned activity is important so that the nurse can advise the therapists and physicians on a patient's compliance, safety, and accuracy. The nurse also gives the patient immediate feedback as he performs the task.

The ability to teach others is mandatory. Every day the nurse encounters situations in which teaching patients and their families is necessary. Quite often instruction is informal and on a one-to-one basis, but formal teaching sessions must also be planned to achieve certain teaching/learning objectives.

The nurse must be able to identify and find solutions to problems as they arise. Long-range planning for nursing goals, as well as helping the patient plan for the future, is imperative. The nurse utilizes resources inside and outside of the facility to assist the patient. Preparing the patient for discharge is done through identifying what knowledge, equipment, and supplies he needs. These requirements are met and, if needed, a referral to a community nursing agency is made. The nurse seeks to provide some continuity of care with personnel and nursing actions not only during the patient's hospitalization, but upon his return to the community.

The nurse must know herself, and she should frequently examine her own attitudes toward disability. The attitudes of the health care providers have a dynamic influence on how a patient views himself and works through the adjustment process. Pity and excessive sympathy have no therapeutic value. Instead, firmness, tempered with humor and kindness, is needed by the nurse to help the patient achieve greater independence. This firmness in encouraging the patient to learn to do things for himself may be interpreted by the patient or others as an insensitivity. In actuality, sensitivity and responsiveness are hallmarks of the rehabilitation nurse, as are flexibility, creativity, and assertiveness.

Maturity to deal with one's own emotions is required in order to handle the overwhelming emotional reactions of many patients. Last, but not least, there must be patience. The results of rehabilitative care are often not seen for weeks, months, and even years. A patient's accomplishments or gains are measured in inches rather than in feet. Often the nurse can help ease the patient's frustration by imparting an attitude of patience. This is especially true during times of the day when the patient is not involved in some meaningful activity. Nursing the rehabilitation patient requires that mutual trust and respect be established and that they be sustained over an extended period of time.

COMMUNICATION AND RELATIONSHIPS WITH OTHER TEAM MEMBERS

The professional nurse shares a collegial relationship with the physician and other professional members of the rehabilitation team. All are partners in health care. Each professional is responsible and accountable for his or her own decisions and actions. There must be mutual respect among the team members. Leadership within an effective team may change periodically, depending on the group and the objectives at hand.

There must be open communication among the individuals representing the various disciplines. These communications may be in the form of bedside rounds, regular conferences, or informal conferences via telephone or personal contact. However, it cannot be overemphasized that regularly scheduled interdisciplinary conferences are a must in the rehabilitation setting. Conferences provide each professional an opportunity to report on the patient's treatment plan and progress or regression, but, most important, it is a time for critical evaluation of the total rehabilitation program. A conference should even allow for patient participation. Documentation of care and results of care are a daily task, but the pooling of weekly summaries or progress notes by members of each discipline are helpful for evaluation.

The importance of maintaining open lines of communication and good interpersonal relationships should not have to be pointed out, but it is added here for emphasis. Teamwork takes effort. If it is neglected, frictions can develop among health care professionals and the patient is often caught in the middle.

EDUCATIONAL PREPARATION

Preparation to enter nursing practice is possible via a hospital diploma program, an associate of arts degree program, or a baccalaureate degree program. The American Nurses' Association supports the position that nursing education should take place in an institution of higher learning, and the minimum preparation for entry into professional nursing should be the baccalaureate degree in nursing.[3]

Basic nursing programs do not include rehabilitation nursing as a separate course. Pertinent concepts of rehabilitation and management of selected conditions are integrated into the total curriculum. Most new graduates, however, have had little or no exposure to patients undergoing a comprehensive rehabilitation program. Therefore, it becomes the responsibility of the treatment facility to provide a comprehensive orientation and training program for newly employed nurses.

A few short courses in rehabilitation nursing, ranging from one to four weeks, are offered throughout the United States for registered and licensed practical nurses. These courses are sponsored by major rehabilitation centers or universities and generally focus on nursing management of selected disabilities and provide for mastery of techniques for positioning, transfers, activities of daily living, and methods of preventing dysfunction. Unfortunately, the frequency of such courses has decreased in the past few years.

Although there are numerous graduate programs available that lead to a master's degree in nursing, only a few programs exist for specialization in rehabilitation nursing. The author believes that there is a greater demand than supply of rehabilitation nurse specialists and that there is a critical need for more formal graduate programs in this area.

Because the availability of programs is limited, the nurse who seeks to become a clinical nurse specialist in rehabilitation or orthopedics may choose to pursue graduate study in a broader-based specialty program, such as medical-surgical nursing, nursing science, or community health nursing. Through a careful combination of elective courses of special interest, individual study, and selected clinical experiences, expertise can be acquired in orthopedics or rehabilitation. Graduates with such expertise are needed in a variety of settings: acute-care hospitals, outpatient clinics, rehabilitation centers, nursing homes, community health agencies, and schools of nursing. The nature of the specialty provides opportunities for the rehabilitation nurse specialist to engage in private practice, serve as a consultant to various types of health agencies and the insurance industry, or become a resource to other nurses and health care providers.

Some of the titles applied to nursing specialists are rather confusing. For clarification, several nursing roles are cited below. The American Nurses' Association Congress for Nursing Practice supports the following three definitions of nursing roles or titles:[2]

A *clinical nurse specialist* (CNS) is a clinician

> with a high degree of knowledge, skill and competence in a specialized area of nursing. These are made directly available to the public through the provision of nursing care to clients and indirectly available through guidance and planning of care with other nursing personnel.

A CNS holds a master's degree in nursing, preferably with an emphasis in clinical nursing.

A *nurse clinician* has

> well developed competencies in utilizing a broad range of cues. These cues are used for prescribing and implementing both direct and indirect nursing care and for articulating nursing therapies with other planned therapies.

Clinicians acquire expertise and ensure ongoing professional development through clinical experience and continuing education. Usually the minimal preparation for this role is the baccalaureate degree.

A *nurse practitioner* has

> advanced skills in the assessment of the physical and psychosocial health-illness status of individuals, families or groups in a variety of settings through health and development history taking and physical examination.

Preparation for these skills is by "formal continuing education which adheres to the American Nurses' Association's approved guidelines, or in a baccalaureate nursing program." Graduates must take a national examination to become certified.

An increasingly popular role in rehabilitation is that of *liaison nurse*. From preadmission assessment to discharge planning and community follow-up, this nurse attempts to ensure continuity of nursing care for the patient. Prior to discharge, a home visit may be made by the liaison nurse. After discharge, contact with the patient via telephone or outpatient clinic visits is sustained as long as is needed.[10] The liaison nurse makes referrals to community nursing agencies when necessary. The importance of continuity of care for rehabilitation patients cannot be overstated. Most often the patient has a permanent disability, must alter his style of life considerably, and must attend to new health needs resulting from the disability. Although patients and families are taught to become responsible for care needs, a health professional who can serve as a point of contact for assistance with problems is a valuable resource to the patient. The liaison nurse can also serve as a resource to other nurses while the patient is in another health care facility or at home. The concepts and practices described for the liaison nurse may be incorporated into the clinical nurse specialist or nurse clinician role. Thus the title is not as important as the fact that continuity of care is being provided. Qualifications and job descriptions for liaison nurses vary throughout the country. Ideally, this nurse should hold a master's degree in nursing and be an expert rehabilitation nurse with experience in community health.

Professional organizations provide opportunities for working toward common goals and for continuing education. In addition to the American Nurses' Association, three national organizations are available for nurses interested in orthopedics and rehabilitation: the National Association of Orthopedic Nurses, the Association of Rehabilitation Nurses, and the American Congress of Rehabilitation Medicine. The first two are exclusively for nurses working within the designated specialty. The third is a multidisciplinary organization with membership open to nurses who meet the membership criteria. Nurses may belong to several organizations or select one that best meets their professional needs.

SUMMARY

Professional nursing is a key therapeutic force in helping patients to recover and become rehabilitated.[1] The foci of rehabilitation nursing are maintenance of the patient's abilities, prevention of further disabilities and complications, optimal restoration of physical and psychosocial health, and fostering independence in self-care.

The basic concepts and practices of rehabilitation nursing are applicable to many health and community settings, yet specialized knowledge and expertise are needed to work in facilities specializing in comprehensive rehabilitation.

The professional nurse exercises autonomy in nursing practice and is accountable for nursing care. The nurse collaborates with other team members to provide coordinated comprehensive care to patients. Effective teamwork among health care professionals is vital for the success of rehabilitation. It works best when each member respects and has an understanding of everyone's roles and responsibilities.

More specialized courses of study are needed in rehabilitation nursing. This applies to undergraduate, graduate, and continuing education programs in nursing.

REFERENCES

1. Alfano, G. J.: The Loeb Center for nursing and rehabilitation—A professional approach to nursing practice. Nurs. Clin. North Am. 4:487–493, 1969.

2. American Nurses' Association: Congress for nursing practice. Definitions. American Nurses' Association, New York, May 8, 1974.

3. American Nurses' Association: Educational preparation for nurse practitioners and assistants to nurses. A position paper. American Nurses' Association, New York, 1965 (#G-83).

4. Christopherson, V. A., Coulter, P. P., Wolanin, M. O., eds.: *Rehabilitation Nursing Perspectives and Applications.* McGraw-Hill, New York, 1974.

5. Dunn, B. H.: Rehabilitation: Philosophy, concepts and principles. In Hilt, N., Ed.: *Manual of Orthopedics,* pp. 444–448. C. V. Mosby, St. Louis, 1980.

6. *Guidelines for the Practice of Nursing on the Rehabilitation Team.* American Nurses' Association, New York, 1965.

7. Orem, D. E.: *Nursing: Concepts of Practice.* McGraw-Hill, New York, 1981.

8. Plaisted, L. M.: The clinical specialist in rehabilitation nursing. Am. J. Nurs. 69:562–564, 1969.

9. Riffle, K. L.: Rehabilitation: The evolution of a social concept. Nurs. Clin. North Am. 8:665–670, 1973.

10. Stewart, P.: Through the webwork: Side by side. J. Neurosurg. Nurs. 6:14–19, 1974.

11. Stryker, R. P.: *Rehabilitative Aspects of Acute and Chronic Nursing Care.* W. B. Saunders, Philadelphia, 1977.

4

The Engineer

Donald R. McNeal, Ph.D.

WHAT IS AN ENGINEER?

To many physicians and allied health professionals, an engineer is the person who maintains the hospital facility or repairs and calibrates instruments and equipment on the wards and in the operating room. In actuality, many of these persons are engineers by title only and not by educational degree. The engineer to be described in this chapter may perform some of the functions just listed, but his contributions to the field of medicine and rehabilitation far exceed this limited role. He is a well-trained professional who will be playing an important part in the future development of the medical field.

An engineer has at least four years of training at an accredited engineering school and receives a bachelor of science degree. Today, about half of the engineering graduates go on to graduate school, generally to obtain either a master's degree or a doctorate, or both.

Just as medicine was subdivided into specialties as the profession became broad and complex, so too has engineering. The engineering school of the University of Southern California, for example, offers degrees in 18 engineering specialties through eight separate departments. Specialties that are particularly involved with the medical field include electrical, mechanical, chemical, industrial, computer science, materials, and biomedical engineering. Biomedical engineering is a relatively new specialty that has developed specifically to create engineers having a physiological or clinical background to supplement their technical training.

The newest branch of biomedical engineering is rehabilitation engineering, which is concerned with the application of science and technology to improve the quality of life of the physically disabled rather than to prolonging or saving of life. In the fall of 1979 the first program offering a master's degree in rehabilitation engineering was initiated at the University of Virginia. This program is specifically oriented toward training engineers to become working members of the rehabilitation team. Because of the diversity of the rehabilitation process, the engineer in rehabilitation must be more of a generalist than a specialist and needs propensities and skills in team participation beyond those required of engineers in other disciplines. Reswick[7] has described the characteristics required of the engineer working in the field of rehabilitation.

Although engineers are generally found designing and building missiles, automobiles, calculators, washing machines, or petroleum facilities, more and more of them are finding their way into hospitals and are working with physicians and allied health professionals to provide better patient care. This chapter focuses on the current and future roles of engineers in rehabilitation and discusses the difficulties to be overcome to integrate them into the rehabilitation team. Much of the material is drawn from our experience at Rancho Los Amigos Hospital in Downey, California.

THE ENGINEER'S ENTRY INTO THE REHABILITATION FIELD

Although the field of rehabilitation engineering is relatively new, engineers have been involved in rehabilitation for a long time. Therapeutic and diagnostic equipment and surgical instruments are products of engineering design. In almost all of these cases, however, the design work was done by engineers working for commercial companies in response to needs expressed by clinical personnel. There was some interaction between engineer and clinician, but the patient was seldom involved in the creative process, and very often the engineer never saw the clinical environment in which the equipment was to be used.

Only after World War II did engineers begin to be involved in treatment programs in any organized fashion. This development came about through the Prosthetics and Sensory Aids Program, started by the Veterans Administration (VA) in 1945. Engineers working with prosthetists helped to design new artificial limbs and significant advances in prosthetic design were made in succeeding years. The thalidomide tragedy also fostered considerable interest in prosthetics among the engineering community, especially in England.

Contemporary rehabilitation engineering really began in 1972 when the Rehabilitation Services Administration (RSA), then an agency of the Department of Health, Education and Welfare, established two rehabilitation engineering centers at Rancho Los Amigos Hospital and the Moss Rehabilitation Hospital in Philadelphia. Additional centers have been added since then, and there are now 15 centers in the United States as well as three international centers. A key element in the selection of each center is that it have a close working relationship with a good rehabilitation hospital or vocational program.

To avoid duplication of effort and help coordinate this very large program, each center is required to concentrate its research and developmental effort on one or more "core areas," each of which is a major problem area related to rehabilitation that might be solved by engineering and technological expertise. Examples of core areas are mobility systems for the severely disabled, sensory aids for the blind and deaf, low-back pain, and internal total joint replacement.

The VA has followed suit and established two centers of its own, although these are called "rehabilitative" engineering centers to distinguish them from the RSA centers. The first center funded by the VA is in Hines, Illinois, and the second is located in Palo Alto, California.

A brief description of the Rancho Los Amigos Rehabilitation Engineering Center is provided to explain what a center is like and how it functions. The center is located on the grounds of Rancho Los Amigos Hospital, which is one of five hospitals of Los Angeles County as well as a teaching hospital for the University of Southern California. The center is co-directed by an engineer and a physician, both of whom have academic appointments with the university. A total of 38 staff members are salaried employees of the center; 13 are engineers and the rest are technicians, research assistants, clerical staff, and students. This number, however, does not truly represent the total effort because an additional 48 physicians and allied health personnel are involved in center projects.

Project work is divided into three core areas: functional electrical stimulation, pathokinesiology, and delivery of rehabilitation services. The goal of the first area is to use electrical stimulation to alleviate problems of patients with chronic disabilities and encourage the commercialization of equipment found to be efficacious in carefully controlled clinical studies. Three projects, focused on scoliosis, stroke, and spinal cord monitoring, are described in the following section. The second core area, pathokinesiology, deals with the objective measurement of human function in physically normal and disabled persons. The pathokinesiology laboratory is unique in that a major portion of staff activity is spent on diagnosis and follow-up of patients, a medical service distinct from research. One of their projects is described in the following section. Furnishing rehabilitation services is the newest core area and is aimed at providing direct engineering service to individual disabled clients. Services include counseling for problems that may be solved by appropriate equipment, prescription of equipment, and fabrication of custom equipment. In each of these areas, close collaboration with industry is strongly encouraged and supported by the rehabilitation engineering center. It is only through the private sector that devices developed within the center can be made available to the disabled population.

THE ENGINEER'S CONTRIBUTIONS TO REHABILITATION

Because the rehabilitation engineer's goal is to apply science and technology to improve the quality of life of the physically disabled, his work revolves around designing and fabricating equipment for patients or for the clinical staff to use in treating patients. Successful application of this equipment is possible only through close interaction among the engineer, the clinician, and the patient throughout the developmental process. It also requires that the engineer be involved in many tasks other than equipment design, including:

> Defining the requirements of the equipment proposed to solve the problem.
> Planning and conducting animal experiments to test instrumentation and equipment prior to human trials and gather basic physiological data required for design.
> Testing patients to gather data to be used for equipment design.
> Evaluation of prototype systems in the clinical environment.
> Collecting and analyzing data during the clinical evaluation.

The involvement of the rehabilitation engineer is best illustrated by example. Four currently active projects at Rancho Los Amigos Hospital will be described. In each case, the engineer's role in the project, the tasks he performs, and his interaction with the clinical staff are discussed.

Scoliosis

The treatment of choice for idiopathic scoliotic curves in the range of 20 to 45 degrees is a Milwaukee, Boston, or low-profile underarm brace. These braces are generally successful in halting further progression of the curve, but they are not accepted graciously by patients because of their uncosmetic appearance and restrictions on extracurricular activities. An alternate treatment currently under investigation is electrical stimulation of back muscles on the convex side of the curve.

Axelgaard et al.[2] have shown that stimulation of the intercostals and the latissimus dorsi through electrodes placed on the skin produces an immediate correction of the primary curve of 5 to 12 degrees. In most cases, the secondary curve is also corrected, although to a lesser extent. The immediate correction is obtained only when stimulation is turned on, but the hypothesis currently under investigation is that chronic, cyclical stimulation will halt or reverse progression of the curve.

Preliminary results from a clinical treatment program begun in October 1977 are encouraging.[1] Sixteen patients with curves ranging from 20 to 39 degrees (average, 29 degrees) have been followed for six months or longer. Typically, these curves progressed from 16 to 29 degrees over a six-month period just before initiating the treatment program. Six months after the program's initiation, the average curve had decreased to 27 degrees. Three of the curves had been corrected by more than 5 degrees, 1 had progressed by more than 5 degrees, and all the rest were within ±5 degrees of the value measured at the beginning of treatment.

In this program, patients are cyclically stimulated each night during the hours of sleep. The stimulus comes on for seven seconds, causing the muscles to contract slowly; then the stimulus is turned off for eight seconds to allow the muscles to relax. This cycle is repeated automatically for approximately eight hours each night. Patients quickly adapt to this routine and report no difficulty in sleeping.

Engineers have played an important role in developing this program. One engineer has been assigned to work with the orthopedic staff and has been instrumental in helping to develop the patient selection criteria and the treatment protocol, as well as the specifications for the stimulation equipment. In the early stage of the program, equipment was designed and fabricated by staff engineers at the rehabilitation engineering center. Later in the program, a company interested in commercialization of the device began working with the engineering and clinical staff at the hospital to develop a more compact unit based on specifications provided by the hospital engineering staff. The original unit and the one now in widespread use are shown in Figure 4-1.

This program originated in the spring of 1976 with work performed by an engineering student while he was serving an internship at Rancho Los Amigos Hospital to complete his requirements for a master's degree in biomedical engineering. Using cats, he investigated the optimal placement of electrodes on the back for maximizing the spinal curvature induced by electrical stimulation. Much greater curvature was induced during stimulation when the electrodes were placed near the mid-axillary line rather than over the paraspinal musculature. Based on these results, a screening program was initiated on idiopathic and spinal cord injured scoliotic patients that confirmed a similar finding in human beings.[2]

Engineering design has also been applied to improving measurement of the spinal deformity. Engineers working with the orthopedists found that the standard technique for measuring the rib hump was not very accurate or repeatable. Two devices, one of which is shown in Figure 4-2, were built and tested and are now being used routinely by the orthopedic staff. The first device measures the vertical difference and the spacing between the high points of the back on either side of the

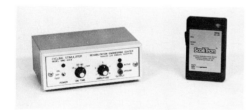

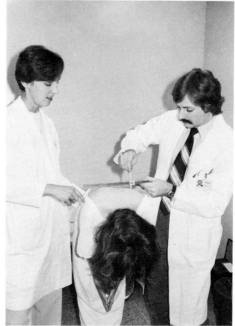

Fig. 4-1. Electrical stimulation devices for correcting scoliosis: the piece of equipment on the left was developed by hospital personnel and the one on the right was made by a private company in cooperation with engineers at the hospital.

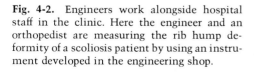

Fig. 4-2. Engineers work alongside hospital staff in the clinic. Here the engineer and an orthopedist are measuring the rib hump deformity of a scoliosis patient by using an instrument developed in the engineering shop.

spine, and the second uses a flexible bar to trace out a complete profile of the patient's back.

When patients come into the clinic, they are seen by the orthopedist, the physical therapist, and the engineer. The engineer's primary responsibility is to ensure that the equipment is functioning properly and to repair or replace any part of the system that may be malfunctioning. He also assists in recording data documenting the current status of the patient and the curve. Although the engineer is often consulted and helps make decisions regarding treatment, he carefully avoids answering any questions about the medical status of the patient. Questions of this nature, if put to the engineer, are referred to the attending physician.

It is important for the engineer not to substitute for the physician, yet it is also essential that he thoroughly understand the medical problem and the related physiology. It is impossible to design a system properly coordinated with the patient that will correct the clinical problem without this understanding. Before beginning the program, the engineer will therefore become acquainted with pertinent literature and throughout the program will continue reviewing journal articles. This background, coupled with his clinical interaction with the patient and physician and frequent discussions with physicians outside the clinic, provides the engineer with the knowledge required to carry out the system design and allows him to talk fluently about the subject matter with medical personnel.

In this program, as in most developmental programs, the responsibility falls most heavily on the engineer early in the program when hardware prototypes are being developed and tested; it shifts gradually to the physician as the program becomes less experimental and more clinical. At all stages of the program, of course, the ultimate responsibility for patient care rests in the hands of the physician, and he may at any time veto a decision he feels is not in the best interests of the patient.

Stroke

Rehabilitation following a serious stroke is a long and tedious process, generally requiring three to six months of intensive therapy. Conventional therapeutic techniques have been supplemented in recent years with innovative ideas, such as biofeedback training and electrical stimulation. Both techniques are extensively used in stroke therapy at Rancho Los Amigos Hospital, and engineering has played a major role in developing the clinical program and fabricating the required equipment.

Electrical stimulation of muscle paralyzed by a stroke will strengthen the muscle and, if the joint is free to move, will prevent contractures and increase passive range of motion.[3] Biofeedback, on the other hand, can be used effectively to increase body awareness and motivate and encourage the patient as he attempts to relearn the use of his extremities. Coupling stimulation with biofeedback therefore has the potential for motivating the patient to maximize his voluntary abilities while simultaneously improving the physical state of muscles and joints.

One system now routinely used in stroke therapy at Rancho Los Amigos Hospital is the positional feedback stimulation trainer (PFST). The basic system consists of a goniometer to measure the position of a joint, an audiovisual display of joint position, and an electrical stimulator to activate the muscles acting on the joint. As an example of how the system is used, consider the case of a stroke patient with impaired wrist extension, but having at least 5 degrees of active extension. When a green light on the display comes on, the patient is asked to extend his wrist as far as he can (Fig. 4-3). As he does so, a meter displays the position of his wrist and an audible tone increases in pitch as the wrist is extended. When the patient exceeds a threshold previously by the therapist close to his maximum active range, electrical stimulation of the wrist extensors is initiated, causing the wrist to extend through its full range. The patient can then relax until the green light signals the beginning of a new sequence.

Operation of the PFST requires no intervention by a therapist after the initial set-up, which takes about five minutes. The therapist must set the threshold and the variable resistance to wrist extension to match the patient's ability and adjust the stimulus level to obtain a strong but tolerable contraction of the wrist extensor muscles. After that, the patient cycles through the exercise regimen under the control of the PFST, which keeps track of the number of successfully completed trials.

In a controlled study of two similar groups of patients, differing only in that the experimental group underwent two 30-minute sessions of PFST therapy daily in addition to the conventional therapeutic program, the experimental group demonstrated significantly greater gains in active range and extension strength than the control group after only four weeks of therapy.[4]

This same system is also used to exercise the fingers and the elbow. Only the goniometer used to measure joint position need be changed. Goniometers for the fingers, wrists, and elbows are shown in Figure 4-4. A unique parallelogram construction provides an accurate measure of joint position without requiring a critical adjustment of the device on the patient.

The PFST is just one of an array of devices that have been or are being developed for use in stroke therapy. The equipment ranges from a simple cycling stimulator used for strengthening to a sophisticated system that requires the patient to position his arm to reach any one of a number of panel switches lighting up in random fashion. A therapy program has been designed that allows a patient to enter the program at a level consistent with the severity of the stroke and to

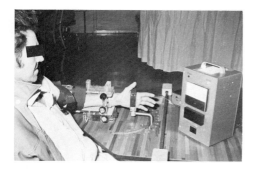

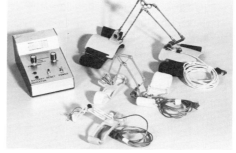

Fig. 4-3. This stroke patient is using a system that simultaneously encourages voluntary extension of the wrist and electrically stimulates the extensor muscles for full ranging of the wrist.

Fig. 4-4. Goniometers for the fingers, wrists, and elbows. The unique parallelogram construction permits accurate measurements without having to make critical adjustments on the patient.

proceed to his highest possible functional level at a rate coinciding with his own rate of recovery.

Development of this therapeutic program was possible only through close interaction among the engineer, therapist, and physician. The engineer in charge of this project spent many hours in the therapy gymnasium working with the therapist to understand the problems of the stroke patient and the needs of the therapist better. These sessions were supplemented by lengthy meetings involving key members of the engineering and clinical staff for planning the therapeutic program and the general nature of the equipment needed. After these determinations were made, interstaff meetings within engineering were held to establish specific design details.

Even after all this planning, the completed equipment often fails to achieve all the intended goals when it is tested in the clinical environment. It is again essential for the engineer to be involved in this stage of applying equipment to the patient, so that he may fully appreciate the need for changes in hardware design. After identifying the problems encountered during clinical evaluation, the engineer goes back to the drawing board to rectify each of the problems. This stage is followed by further testing, and the process is repeated until the equipment functions correctly.

Spinal Cord Monitoring

Surgery of the spine carries a small but potentially catastrophic risk of damage to the spinal cord. The only test available to the surgeon today to check spinal cord function during surgery is the "wake-up" test, in which anesthesia is lightened and the patient is asked to move his toes.

Another approach that offers the possibility of monitoring cord function continuously during the procedure and the postoperative period is the use of spinal-evoked potentials.[5] Electrical stimulation of nerves in the extremities evokes nerve impulses that are conducted up the spinal cord. Although these signals are very small, they can be recorded by using sophisticated digital processing techniques. Damage to the cord produced by mechanical trauma or anoxia alters the conduction properties of the spinal nerves and produces a measurable change in the recorded evoked potential. If the surgeon is made aware of these changes at an early stage, there is a good possibility that he can take action to reverse or prevent further damage to the spinal cord.

The purpose of this project is to develop a sophisticated instrument that will be used during operations. The project is primarily an engineering task, and it will be up to the engineer to determine the appropriate bandwidth and gain of the amplifiers, sampling rates for digitizing the analogue signals, the best techniques of digital processing to obtain a signal not obscured by electrical interference, and other technical matters.

However, the surgeon and the surgical staff will be the ultimate users of the equipment. They must therefore offer early advice on such questions as how and where the recording electrodes will be placed on the spine, how the data should be displayed, how long monitoring should be continued, and many other issues relating to the use of the instrument and interpretation of the data. Once again, it is imperative that the engineers and clinicians work closely together through all

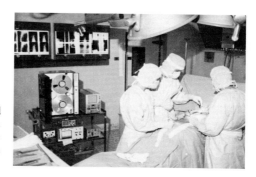

Fig. 4-5. When necessary, engineers scrub and assist in data collection during an operation. In this case, the viability of the spinal cord is being monitored during surgical correction of a scoliotic curve.

phases of the project to ensure that the final design will satisfactorily solve the problem. The engineers must have a good understanding of the clinical problem, and the surgeon must have some understanding of the technical difficulties to be overcome and the design concepts to be tested. In this project, the engineers go into the operating room frequently. Therefore all must, of course, be trained in sterile technique and in the rules and etiquette of the operating room (Fig. 4-5).

The engineering staff also has been significantly involved in supportive animal studies for the purposes of developing hardware to be used in the operating room and for testing the feasibility of using evoked potentials to detect early damage to the spinal cord. This, too, is a joint effort between engineer and surgeon to plan the experimental protocol, carry out the experiments, and analyze the data that are obtained. Most engineers with a master's degree or doctorate in biomedical engineering will have had training and experience with animal surgery and can assist the surgeon or independently perform many of the surgical procedures.

The Foot-switch Stride Analyzer

The pathokinesiology laboratory at Rancho Los Amigos Hospital is used to assess function in normal and impaired individuals. One of the principal areas of interest is gait analysis, and a number of instrumentation techniques are available to quantify the gait pattern. Among these are the foot-switch definition of stride characteristics and foot support pattern, dynamic electromyography and goniometry, energy measurement, and foot-floor reaction vector generation.

Instrumentation and associated equipment required for these measurements and for processing of the data are very costly. The purpose of the project to be described is to develop a low-cost, compact, clinically convenient instrument (the foot-switch stride analyzer) to record, calculate, and display certain characteristics of gait that have been found to be clinically significant in evaluating pathological gait. These variables are velocity, single- and double-limb support durations, stride length, cadence, gait cycle duration, and swing-stance ratio. This instrument is intended to be used in a standard clinical environment, thereby making quantitative gait analysis available to everyone.

The stride analyzer system consists of a pair of foot switches, a start and stop controller, a recorder, and a calculator. The foot switches are contained in insoles and indicate the total time the patient is bearing weight on each of four areas of each foot: heel, first and fifth metatarsal heads, and great toe. These data are stored during a 6-m walk in the recorder that is supported at the patient's waist. Two triggering lights placed 6 m apart activate a light-sensitive switch placed on the patient's arm that starts and stops data acquisition. Following the walk, data are transferred from the recorder to the calculator (Fig. 4-6). Gait characteristics are then calculated and printed out to provide a permanent record of the walk. Each is printed in absolute value and as a percentage of normal. Males and females are considered separately.

This is another good example of a project requiring close collaboration between engineers and clinicians. The first unit that was built was much simpler than the present one. That instrument calculated only velocity and single-limb support times of the right and left feet. Each of these variables was calculated and displayed at the end of the run on a digital display. The displayed value then had to be copied down on the patient's data sheet. The design of that instrument was dictated by the desire to keep its operation simple and to restrict the number of characteristics presented to the clinician in order to simplify interpretation of the data.

Trial use of this initial device at Rancho Los Amigos Hospital and other evaluating medical centers determined that two major design changes would be highly desirable. First, it became clear that calculation of additional variables would not confuse, but rather would provide much greater understanding of the gait pattern. Secondly, direct hard copies of the results were needed. Hand copying the gait characteristics onto the patient's permanent record was often done incorrectly, and after erasing the data from the recorder/calculator, it was impossible to go back and recheck the values recorded in the chart.

Intensive discussions between engineers and clinicians resulted in a new design that permitted calculation of additional variables and provided a hard copy printout. A key factor in this redesign was the emergence of a major new technological advance (low-power microprocessors), which permitted calculation of the additional gait variables without increasing the size or power consumption of the recorder.

It was also essential that the second system, although now more complex and sophisticated than the first, be at least as easy for the user to operate. Special features were therefore built into the second system to simplify operation. For example, the calculator is designed so that it is reset automatically when the recorder is disconnected. This obviates the necessity of a separate reset button

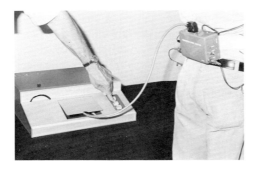

Fig. 4-6. Following a 6-m walk, foot-switch data are transferred from the recorder at the patient's waist to the calculator, where the data are processed and results printed out for inclusion in the patient's medical record.

and eliminates one more task for the operator. This may seem like a trivial design feature, but the combination of many such features in the same instrument simplifies the operation considerably.

The second version of the stride analyzer is also a more intelligent machine than the first. During trial use of the first instrument, it became obvious that "foot scuff" was a problem. If the subject scuffed his foot during the swing phase just prior to the beginning of the stance phase, the analyzer was unable to determine if the scuff should be considered part of the stance or swing phase. The new machine has a built-in decision-making capability to answer this question.

Development of the stride analyzer is typical of all programs in medical device development. The first prototype may come close to the desired specifications, but there are always problems that were not expected or improvements that become obvious only after repeated clinical trials. A second generation system must then be designed, built, and tested. Often this cycle must be repeated several times before a satisfactory system is achieved. This process requires patience and good communication between engineer and clinician. The engineer must understand why the clinician is unable to state precisely what the system must do before having an opportunity to evaluate a prototype system, and the clinician must understand the complexity of the design/fabrication phase to appreciate the time required for each step. An excellent discussion of the design/fabrication/evaluation/redesign process inherent in medical equipment development is provided by Reswick.[6]

INTEGRATION INTO THE TEAM

As illustrated in the previous examples, the engineer has become an active member of the rehabilitation team. This is a major departure from the past, when the engineer worked in his own company or laboratory and depended completely on the clinical staff to define the patient's problem for him. Based on the information they provided, he built equipment and then handed the "finished product" back to the clinicians for testing. It is not surprising that in many instances the results were disappointing. The process of developing a medical device requires frequent clinical trials and redesigns, close interaction between the engineer and the clinician, and an appreciation of the difficulties to be encountered by each in building the device and in applying it to the patient.

Successful device development depends upon the engineer being a working member of the team, yet the process of integrating the engineer into the team is not a simple one. Although the number of examples of successful integration is growing, they are still few because of the many barriers that block the engineer's being accepted as part of the team.

One of these barriers is physical isolation from the rest of the team members. The physician, the nurse, the physical therapist, the occupational therapist, and other members of the rehabilitation team are all located within the hospital or medical center, but the engineer is generally found in the engineering school or at a company that may be located several miles away. This isolation effectively prevents frequent interaction and discourse with other team members, and it places the engineer in the role of an outsider. It is imperative that the engineer have an office or laboratory within the rehabilitation center if he is ever to be truly accepted as a member of the team.

However, it can be a mistake for an engineer to work full time within the rehabilitation center without contact with other engineers. The engineer needs constant interaction with the allied health personnel, but he also needs to continue to work among his engineering peers. Such interaction is essential for his professional development and for the maintenance and expansion of his technological competence and it is why the concept of engineering centers located at major rehabilitation facilities is so important. A center provides space and adequate equipment for a number of engineers to work with each other and with the other members of the rehabilitation team.

A second barrier that impedes acceptance of the engineer as a team member is the lack of a common language. Both the medical and engineering fields are filled with terminology known only to those who have paid the price of many years of study and training. While the engineer is trying to fathom the meaning of myelodysplasia and osteochondrosis, the clinician is equally perplexed by 16-bit A/D converters, bubble memories, I/O buffer storage, and FET-input devices with low bias current and low offset-voltage drift. Is it surprising that these two have difficulty in communicating?

Communication is possible only if both parties are willing to drop the jargon of their professions and speak in plain language as much as possible. When a term is used that is unintelligible to one or the other, they must be willing to swallow their pride and ask what it means. The main point to keep in mind is that the object of the conversation is not to impress, but rather to communicate.

Acceptance of the engineer as a professional who can contribute to the rehabilitation effort in a judgmental as well as technical way is also essential in attracting and holding good engineers on the team. Treating the engineer as a technician and prescribing a specific device for him to build is using only a part of his competence. By explaining the clinical problem and stating the intended purpose of the proposed device, the clinician gives the engineer the opportunity of drawing upon his knowledge of materials and design to suggest one or more ways of solving the problem. Very often these initial ideas will not be acceptable because of medical or physiological considerations that did not occur to the engineer or of which he was unaware. Through this exchange of ideas, however, a far better solution will often emerge than the one that initially seemed obvious to the clinician. The engineer, of course, has a similar responsibility to listen to comments and suggestions from the clinical staff in order to ensure that the equipment that he designs will meet their expectations.

Finally, the clinician and the engineer must become comfortable with questioning and challenging each other. When first entering a clinical environment, the engineer usually is somewhat awed by being in alien territory and is easily intimidated by the clinician. At first he tends to accept unquestioningly all statements made. A comment by the physician, such as "we really need to have a brace that does such and such" may be literally true. He may actually know one or two patients who would appreciably benefit from such a brace. The engineer, however, may assume that the application is much broader and may spend an inordinate amount of time (and therefore money) on developing a brace with really a very limited application. Another potential pitfall is the engineer's question, "How good should this amplifier be?" Of course the clinician answers, "It should be as good as possible!" The engineer then expends great effort to design an amplifier with extremely high performance specifications when, in fact, a commercially available amplifier may very well have been more than adequate for this application at a fraction of the cost. In each of these cases, it is the engineer's responsibility to ensure that the work he is performing is consistent with the job requirements.

The clinician may also be reluctant to question technical solutions proposed by the engineer. When the engineer states, "A telemetry system must be built to transmit the data from the subject to the recorder," the clinician may accept it even when, in some cases, a direct wire connection might work just as well and would be far cheaper and more reliable. The clinician may not appreciate that the engineer suggested the telemetry system because it would be more challenging and exciting to build.

PROSPECTS FOR THE FUTURE

In the previous section, some of the barriers restricting the engineer's involvement in the rehabilitation effort were discussed. These barriers will not be broken down easily, but gradually, over the next few years, they will be, and the engineer will be accepted as an essential member of the rehabilitation team.

Education is the key to achieving this end. An increasing number of students entering medical school in the United States are graduates of engineering schools. Just as future generations of doctors graduate with a background of engineering training, more and more engineers have had courses in anatomy and physiology as well as clinical experience through internship programs. Biomedical engineering programs at the undergraduate and graduate level now offer courses in the basic health sciences and medical instrumentation in addition to the standard engineering curricula, and programs or electives in rehabilitation engineering will become more readily available. Through these educational programs, the problems of communication and lack of understanding between engineer and clinician will gradually be overcome.

As this happens, the influx of technology into the rehabilitation field will certainly produce some marvelous innovations in the coming years. Cardiac pacemakers and heart valves are now used routinely to prolong life. Total replacement of hips, knees, and other joints has become commonplace. Communication devices for cerebral-palsied children with normal or better than normal intelligence but who have serious speech defects will offer opportunities for human interaction that are unheard of today. Modified vans with a joystick control will allow quadriplegics to drive independently and provide them with a freedom that all of us take for granted. The stimulation system described previously for correcting scoliosis is another example of a major improvement in available treatment made possible by technology. Work in progress today on artificial hearts, kidneys, and other organs has the potential of offering significant extensions in lifespan for thousands of people. Visual prostheses for the blind and auditory prostheses for the deaf offer a new world for those with sensory loss

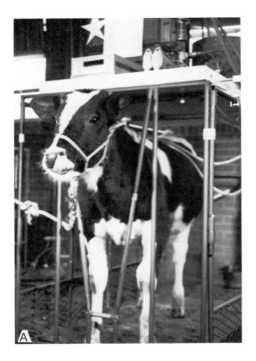
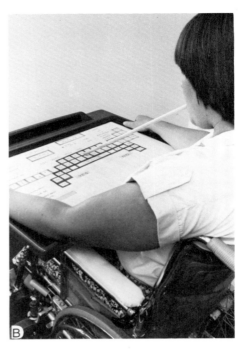
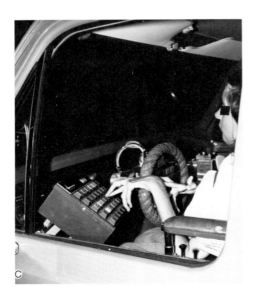
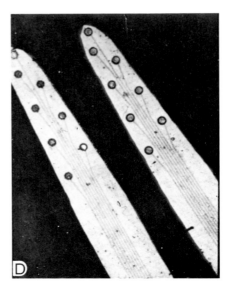

Fig. 4-7. Engineering technology holds great promise for the future: (A) A calf, Fumio Joe, seven months after implantation of a total artificial heart; (B) communication for nonspeaking persons will be possible with the aid of portable computer-assisted systems; (C) special controls for cars and vans will allow quadriplegics to drive; (D) a highly magnified view of microelectrodes that will be inserted into the eighth cranial nerve of totally deaf persons to produce useful sound.

(Figures 4-7A–D). Technology, applied by the engineer working closely with the clinical team, truly offers new hope for helping to restore victims of trauma and disease to near normal function.

REFERENCES

1. Axelgaard, J., Brown, J. C., Nordwall, A., and Swank, S. M.: Transcutaneous electrical muscle stimulation for the treatment of idiopathic scoliosis—preliminary results. J. Bone Joint Surg. 4A(1):29–30, 1980.

2. Axelgaard, J., Nordwall, A., Harada, Y., et al.: Lateral surface stimulation for the correction of scoliosis. J. Bone Joint Surg. 2A(2):267, 1978. (abstract)

3. Baker, L. L., Yeh, C., Wilson, D., and Waters, R. L.: Electrical stimulation of the hemiplegic hand for treatment of contractures. Phys. Ther. 59(12):1495–1499, 1979.

4. Bowman, B. R., Baker, L. L., and Waters, R. L.: Positional feedback and electrical stimulation: An automated treatment for the hemiplegic wrist. Arch. Phys. Med. Rehabil. 60(11): 497–502, 1979.

5. Nordwall, A., Axelgaard, J., Harada, Y., et al.: Spinal cord monitoring using evoked potentials recorded from vertebral bone in cat. Spine 4(6):486–494, 1979.

6. Reswick, J. B.: The design-development-production process in rehabilitation: or technology for the disabled in the free enterprise system. Presented at the 141st meeting of the American Association for the Advancement of Science, New York, January 29, 1975.

7. Reswick, J. B.: Some thoughts relative to the rehabilitation engineer. The Bridge 8:7–9, 1978.

5

Kinesiology—Its Measurement and Importance to Rehabilitation

Sheldon R. Simon, M.D.

It is generally agreed that the ultimate goal of a rehabilitation program is to restore human function. However, because of differences in the nature, severity, and degree of irreversibility of the underlying disease that creates functional incapacity, various medical specialists differ in their definition of what constitutes human function and the bodily mechanics required for its performance, and, hence, in the therapeutic regimen advocated for use in the rehabilitation process. Further, if one looks beyond the simple idea of "restoring function" and considers any relatively complex illness, one immediately realizes the difficulties, degree of complexity, and uncertainty involved in establishing an appropriate rehabilitation program.

For example, a person who has sustained a fractured tibia and has been treated in a short-leg walking cast for 16 weeks has sustained a curable "disease." However, the person is still functionally disabled if secondary muscle atrophy and ankle joint stiffness are not treated; a rehabilitation program is, therefore, indicated. Here the goal of therapy is to return the individual to the same functional level existing before the fracture; the treatment program and anticipated time to reach that goal are clear. Yet the goal of a rehabilitation program for a professional athlete who has sustained tears of multiple ligaments and the meniscus of one knee is different. Therapy is directed toward rapid restoration of the individual to an extremely high level of performance. But even if surgery is performed to correct the deficit, the individual may be left with an unstable knee. The goal in this case is less clear. A rehabilitation program may be instituted to strengthen muscles, restore joint motion, and seek to return the player to a functional level of unrestricted athletics quickly enough so that he or she may participate in professional sports for the remainder of the season. However, such swift restoration of motion may jeopardize the long-term status of the knee.

If the rehabilitation goal and therapeutic program appear somewhat uncertain in the latter example, they can be even more ambiguous for an adult who has suffered a cerebrovascular accident or a child with cerebral palsy. For the adult, restoration of normal function often means a return to all previous activities as effortlessly, quickly, and cosmetically as before; for the child, it implies the performance of all functions in the same manner as his or her peers. For the majority of both categories of patients these goals are unattainable. The basic disease process is irreversible, and it affects not merely one single area or even multiple areas of the mechanical system. It also involves the nervous system, which controls the mechanical system. In such cases the goal of rehabilitation becomes extremely complex. It is difficult to determine what new "functional" level can be achieved. It is even more difficult to ascertain how this level will be attained, and if it is attained, whether the benefits accruing to the patient will be the same as those for an unaffected individual. A specific rehabilitation program may succeed in teaching an individual to walk without crutches. However, it is possible that achieving such a goal would make the individual walk at a slower speed, consume more energy, appear more awkward, be more subject to tripping, and/or utilize muscles and joint motions in such a manner that over a long period of time deleterious effects would be noted in local regions of the body.

Knowledge of a given pathological process and how the body can compensate for it leads to a better understanding of why function in some disorders is more readily restored than in others and what must or can be done to any aspect of the physiological system to rehabilitate the individual properly. A person usually attempts to compensate for knee joint damage during walking by reducing the joint's load by decreasing walking speed, decreasing quadriceps activity,[44,65] and (if necessary) leaning the trunk forward over the knee in the stance phase. If the individual then sustains a cerebrovascular accident, some of the control mechanisms of compensation may not be able to be invoked, and knee damage may increase if an alternate treatment program is not initiated. If such individuals are still capable of performing active jobs on their feet all day, they may need some reduction in their normal functional activities. They may require continued use of a cane or a reduction in the total number of "poundings" the joint will feel in a given day, month, or year. The need for caution and an awareness of the detrimental effects that multiple disease states can exert must be understood by the practitioner and conveyed to the patient. How severe and chronic the initiating cause is, how effectively medical treatments produce remission or cure, whether available compensatory mechanisms are adequate, whether an individual can sufficiently invoke such mechanisms or whether he or she is limited by physical, neurological, psychological, or social factors, are all necessary for the practitioner to understand so as to relate to the patient what can realistically be achieved. Dealing with all these variables is indispensable to the success of a rehabilitation program.

The practitioner involved in the rehabilitation process can control only some of these factors yet must be aware of all of them and understand their interaction.

In most instances, in order to formulate a rehabilitation program properly, it is clinically important to understand how human movement occurs and how it is disturbed by a given pathological process. The systematic understanding of human movement constitutes kinesiology.

KINESIOLOGY: THE STUDY OF MECHANICAL AND ANATOMICAL PRINCIPLES OF MOVEMENT

"Kinesiology is an indispensable background for the prevention, treatment, and rehabilitation of locomotor disorders," Arthur Steindler has written. Although, in his words, "practical conclusions could be attained more directly by observation and empiricism without any tedious preambles," this "short-cut method based entirely on impressions . . . summersaults over the hard facts of basic sciences in order to arrive at quick and usually superficial practical conclusions."[56]

Segmental body rotational movements and the muscular effort needed to control them combine to create the multitude of functions an individual performs. In the human, the primary function of the upper extremities is to transport and manipulate objects; that of the lower extremities is to facilitate locomotion.

Joint motions allow limb positional changes. True joint movement is the relative change in position of a skeletal member in relation to its adjacent one. Although at any joint there are six possible types of motion (three rotational and three translational), each joint is distinct with regard to both the types of motions that exist and the degree to which each is allowed.[1,6,24,40] Some joints have grossly similar movements—e.g., hip and shoulder, knee and elbow, and ankle and wrist, but the combination of the structural units comprising them are different and appear related to the external force demands and functional requirements imposed upon them.

To provide for the wide sphere of influence an extremity can encompass, the most proximal joint must have the widest range of motion and allow rotatory motions of large degrees in all three planes (Fig. 5-1).[11,45] Because most of the external forces on the extremity are exerted at some distance from the joint, muscles about these joints must be large and strong. In the human, the hip joint established to suit these demands is a ball and socket joint. The stable, enclosing, bony contoured joint and large muscle mass about it appear necessary to balance the trunk (body weight), shifting its position at very frequent intervals above it.[22,26,46,47] The shoulder, with its reduced demand for weight bearing and repetitive use, relies less on bony stability. However, it retains its muscle mass.[48–50]

In order for an extremity to cover all areas within the range allowed, a means must be provided to alter its length. It would not be advisable to have the bones of the upper and lower arm or leg extend and shorten in a piston-like manner, because a number of repetitions in combination with high imposed loads would place too great a strain on the bony structures.[29–31] By having both adjacent limb segments move, the elbow and knee joints allow overall limb length changes, often necessitating movement at an adjacent proximal joint (Fig. 5-2).

When a person picks up a glass and brings it to the mouth, the wrist moves from a position on the table to one adjacent to the face. By means of muscular

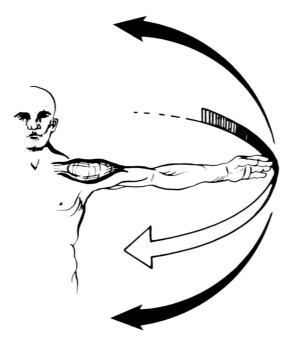

Fig. 5-1. Changes in rotation of an extremity's most proximal joint in any direction allows the limb to be positioned within a vast circumscribed area of space.

effort, coordination and synchronization of the various limb segments are maintained via the neurological system. In circumstances in which muscles spanning a single joint are employed, neurological control coordinates separate muscles about each joint involved in the task. In other circumstances, when it would be more efficient to provide control with two-joint muscles, one joint moves while the other joint is maintained in a stable position. At other times, the existing mechanism for control between two joints can be a passive one, and the neurological

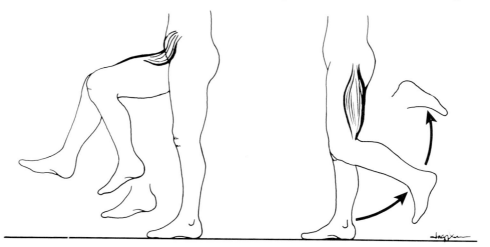

Fig. 5-2. Shortening of the lower extremity is primarily accomplished through changes of rotation of the knee joint, but to effect it in certain spatial areas, simultaneous rotations at the hip must occur.

control must "know" that no muscle should be activated. During the initiation of the swing phase of walking or while climbing stairs, hip flexors flex the hip, whereas the knee flexes without controlling the muscles about this joint. The inertia of the shank lagging behind that of the actively mobile femur creates knee flexion and a relative shortening of the limb's length occurs, providing floor or step clearance.[2,7,16,23,31]

Muscles, then, do not act continuously. To do so with the same degree of forceful contraction at all times would be inefficient either in performing an activity or in preserving energy. Rather, the magnitude of the muscular effort as well as the total time a muscle is active depends upon what the specific functional activity is, how the activity is performed, and how fast it is completed. At the knee joint, 15–20 degrees of knee flexion occur in the early support phase of walking. The quadriceps muscle attempts to prevent collapse of the leg under the body's weight as the leg is decelerating. If the individual walks faster, greater muscle activity is needed (Fig. 5-3). Activity increases even more during the act of running. It also increases in rising from a chair or climbing stairs to lift the body to a higher height rather than to control deceleration.[2,23] The activity of this and other muscles during repetitive cyclical activities in which overall efficiency and energy are prime considerations in the type of control needed appears to be dictated by single, fixed, pre-programmed, neurological responses.

When activities involving less repetitive motions are considered, the manner in which they are performed varies from person to person and from time to time in the same person. As an example, someone wishing to bend over and pick something up may accomplish this task by keeping the legs straight and bending from the back and hips (Fig. 5-4A). To do so, the person must have adequate strength in the back muscles to withstand the brunt of the lifting that will be required of these tissues. Alternatively, the person may keep the back straight and bend at the hips, knees, and ankles, and lift the object by utilizing the leg muscles (Fig. 5-4B). If this method is chosen, sufficient strength in the leg muscles must be present.[33] A person may also choose to utilize a combination of these two methods, employing both back and lower extremity muscles (Fig. 5-4C).

Whatever combination is used, the act should still be done with "good form." Proper form not only utilizes the "appropriate" number of joints and body segments, but relates to the speed and frequency with which any particular part

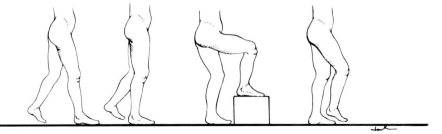

Fig. 5-3. Positions of the lower extremity that seem to need quadriceps activity. Walking, jogging, and going up stairs (left to right) need progressively increasing amounts of quadriceps activity during stance. However, if the leg is in swing (far right) during any of these activities, no quadriceps activity is required.

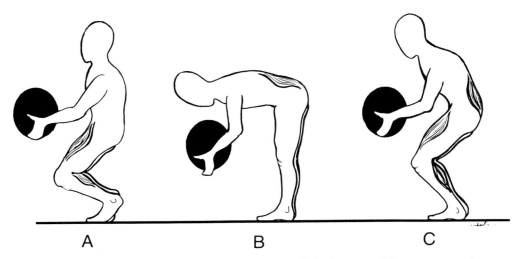

Fig. 5-4. Lifting an object off the floor can be accomplished in many different ways. Each pattern requires the use of different muscles and/or different degrees of effort within any given muscle.

moves (Fig. 5-5). One could liken this situation to viewing someone swinging a golf club or tennis racket. Prior to hitting the ball, the person might be swinging rapidly at the onset of the stroke, and minimizing the follow-up after the ball is hit. This type of movement would cause increased stresses in certain muscles and at

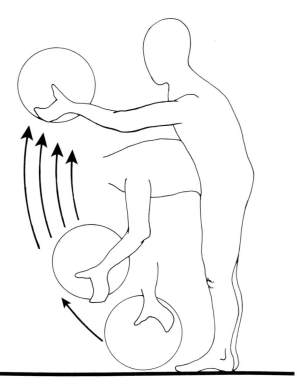

Fig. 5-5. When an object is lifted off the ground, slow movements in the early stages of the movement and rapid movements later may place unnecessary stresses on muscles, bones, and joints.

certain arcs of joint motion in the initial part of the stroke while reducing those that would occur normally during the latter part of the stroke.

Many other factors contribute to how a particular function will be performed. Of importance is the fact that in normal subjects the same non-repetitive function utilizing an intact neurological control system can produce different forces in different muscles and joints in the same individual at different times and in different individuals acting at the same time. Although one method may be considered to be the "best," in most circumstances, for one of many reasons, each individual performs the same task in a unique way.

KINEMATICS: THE STUDY OF MOTION ISOLATED FROM ITS CAUSES

In normal, healthy persons, this entire system, created to be adaptable and allow a variety of functional movement, is itself delicately balanced and not very adaptable after all when loss of some functional component is irreversible or chronically present. When such a loss occurs, the balance may be so upset as to lead to an inability of a rehabilitation program to restore easily all "normal" functions in the "best" possible way. A thorough understanding of what a rehabilitation program can restore and how best to do it requires a basic knowledge of kinesiology. But while such knowledge is necessary, it is often not sufficient. Some means by which each individual's functional performance can be adequately evaluated must be provided. For centuries clinicians have relied on a subjective evaluation of a patient's kinematics—those aspects of motion that are separate from considerations of mass and force.

Kinematics provides one means by which overall performance as well as localized bodily movements can be evaluated. However, the clinician cannot directly obtain information of how a pathological movement is created from kinematics. That would require knowledge of how body movements are the end product of the interaction of forces arising from segmental inertial and gravitational forces and intersegmental muscle forces. Kinematics thus does not explain the number of forces and the intensity with which each force acts at any instant. Despite this limitation, clinicians have empirically identified patterns or rules of movement existing in many pathological states. Applications of such rules have allowed proper inferences to be made about how a movement is produced merely from observing the movement itself. This method of evaluation (subjective kinematic study) has been the most widely taught and most clinically used aspect of kinesiology.

Unfortunately, in many instances, too many movements need to be viewed in too short a period of time. They are usually seen by relatively untrained observers, and comparative observations must often be made at some later time. All these factors may make subjective interpretation of the information that can be gained from kinematics imprecise and inconsistent. Therefore, objective measurement and recording of motion data are of great value. A brief look at how our ideas of the treatment of back pain have changed as a result of kinematic measurement will illustrate the importance of such measurements of human movement.

For patients to maintain function while minimizing back pain, physicians have been recommending since the mid-1930s that all lifting activities be carried out with the back near vertical and the knees and hips bent.[33] The advocates of this method have been so enthusiastic and persistent in regard to training programs that nearly every major industry has adopted this method to the exclusion of any other, regardless of the size, shape, or weight of the object to be lifted, the worker's ability to lift, or the number of times a worker needs to lift an object in any given day. In view of the popularization of the theory of correct lifting methods, it was expected that the incidence of low back injury would be significantly reduced. However, studies conducted in Britain and Canada offer clear evidence that no such reduction followed in the number of back injuries due to lifting and handling activities.[9]

A skepticism of the proper way to lift emerged from these and similar studies, and some investigators sought the reasons for the apparent failure of the instructional programs that had been designed to promote correct lifting. A kinematic (photographic) study of the lifting techniques of industrial workers showed that a wide variety of lifting methods was employed, and that the prescribed manner of lifting with a straight back and bent knees was seldom used.[9] Results indicated either that the indoctrination was insufficient, or that the workers preferred to use another method even though they understood the "proper" lifting technique. Since the proper lifting method was not used consistently, it could not be expected to contribute to a reduction in the incidence of low back injuries even if it were a truly superior technique. This and other studies have led to new approaches toward reducing the incidence of low back pain.[54]

Despite the importance kinematic measurements can have in better understanding and documenting a patient's condition, clinically their application has been largely limited to evaluating walking dysfunction and, more recently, to evaluating sports performance.

Almost all aspects of the motion patterns of human gait, from the motions of a single point to the changes in joint angles and the overall positions of various limb segments, have been subjectively considered to be clinically important. Thus at one time or another each has been objectively measured.

Perhaps the simplest motion that can be measured is that of a single point traversing space. Monitoring the location of a point on the foot during swing phase will provide information about when and to what degree an individual might have problems in clearing his foot from the ground. Observing such motions will only provide information demonstrating that an abnormality exists at a certain time in a given function. Too little information has been furnished to allow the clinician to determine how various limb motions cumulatively have resulted in functional impairment. Accurately defining a point on the foot to determine when and if foot clearance is insufficient does not allow one to know if the abnormality is created by insufficient ankle dorsiflexion or knee or hip flexion.

Therefore, facts about the motions of multiple points are necessary and are obtainable. Graphing the translational data derived from these multiple points by connecting them in a way to represent the body as a series of "stick figures," although qualitative in nature, is often very valuable. Clinicians inexperienced in biomechanics and kinesiology can easily utilize data presented in this way to evaluate overall gait abnormalities and/or abnormalities present at specific areas (Figs. 5-6A and 5-6B).[36,52]

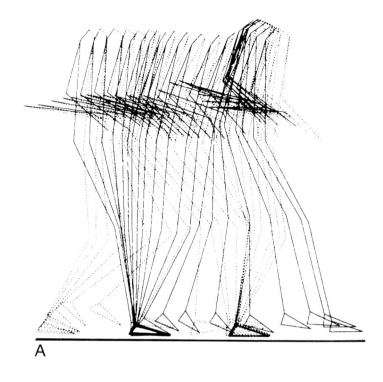

A

Fig. 5-6. Stick figure representations of a gait cycle of the motions of an individual with lower extremity spasticity. (A) During right leg (solid lines) stance, note the persistence of ankle plantarflexion associated with right knee recurvatum and a slight forward trunk lean. During left stance (dotted lines), the cessation of ankle dorsiflexion later in stance is not associated with knee recurvatum but with vaulting upward of the trunk and increased transverse rotation of the trunk. (B) After a solid ankle-foot orthosis is placed on the right leg, abnormalities of right-leg stance are corrected while step length is unchanged; left stance abnormalities are still present.

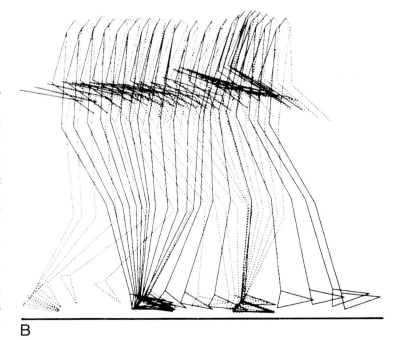

B

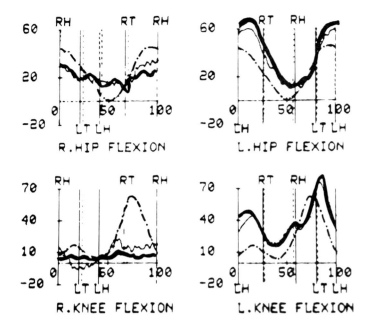

Fig. 5-7. Graphs of sagittal plane flexion/extension motions of an individual's left and right hips and knees during one gait cycle determined during two measurement sessions a year apart (light and heavy solid lines). The dotted solid line in each graph depicts normal hip and knee flexion/extension. Increased extension (hyperextension) of the right knee during right stance is noted clearly, pinpointing the time and degree of the amount of gait deterioration that has occurred.

Another method of combining the information derived from monitoring the movements of several points consists of calculating and graphing the angular rotations of the various joints of the lower extremities during walking. Since human locomotion is produced by the movement of various limb segments rotating about respective adjacent segments, describing the motion of these angles yields valuable information on normal and pathological gait.[15,20,25] All forces, be they muscular, inertial, or gravitational, are reflected in "joint movement" and most clinical problems and treatments are manifested and directed toward altering joint motion (Fig. 5-7).

KINETICS: THE STUDY OF THE EFFECTS OF FORCE UPON MOTION

"Kinesiology is that part of the physiology of motion which describes and analyzes locomotor events so far as they reflect the action of mechanical forces. It presents bodily motion as a special case in mechanics," wrote Steindler as he described the orientation of the specialty. He could not help but question, "Can human motion with its boundless variability and being the product of a multitude of only partially known factors, be forced into the narrow frame of precise and austere mathematical and physical laws? . . . This is the very point which ultimately decides whether or not there is enough practical value in the undertaking to warrant this line of investigation."[56]

Although valuable, the study of kinematics alone is often incapable of allowing the clinician to establish a proper rehabilitation program. As long as the clinician understands how human motions reflect the action of mechanical forces, kinematic measurements are adequate. Unfortunately, for the majority of patients needing rehabilitation this is not the case. Muscles are the body's engines of movement, the force generators through which the neurological system creates or controls movement. The nature of the movement depends upon whether the force of a muscle is assisted or opposed by the forces of other muscles and/or adjacent limb segment and bodily inertial and gravitational forces. It is understandable that clinicians, only being able to perform a history and physical exam, find it difficult to define and utilize the kinetics of movement. Yet modern technology has brought forth many instruments applicable for such purposes. Again, these instruments clinically have had limited use, mostly in the area of bipedal locomotion.

At any instant during human support, a force is generated between the foot and floor. Equal and opposite to the sum total of the body's weight and inertial forces, this external reaction force can be represented as acting at a single point with a certain magnitude and direction. In healthy persons the pattern of how the direction, magnitude, and point of application change during the stance phase of gait or during normal standing is quite constant from person to person, and it can be utilized to evaluate abnormalities (Figs. 5-8A and 5-8B).[5,35] This external force produces a torque about each joint. The magnitude of this torque is equal to the force times the perpendicular distance from its line of action to the joint's center of rotation (Figs. 5-9A and 5-9B). The component of the torque acting perpendicular to any given anatomical joint axis would cause rotational motion if it were not counteracted dynamically by muscle effort or passively by the joint's capsule or ligaments.[8,15,34,52,53] Over three decades ago, Elftman[17,18] observed that during walking such torques seem to be the main cause of limb segment motions and joint angular rotations. Muscle and ligamentous efforts merely control the rate and degree of such motions. Thus to describe the kinetics of walking, clinicians must be provided with information about the external torques produced about each joint and the muscular forces utilized to counteract them.

There are many ways to establish a system for clinically determining the body's changing external force vector and quasi-statistically measuring the torques it produces about each joint. All methods use a force platform substituted for the floor in a given area of a walkway. From the platform, the magnitude, direction, and point of application of the body's external reaction force at every instant during the stance phase can be obtained. The measuring devices of the platform consist of either piezoelectric load cells or strain gauges. These measuring devices are arranged within the platform to obtain the magnitude of the forces in the vertical, fore-aft, and medial-lateral directions. Electronic hardware devices or computer processing can then be utilized to sum vectorally all three reactions of the body's external reaction force.

Currently, all commercial varieties of force platforms use at least three measuring devices in the vertical direction at any instant. Knowing the magnitude of the force in each of the three vertical measuring devices and the distance between each of the three devices themselves allows for the center of pressure to be readily determined.

To interpret muscle action and joint motions correctly, the clinician needs to know the magnitude of the component of the external reaction torque acting perpendicular to a desired anatomical joint axis. If a means for monitoring a desired joint's translational movement is provided and such information is synchronized with information from the force platform, the calculation of the torques

Text continues on p. 58

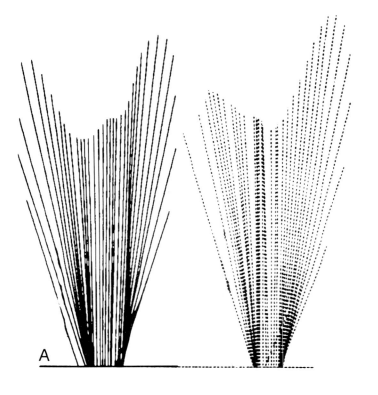

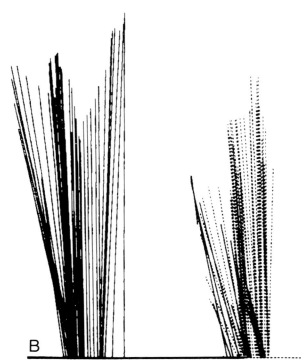

Fig. 5-8. (A) The normal sagittal plane patterns of the foot-floor ground reaction forces during the stance phases of the right and left legs during one complete gait cycle. As the center of pressure moves forward, the magnitudes of the vertical and fore-aft forces change, producing a butterfly-shaped pattern. (B) The patterns of a patient in whom weakness exists diffusely in both lower extremities. A cane is used to supplement support of one leg.

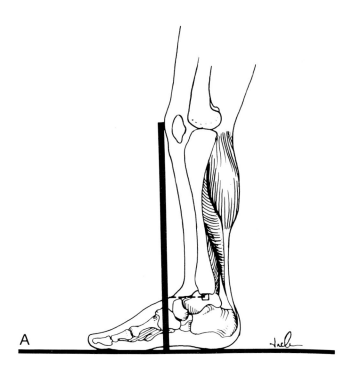

A

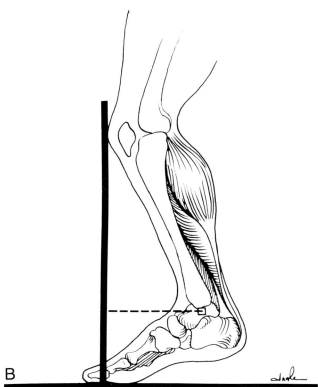

Fig. 5-9. When a person is walking with only single-limb support, body weight and momentum of all limb segments above the ankle tend to cause rotation of the shank about the foot. While the magnitude of the external torque about the knee is the same in mid-single-limb stance (A) and slightly later on (B), the torque about the ankle continues to increase, owing to the progressively increasing moment arm. If the ankle is to maintain the same degree of dorsiflexion, the posterior calf muscle must increase its restraining force.

B

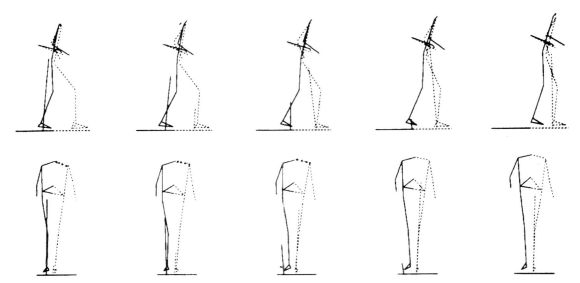

Fig. 5-10. Side and front stick-figure views of a double-limb support phase of a subject walking. This subject had a locomotor disorder secondary to spastic diplegia. Note that although the limb segment motions and foot-floor reaction vector producing abnormal torques about each joint are abnormal, the transfer of total weight is smooth (height of foot-floor reaction vectors) from one leg to the other.

produced by the external reaction force about that joint can be made. If only a qualitative measure of the generated torque is desired, the force vector data derived from the force plate electronically can be transferred and superimposed upon a videotape of movie film of the individual walking, or on a computer-generated representation of motion data digitally recorded (Fig. 5-10).

To visualize more accurately or define the body's external reaction torques produced about each joint, a means of measuring the motion of each joint in three dimensions must be obtained. In addition, a three-dimensional coordinate system of joint axes based on a coordinate system internal to the moving body and referenced to the laboratory must be prescribed. These calculations can be done in a variety of ways, and they have been well documented.[2,15,25,52,53]

DYNAMIC ELECTROMYOGRAPHY (EMG): THE RECORDING OF AN ACTIVE MUSCLE'S ELECTRICAL ACTIVITY DURING MOVEMENT

The clinician, having a basic knowledge of the anatomical origins and insertions, the fast- and slow-twitch properties, and the isolated independent actions of each muscle in the body, is still limited in understanding the timing and magnitude of the force that each muscle generates in performing a given task in normal and pathological states. Clinical knowledge of the pathological state and observational acumen during the physical examination are only superficially helpful in evaluating the role that each muscle plays in a given movement. But as clear as the need for objective measurement of muscle forces is, it is equally clear how difficult such measurements are. Muscles and tendons are soft tissues, blending well into their surroundings and changing little in shape and length when they are activated. They are thus difficult to "see from the outside" and hard to analyze for stress from the inside by classical mechanical techniques. Further, when we consider that over 39 muscles exist in one leg alone, the task of measuring and recording muscle forces during human movement is formidable.

Although many approaches to solving this problem are now being investigated,[10,13,51] the single most useful technique currently providing the clinician information about muscle activity relates to the use of dynamic electromyography. Although no clear relationship exists between a muscle's electrical activity and the force it generates during movement,[21,27,32,58,66] the ability of electromyography to record the presence of muscular activity and the relative changes in that activity over time has been found very useful.[37-39,57] According to Basmajian, its power is clinically unique: "Electromyography is unique in revealing what a muscle actually does [electrically] at any moment during various movements and postures. Moreover, it reveals objectively the fine interplay or coordination of muscles . . . patently impossible by any other means."[3]

The recording of the electricity generated by muscle activity during human performance is similar to routine diagnostic EMG, although the former is technically more difficult to obtain. The major clinical difference among dynamic EMG systems currently available is whether surface electrodes or fine-wire electrodes serve as the monitoring device. Surface electrodes are widely employed because of their non-invasive nature. They are utilized when information from a muscle group is needed and/or in areas where a needle's insertion of fine-wire electrodes may preclude the subject from subsequently acting "normally." Surface electrodes have the disadvantages of frequently being unable to isolate the activity of a single superficial muscle, or being completely unable to isolate a deep muscle's activity, of requiring large signal amplification (there is a great distance between muscles and electrodes, and a poor conductor—skin—is between them), and of having a large noise component (from skin movement) as part of the signal. The use of fine-wire electrodes minimizes these problems. Because fine-wire electrodes are directly in contact with a small portion of one single muscle, and because many motor units are represented throughout a muscle, fine-wire electrodes yield representative recordings of a single muscle with a minimum of secondary amplification and noise interference.

Whether or not fine-wire or surface electrodes are used, a large variety of dynamic EMG systems are commercially available or can be built in-house. Yet it is important to realize that no single system can provide information about all the muscles acting during a specific function. With the large number of muscles existing in one leg alone, and with only 8–16 muscles capable of being monitored at any one time, the clinician must choose a representative quantity. Should a large number of muscles in a localized area be monitored, or is it more appropriate to select a group of muscles that best represents one leg, both legs, or the back and one leg? The clinical problem then dictates not only the proper sampling mode (surface or fine-wire electrodes), but the proper sampling group.

EMG recordings cannot be utilized to determine directly forces produced by muscular effort. But they can be used to identify the times when a muscle is active and its relative "effort" during those times. Such information has been clinically

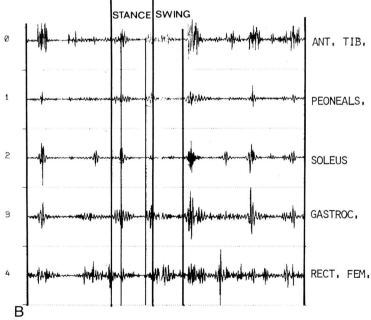

Fig. 5-11. Sample EMG recordings obtained during walking of a patient with ALS. The original raw signal (A) shows no obvious patterns of muscle activity. After appropriate data filtering to eliminate artifacts, a recognizable pattern of muscle activity can be noted (B).

useful in understanding how a given pathological disorder has produced dysfunction, and, more importantly, in many instances how individualized the pattern of muscular activity can become from subject to subject within any given disorder.[15,36,38,39,52,57,59] Although the use of dynamic EMG in planning a rehabilitation program is becoming well recognized, knowledge of its limitations and proper interpretation is less well appreciated. The nature of a subject's movement disorder, the desired muscles monitored, and the amount of non-EMG signal allowed by a given instrument to remain in the final recorded signal often make EMG recordings very difficult to interpret (Figs. 5-11A and 5-11B). Even if the appropriate muscles have been selected for study and the EMG signals obtained have been properly interpreted, the clinical meaning of these recordings still requires an understanding of mechanics, and in some cases, some additional kinematic or foot-floor reaction information. If agonist-antagonist EMG muscle activity is noted, but without a knowledge of the force each muscle produces, one would need to know if joint rotation favors movement toward the agonist, the antagonist, or neither, to interpret the EMG signal. If the function is performed either against gravity or in a standing position, additional antagonist forces will be present: limb segment gravitational and inertial forces and/or foot-floor reaction forces. Taking these forces into account is invaluable in many cases for a proper interpretation of the EMG recordings obtained (Fig. 5-10).

ENERGY EXPENDITURE: THE EXERTION OF FORCE ALLOWING WORK TO BE DONE

Many bilateral above-knee amputees have had intensive, prolonged, and expensive rehabilitation programs to restore them to walking in a bipedal fashion. Yet many of them eventually abandon this mode of locomotion in favor of a wheelchair. Only recently[59] have we learned that this change appears due to the higher energy expenditure utilized by these individuals in bipedal versus wheelchair ambulation.

This research by Waters and his colleagues[59] illustrates the importance of measuring the amount of energy consumed by an individual performing a task in a given way. Energy so consumed is defined as the amount of aerobic and anerobic metabolism occurring in muscles as a given function is performed. The amount of energy consumed is dictated by the mechanical changes each segment of the body has undergone to move from one position to another, by the efficiency by which segmental potential and kinetic mechanical energy can be exchanged during the function, by the manner by which the neurological system activates and controls the additional muscular activity needed to perform the given task, and by the efficiency by which individual muscles translate their metabolic work into mechanical work.[19]

Ultimately, this means that the mechanical and metabolic work done by each individual muscle must be measured. Unfortunately, such measurements cannot be made in living human beings. The mechanical energy expended by individual body segments in performing a given task can be obtained from kinematic measurements and knowledge of the inertial properties of the various segments.[41,43,61,63,64] The measurement of oxygen consumption can be utilized to determine the total amount of aerobic metabolic work involved in doing a specific task.[4,12,14,28,42] This requires a minimal degree of equipment and for certain functions can be relatively easily performed. (Alternatively, a patient's heart rate can be monitored to compare relative energy expenditures in the same subject under varying conditions. It has been found to be linearly related to metabolic energy expenditure at submaximal levels of work.[55]) Oxygen consumption and heart rate measurements generally can only be utilized for steady-state, predominantly aerobic repetitive functions in which the 1–2 minutes of start-up time have little bearing on the overall energy expended on the activity. Such measurements are valuable in determining the overall performance capabilities but are limited in explaining at the localized level why a given individual is inefficient and in determining energy consumption for tasks that are not steady-state functions. One can also obtain the time of muscular activity and some relative idea of the change in an active muscle's intensity from EMG signals. While to date only a general indication of aerobic steady-state metabolic work, overall and individualized segmental-mechanical energy changes, and muscular activation (but not individualized mechanical nor metabolic work) can be measured, much useful clinical information can be obtained from such measurements.[59,60,62]

SUMMARY

"The analysis of human motion is primarily the job of the biologist, and only secondarily that of the physicist or engineer. All motion events are the end result of a long chain of cause and effect. . . . The study of kinetics taps this chain at a point behind the clinical manifestation while the biologist tries to penetrate much further into the background. In other words kinetics explains only the physical events which led immediately to the local performance and it is not concerned with the more remote causes of human motion."[56]

In the past decade, a plethora of instruments has been developed to allow the clinician to record and evaluate various aspects of many human functions objectively. Although much work still needs to be done by engineers and physicists to harness the exploding electronics and computer fields to suit kinesiological rehabilitation needs, even more work needs to be done by biologists to utilize such information to determine the true causes of human motion and understand how best to formulate an optimal rehabilitation program. After first realizing the value of kinesiology, the clinician must then gain sufficient knowledge of this field, incorporate human performance testing procedures as part of a subject's evaluation, properly interpret the results obtained, and channel all this information into a formulation of the pathodynamics of a given subject's movement disorder. Steindler's words are as true today as when first said 30 years ago.

REFERENCES

1. American Academy of Orthopaedic Surgeons: *Joint Motion: Method of Meaning and Recording.* American Academy of Orthopaedic Surgeons, Chicago, 1965.
2. Andriacchi, T. P., Anderson, G. B. J., Fermier, R. W., et al.: A study of lower limb mechanics during stair climbing. J. Bone Joint Surg. 62A:749–757, 1980.

3. Basmajian, J. V.: *Muscles Alive,* 3rd ed. Williams & Wilkins, Baltimore, 1974.

4. Bobbert, A. C.: Energy expenditure in level and grade walking. J. Appl. Physiol. 15:1015–1021, 1960.

5. Boccardi, S., Chiesa, G., and Pedotti, A.: New procedure for evaluation of normal and abnormal gait. Am. J. Phys. Med. 56(4):163–182, 1977.

6. Boone, D.C., and Azen, S. P.: Normal range of motion of joints in male subjects. J. Bone Joint Surg. 61A(5):756–759, 1979.

7. Brand, P. W.: Biomechanics of tendon transfer. Orthop. Clin. North Am. 5:205–230, 1974.

8. Bresler, B., and Frankel, J. P.: The forces and moments in the leg during level walking. Trans. Am. Soc. Mech. Eng. 72:27–36, 1950.

9. Brown, J. R.: *Manual Lifting and Related Fields: An Annotated Bibliography.* Labour Safety Council of Ontario, Ontario Ministry of Labour, Ottawa, 1972.

10. Cappozzo, A., Figura, F., Marchetti, M., and Pedotti, A.: The interplay of muscular and external forces in human ambulation. J. Biomech. 9:35–43, 1976.

11. Cleland, J.: The shoulder girdle and its movements. Lancet 283, February 19, 1881.

12. Cotes, J. E., and Meade, F.: The energy expenditure and mechanical energy demand in walking. Ergonomics 3:97–119, 1960.

13. Crowninshield, R. D., Johnston, R. C., Andrews, J. G., and Brand, R. A.,: A biomechanical investigation of the human hip. J. Biomech. 11:75–85, 1978.

14. Dean, G. A.: An analysis of the energy expenditure in level and grade walking. Ergonomics 8:31–47, 1965.

15. Demottaz, J. D., Mazur, J. M., Thomas, W. H., et al.: Clinical study of total ankle replacement with gait analysis—A preliminary report. J. Bone Joint Surg. 61A:976–988, 1978.

16. Eberhart, H. D., Inman, V. T., and associates: Fundamental studies of human locomotion and other information relating to design of artificial limbs. Subcontractor's Report to the Committee on Artificial Limbs, National Research Council. Prosthetic Devices Research Project, College of Engineering, University of California, Berkeley, Serial No. CAL 5, 2 vols. Berkeley, Calif., The Project, 1947.

17. Elftman, H.: Forces and energy changes in the leg during walking. Am. J. Physiol. 125:339–356, 1939.

18. Elftman, H.: The basic pattern of human locomotion. Ann. N.Y. Acad. Sci. 51:1207–1212, 1951.

19. Fenn, W. O.: Work against gravity and work due to velocity changes in running. Am. J. Physiol. 93:433–462, 1930.

20. Gore, D. R., Murray, M. P., Sepic, S. B., and Gardner, G. M.: Walking patterns of men with unilateral surgical hip fusion. J. Bone Joint Surg. 57A:759–765, 1975.

21. Inman, V. T., Ralston, H. J., Saunders, J. B., et al.: Relation of human electromyogram to muscular tension. Electroencephalogr. Clin. Neurophysiol. 4:187–194, 1952.

22. Johnston, R. C.: Mechanical considerations of the hip joint. Arch. Surg. 107:411–417, 1973.

23. Joseph, J., and Watson, R.: Telemetering electromyography of muscles used in walking up and down stairs. J. Bone Joint Surg. 49B:774–780, 1967.

24. Kapandji, I. A.: *The Physiology of Joints,* 2nd ed. Churchill Livingstone, Edinburgh, 1970.

25. Mazur, J. M., Schwartz, E., and Simon, S. R.: Ankle arthrodesis. Long-term follow-up with gait analysis. J. Bone Joint Surg. 61A:964–975, 1979.

26. McLeish, R. D., and Charnley, J.: Abduction forces in the one-legged stance. J. Biomech. 3:191–209, 1970.

27. Milner-Brown, H.S., and Stein, R. B.: The relation between the surface electromyogram and muscular force. J. Physiol. 246:549–569, 1975.

28. Molen, N. H., Rozendal, R. H., and Boon, W.: Graphic representation of the relationship between oxygen consumption and characteristics of normal gait of the human male. Proc. Kon. Ned. Akad. Wet. C75:305–314, 1972b.

29. Morrison, J. B.: Function of the knee joint in various activities. Med. Biol. Eng. 4:573–581, 1969.

30. Morrison, J. B.: The mechanics of the knee joint in relation to normal walking. J. Biomech. 3:51–61, 1970.

31. Murray, M. P.: Gait as a total pattern of movement—including a bibliography on gait. Am. J. Phys. Med. 6:290–333, 1967.

32. Nelson, A. J., Moffroid, M., and Whipple, R.: Relationship of integrated electromyographic discharge to isokinetic contractions. In Desmedt, J. E., Ed.: *New Developments in Electromyography and Clinical Neurophysiology,* Vol 1, pp. 584–595. Karger, Basel, 1973.

33. Park, K. S., and Chaffin, D. B.: *Methods of Manual Load Lifting: A Biomechanical Evaluation of an Old Problem.* Ann Arbor, University of Michigan, Department of Industrial and Operations Engineering, 1973.

34. Paul, J. P.: Force actions transmitted in the knee of normal subjects and by prosthetic joint replacements. Proc. Inst. Mech. Eng. 184:126–131, 1974.

35. Pedotti, A.: Simple equipment used in clinical practice for evaluation of locomotion. IEEE Trans. Biomed. Eng. BME-24:456–461, 1977.

36. Perry, J.: The mechanics of walking. A clinical interpretation. Phys. Ther. 47:778–801, 1967.

37. Perry, J., Fox, J. M., Boitano, M. A., et al.: Functional evaluation of the pes anserinus transfer by electromyography and gait analysis. J. Bone Joint Surg. 62A:973–980, 1980.

38. Perry, J., Hoffer, M. M., Antonelli, D., et al.: Electromyography before and after surgery for hip deformity in children with cerebral palsy. A comparison of clinical and electromyographic findings. J. Bone Joint Surg. 58A:201–208, 1976.

39. Perry, J., Hoffer, M. M., Giovan, P., et al.: Gait analysis of the triceps surae in cerebral palsy. A preoperative and postoperative clinical and electromyographic study. J. Bone Joint Surg. 56A:511–520, 1974.

40. Plagenhoff, S.: *Patterns of Human Motion.* Prentice-Hall, Englewood Cliffs, N.J., 1971.

41. Quanbury, A. O., Winter, D. A., and Reimer, G. D.: Instantaneous power and power flow in body segments during walking. J. Human Movement Stud. 1:59–67, 1975.

42. Ralston, H. J.: Energy-speed relation and optimal speed during level walking. Int. Z. Angew. Physiol. 17:277–283, 1958.

43. Ralston, H. J., and Lukin, L.: Energy levels of human body segments during level walking. Ergonomics 12:39–46, 1969.

44. Reilly, D. T., and Martens, M.: Experimental analysis of the quadriceps muscle force and patellofemoral joint reaction force for various activities. Acta Orthop. Scand. 43:126–137, 1972.

45. Rowe, C. R.: Re-evaluation of the position of the arm in arthrodesis of the shoulder in the adult. J. Bone Joint Surg. 56A:913–922, 1974.

46. Rydell, N. W.: Forces acting on the femoral head-prosthesis: A study of strain gauge supplied prostheses in living persons. Acta Orthop. Scand. 37, Suppl. 88, 1966.

47. Rydell, N. W.: Biomechanics of the hip joint. Clin. Orthop. 92:6–15, 1973.

48. Saha, A. K.: *Theory of Shoulder Mechanism.* Charles C Thomas, Springfield, Ill., 1961.

49. Saha, A. K.: Dynamic stability of the glenohumeral joint. Acta Orthop. Scand. 42:491–505, 1971.

50. Saha, A. K.: Mechanics of elevation of glenohumeral joint. Its application in rehabilitation of flail shoulder in upper brachial plexus injuries and poliomyelitis and in replacement of the upper humerus by prosthesis. Acta Orthop. Scand. 44:668–678, 1973.

51. Seireg, A., and Arvikar, R. J.: The prediction of muscular load sharing and joint forces in the lower extremities during walking. J. Biomech. 8:89–109, 1975.

52. Simon, S. R., Deutsch, S. D., Nuzzo, R. M., et al.: Genu recurvatum in spastic cerebral palsy. Report on findings by gait analysis. J. Bone Joint Surg. 60A:882–894, 1978.

53. Simon, S. R., Mann, R. A., Hagy, J. L., and Larsson, L. J.: Role of the posterior calf muscles in normal gait. J. Bone Joint Surg. 60A:465–472, 1978.

54. Snook, S. H., Campanelli, R. A., and Hart, J. W.: A study of three preventive approaches to low back injury. J. Occup. Med. 20(7):478–481, 1978.

55. Stallard, J., Rose, G. K., Tait, J. H., and Davies, J. B.: Assessment of orthoses by means of speed and heart rate. J. Med. Eng. Technol. 2:22–24, 1978.

56. Steindler, A.: *Kinesiology of the Human Body,* 4th ed. Charles C Thomas, Springfield, Ill., 1973.

57. Sutherland, D. H., Schottstaedt, E. R., Larsen, L. J., et al.: Clinical and electromyographic

study of seven spastic children with internal rotation gait. J. Bone Joint Surg. 51A:1070–1082, 1969.

58. Vredenbregt, J., and Rau, G.: Surface electromyography in relation to force, muscle length, and endurance. In Desmedt, J. E., Ed.: *New Developments in Electromyography and Clinical Neurophysiology,* Vol. 1, pp. 607–622. Karger, Basel, 1973.

59. Waters, R. L., Perry, J., Antonelli, D., and Hislop, H.: Energy cost of walking of amputees: The influence of level of amputation. J. Bone Joint Surg. 58A:42–46, 1976.

60. Winter, D. A.: Energy assessment in pathological gait. Physiother. Can. 30:183–191, 1978.

61. Winter, D. A.: A new definition of mechanical work done in human movement. J. Appl. Physiol. 46:79–83, 1979.

62. Winter, D. A., Loughram, A., and Reimer, G. D.: Detailed kinematic analysis of gait of a hip disarticulation amputee with special reference on output mechanical work. Paper presented at Fifteenth Anniversary of the International Conference of the Biological Engineering Society, Edinburgh, August 1975.

63. Winter, D. A., Quanbury, A. O., and Reimer, G. D.: Analysis of instantaneous energy of normal gait. J. Biomech. 9:253–257, 1976.

64. Winter, D. A., and Robertson, D. G.: Joint torque and energy patterns in normal gait. Biol. Cybernet. 29:137–142, 1978a.

65. Zdravkovic, D., and Damholt, V.: Knee and quadriceps function after fracture of the femur. Acta Orthop. Scand. 42:460, 1971 (Abstract).

66. Zuniga, E. N., and Simons, D. G.: Non-linear relationship between averaged electromyogram potential and muscle tension in normal subjects. Arch. Phys. Med. 50:613–620, 1969.

6

The Physical Therapist

Marilyn J. Lister, B.S.

The orthopedic physical therapist aids in rehabilitation by assessing the extent of the patient's disability or the remaining disabilities, relieving pain, preventing deformity and further disability, developing or improving muscle strength or motor skills, and restoring or maintaining maximal functional abilities. Physical therapists practice prevention, restoration, or substitution in a variety of settings, including general and specialized hospitals, nursing homes, rehabilitation centers, schools, private offices, and industrial clinics.

This growth in the physical therapist's responsibilities resulted from the profession's early efforts to counteract tragedy. Two catastrophic episodes in the history of our country are especially relevant—World War I and epidemics of poliomyelitis. Although many of the old problems have been solved or no longer exist, new disabilities and public health problems have taken their place.

As our profession's experiences have accumulated and our body of knowledge has grown, we are now able to turn our attention to the preventive concerns of our profession. We no longer function just to help with the tragedies in life but to provide for the preventive care of all individuals.

HISTORY AND EMERGENCE
OF THE PROFESSION

The physical therapy profession became solidly established in the United States at the time of World War I with the organization of the program for Reconstruction Aides. When war was declared in 1917, the Surgeon General instituted the

Division of Special Hospitals and Physical Reconstruction for the physical rehabilitation, education, and vocational programs for the war-injured. Several orthopedic surgeons assigned to this division were responsible for organizing and developing the program for Reconstruction Aides in physical therapy. Assisting in the original planning was Marguerite Sanderson, a college graduate with gymnastics training, who was associated with one of the orthopedic surgeons. In 1918 Mary McMillan was appointed by the Surgeon General as the first Reconstruction Aide in our country and was assigned as Head Reconstruction Aide at Walter Reed General Hospital. Later in 1918, on leave from the army, McMillan was instrumental in developing and directing one of the first emergency training programs for aides. During the war there were seven such emergency training programs throughout the country. Nearly 800 aides were in service during the course of the emergency; almost 300 of them were overseas. From the very beginning it was the close collaboration and mutual respect between the orthopedic surgeons and the Reconstruction Aides that led not only to the development of physical therapy but to the acceptance of physical therapy as a profession. Orthopedic surgeons continued to make a profound and positive contribution to the course of events that shaped the future of physical therapy.

The incidence of epidemic proportions of poliomyelitis in the United States during 1914 and 1916 also greatly influenced the growth of the physical therapy profession. The first statewide program in Vermont for the aftercare of the patient involved teams of health workers, including what were generally referred to as "physician's assistants" or physiotherapists. A Boston orthopedic surgeon was instrumental in developing the plan and providing special training for a number of young women in muscle training, corrective exercise, and massage. Among them were Wilhelmine Wright, Janet Merrill, and Alice Lou Plastridge. The contributions that these women made as a result of their training and work during the epidemics led to the further recognition and acceptance of the profession and the establishment of major schools and departments of physical therapy. In 1922 the first postwar course in this country for physical therapists was established by Emma Vogel during her service at Walter Reed General Hospital. Vogel later was commissioned and became the first physical therapist to be accorded military status.

The epidemics of poliomyelitis also led to the establishment of the National Foundation for Infantile Paralysis in 1938. This foundation played an important part in continuing the profession's growth. Nearly 1000 physical therapists participated in the emergency work provided by the Foundation between 1948 and 1960. During the Salk vaccine trials in the 1960s, 38 physical therapists performed more than 2500 muscle tests and traveled more than 100,000 miles. Over the years the Foundation also provided grant support and funding to the American Physical Therapy Association, the official national organization for physical therapists. Service programs for patients and undergraduate and graduate educational programs for physical therapists were strengthened by this support.

In 1921, the American Physical Therapy Association was started by the same nucleus of people who served as Reconstruction Aides and who were responsible for the development of physical therapy in this country. The standards these individuals set for themselves, their work, and their profession were the keystones from which the Association has developed. In 1930, the Association was incorporated in Illinois, and the first constitution stated the practice of physical therapy consisted of "massage and therapeutic exercise with some knowledge of electrotherapy or hydrotherapy."

The practice of physical therapy changed a great deal, especially in the late 1940s, and particularly under the guidance of orthopedic surgeons. Rehabilitation centers were established that emphasized the *total* rehabilitation of the patient. Under the direction of a physician, physical therapists cooperated with other professional groups and developed a greater awareness of what total rehabilitation meant. Emphasis was increasingly placed on functional exercises and activities. The scope of techniques in physical therapy also widened to include new treatment methods for strengthening muscles, regimens for treating peripheral vascular conditions, body mechanics exercise for posture and back conditions, and exercises for chest conditions.

Physical therapists also began to conduct research in the late 1940s; since then, research papers have been presented routinely at the annual conferences of the Association. This demonstration of an active participation in research has increased, not only as required work for an advanced degree, but as a result of personal endeavors to study the clinical applications of physical therapy.

THE PROFESSION TODAY

The physical therapy profession has become accountable for the quality and integrity of its practice through the activities of the American Physical Therapy Association,[3] which has more than 30,000 members. The Association is now responsible for establishing educational standards and accrediting programs for physical therapists and physical therapist assistants. There are approximately 90 Association-accredited entry-level professional programs for physical therapists and approximately 52 programs for physical therapist assistants. For physical therapists, there are now at least 25 graduate-level programs leading to a master's or doctoral degree. Many therapists have an advanced degree in related subjects, such as physiology, neurophysiology, neuroanatomy, education, anatomy, or hospital administration.

The qualifications to practice physical therapy are established by law in each state and include attainment of at least the bachelor's degree, graduation from an accredited program, and successful completion of a licensure examination. Advanced degrees are usually needed to obtain administrative or faculty positions. In general, the physical therapist has a background in the biological and physical sciences, the social and behavioral sciences, the humanities and liberal arts, the science and art of physical therapy, plus clinical experience.

In many situations, the skills and clinical knowledge of the therapists have advanced beyond those required in entry-level physical therapy education. Recently, formal programs of the American Physical Therapy Association were organized to certify advanced clinical competence in the specializations of cardiopulmonary, neurological, orthopedic, and pediatric physical therapy. The advanced clinical competence will be determined by a competency-based evaluation. The Association has also worked to develop methods for increasing clinical research to assess the effectiveness of care and ensure that growth is based on sound scientific principles.

Other activities on behalf of improving the quality of the physical therapist's care, knowledge, and skills are emphasized by the Association. Continuing education programs in the form of conferences, seminars, publications, and workshops are sponsored regularly, as are quality assurance programs.[2] In 1977, the Association completed the analysis of competencies for the basic entry level of physical therapists.[4]

CONTRIBUTIONS AND FUNCTIONS THERAPISTS OFFER TO REHABILITATION

Physical therapists assume responsibility for evaluating the physical limitations of the patient, planning a treatment program, implementing the treatment plan, modifying and terminating treatment, communicating pertinent information, and delegating appropriate tasks.

The physical therapist is not only concerned with the orthopedic problems of the patient but with related problems as well. Most therapists use the same organized approach to solving these related problems and adapt their treatment principles and techniques to each individual case. Two primary examples are the management of certain pulmonary problems involving the muscles of respiration and neurological disabilities involving the cranial nerves. For purposes of brevity, this chapter will contain information more applicable to orthopedic rehabilitation.

By law in several states, patients must be referred to the therapist by a physician. Physical therapists are professionals who need only a referral for evaluation and treatment that includes a summary of the diagnosis of the patient and any extraordinary precautions or complications. It is not only unnecessary but inappropriate to provide a specific prescription clarifying how to treat the patient. Physical therapists are independently able to determine if the patient has a physical problem that can be ameliorated by physical therapy, estimate the time needed to achieve the treatment goal, know the most effective approach to solve the problem, determine when treatment is no longer effective or indicated, and recognize problems that need the attention of the physician. The physical therapist will keep the physician informed about the evaluation findings, treatment plans, and patient's response.

Evaluating the Patient

The physical therapist initially screens the patient to obtain general information about any current or potential physical limitation that can be improved with physical therapy (Fig. 6-1). This information provides a baseline from which immediate priorities and short-term goals are defined, specific needs for further testing are clarified, immediate needs for assistive equipment are identified, plans for an initial treatment program are made, and educational needs of the patient, family, and staff are determined.

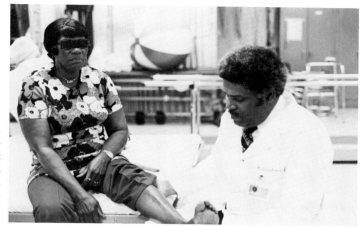

Fig. 6-1. Initial screening of patient by physical therapist to detect current or potential physical limitations. (Courtesy of the American Physical Therapy Association.)

Specific evaluations are then performed by the therapist. The unique disability demonstrated by the patient determines the assessment the therapist will use to test, measure, or evaluate the patient. Not all tests can or need be done on all types of patients. Testing usually provides the medical history with timely documentation, unique to physical therapy, about the physical status of the patient; establishes a source of baseline information for comparing the patient's status on an ongoing basis, even from admission to admission; supplies information that will assist the physician in making a diagnosis or establishing a prognosis; and helps the physical therapist define the magnitude of the patient's physical limitations.

The list of tests, measurements, or evaluations the physical therapist can administer is long and varied. Some of the tests are unique to physical therapy and require special training to perform them. In addition, not all therapists are able to make all of the specialty evaluations. Examples of different evaluations are joint range of motion;[1] muscle function,[6,10] including manual muscle tests, motor control tests, and electroneuromyography; sensation, including tests for tactile, proprioceptive, and perceptual senses; functional capacity; neurodevelopment;[8] respiratory function; cardiovascular and cardiorespiratory endurance; postural alignment; nerve function, including strength-duration curve, galvanic tetanus ratio, and reaction of degeneration; cranial nerve; and even the physical environment of the home. All physical therapists can be expected to evaluate patients for muscle strength, joint range of motion, and functional capacity.

The physical therapist evaluates the gait of a patient by providing an observational analysis of the problems, their causes, and their possible solutions. The use of electronic instruments, including the electromyograph, has furnished all interested health professionals, including physical therapists, the opportunity to obtain more precise information about gait. Many physical therapists work directly in the kinesiology laboratories providing these services. In some cases they carry out their own research projects.

Evaluating the patient's need for certain assistive and adaptive equipment is also the concern of the physical therapist. Unique to the domain of physical therapy are usually those items related to mobility. The list of equipment includes canes, crutches, grab bars, wheelchairs (manual or electric), wheelchair cushions, walkers, tub seats, corsets, lower extremity orthoses, transfer aids, commode chairs, portable lifts, and hydraulic lifts for vans.[11,12] By analyzing the data from all the routine physical therapy evaluations, therapists determine which equipment can best meet the needs of the patient. Later they will evaluate the equipment for fit and then train the patient in its use. Therapists also determine if equipment is needed temporarily or permanently, if equipment is needed in the home to assist someone taking care of the patient, and who needs to be trained to use the equipment.

In summary, the greatest value of the physical therapy evaluation is the clarification and documentation of the extent of the patient's physical disability, which aid in establishing the diagnosis, prognosis, and treatment goals.

Planning A Treatment Program

The treatment program for each patient is an individually tailored plan formulated after analyzing the results of the evaluations performed by the physical therapist and other health care professionals. Some generalizations can be made about problem selection and the resulting treatment goals and plans.

> Not all problems interfering with a patient's functioning can be solved by physical therapy. Therefore the therapist needs to recognize the limitations of treatment.
>
> Not all problems act as a negative influence on the patient's functioning. Therefore the therapist analyzes which of the small problems contribute to an overall loss of function.
>
> Not all of the patient's problems selected by the physical therapist to solve will be solved. Therefore every attempt should be made to clarify the expectation of achievement or the reasonable trial period needed for a treatment.
>
> Not all physical deviations interfere with a patient's functioning. Therefore the therapist must select for treatment only those factors that have a negative influence.
>
> Not all of the patient's problems designated to be solved by other health professionals can be solved. Therefore, because of these unresolvable difficulties, the therapist may ultimately be thwarted in achieving specific physical therapy goals that are usually attainable.
>
> Not all of the patient's problems within the physical therapist's realm need only a physical therapist's treatment. Therefore, the therapist may need to see that an activity is carried out by ancillary personnel in the therapy department or by those in other health disciplines.

The treatment plans usually contain both short- and long-term goals. The immediate steps, such as gaining a specific amount of muscle strength or range of motion, lead to the ultimate long-range or functional goal, such as wheelchair independence or ambulation with assistive devices. Specific long-term goals for patients with certain diagnoses tend to be established from observing the functional accomplishments of many other patients with the same diagnoses or physical findings. For example, expectations for certain functional achievements for one patient with a spinal cord injury are derived by comparisons with others similarly disabled.

Selecting the Treatment Plan

Selection of treatment depends upon the unique problem itself, how long it has existed, and the situation in which it exists. For example, the kind of disability considered as especially responsive to physical therapy is a movement deficit.[7] Human movement problems, however, are complicated to analyze and solve because they usually involve several systems of the body, including the lever (force) system, the control-guidance system, and the energy system. Therefore the great variety of possible problems and influences of all these systems are carefully analyzed by the therapist before selecting a treatment.

Another factor that influences the choice of physical therapy is the known effectiveness of a specific treatment or modality. Many guidelines for management of patients have come from experienced therapists who have worked with large numbers of patients with the same diagnosis or in the same age range. Such therapists have also worked closely with all the health care professionals involved with such cases and the team has been able to evaluate the clinical effectiveness of their care as well as learn to solve problems common to many of the patients. The result is an organized and systematic approach to patient care. When applying such a philosophy of care, it is important that the therapist does not simply apply the same treatment to each patient having the same diagnosis but does adapt the overall concepts of care for each individual.

Still other factors that influence the treatment selection are the experience and training of the physical therapist, the size of the department, the type of facility providing service to the patients, and the financial circumstances of the patient and the health care provider. For instance, a rehabilitation center having little or no need to provide physical agents will influence a physical therapist's selection of treatment.

The following discussion presents each of the overall goals for physical therapy and the more common procedures used in a rehabilitation setting to accomplish them. Most physical therapy includes therapeutic exercise, techniques to increase or maintain mobility, training in activities of daily living and in management of devices and equipment, gait training, procedures for improving cardiac and respiratory function, and, at the time of discharge, ways to overcome architectural barriers.

Relieving Pain. The procedures and techniques used to relieve pain vary according to many factors. Two critical determinants of the effectiveness of any treatment are the accurate identification of the source of pain and a thorough understanding of the physiological effects of the possible treatment.

Once the source of pain has been determined, physical therapy may be directed to relieving the symptoms as well as alleviating the cause. For some conditions, it may be necessary to relieve the pain before being able to correct the cause, and in other cases the opposite may be true. It is important to have the therapist and the physician recognize how each condition can be best approached, know when the primary cause of pain cannot be corrected by physical therapy, and know the period of time in which to expect results. For example, although the symptoms are similar, not all patients with an acute low-back problem can be placed on the same regimen and be expected to demonstrate the same degree of progress.

If the source of pain cannot be determined, the physical therapist may be able to provide relief by using short trials of different techniques. One technique that has been demonstrated clinically to offer pain relief for both acute and chronic conditions is transcutaneous electrical nerve stimulation (TENS).[13] One advantage in using TENS is that the patient with chronic pain can undergo effective treatment at home, outside the medical setting. Other sources of pain relief, some of which are not commonly used, are heat, cold, electricity, sound, exercise, traction, and water. In a rehabilitation setting, examples of pain relief treatments are moist heat for an acutely inflamed joint caused by rheumatoid arthritis and assistive and active exercises for painful joint motion after prolonged immobilization.

Preventing Deformity and Further Disability. One of the major contributions orthopedic physical therapists make to a patient's rehabilitation is the prevention of deformity and further disability (Fig. 6-2). Alleviating the loss of range of joint motion, one of the key factors contributing to pain and the loss of function, is one of the most challenging aspects of physical therapy. The problem is complex because it may have occurred for a variety of reasons and may have involved different anatomical structures.

The physical therapist prevents deformity by providing the best exercise and positioning program for the physical status of that individual patient. For a severely paralyzed patient, the program may include the use of resting splints. The therapist will adapt or modify the program according to the response of the patient and the limitations imposed by the symptoms of the condition.

Many general procedures and techniques are used by physical therapists to restore joint mobility, including positioning, stretching, use of equipment, exercise, and education. The effectiveness of this particular combination of treatments

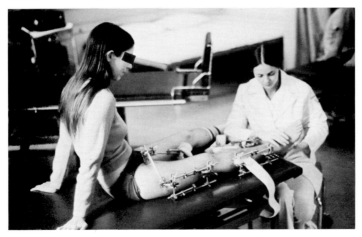

Fig. 6-2. Preventing deformity and further disability through the use of passive and active exercise. (Courtesy of the American Physical Therapy Association.)

is far more dependent than any other regimen upon the cooperation of the patient and the personnel from the other health care disciplines. If it is not plausible to implement the treatment program with the utmost degree of cooperation, then the ultimate functional achievements attained are compromised. Many times the intervention of surgery may temporarily correct the deformity, but long-term results can depend upon the follow-up care preventing the recurrence of the problem.

The use of *positioning* as an adjunct to gaining range of motion requires that the disabled part of the body be held in the new, more desirable position at the extreme end of the range for the length of time that is necessary to counteract the deforming forces that have caused the contracture. For example, 24 hours a day of proper positioning in the prone position would probably be required to gain hip and knee extension range of motion in a patient who has developed hip and knee flexion contractures from sitting all day. Another less extreme example is that of providing a resting extension splint solely for night-time use for an elbow with a flexion contracture, innervated flexors, and no active extensors.

For a positioning program to succeed in restoring mobility, the patient must only be expected to tolerate the new positions and the pressures from any restraints if there is no discomfort, the position must be changed frequently to take up the slack in the range of motion that has been gained, and the patient, as well as all personnel involved, must understand the concept and principles of the treatment. Moreover, the positioning program, to be most effective, should be accompanied by an exercise program and periods of static stretch.

Stretching, as a means of restoring joint mobility, can be done manually or by using equipment. Generally, intermittent stretching done manually does not reduce contractures of long duration.

Mobilization and manipulation are techniques requiring special advanced training to increase joint motion in certain cases. Restoring normal range of motion by these techniques can result in reduced pain as well as increased function.

The static, prolonged stretch applied to help relieve contractures need not be done with an elaborate arrangement of *equipment.* Many times a simple sling and pulley arrangement with weight applied twice daily for 20 minutes can be effective if the treatment is followed up with a positioning program to maintain the body part at the end of the newly acquired range. What is critical is stabilizing the part to ensure that stretch occurs at the designated joint.

Exercise to help restore motion emphasizes strengthening the muscles opposing the contracture. This approach builds in a 24-hour-a-day mechanism for combating contracture formation.

Patient *education* concerning prevention of the reoccurrence of the deformity requires special attention. The physical therapist provides practical guidelines and suggests adaptive equipment for maintaining joint mobility to be used by patients or their families. The therapist, by knowing where unopposed muscle action occurs, how the patient has responded to previous treatment, the patient's usual resting postures, and the functional uses of the extremities, can pinpoint potential areas for tightness and make preventive plans.

The prevention of pressure sores is one of the major regimens in which the orthopedic physical therapist participates to prevent further disability for the patient. Just as members of the other disciplines are responsible for preventing sores while carrying out their treatment procedures and plans, physical therapists are involved during their phase of care. When they oversee the ordering, fitting, or applying any piece of equipment, therapists vigorously protect the patient from pressure that could cause a sore. Therapists also help plan special positioning programs and devise unique equipment for the relief of pressure. In addition, each patient receives individual instruction on pressure relief as part of routine patient education conducted by therapists. Therapists also help patients develop the tolerance needed for wearing or using equipment.

Developing or Improving Muscle Strength or Motor Skills. Various exercises are used to influence movement related to strength, tone, and control of muscle action. Therapeutic exercise is the broad term used by physical therapists to designate the various types of exercises. For each patient and exercise, there is an optimal technique of application comprised of frequency, speed, duration, and position. Also of importance is the skill of the person who performs the treatment, whether it be the therapist, physical therapist assistant, or the patient himself. Physical therapists can advance or modify the patient's exercise program independently without having to check with the physician before each step.

One of the most important kinds of exercise used in the rehabilitation of a patient is progressive resistive exercise. In general, any exercise for increasing muscle strength must involve work by having a muscle contract against a resistance. Therapists apply the resistance in different forms, such as disk weights, springs, gravity, manually applied pressure, or body weight. The three common terms therapists use to describe the types of resistive exercise that take place during different methods of application are *isotonic, isometric,* and *isokinetic* exercise. In applying resistance, the muscle must really be made to work and not just perform a mild repetitious exercise. Therapists take great care in making the proper selection of muscles to be exercised, such as the specific muscles used to perform a certain task (Fig. 6-3). There are also times when it is advantageous to apply resistive exercises to isolated muscles rather than muscle groups.

Many exercise regimens are specifically designed for patients with motor control problems from deficits in the central nervous system, such as cerebral palsy or a cerebrovascular accident (Fig. 6-4). In general, the procedures used by the therapist in an attempt to alter the patient's motor control involve changing the patient's body position, using facilitatory techniques, and emphasizing sequential progression of performance based on neurodevelopmental theory. The treatment goals are the same as for orthopedic cases, but the methods of treatment are different.

Many orthopedic physical therapists have great expertise in exercising patients who have had tendon transfers, soft tissue repairs, and athletic injuries needing surgery. Therapists pay careful attention to muscle re-education and strengthening, based on their knowledge of what the surgeon has done and the functional goals of the patient. One technique some physical therapists find useful as an adjunct to their exercise programs is electromyogram biofeedback to improve motor control.[5]

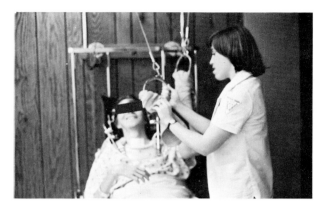

Fig. 6-3. The overhead pulley setup provides progressive resistive exercises in a functional pattern of motion for a patient with quadriplegia. (Courtesy of the American Physical Therapy Association.)

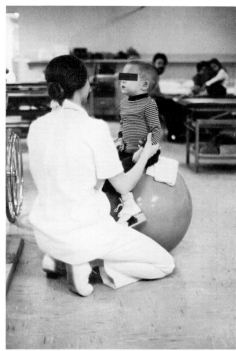

Fig. 6-4. A child with a central nervous system deficit participates in a special program designed to improve motor control. (Courtesy of the American Physical Therapy Association.)

Restoring or Maintaining Maximal Functional Abilities. Orthopedic physical therapists specialize in teaching activities necessary in the patient's daily living, including categories for bed, wheelchair, standing, and ambulation.[9] In preparation for teaching the patient each functional act, the therapist must know the physical requirements involved in the act, the degree of potential the patient has in meeting those requirements, and the assistive or adaptive devices that might be helpful. This analysis calls for an understanding of kinesiology, anatomy, biomechanics, and teaching techniques combined with knowledge of the patient's present and potential physical status. The therapist knows the tasks the patient needs to learn, the best sequence for learning, when the patient is ready for the next step, and the predicted amount of time it will take to learn the task (Fig. 6-5).

Physical therapists specialize in knowing about the assistive and adaptive devices related to wheelchairs and ambulation. For example, therapists are able to select whatever crutch, walker, wheelchair, seat cushion, or orthosis a patient needs,[12] teach the patient how to don or use the equipment, determine if the devices fit or need repair, and recognize when the patient no longer needs the device. Of special significance is the choice of a wheelchair to provide maximum functional use and the custom selection and contouring of a wheelchair cushion to relieve pressure.

Many physical therapists also develop expertise in and become responsible for determining the patient's potential to drive and providing the specific driver

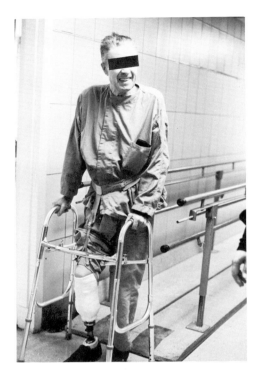

Fig. 6-5. Ambulation with assistive devices is a functional goal for this patient with an amputation. (Courtesy of the American Physical Therapy Association.)

training. Therapists are often consulted about the transportation needs for specific patients, such as giving specifications of an automobile or van suitable for a patient and his wheelchair or the best type of portable lift for an automobile.

A relatively new teaching responsibility for physical therapists is in advising patients about positions for sexual functioning that are compatible with their disability or postoperative limitations. For example, therapists teach the patients essential limitations in hip motion following total hip replacements or help a patient with severe arthritis to find comfortable positions and pillow arrangements.

Gait training is the one specialty for which physical therapy is renowned. Many requests, however, for helping the patient walk are not always realistic or feasible. The most important role for therapists in regard to ambulation is to determine for themselves, their patients, and other health care professionals if the patient is a candidate for ambulation. That decision must take into account such variables as the objective evaluation of what strength, range or motion, and endurance the patient has and what he needs, the significance that walking has for the patient, and the physical barriers to be encountered in the patient's environment. One example of false hope and unrealistic functional goals is to have a patient walk in the parallel bars day after day when maximal help is needed for the physical support of the patient, who thus will never be able to progress to walking out of the bars.

Modifying and Terminating Treatment

Physical therapists modify their treatment programs when the patient's response indicates a need for change. The therapist also knows when to terminate a treatment if the goal has been achieved or if a problem arises that needs the attention of the physician. The therapist can discern when there has been an adverse change in the patient's response, when the patient does not respond as expected, or when the patient no longer demonstrates the need for continued therapy.

Communicating

The physical therapist communicates with the physician, other health care professionals, and the patient's family about the physical therapy program plans, the patient's progress in therapy, and any problems encountered. The initial plans for treatment are discussed with the physician and the rest of the rehabilitation team to inform them about the results of the physical therapy evaluation, the problems to be worked on in therapy, the goals to be achieved, the general plans for treatment, and the estimate of the time that it will take to achieve the goals. The details of the evaluations and ongoing written progress notes are documented in the patient's medical history. And, of course, informal discussions are routine in regard to progress toward goals, remaining difficulties to overcome, the patient's current goals, the functional level at the time, and any problem needing attention of the team. Of particular importance is the almost daily up-to-date communication with all the personnel about the latest functional abilities of the patient and the equipment or assistance required.

Before a patient's discharge, the therapist works closely with the appropriate team members to coordinate the plans and clarify the needs of the patient as well as establish contact with the family for necessary training or information. If the patient is transferred to another facility, the therapist can prepare a special report about the patient's physical status and functional level for the new medical personnel.

Delegating Tasks

Physical therapists rely on others to assist them in providing treatment because it is not feasible, practical, or necessary for them to use their professional skills for all degrees of care. The essential responsibilities of routine patient care that therapists do not usually delegate are evaluation, program planning, and certain exercise regimens requiring advanced training or expertise.

Available to assist in providing care are a variety of unlicensed physical therapy aides, most of whom are trained on the job in a hospital or clinical facility. A *physical therapy aide's* primary function is to perform designated routine tasks related to the operation of a physical therapy program, such as preparing the patient for treatment, assisting the patient with routine practice of an activity, and helping to maintain the equipment and space of a department.

The *physical therapist assistant* is a more highly trained health technician who works within a physical therapy service under the direction and supervision of the physical therapist. The extent to which an assistant works with the patient depends on the organization of the facility, the supervising therapist, and the individual patient. Physical therapist assistants take education programs in community and junior colleges. The course of study includes physical, biological, and social sciences, physical therapy technical courses, and clinical experiences. Graduates receive an associate degree as a physical therapist assistant. Assistants help carry out the physical therapy program by training patients in exercise and activities of daily living, conducting treatments using special modalities, assisting in complex treatment procedures, and observing and reporting to the physical therapist the patient's responses to the treatments.

Many times the physical therapist relies on the patient as well as the other health care professionals to carry out the routine practice of certain activities the patient needs to do. After the therapist provides the equipment and the instructions, the patients can exercise frequently and alone. They can, for instance, use pulley and sling exercise equipment attached to the overhead frame of the bed or practice using a walker to build up endurance in preparing to go home. The nursing aides can help patients by placing them in a position to exercise or practice.

FUTURE DIRECTIONS IN PHYSICAL THERAPY

The future provision of care by the physical therapist will be greatly influenced by the same government standards and directives that effect all other health professions. In particular, the scope of practice and methods of reimbursement will be influenced directly by predicted changes in our insurance structure.

That physical therapy can be considered a primary source of health care for society is not yet firmly established or obvious to all who make decisions regarding our practice. Yet the growth of the profession has been noteworthy in leading to ethical and high-quality care, accountability, research providing a body of knowledge, educational standards, and well-defined competencies. A few of our many new challenges could involve extending our services and contributing even more to the aspect of preventive medicine by participating in the screening of patients, determining the actual efficacy of established treatments, and finding new treatments based on sound scientific investigation and extensive knowledge about specific disabilities.

REFERENCES

1. American Academy of Orthopaedic Surgeons: *Joint Motion: Method of Measuring and Recording.* American Academy of Orthopaedic Surgeons, Chicago, 1965.
2. American Physical Therapy Association: *Physical Therapy Patient Care Audit Manual.* American Physical Therapy Association, Washington, D.C., 1978.

3. American Physical Therapy Association: *Standards for Physical Therapy Service Evaluation Forms.* American Physical Therapy Association, Washington, D.C., 1979.

4. American Physical Therapy Association and Courseware Incorporated. *Competencies in Physical Therapy: An Analysis of Practice.* Courseware Incorporated, San Diego, 1977.

5. Baker, M., Regenos, E., Wolf, S. L., and Basmajian, J. V.: *Developing Strategies for Biofeedback Applications in Neurologically Handicapped Patients.* American Physical Therapy Association, Washington, D.C., 1977.

6. Daniels, L., and Worthingham, C.: *Muscle Testing: Techniques of Manual Examination,* 3rd ed. W. B. Saunders, Philadelphia, 1972.

7. Daniels, L., and Worthingham, C.: *Therapeutic Exercises for Body Alignment and Function,* 2nd ed. W. B. Saunders, Philadelphia, 1977.

8. Hoskins, T., and Squires, J.: Developmental assessment: A test for gross motor and reflex development. Phys. Ther. 53:117–126, 1973.

9. Lawton, E.: *Activities of Daily Living for Physical Rehabilitation.* McGraw-Hill Book Co., New York, 1963.

10. Kendall, H., and Kendall, F.: *Muscles, Testing, and Function,* 2nd ed. Williams & Wilkins, Baltimore, 1971.

11. Perry, J., Ed.: *Upper Extremity Orthotics—A Monograph.* American Physical Therapy Association, Washington, D.C., 1978.

12. Perry, J., and Hislop, H. J., Eds.: *Principles of Lower-Extremity Bracing.* American Physical Therapy Association, Washington, D.C., 1972.

13. Wolf, S. L., Ed.: *Transcutaneous Electrical Nerve Stimulation—A Monograph.* American Physical Therapy Association, Washington, D.C., 1979.

7

Occupational Therapy

Mary W. McKenzie, B.S., L.O.T.R., F.A.O.T.A.

Occupational therapy employs functional evaluation and treatment to minimize the disabling effects of developmental deficits, aging, physical illness, injury, psychological and social disability, poverty, and cultural differences.[1]

The goals of occupational therapy as it applies to rehabilitation are to prevent further loss to the individual and restore his functional ability to the optimum in tasks of daily life. The potential level of function depends upon the degree of disability that results from specific injury or disease, and the patient's psychological acceptance of his condition. Occupational therapy attempts not only to help correct and overcome pathology, but to understand the psychological effects of illness and disability and incorporate into treatment the support that assists the person in developing adaptive skills to cope with his disability.

SPECIAL QUALIFICATIONS OF THE OCCUPATIONAL THERAPIST

Educational preparation for entry into occupational therapy is a four-year bachelor's degree that provides a theoretical base in behavioral, biological, and physical sciences. In addition, a minimum of six months' supervised clinical training is required for the purpose of applying the theoretical knowledge.

Following completion of these basic educational requirements, the student therapist is eligible to take the American Occupational Therapy Association's certification examination. Additionally, several universities offer advanced degrees in occupational therapy.

From their preparation as generalists, occupational therapists specialize, just as do other health care professionals. Broad specialty areas include physical dysfunction, psychiatry, and pediatrics. Others further specialize in such areas as developmental disabilities, sensory integration, hand rehabilitation, and spinal cord injury. The individual therapist pursues additional learning experiences through formal education, independent study, and continuing education to develop competency in a specialized practice area.

HISTORY AND EMERGENCE OF THE PROFESSION OF OCCUPATIONAL THERAPY

The National Society for the Promotion of Occupational Therapy was formed in March 1917. Occupational therapy's initial growth came as a result of World War I. Patients on orthopedic and surgical wards were treated as well as those suffering from nervous and mental disorders. Following World War I, development of occupational therapy remained stationary. With the advent of World War II and the influx of wounded veterans, occupational therapy experienced renewed growth. As a result of the war, occupational therapy techniques and knowledge were expanded, especially in the area of physical disability.[4]

Occupational therapy's emergence somewhat parallels that of rehabilitation. The term "rehabilitation" did not exist before World War II. The popular term during World War I was "reconstruction."[3] Many occupational therapists received their training as Reconstruction Aides.[4]

ROLE AND FUNCTION OF THE OCCUPATIONAL THERAPIST

Occupational therapists, like other health care professionals, are trained to perform as independent practitioners. Detailed, written prescriptions to the occupational therapist by the physician are not necessary. In 1968, Nickel[7] suggested abandonment of the detailed written prescription, suggesting instead a program in which the physician maintained general medical direction.

In this paradigm, the professional occupational therapist functions as an independent practitioner contributing knowledge and skill, making independent decisions within the scope of occupational therapy practice and boundaries determined in consultation with the interdisciplinary team. Composition of the team may vary according to the patient's need. Members most often include the physician, occupational and physical therapists, nurse, medical social worker, speech and language pathologist, and chaplain. Within this framework, it is the occupational therapist's responsibility to:

1. Become acquainted with the patient's diagnosis, current medical status, complications, or precautions.
2. Evaluate the patient by using appropriate testing procedures.
3. Assist the team, patients, and families in establishing realistic goals, estimate the length of time required for the accomplishment of these goals, keep the patient and his family apprised of progress, and be involved in discharge planning.
4. Plan and execute a treatment program by constantly re-evaluating, updating, and making changes in the program as progress or regression dictates.
5. Identify, prescribe, adapt, or fabricate specialized equipment that will enable the patient to function independently or with assistance after discharge.
6. Discuss regularly with team members the progress, regression, changes in the occupational therapy goals, problems encountered, and discharge planning status.
7. Record on a routine basis all pertinent information in the patient's medical chart.

To plan and implement effective treatment, the occupational therapist must first establish a baseline. *Subjective* information is gathered from the patient and family regarding previous lifestyle, accomplishments, work and leisure time interests, education, coping mechanisms, and, most importantly, their expectations of the outcome of therapy. *Objective* information includes skeletal muscle strength, joint range of motion, cognitive, perceptual, and sensory function, performance in self-care skills, vocational and prevocational interests, and home and community environment. Once the baseline information is secured, an *assessment* is made of the individual's physical, cognitive, educational, social, and environmental assets and liabilities based on the subjective and objective data collected. A *plan* for treatment and an estimated length of stay are established, and goals the patient may be expected to accomplish are identified.

INTERVENTIONS FOR OCCUPATIONAL THERAPY

Occupational therapists practice in many settings. Among them are public schools, community centers, psychiatric settings, general hospitals, rehabilitation centers, and outpatient clinics.

Equally diverse are the conditions with accompanying orthopedic problems for which occupational therapy intervention may be indicated: cerebral palsy, neurodevelopmental disability, congenital and traumatic amputations, burns, neurological diseases and injuries, degenerative diseases, and low back pain, to name a few.

Objectives for occupational therapy treatment vary with the person's age and the resulting disability. In general, treatment goals for persons with acquired orthopedic and neurological conditions are: achievement of the highest level of functional performance in activities of daily living, including eating, self-care, vocational and avocational pursuits; improvement of upper extremity function through the use of exercises, activities, splinting, orthotic devices, and adapted equipment; education of the patient and family; socialization and adaptation to new life patterns; and participation in the pre- and postoperative management of upper extremity surgical procedures.

Space does not permit an in-depth discussion of all conditions for which occupational therapy may be indicated or possible treatment techniques that might be used. The following diagnostic groups have been chosen because of the frequency in which they are seen in rehabilitation centers: arthritis, cerebrovascular accidents, spinal cord injury, and hand rehabilitation.

The purpose of the discussion that follows is to illustrate occupational therapy's function and ways in which the occupational therapist participates in rehabilitating persons with disabling conditions. Techniques described are intended to serve as examples of treatment.

Arthritis

Persons with arthritis have limited function, which results from pain, muscle weakness, and deformities imposed by the disease process. Early diagnosis and treatment can often prevent or delay the disabling effects of deformity.

An essential component in the successful management of arthritis is patient and family education. Everyone involved must understand the process of the disease, joint protection techniques to be used in daily activities to decrease the joint stress that may damage joints even more, exercises that maintain joint mobility best while minimizing stresses that increase the possibility of joint damage, and the importance of a proper balance between rest and activity. The occupational therapists assist the patient in evaluating daily activities, that is, self-care, homemaking, and employment. Alternate methods for performance and adaptive devices are demonstrated or provided, which help minimize deforming forces.[6]

An adjunct of treatment of arthritis by occupational therapy is handsplinting. Three types of splinting are generally used. Positioning splints are used to rest inflamed, painful joints during periods of exacerbation. Functional splints are worn to stabilize a painful joint during activities that increase pain. Postoperative splints are used postoperatively.

Surgical procedures have long been included in the management of severely destroyed, painful arthritic joints. With the advent of joint replacements, surgery has become a more common approach. Preoperatively, occupational therapists work closely with both patient and physician in evaluating upper extremity and hand function, contributing information to the overall plan for surgical reconstruction. Preoperative measurements provide a basis on which to evaluate postoperative results. Pre- and postoperatively, exercises to improve joint mobilization and splinting for correct positioning are prescribed.

In summary, occupational therapy helps the person with arthritis by evaluating his activities, introducing him to alternate methods of functioning, and assisting him in restructuring his life and modifying his behavior to reach a balance in activity.

Cerebrovascular Accidents

The primary objectives of occupational therapy with the stroke patient are to:

1. Prevent or correct deformity.
2. Increase motor function and control in the affected upper extremity for purposeful activity.
3. Teach compensation for sensory deficits.
4. Improve levels of self-care.
5. Evaluate, preoperatively, with the physician, the deforming forces in the upper extremity.
6. Participate in postoperative upper extremity positioning, splinting, and treatment.

It is important to establish the extent to which the stroke has affected the patient's physical, intellectual, social, and psychological functioning before beginning treatment. Numerous factors influence the outcome of rehabilitation in persons who suffer a stroke.

Sensory impairment is a major factor in determining the use a person will make of functional return in the affected extremity. If the patient has no awareness of the affected side or an inability to distinguish objects or stimuli on that side, the prognosis for functional use of the extremity is poor, even in the presence of selective motor control.

To prevent deformities, exercises are prescribed and demonstrated to the patient for maintaining range of motion in the upper extremity. Devices such as wheelchair suspension arm slings for the nonambulatory patient, may be ordered by the occupational therapist to be used for upper extremity positioning to decrease the potential for hand edema, shoulder subluxation, and loss of range of motion in the shoulder. Positioning handsplints may be prescribed or constructed by the occupational therapist to overcome the force of gravity and diminish the effects of increased tone in the flexor groups, which potentiate flexion contractures in the wrist and hand of the stroke patient.

Motor control must be analyzed to determine the amount and strength of selective or patterned motion. Spasticity limits functional use in the upper extremity by decreasing the speed and control of motion or causing the arm to assume a nonfunctional position. Neuromuscular facilitation techniques are used to inhibit spasticity and increase voluntary control in the affected upper extremity.

Residual function in the affected upper extremity ranges from nonfunctional—merely used as an assist in the gross, stabilizing motions—to the highest level, that is, precise motor control in fine activities.

Activities that encourage sensory, perceptual, and cognitive integration are incorporated into training for daily life tasks. One-handed methods for dressing, grooming, feeding, homemaking, work, and leisure skills are learned. Adapted equipment that increases the patient's independence in activities of daily living is recommended or provided by the occupational therapist.

Before surgical intervention on the hemiplegic upper extremity, the occupational therapist collaborates with the physician in evaluating the deforming forces that are present and the prognosis for effective use of the impaired extremity following surgery. After the operation, an active program of splinting, exercises, and use training is initiated to augment the surgical results.

Other factors influencing the outcome of rehabilitative measures are emotional lability, perceptual disturbances, speech, language, and visual impairment, impaired body image, and problems involving both cognitive and intellectual functioning.

To summarize, the occupational therapist evaluates the person who has suffered a cerebrovascular accident to determine the extent to which the stroke has affected functional abilities. Programs are individually tailored to the constraints of the patient's motor, sensory, and cognitive impairment.

Spinal Cord Injury

Ideally, occupational therapy for the spinal cord injured person should begin during the acute stage. For the purpose of this discussion, the acute stage can be defined as the one or two days immediately following the injury, when care is directed toward stabilization of the patient's physical condition through management of life-threatening complications and the achievement of adequate spine immobilization.

As soon as spine immobilization is accomplished, there are three *immediate* functions the occupational therapist should perform: evaluate passive joint range of motion, skeletal muscle strength, and sensory modalities; establish an upper extremity positioning program; and provide psychological support for the patient and family members.

It is important for the occupational therapist to evaluate the patient immediately and document the muscle and dermatome levels so that improvements or deterioration in the neurological condition can be monitored. Additionally, the information can contribute in establishing a prognosis.

In this author's experience, joint tightness has been noted to occur within 48 hours following injury. Prompt attention should be given by the therapist to proper upper extremity positioning and passive range of motion.

Normal range of motion in the shoulder and elbow is critical to the quadriplegic patient with the physical capacity to transfer independently and drive a vehicle. An elbow flexion contracture will prevent the patient from mechanically locking the elbow in extension to substitute for triceps, which is absent in lesions above the C6 neurological level. Joint contractures often take months to resolve, frequently require surgical release, and may necessitate a complete alteration in goals the patient should achieve. Prompt treatment intervention can prevent these complications.

The time immediately following the injury is a time of shock and disbelief. Both the patient and family are in a dreamlike state, hearing little of what is said. It is necessary, especially during this period, for all who come in contact with the patient to provide psychological reinforcement while explaining simply and frequently what is being done and the reason why. It is essential during this time that the patient and family be guided in setting realistic, attainable goals that are in keeping with the level of injury.[5,12]

As soon as the physician determines spine stability and gives clearance for the patient to begin sitting upright, the therapist begins a more aggressive treatment program that progressively moves through strengthening and balance activities, transferring to and from the wheelchair, self-care, and exploring all functional, vocational, and avocational areas.

Adaptive equipment needs are assessed and prescribed. Orthotic devices, such as handsplints and mobile arm supports, are important for quadriplegics for preventing deformity and increasing function.[13]

Three major types of upper extremity equipment are prescribed by the occupational therapist for the quadriplegic patient: *positioning splints* support the wrist and position the thumb in abduction and opposition, *functional splints* provide palmar prehension for function, and *mobile arm supports* eliminate the gravitational pull and assist weak shoulder and elbow muscles.

There are references in the literature describing tendon transfers to increase prehension and grasp in the quadriplegic hand. Perry[8] points out that how the patient will use his hands during functional activities should strongly influence the decision for hand surgery. Transfers that require the patient to support his full body weight on the extended wrists and hands are particularly damaging to tendon transfers. Freehafer et al.[2] discuss the importance of the following prerequisites to hand surgery in spinal cord injured patients: the patient's having completed his rehabilitation program, a plateau in neurological return has occurred, as have an absence of or a minimum of spasticity, adequate sensation and motor power, and a sincere desire on the patient's part to improve himself. The authors further state: "for these reasons tendon transfers done less than one year after spinal cord injury may not give optimum results and may actually cause more problems for these patients."[2]

Occupational therapists can help evaluate candidates for operative procedures and provide information with regard to the effect the procedure will have on the patient's overall functional ability.

The degree of neurological return will determine the projected functional level the patient can be expected to reach as well as the kinds of assistive devices required.

Because each patient's requirements vary, the occupational therapist provides or fabricates equipment based on individual needs.

In summary, occupational therapists help the patient and family define realistic goals. They also provide the necessary training and guidance in attaining the highest functional levels possible.

Hand Rehabilitation

Perry[9] has also observed that "effectiveness of the upper extremity is judged by the hand's ability to manipulate, position, or use objects." When disease, injury, or direct trauma result in loss of hand function, that person's function, to whom disease or injury has occurred, is critically affected.

Rehabilitation of traumatic hand injuries is challenging to both the surgeon and the occupational therapist. Management of hand treatment can best be accomplished by their cooperative efforts. Successful management of hand problems is dependent on accurate preoperative assessment, skilled surgery, and diligent postoperative treatment.[10]

Standard evaluations include the manual muscle test, active and passive joint range of motion, sensory examination, pinch and grasp strength, and the ability to perform self-care. Individual problems may require that the therapist perform such additional evaluations as volumetrics and dexterity tests.

Preoperatively, the occupational therapist can provide the surgeon with valuable information regarding how the patient feels about himself, his overall goals, work habits, the importance of cosmesis, the specific functions he needs to perform with his hand, motivation, and the degree of *active* participation by the patient in the preoperative treatment program. All are critical factors in the outcome of that individual's hand rehabilitation. Early occupational therapy referral can reduce the possibility of the joint stiffness and scarring that so often complicate the recovery of the hand-injured patient.

Techniques used in occupational therapy for hand injuries include mobilization of scar tissue, muscle re-education using biofeedback, desensitization, active exercises, and activities to increase strength and joint range of motion. Static and dynamic hand splinting is directed toward protecting and assisting weak muscles and preventing and correcting deformities.

THE INTERDISCIPLINARY TEAM

The interdisciplinary team is the most effective approach for managing persons with chronic disabling diseases and injuries. Health professionals must become specialists in treating the problems manifested in the disabling conditions of persons with whom they work. They cannot minister to all problems themselves. Accordingly, they must develop a working knowledge of the roles of the other professionals in the rehabilitation setting in order to relate to and participate in the total care of patients needing specialized treatment. Implicit in this concept is the freedom of one discipline to call upon the other for mutual problem-solving.

Within the team, an overlapping of professional roles will frequently occur. Leadership on the team may shift when dealing with any given patient, depending upon the circumstances and the understanding that develops between a particular patient and health professional. Both formal and informal communication contributes to effective team work. Open communication among the interdisciplinary team serves to improve the outcome of the person's rehabilitation program.

Four specific areas for which team treatment is essential are goal setting, patient and family education, discharge planning, and outpatient follow-up. Each member of the team should establish mutual goals with the patient, family, and other disciplines. Clear and simple explanations are necessary for the patient and family to understand the disability and its implications on the remainder of the patient's life. Family members are encouraged to participate in all aspects of the person's care. This approach does not necessarily ensure follow-through after discharge. Odds, however, are increased that the person will experience fewer complications and maintain a higher level of performance. Discharge planning begins shortly after admission. The patient and family are encouraged to consider vocational plans and living arrangements as early as feasible so that treatment can be directed toward the new home and work situations that must be created. Weekend passes during the hospital stay are encouraged in order to spot potential problems that might increase stress in the family unit after discharge. Actual visits to the home are made by members of the team whenever possible to make suggestions for personal care and alterations in architectural barriers. Outpatient follow-up allows the team to evaluate the results of rehabilitation and assess how the patient and family are managing post-discharge, suggest needed changes, and provide emotional support.

FUTURE DIRECTIONS

Since its founding in 1917, occupational therapy has expanded its professional services in response to the needs of society. One of the most recent examples is the demand for occupational therapy services for handicapped children in the public school systems brought about by the enactment of Public Law 94-142 in 1975. Occupational therapy will continue to expand its body of theoretical knowledge, skills, roles, and services to provide necessary remediation and resources to those persons who can benefit from these special services.

SUMMARY

Occupational therapy's role in rehabilitation is varied. The central focus of concern is evaluating the effect the disease, injury, or disability has on a person's ability to participate in his chosen way of life. Remediation includes a treatment plan that encompasses realistic goals and adaptive skills that enable a person to realize his potential.

As a member of the rehabilitation team, the occupational therapist formally and informally communicates assessment, goals, progress, regression, and problems. The cooperative efforts of the interdisciplinary team support the patient and family. Our common goal in rehabilitation is, as one definition states, "the restoration of the handicapped to the fullest physical, mental, social, vocational and economic usefulness of which they are capable."[11]

REFERENCES

1. American Occupational Therapy Association, Representative Assembly, Resolution 500, April, 1977.
2. Freehafer, A. A., Vonhaam, E., and Allen, V.: Tendon transfers to improve grasp after injuries of the cervical spinal cord. J. Bone Joint Surg. 56A:951–959, 1974.
3. Gullickson, G., Jr., and Licht, S.: Definition and philosophy of rehabilitation medicine. In Licht, S., Ed.: *Rehabilitation Medicine,* pp. 1–14. Elizabeth Licht, New Haven, 1968.
4. Hopkins, H. L.: An historical perspective on occupational therapy. In Hopkins, H. L., and Smith, H. D., Eds.: *Willard and Spackman's Occupational Therapy,* 5th ed., pp. 3–21. J. B. Lippincott, Philadelphia, 1978.
5. McKenzie, M. W.: The role of occupational therapy in rehabilitating spinal cord injured patients. Am. J. Occup. Ther. 4:257–263, 1970.
6. McKenzie, M. W., Hennig, L. M., and McGill, M. M.: *The Arthritis Learning Notebook.* Mississippi Methodist Rehabilitation Center, Jackson, Miss., 1976.

7. Nickel, V. L.: The orthopedic surgeon and the occupational therapist. Am. J. Occup. Ther. 2:86–88, 1968.

8. Perry, J.: Surgical treatment of the paralytic hand. In Pierce, D. S., and Nickel, V. L., Eds.: *The Total Care of Spinal Cord Injuries,* pp. 103–133. Little, Brown, Boston, 1977.

9. Perry, J.: Normal upper extremity kinesiology. Phys. Ther. 58:265–281, 1978.

10. Pulvertaft, R. G.: Foreword. In Hunter, J. M., Schneider, L. H., Mackin, E. H., and Bell, J. A., Eds.: *Rehabilitation of the Hand,* p. ix. C. V. Mosby, St. Louis, 1978.

11. Reggio, A. W.: Rehabilitation—what is it. Am. J. Occup. Ther. 1:149–151, 1947.

12. Stauffer, E. S.: Long term management of traumatic quadriplegia. In Pierce, D. S., and Nickel, V. L., Eds.: *The Total Care of Spinal Cord Injuries,* pp. 81–102. Little, Brown, Boston, 1977.

13. Wilson, D. J., McKenzie, M. W., and Barber, L. M.: *Spinal Cord Injury, A Treatment Guide for Occupational Therapists,* pp. 36–73. Charles B. Slack, Thorofare, N.J., 1974.

8

The Prosthetist

Ernest M. Burgess, M.D.
Shirley M. Forsgren

The word "prosthetist" is derived from the Greek *pros* (to) and *thesis* (place). In terms of amputee rehabilitation, the prosthetist replaces that part of the limb that is missing. The ideal prosthesis would replace all of the function of the missing structure.

In the light of present knowledge, this goal is not now attainable. Certain life forms are able to regenerate the missing limb. It is also possible with modern microsurgical techniques to reimplant the amputated part with restoration of some or all of its functional capacity. In practical terms, limb regeneration and even major limb reimplantation lie in the far horizons of biological science and technical skills. The prosthetist then must use inert, non-living materials to "put in place" that which has been lost by amputation.

The first requirement for the prosthetist who would provide an artificial limb is a knowledge of the anatomy and function of the missing part. The more he understands the anatomy and function of that portion of the limb that he is replacing, the more qualified he is to design, fabricate, and fit a substitute device. This area of knowledge is included in the broad term, biomechanics.

The second basic requirement for the prosthetist is a knowledge of the materials used in prosthetics fabrication. The physical characteristics and appearance of the materials that make up the prothesis are critical to its use. This area of knowledge includes materials engineering and biological compatibility.

The third requirement of the prosthetist is fabrication. Having determined what degree of function he can successfully replace and selected the materials and components that will make up the prosthesis, he must then fabricate and assemble the substitute limb and fit it for successful and comfortable operation.[2] He must also be in a position to provide continuing service to assure maximum mechanical performance and wear.

Finally, the prosthetist needs to establish a personal, caring relationship with his patients. The prosthetist is a key and indispensable member of the amputee rehabilitation team. Recent studies indicate that amputees list prosthetic deficiencies as their greatest hurdle to improve function and quality of life.[4] It is natural that this should be so: no artificial substitute can replace what has been lost. Frustrations are often directed toward the prosthesis. The prosthetist's responsibility extends to a communication and support level equal to that of other team members. Competence in these four major areas of knowledge qualifies the prosthetist as a professional health care specialist. Continuing education will keep him abreast of research and new developments in the field.[3]

HISTORY

Survival following untreated limb loss will on occasion occur among all living things whose body form includes the appendages we refer to as extremities, or limbs. Human beings are no exception. The earliest crude records of our ancestors depict members of those ancient social orders with both acquired and congenital amputations. Natural selection and survival of the fittest often condemned primitive human beings to death as a result of inability to move about and cope effectively with the environment. This same fate still befalls most animals who live in their natural setting.

Self-survival undoubtedly prompted early man's ingenuity to acquire some form of substitute for a lost limb. The availability of wood throughout most of the earth makes it a natural material for the construction of limb substitutes. Primitive but ingenious wood crutches and walking sticks permitted the leg amputee a substitute function to some degree by using the arms. These compensating devices are referred to as mobility aids. We have come a long way from these primitive wood crutches to motorized mobility devices that can allow a quadramembral amputee to move about with a minimum of human input. On occasion nothing more is needed to activate them than respiration or head and neck movement.

The Spartans record use of wooden peg legs and feet as early as 400 B.C. and Roman leg substitutes were in use as early as 300 B.C. The Royal College of Surgeons' Museum in London had in its collection a bronze and wood above-knee prosthesis of this era with thigh and calf components shaped to resemble normal anatomy. It was lost when the museum was destroyed by bombing during World War II.

The wooden peg leg is the precursor to modern artificial limbs (Fig. 8-1). It was practical, durable, and could be fabricated by the amputee himself or by artisans. Leather and woven or braided fabrics, such as linen and hemp, increased comfort and efficiency. A variety of functional end-bearing devices were used, mostly of peg configuration. Stability, durability, and ease of maintenance and application generally dictated design. Many of these substitute devices were

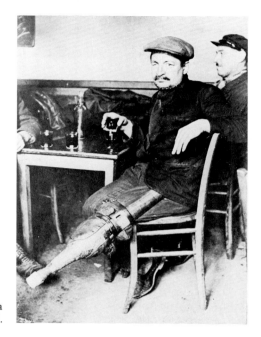

Fig. 8-1. A below-knee amputee wearing a prosthesis commonly used before World War I.

surprisingly functional, especially when the residual limb could be used for end-bearing, as with a knee disarticulation or below-knee amputation fitted in the bent knee position.

During the Middle Ages, metal gradually replaced wood as a prosthetic material. It was natural that metalworkers who made the armor would turn their skills to prosthesis for both upper and lower limbs. Many of these devices were fully articulated and cosmetically quite acceptable, but they were very heavy. Although some function was provided, many of these substitute devices were designed to improve appearance for those amputees able to afford them. These limbs can be seen in museums throughout the world. Some of them demonstrate a remarkable degree of design ingenuity as well as art.

The industrial revolution carried the field of prosthetics into the modern era (Figs. 8-2A–C). Wood, leather, and metal continued to be the materials of choice. The prosthetist-orthotist-orthopedic bootmaker emerged as a highly skilled craftsman. Training was by apprenticeship. Amputees often entered the trade to become the clinical source for their own prosthetic experimentation. Most amputations were the result of trauma, many of them war-incurred. The limb maker and limb fitter held a position of some importance in the military order.

An area of particular historical interest relates to upper limb prostheses. Simple, functional hooklike devices had been used for centuries prior to the Middle Ages. Prostheses resembling a hand were not used in any numbers until the Middle Ages when metal arms and hands with complicated articulations including all of the digits were used. Control of the articulated joints was passive.

Early in the 19th century, functional harnessing for terminal device, upper limb prosthetics appeared in Germany. This use of shoulder girdle harnessing for voluntary hook and hand function revolutionized arm prosthetics.

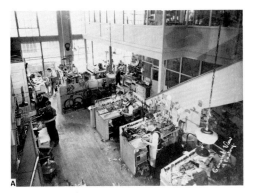
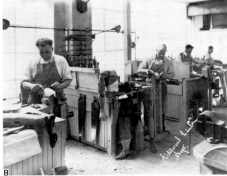
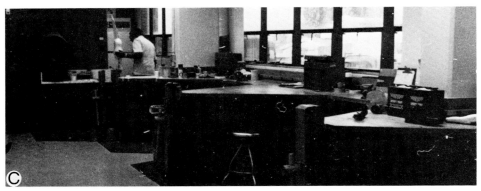

Fig. 8-2. (A) Artificial limb department of a leading San Francisco prosthetics facility, 1930. (B) Skilled handcraftsmanship is demonstrated in this 1930 prosthetics-orthotics factory. (C) A modern prosthetics facility in a Veterans Administration hospital.

Historically, war has been the driving motivation for prosthetic progress. World War I proved to be the turning point not only for the surgery of trauma and infections of the musculoskeletal system, but also for prosthetic development. When the battlefields were stilled, hundreds of thousands of combat casualties with limb loss returned to their homes all over the world from hospitals and prison camps. The empty sleeve and empty pant leg on city streets and in the towns and countryside throughout the world provided the political and humanitarian pressure for modern prosthetics. The prosthetist gradually moved into the ranks of the professional. World War II further ignited a demand for improved limb substitutes that continues today.

Backed by substantial government funding for research and challenged by the complexity of functional restitution in the presence of limb loss, the field of prosthetics is today intermingled with many engineering disciplines, sophisticated surgical techniques, and exciting methods of training and rehabilitation. Whether in the private enterprise sector or as a function of government, the prosthetic profession is hard-pressed to meet demands. Still severely undermanned, it has responded locally, nationally, and worldwide in a commendable manner. As this profession continues to move into the broad, almost boundless, horizon of science and technology, it is important to look back over its history. Great value can be gleaned from a knowledge of those concerned and hardworking artisans of the past.[7]

STATE OF THE FIELD

The field of prosthetics is undergoing rapid transition. As indicated in the section on the history of prosthetics, World War I initiated a major revolutionary change with a profession emerging from what for centuries had been a guild or craft. Amputees coming out of World War II placed further heavy demands on prosthetics and accelerated their position and responsibility as a legitimate and vital segment of professional health care services. Major change is never easy and rarely smooth. This is particularly true when the changes involve traditional, long-standing, established systems. There is no better simple example than the introduction of suction as a means of above-knee prosthetic socket suspension. When a small team of American surgeons and prosthetists returned from Germany at the end of World War II and introduced to the United States the revolutionary idea of suction socket suspension, it was greeted incredulously. The floodgates of change opened. Demands mounted for improved limb substitutes incorporating modern science and technology. The Veterans Administration (VA) deserves the major credit for transformation of the prosthetics field in America at the end of World War II. A VA document published in 1977 recounts the history of these years.[6]

The rapid evolution of prosthetics as a profession continues. Older prosthetists trained entirely by preceptorship continue to work side by side with institutionally trained individuals graduated from universities with bachelor of science degrees in prosthetics. Each respects the other's abilities. Both share knowledge and experience that combine to serve the amputee more effectively.

The urgent need to establish the field of prosthetics as a profession has generated heavy demands for leadership. Prosthetists called upon the experience of other health professionals to assist in directing their course. The American Academy of Orthopaedic Surgeons has been particularly supportive at the organizational level. Its modes of certification, education, research, and patient service assisted in directing this emerging profession along established, proved lines of excellence. The American Orthotics and Prosthetics Association, the American Board for Certification in Orthotics and Prosthetics, the American Academy of Orthotists and Prosthetists, the International Society of Prosthetics and Orthotics, the International Association of Orthotists and Prosthetists, and other organizational activities are filling the need to provide better prosthetists and better substitute limbs. A national and worldwide organizational framework now exists to complete the transition of prosthetics from a craft to a profession.

In caring for amputees, a shortage of qualified prosthetists is perceived by professionals to be the single greatest medical need in the United States and throughout the world. There are at this time only two universities offering baccalaureate degrees and four colleges and universities providing certificate programs in prosthetics and orthotics that are accredited by the American Board of Certification. Only 1242 certified prosthetists were practicing in the United States as of 1980, and there were 1400 certified orthotists. Of these two groups,

804 individuals were certified prosthetists-orthotists.[1] On a professional visit to Zaire a few years ago, the senior author learned that there was but one prosthetist available for a population of approximately 20 million people. The challenge and the opportunities presented by the prosthetic profession should attract young men and women motivated to serve the health care needs of others. As with any vocation, its appeal includes not only a dedication to serve others and the availability of positions but appropriate economic reward. The prosthetist's income should be reasonably commensurate with his responsibilities. Looking back over the recent past, it is evident that prosthetists have been underpaid. This is now being rectified so that those entering the field of prosthetics can expect income and economic security appropriate to their training and importance in the field of health care. Improved methods of limb design and fabrication, cost-effectiveness, and quality control measures will also extend the ability of the prosthetists to provide more service per individual.

SPECIAL QUALIFICATIONS

The prosthetist fabricates, fits, and services limb substitutes. He is primarily a member of the amputee team. This team consists first of the amputee, and then the surgeon, the prosthetist, and other rehabilitation personnel. The number and qualifications of the rehabilitation team members will vary depending upon the individual needs of each amputee. Physical, social, psychological, and medical rehabilitation are all required in varying degrees of importance. If the amputee is to regain any degree of missing function, however, he will need a limb substitute. It is important that all members of the team, including the amputee himself, understand the nature and function of the artificial limb. Unfortunately this is an area in which members of the team other than the prosthetist are insufficiently informed. Most surgeons and rehabilitation workers have never been inside a prosthetics facility. They have no knowledge of the details of mechanical substitute limb fabrication. Some few have attended courses on prosthetic rehabilitation, but most are without a useful working knowledge of the field of prosthetics. The education of surgeons and other health care professionals is proceeding slowly. In particular, physical therapists are to be commended for their educational effort in teaching and understanding prosthetic design and use. Since the prosthesis is by far the most common source of complaint and frustration on the part of the amputee, the prosthetist faces a continuous struggle to overcome the inadequacies of his product, fully realizing that he can never completely succeed. It is often difficult for the prosthetist to keep up with new developments and improvements, yet it is evident that the other team members have to depend largely on the prosthetist to assist in prosthetic prescription and limb critique.

The general practitioner of prosthetics is gradually disappearing. Nevertheless, for some time to come, one person will be able to design, fabricate, and assemble the prosthesis, as well as fit and service it. It is inevitable, however, that responsibility will be divided and that some prosthetists will be involved primarily in research, some in teaching, some in immediate postoperative care[8] and the early phase of prosthetic rehabilitation, and some in the basic areas of limb fabrication and fitting. This specialization is occurring because of the increased complexity of materials and design. It will be delayed by the use of prefabricated units and by the decreasing need for individual craftsmanship. This trend, too, is inevitable if for no other reason than economy. Prosthetists themselves recognize the need to delineate divisions of responsibility. Specialization need not remove the satisfaction of patient contact and of a service well performed. Nonetheless, the role of the general prosthetist will gradually be restricted to smaller facilities. Many larger organizations now have prosthetists specializing in upper limbs, lower limbs, or selected materials or for special patient populations, such as children and old people. The direction is one of gradual specialization rather than fragmentation. In-depth general knowledge of prosthetic principles and patient service is the base upon which specialization in prosthetics can successfully grow. Direct patient contact must continue to be the center of professional action. In the past, many prosthetists were themselves amputees. There is no reason why this should not continue. Limb loss is a unique physical experience. The prosthetist who is himself an amputee certainly has the opportunity to relate his rehabilitation needs to those he serves.

Until 1975 there were only five certified women prosthetists in the United States; by the end of 1980 there were 17. The prosthetics and orthotics profession has all the ingredients to make it attractive to women. Recruiting efforts must specifically include and emphasize the need for women as full participants in the field.

Because prosthetics, like surgery, requires manual skill, a significant degree of technical proficiency is a necessary requirement. The abilities to operate machines skillfully, to construct, and to understand form as it relates to function are all necessary. The prosthetist also needs a knowledge of body form in the

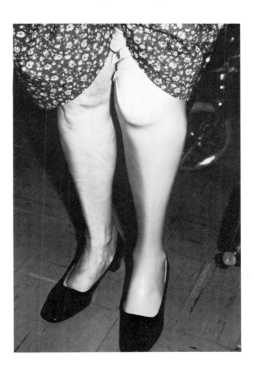

Fig. 8-3. An example of modern prosthetic design. Note the cosmetic features incorporated into lightweight, functionally adaptable materials.

artistic sense as well as in its anatomical make-up. Reproduction of form, referred to as cosmesis, will be appreciated almost as much as function by many amputees. Graceful, symmetrical artificial limbs reflect the sensitivity and character of the prosthetist who fabricates them (Fig. 8-3).

Lastly, the prosthetist often needs to have some knowledge of business management. Most facilities throughout the United States, Canada, and the western world are privately owned and maintained. The business success of prosthetics in the private setting will largely determine its success as a profession. It is neither demeaning nor materialistic to be concerned about the economics of prosthetics. Until recently, prosthetists have been an underpaid segment in our health care services. The rules of the marketplace—in particular, supply and demand—have largely rectified this inequity. This profession cannot be expected to grow with excellence unless compensation for services is commensurate with responsibility.

THE PROSTHETIST AND THE AMPUTEE TEAM

The multidisciplinary nature of amputee rehabilitation is most effective in a team setting. The indispensable individuals on this team are the surgeon, the prosthetist, and the physical therapist. The administrative coordinator (prosthetic representative), nurse, social worker, occupational therapist, psychologist, vocational specialist, and physicians caring for additional health needs are all called on when their advice is required. As a primary team member, the prosthetist's position relative to other team members is one of equality. The director of the amputee team should recognize this relationship (Fig. 8-4A). The team exists for the single purpose of obtaining maximum rehabilitation potential for each amputee coming before it.[5] The dignity and needs of the amputee are best served in a setting of

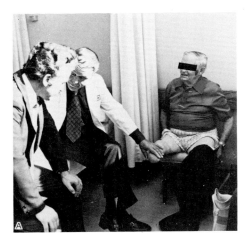 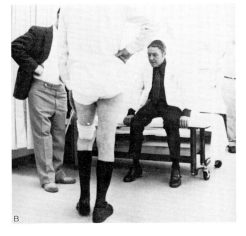

Figs. 8-4A, B. Views of an amputee prosthetic clinic with patient and members of the amputation service team.

quiet team discipline, knowledgeable participation of the several team members, and prompt accomplishment of team directives. When the prosthetist accepts his responsibility in a position of equality as a team member, he can be expected to respond with efficiency and results (Fig. 8-4B).

FUTURE DIRECTIONS

The future course of the prosthetics profession is linked directly to health care needs. The industrialized nations of the world in which modern health care standards prevail already are critically short of prosthetists who can fill present needs. For millions of amputees residing in areas with marginal medical care, few can even hope to obtain modern limb substitutes. Trauma and peripheral vascular disease are presently a major cause for amputations. Congenital limb deficit, neoplasms, and infections unrelated to trauma result in a small but statistically constant number of amputations.

Vascular disease is the greatest health challenge throughout the industrialized world today. Strokes, aneurisms, coronary artery occlusion, hypertension, and ischemia of the extremities are varying clinical manifestations of the occlusive vascular pathology. Degenerative blood vessel changes are the hallmark of a variety of systemic pathological states, such as diabetes and rheumatic fever. The American Diabetes Association reports that 1.2 million new cases of diabetes mellitus were added in the year 1979 to the already known American diabetes population of nearly 9 million persons. A great many individuals with diabetes are undiagnosed.

The number of amputations caused by limb ischemia is increasing and can be expected to continue to increase until medical research directs the way to more effective prophylaxis and therapy. Aging populations add to the problem.

During the last two decades surgeons have developed successful means of mechanical vascular reconstruction. Large numbers of limbs at risk for amputation can be salvaged by skillful and ingenious surgical revascularization. These operations do not influence the underlying pathological process. The functional life expectancy of vascular reconstruction will vary, depending upon many circumstances. Whether of short- or long-term benefit, people are now surviving due to the effectiveness of the surgery, but once again the operated limb is at risk for amputation and, unfortunately, no further reconstruction is available with present techniques. The causes for failure of the reconstruction to maintain continuing limb viability are many. The occlusive disease may have progressed in extent and severity to unreconstructed parts of the vascular tree, further occluding blood flow. Clotting, embolization, aneurism formation, infection, and other complications can occlude or diminish flow through the re-established channels. Some of these patients have actually outlived the life expectancy of the mechanical revascularization.

The second large group of prospective amputees results from trauma and its complications. Here also, refined and improved methods for vascular surgical reconstruction can be expected to salvage many severely traumatized arms and legs. Even with microsurgery, however, and an occasional successful limb reimplantation, most severely damaged and severed limbs will still require prosthetic substitutes. This is the accepted price we pay for mechanization and high-speed transportation.

Patterns of human social behavior remain unpredictable. Weapons capable of unbelievable mass destruction cover the earth. Another major war is not unthinkable. It has been estimated that at the end of World War II there were 50,000 major amputees in what remained of the city of Warsaw, Poland. It is the prayer and hope of all thinking persons that such devastation will not be revisited on mankind.

For some time to come, the demand for prosthetic services will far outstrip supply. This profession can be expected to grow in numbers, in technical competence, in sophistication of replacement devices, and in stature. It must continue to attract qualified, dedicated candidates in increasing numbers. A high level of enlightened leadership will continue to be required. State and international support, particularly in the areas of research and education, will be an increasing necessity. Prosthetics in the private sector can be expected to grow efficiently. Cooperation with other medical and engineering disciplines will increase.

The problems, challenges, and opportunities facing prosthetists are shared in common with many other areas of humanitarian service. Unique to this field is its relative youth as a profession. This circumstance enhances opportunity and makes the problems and obstacles in the way of progress less formidable.

REFERENCES

1. American Orthotics and Prosthetics Association, Alexandria, Virginia: Personal communication, January 2, 1981.
2. Byers, J. L.: X-rays: A ''fitting tool'' for the prosthetist. Orthop. Prosthet. 6(4):55–57. 1974.
3. Foort, J.: Amputee management procedures. In Mastro, B. A., and Mastro, R. T., Eds.: *Selected Reading: A Review of Orthotics and Prosthetics,* pp. 1–11. American Orthotics and Prosthetics Association, Washington, D.C., 1980.
4. Kegel, B., Carpenter, M., and Burgess, E. M.: Functional capabilities of lower extremity amputees. Arch. Phys. Med. Rehabil. 59:109–120, 1978.
5. Kegel, B., Webster, J. C., and Burgess, E. M.: Recreational activities of lower extremity amputees: A survey. Arch. Phys. Med. Rehabil. 61:258–264, 1980.
6. Stewart, R. E., and Bernstock, W. M.: *Veterans Administration Prosthetic and Sensory Aids Program Since World War II.* Prosthetics and Sensory Aids Service, Department of Medicine and Surgery, U.S. Veterans Administration, Washington, D.C., 1977.
7. Wilson, A. B.: Limb prosthetics—1970. Artif. Limbs 14:1–52, 1970.
8. Zettl, J. H.: Immediate postsurgical prosthetic fitting: The role of the prosthetist. J. Am. Phys. Ther. Assoc. 51(2):152–157, 1971.

9

The Orthotist

Maurice D. Schnell, M.D.
John H. Bowker, M.D.
Wilton H. Bunch, M.D., Ph.D.

DEVELOPMENT OF THE PROFESSION OF ORTHOTICS

Orthotics is the allied health profession devoted to the management of musculoskeletal deformities by the application of externally applied force systems known as orthoses (braces). The word "orthotics" is a contraction of the Greek *ortho,* straight, and *statikos,* to cause to stand. The orthotist designs, fits, and services orthoses, which can be made to control, compensate for, or correct a variety of impairments of the movable segments of the musculoskeletal system.

Orthotics has been known since antiquity in the form of splinting for fractures and bracing of spinal deformities, rachitic limbs, and diseased joints. Beginning with armor makers, brace-making became an art passed from one generation to the next by the apprenticeship system. In the nineteenth century, when surgical correction of skeletal deformities was rarely attempted, it was common for an orthopedist to employ a bracemaker in his office. In contrast, most modern orthotists work in private facilities but a significant number are hospital-based.

The modern orthotist is a highly qualified professional who has completed stringent courses at one of several university-affiliated orthotic programs followed by written, oral, and fabrication examinations designed to assess competence in this increasingly complex field. These examinations are administered by the American Board for Certification in Orthotics and Prosthetics, Inc., established in 1948 through the combined efforts of the orthotics/prosthetics industry and the

American Academy of Orthopaedic Surgeons. As the field of orthotics becomes more demanding, Associates of Arts and Baccalaureate programs in orthotics are being more widely offered.

Ideally, the orthotist works closely with the physician and physical therapist or occupational therapist in the formulation of the prescriptions as well as the functional evaluation of the completed orthosis. In the case of hand therapists, mostly drawn from the ranks of occupational therapy, there may be an overlap of function with the orthotist, in that the hand therapist often makes special hand orthoses from easily formed thermoplastic materials.

INDICATIONS FOR THE USE OF ORTHOSES

Many orthopedic surgeons view an orthosis as a device to be used as a last resort when a surgical procedure does not seem feasible. Actually, orthotics and surgery are not the polar extremes of orthopedic care: indeed, they are closely allied. When combined in a total treatment program, the blend can frequently provide better results than either one alone.

For example, use of an orthosis after repair of a major knee ligament disruption can provide mediolateral stability while quadriceps/hamstring strength and joint range of motion are improving. This support, used during collagen maturation, may lead to an improvement in late joint stability. The hemiplegic patient with equinovarus present in the stance as well as swing phases of the gait cycle may often be helped by a combined operative–orthotic approach. This foot deformity is often caused by a spastic/contracted triceps surae and spastic anterior tibial muscle. A split anterior tibial tendon transfer and Hoke percutaneous heel cord lengthening will make the postoperative use of an ankle-foot orthosis (AFO) much more efficient and comfortable.[12,19] These and other examples are listed in Table 9-1. The ingenious orthopedist can and will discover many more combined surgical/orthotic approaches to enhance patient management.

HOW ORTHOSES FUNCTION

Orthoses function in one of three basic ways, as emphasized by Bunch and Keagy in their concise text on orthotic treatment.[1]

The first is the control of movable segments of the musculoskeletal system. Control may be necessary for a variety of reasons. For example, patients with late instability of the knee joint not suitable to reconstruction may prefer a knee-ankle orthosis (KAO) for prevention of abnormal stance phase motion rather than a knee fusion, which is awkward when sitting. When pain is felt in a major joint of the lower limb during weight-bearing, but not during range of motion, it may be ameliorated by an orthosis that transfers body weight to a more proximal normal joint or to the pelvis.[2,8,22] An example of an orthosis for a painful arthritic ankle would be one with a prosthetic type patellar-tendon-bearing (PTB) top and a solid ankle–cushion heel (SACH) lower portion. Patients with joint pain at the extremes of the normal range of motion, but not during weight-bearing per se, may often be relieved by an orthosis limiting motion to the pain-free arc.

Table 9-1. Common Combined Surgical-Orthotic Treatment Approaches

SURGERY	ORTHOTICS
LOWER LIMB	
Split anterior tibial tendon transfer for equinovarus gait in hemiplegics.	Postoperative thermoplastic ankle-foot orthosis to maintain functional position of foot during gait and prevent recurrence of deformity.
Repair of major knee ligament disruption.	Postoperative knee-ankle orthosis or knee orthosis to provide mediolateral stability while quadriceps/hamstring strength and range of motion improve.
Open reduction and internal fixation of femoral fractures with residual rotational instability.	Postoperative supplementation of internal fixation with hip-knee-ankle orthosis until fracture heals.
Release of hip, ankle, and foot contractures in children with progressive muscular dystrophy.	Knee-ankle-foot orthosis to stabilize joints for walking and prevent recurrent deformity.
UPPER LIMB	
Moberg transfer of brachioradialis into extensor carpi radialis brevis with flexor pollicis longus tenodesis for quadriplegia.	Flexible C-bar to hold thumb in abduction during postoperative phase or permanently.
Transfer of spastic wrist flexors to wrist extensors with Z-lengthening of finger flexors.	For the hemiplegic hand with flexed wrist and fingers, a preoperative, orthokinetic cock-up splint.
Split-thickness skin grafting to areas of full thickness skin loss in the burned hand.	Static positioning of hand with wrist extended, fingers flexed at MP joints and extended at IP joints and thumb abducted, beginning immediately post-burn and continuing throughout grafting and mobilization phases.
Release of thumb adduction contracture.	Postoperative orthotic management consisting of C-bar or dynamic thumb abductor attached to volar wrist-hand orthosis.
SPINE	
Cervical spine fusion for instability secondary to trauma or disease.	Halo-jacket pre- and/or postoperatively to enhance stability and protect spinal cord until fusion occurs.
Stabilization of thoracolumbar spine fractures with Harrington rods and fusion.	Thoracolumbosacral orthosis (bivalved thermoplastic jacket) to reduce motion in all planes.

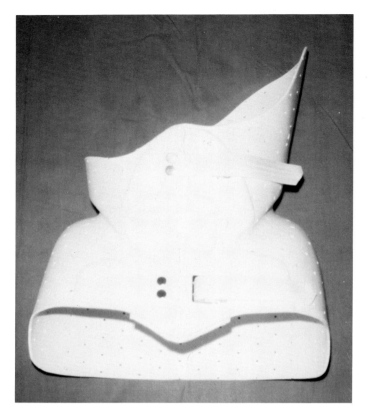

Fig. 9-1. Polypropylene Boston orthosis for scoliosis.

A second type of orthosis is designed to compensate for absent function, usually partial or complete paralysis of key antigravity muscles. With the decline in poliomyelitis in this country, the most commonly prescribed compensatory orthoses are for patients sustaining equinovarus from stroke, paralysis at the first lumbar level or below in spinal cord injury or spina bifida, or muscular dystrophy. In these situations, loss of antigravity function is compensated for in the orthosis by combinations of joints with limited arcs of motion, joints that lock, and joints with purposely designed antigravity assists, such as springs.

Orthoses designed for correction of limb or spinal deformities have important but circumscribed indications. Reduction of joint contracture may be accomplished wholly or partially by use of orthoses with dial lock joints or turnbuckles. The other major classification of corrective orthoses depends on the plasticity of the growing skeleton. Examples are the Boston (Fig. 9-1) or Milwaukee (Fig. 9-2) scoliosis orthoses, which are only effective in producing correction of lateral spinal curvature if sufficient skeletal growth remains.

PRESCRIBING AN ORTHOSIS

The foundation of a sound orthotic prescription is an accurate determination of the patient's functional impairment. The exact medical diagnosis is of somewhat less importance since a number of conditions may produce the same loss of function. It

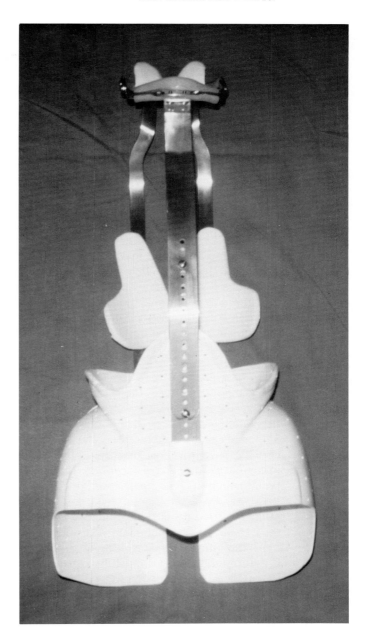

Fig. 9-2. Milwaukee brace with a thermoplastic molded girdle and metal superstructure.

is useful, however, to know if the disease is evolving, static, or resolving in order to attain proper orthotic management.

To determine functional impairment of the lower limb, gait analysis is essential.[2,10,12,17,19] For proper gait observation, the patient should wear a minimal amount of clothing and be viewed from the side, front, and rear during several complete gait cycles. Attention should be directed serially to each limb segment beginning at either the foot or the pelvis and progressing proximally or distally, respectively. Evidence of flaccid or spastic paralysis and major joint malalignments or contractures becomes readily apparent when gait is observed in this organized manner. It is important to examine for limb spasticity in supine and sitting positions, as well as standing, since it may be quite different in each due to postural reflexes. Joint range of motion, both active and passive, as well as joint stability are determined. Any pain elicited during the examination must be noted, because it is often the patient's chief complaint and may be correctable orthotically. The services of a physical therapist are highly recommended in the pre-orthotic assessment of lower limb problems. In devising an orthosis for upper limb impairment, a careful analysis of the patient's function and needs in such daily activities as feeding, grooming, hygiene, and dressing will lead to prescription of a more useful and acceptable device.[11,12,18] An occupational therapist can be of great assistance in making this assessment.

After carefully determining the functional impairment, the next step in prescription of an orthosis is the complete description of a device that will substantially reduce the impairment. Until very recently, there was no standardized, easily comprehensible method of writing an orthotic prescription. Prior to that time, many orthoses were known by the name of their inventor, yet significant variations resulted in no eponymic change. To provide a standardized vocabulary and improve communication between the two professions, in 1971 the American Academy of Orthopaedic Surgeons, the American Orthotics and Prosthetics Association, and the Committee on Prosthetic Research and Development of the National Research Council devised a nomenclature that has since been accepted internationally.

There are two basic concepts regarding description of an orthosis inherent in the new nomenclature. First, the orthosis is named by the joints or body segments that it crosses or encompasses. Thus, a lower limb orthosis with controls at the hip, knee, and ankle is called a hip-knee-ankle orthosis (HKAO). If it crosses the ankle only, it is an ankle-foot orthosis (AFO). Similarly, an orthosis controlling the cervical spine by engaging the chin, occiput, and thorax is a cervico-thoracic orthosis (CTO). The description is then secondarily developed by adding the type(s) of control, compensation, or correction to be applied to the body segments involved. For example, an ankle joint may be left free, stopped at 90 degrees or fitted in 5-degree dorsiflexion, each for specific indications determined during the evaluation of functional impairment.

All that remains is consideration of the exact form the orthosis should take. This is determined by the availability of the specific materials, the particular skills of the orthotist, and the vocational, social, and psychological needs of the patient. At times, if financially feasible, the patient may benefit from two orthoses with similar functions, but of different materials. An example would be a rugged steel double-upright ankle-foot orthosis (AFO) for heavy work and a lightweight, molded thermoplastic AFO for social occasions. It is therefore strongly recommended that the orthotist assist in determining the exact orthotic design necessary and evaluating the functional value of the completed orthosis.

Standard forms for prescription of lower limb, upper limb, and spinal orthoses have been developed. When completed as designed, the orthotist will have a summary of the functional disability, the treatment objectives, and the orthotic recommendation from which to begin measurement, fabrication, and fitting. Three common orthotic prescriptions using the new forms are shown in Figures 9-3–9-5.

Text continues on p. 112

Summary of Functional Disability <u>Loss of active wrist and finger extension. Radial nerve injury associated</u>

<u>with humeral shaft fracture.</u>

Treatment Objectives: Prevent/Correct Deformity ☒   Improve Function ☒
                       Relieve Pain ☐   Other _____

ORTHOTIC RECOMMENDATION

UPPER LIMB			FLEX	EXT	ABD	ADD	ROTATION Int.	ROTATION Ext.	AXIAL LOAD
SEWHO	Shoulder								
EWHO	*Humerus*								
	Elbow								
	Forearm						(Pron.)	(Sup.)	
WHO	Wrist		S	30° S	(RD) H	(UD) H			
HO	Hand								
Fingers 2-5		MP	F	A					
		PIP	F	F					
		DIP	F	F					
Thumb		CM	F	A	F	F	F	(Opposition) F	
		MP	F	A	F	F	F	F	
		IP	F	F					

REMARKS: Basic long opponens orthosis with rubber band extension assists to proximal phalanges from dorsal outrigger.

Signature   Date

KEY: Use the following symbols to indicate desired control of designated function:

F = FREE   — *Free* motion.
A = ASSIST   — Application of an external force for the purpose of increasing the range, velocity, or force of a motion.
R = RESIST   — Application of an external force for the purpose of decreasing the velocity or force of a motion.
S = STOP   — Inclusion of a static unit to deter an undesired motion in one direction.
v = Variable — A unit that can be adjusted without making a structural change.
H = HOLD   — Elimination of all motion in prescribed plane (verify position).
L = LOCK   — Device includes an optional lock.

Fig. 9-3. Upper limb prescription form for a wrist-hand orthosis (WHO). The form includes a summary of the patient's functional disability, treatment objectives, and orthotic recommendations.

Summary of Functional Disability: ___Fracture-dislocation T-10 - T-11, post-operative___

___Harrington rod fixation. Complete paraplegia T-11.___

Treatment Objectives:

Spinal Alignment ☐   Motion Control ☒
Axial Unloading ☐   Other _____

ORTHOTIC RECOMMENDATION

SPINE		FLEX	EXT	LATERAL FLEXION		ROTATION		AXIAL LOAD
				R	L	R	L	
CTLSO	Cervical							
(TLSO)	Thoracic	R		R	R	R	R	
LSO	Lumbar							
	(Lumbo sacral							
SIO	Sacroiliac	▓▓▓	▓▓▓	▓▓▓	▓▓▓	▓▓▓	▓▓▓	

REMARKS: Plastic body jacket, anterior and posterior halves joined by Velcro straps.

KEY: Use the following symbols to indicate desired control of designated function:

F = FREE   – Free motion
A = ASSIST   – Application of an external force for the purpose of increasing the range, velocity, or force of a motion.
R = RESIST   – Application of an external force for the purpose of decreasing the velocity or force of a motion.
S = STOP   – Inclusion of a static unit to deter an undesired motion in one direction.
v = Variable – A unit that can be adjusted without making a structural change.
H = HOLD   – Elimination of all motion in prescribed plane: specify position, e.g. in degrees or (+) (–).
L = LOCK   – Device includes an optional lock.

Fig. 9-4. Prescription form for ordering a thoracolumbosacral orthosis (TLSO). Indicated orthosis would resist those motions marked; others are left blank.

Summary of Functional Disability __Loss of toe clearance during swing phase of gait, secondary to drop foot__

__from anterior compartment syndrome. No heel cord tightness or peroneal muscle weakness.__

Treatment Objectives:

Prevent/Correct Deformity ☒	Improve Ambulation ☒
Reduce Axial Load ☐	Fracture Treatment ☐
Protect Joint ☐	Other_____

ORTHOTIC RECOMMENDATION

LOWER LIMB			FLEX	EXT	ABD	ADD	ROTATION Int.	ROTATION Ext.	AXIAL LOAD
HKAO	Hip								
KAO	Thigh								
	Knee								
(AFO)	Leg								
	Ankle		(Dorsi) F	(Plantar) 90° S					
		Subtalar					(Inver.) H.	(Ever.) H.	
FO Foot	Midtarsal	H.	H.						
		Met.-phal.	F	F	F	F			

REMARKS: Polypropylene with Velcro closure.

Signature   Date

KEY: Use the following symbols to indicate desired control of designated function:

F = FREE — *Free* motion.

A = ASSIST — Application of an external force for the purpose of increasing the range, velocity, or force of a motion.

R = RESIST — Application of an external force for the purpose of decreasing the velocity or force of a motion.

S = STOP — Inclusion of a static unit to deter an undesired motion in one direction.

v = Variable — A unit that can be adjusted without making a structural change.

H = HOLD — Elimination of all motion in prescribed plane (verify position).

L = LOCK — Device includes an optional lock.

Fig. 9-5. Completed prescription form for a polypropylene ankle-foot orthosis (AFO) to correct a drop foot deformity.

Once understood, they are the simplest and clearest prescriptions that a physician can write. In each chart, the gray boxes represent motions not present or potentially present in that segment or joint. The white boxes represent motions that may need orthotic control, compensation, or correction. It is completed by merely circling the abbreviation for the appropriate orthosis (e.g., KAO) and indicating the desired functional joint controls, as shown in the key.

The Cervical Spine

Cervical spine orthoses are all designed to provide stability and immobilization. Their contribution to increased function of the patient is better placement of the head or reduction of pain by restricting neck motion. The choice of a cervical orthosis is determined by the degree and extent of immobilization desired.

Studies of neck motion with a cervical orthosis are in general agreement regarding immobilization efficacy.[3,6,7] However, these studies suffer from the limitation of using healthy subjects tested in the upright position. It is probable, therefore, that orthotic control might be decreased with changes of position, abnormalities of spinal stability and alignment, spasticity, or weakness of cervical muscles.

Soft cervical collars limit about 25 percent of the flexion-extension motion of the lower cervical vertebrae, yet they fail to restrict rotation. Rigid or semi-rigid collars (Fig. 9-6) limit both motions 40–50 percent more.[6,7] Since these devices

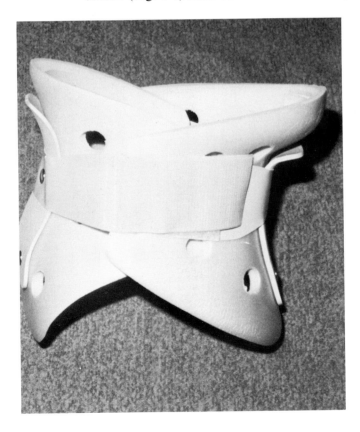

Fig. 9-6. Polyethylene foam (Plastazote) cervical collar.

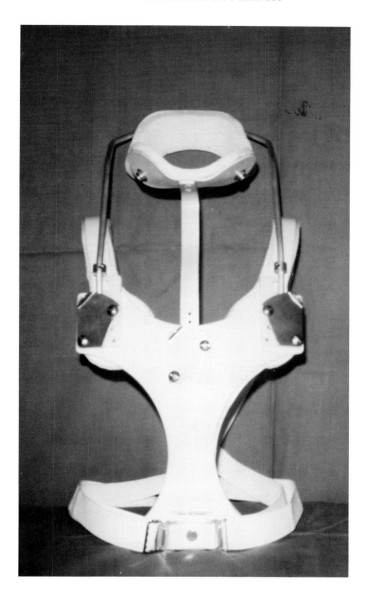

Fig. 9-7. Prefabricated cervicothoracic
orthosis (SOMI brace).

provide minimal support, their role in rehabilitation is to assist in head control
where some strength is present or where a reduction in motion will give pain relief.
Examples would be the arthritis patient with pain at the extremes of motion or the
patient with a neuropathy or myopathy who has marginal neck control.

The various forms of cervicothoracic orthoses (Fig. 9-7) provide considerably better immobilization. Up to the C3 vertebrae level, this group controls
about 90 percent of the flexion-extension and only slightly less rotation.[6] As such,
except in circumstances of highly unstable fractures and/or dislocations, they may
be used with confidence for postoperative and post-traumatic stability in the lower
cervical spine. This degree of immobilization is seldom needed for pain relief.

Immobilization of C1 and C2 deserves special consideration. No orthosis of conventional design is effective. A halo cast is the only device providing immobilization above C3 and is the orthosis of choice for control of markedly unstable fractures/dislocations of the cervical spine. The halo cast may also be attached to a plastic vest (Figs. 9-8A and 9-8B) when a slight amount of motion is acceptable.

The Thoracic and Lumbar Spine

There is virtually no place for any of the multitude of conventional thoracolumbar orthoses in rehabilitation. Most of these have areas of high pressure that cannot be tolerated by anesthetic skin or the immobile patient. Nearly all of them severely limit upper limb placement. To make matters worse, they often fail to provide effective immobilization.

Effective control of thoracolumbar motion is available with the molded plastic bivalved body jacket. This orthosis provides total contact, which permits excellent force application as well as acceptable soft tissue pressure. The foam padding allows for adjustments in size or contour and provides volumetric control. Skin inspection is possible by removing first one half of the jacket and then the other. The patient may be upright in the jacket even after extensive surgery.

Very rarely is an orthosis indicated in the management of low-back pain.[1,14] When one is used in this manner, it provides little more than relative immobility and acts as a reminder to avoid certain positions during physical activities. With the aid of an adequate exercise program, the patient should rapidly progress beyond an orthosis.

The Lower Limb

The Hip. Orthoses for hip disease are commonly used in pediatric orthopedics but only rarely in rehabilitation. When they are indicated it is either for directional control or weight relief.

Directional control orthoses are nonstandard and custom-designed. They have occasional use in patients with unstable total hip replacements or similar problems.

Weight relief is a more common indication for a hip orthosis. With ischial bearing, it is possible to relieve a portion of the force across the hip joint.[8] Orthoses used for this purpose should be as light as possible so as to avoid increasing the hip's force during the swing phase. The lightest orthosis that will relieve the force across the hip joint remains a cane used in the opposite hand.

The Lower Limb

The Knee. In contrast to the hip, there are many indications for orthotic management of the knee: weight relief, mediolateral stability, anterolateral stability, motion control, and combinations of weight relief and stability.

Weight relief may be accomplished by loading the soft tissues of the thigh with a large total contact device. This is most useful for arthritis patients of any type who experience pain during stance phase.

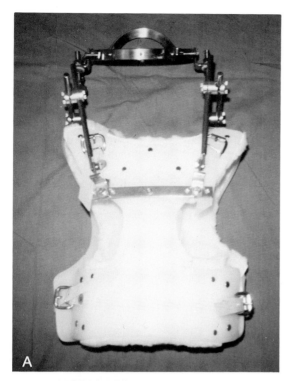

Fig. 9-8A. Front view of a halo-vest orthosis.

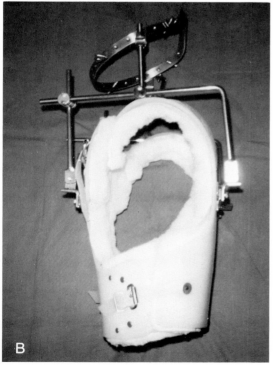

Fig. 9-8B. Side view of a halo-vest orthosis.

The control of mediolateral stability is necessary in treating many forms of disease and trauma. It is usually required for rehabilitation of ligamentous injuries and for "salvage" of loose total knee replacement units, and it should be strongly considered as a part of the postoperative phase of the total joint replacement. When used this way, the implant is protected from high stresses and loosening while muscle strength and range of motion are regained.

Mediolateral stability is easily accomplished by the rigidity of the hinges in a standard knee-ankle orthosis (Fig. 9-9). Some of the newer devices such as knee orthoses provide somewhat less mediolateral stability without the need of the foot-piece or shoe attachment. Obviously, suspension is the major problem here, and exact measurements in casting are required.

Anteroposterior stability is determined by the placement of the knee-hinge axes. If these are offset posteriorly, the weight line is quickly shifted anteriorly at heel-strike. When the center of gravity passes anterior to the axis of the knee, it

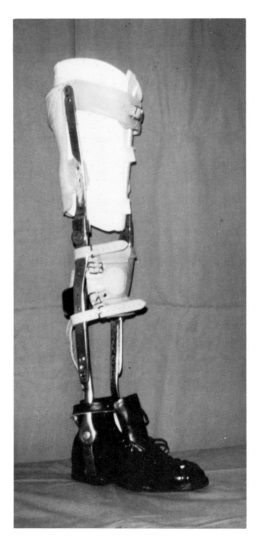

Fig. 9-9. Knee-ankle-foot orthosis with a nonstandard thermoplastic thigh component to protect burn scars of the skin.

becomes stable. Weakness of the quadriceps from any cause is an indication for assisting knee extension with offset knee hinges.

Knee extension can also be aided by an ankle-foot orthosis of the "floor-reaction" type.[1,22] In this kind of orthosis the ankle is rigidly set in a few degrees of equinus so that at foot flat, the force of the rigid ankle is transmitted to the anterior leg, pushing the tibia posteriorly. This type of extension assist is most valuable in upper motor neuron lesions in which voluntary control of the limb is limited or absent.

Genu recurvatum in patients with upper motor neuron damage is often caused by equinus deformity of the ankle and foot due to Achilles tendon contracture, or more frequently, spasticity of the calf muscles. If the spasticity is relatively mild, control of the knee can be influenced by the type of orthotic control provided at the ankle. A flexion moment at the knee created by stabilizing the ankle in 10–15 degrees of dorsiflexion tends to reduce the degree of hyperextension of the knee during stance phase. This may be accomplished by prescribing a polypropylene ankle-foot orthosis fabricated with sufficient fixed dorsiflexion of the foot, or applying a double upright ankle-foot orthosis with a bichannel adjustable ankle mechanism.[2,10,12] Should the equinus deformity be associated with heel cord contracture or severe calf muscle spasticity, it may be necessary to correct the deformity by careful lengthening of the heel cord combined with lengthening of the toe flexors to prevent postoperative curling of the toes.[2,10,12,19]

An orthosis may control motion as a means of reducing contractures. Orthotic correction of flexion contracture of the knee is slow and usually inadequate. Casts, preceded by surgical releases if necessary, make a better correction; the orthotic device can be employed to maintain the correction (Figs. 9-10A and 9-10B).

The Ankle. Orthotic applications about the ankle, as at the knee, may relieve weight, provide stability, and supply power for toe pick-up. The greatest advances have been in ankle immobilization (Fig. 9-11). The solid-ankle, molded, posterior leaf orthoses do a reasonably good job of controlling ankle and subtalar motion and, when combined with a solid-ankle cushion heel (SACH) and rocker sole modifications of footwear, can provide very comfortable ambulation for arthritic and post-traumatic conditions.

In cases of this type—in which weight relief is helpful—the ankle can be partially unloaded by utilizing a total contact device (Fig. 9-12) similar to the proximal part of the patellar tendon-bearing prosthesis. This permits some of the weight to be transmitted to the shoe, thereby bypassing the ankle.[8]

Articulated ankle orthoses serve two functions. They may be used to provide mediolateral stability while maintaining range of motion, or they may be used as a means of providing dorsiflexion assistance, as in one-direction, spring-loaded ankle joints. Plantar flexion assistance in the late stance phase to substitute for the triceps surae is easily achieved merely by limiting dorsiflexion.

The conflicting needs for stability versus motion at the ankle in an ambulating paraplegic have been the source of some debate. In the past, orthoses for paraplegics usually were prescribed with ankle components having unlimited motion or a posterior 90-degree stop with free dorsiflexion. Ankle motion was considered necessary for donning and doffing the orthoses, negotiating stairs, and rising from a sitting position. However, during the last two decades, clinicians have learned that improved standing balance and reduced energy consumption can result from

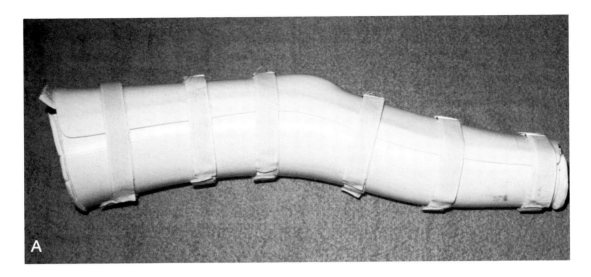

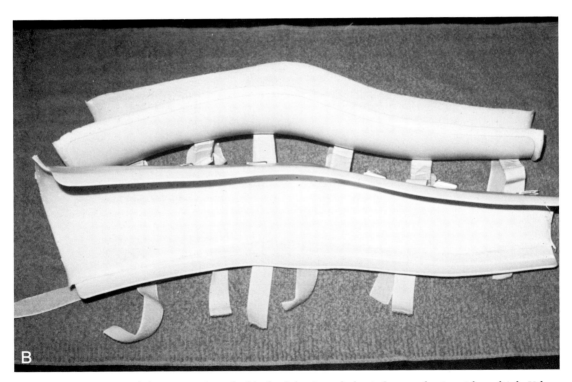

Fig. 9-10. (A) Exterior view of a bivalved, laminated plastic knee orthosis, with multiple Velcro straps for closure. (B) Interior view of bivalved plastic knee orthosis demonstrating a complete Plastazote lining.

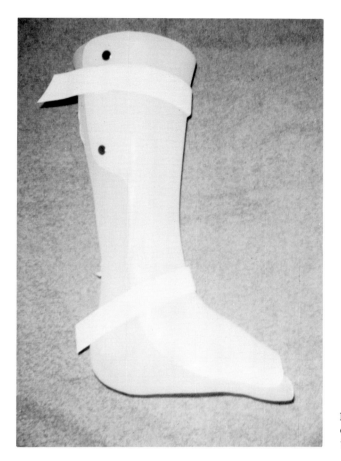

Fig. 9-11. A rigid, thermoplastic ankle-foot orthosis designed to restrict all motion of the ankle and the major part of the foot.

conversion to a dual-channel, adjustable ankle joint locked in 5–10 degrees of dorsiflexion combined with a rigid steel plate for the sole extending to the metatarsal head area.[8,9] This modification of ankle function has no detrimental effect on donning and doffing the orthoses or on transfer activities. Moreover, adjustment of the two channel stops allows quite precise control of orthotic alignment, thus improving the device's efficacy during standing and walking.

The Foot. Although the foot is highly integrated biomechanically with the proximal segments of the lower limb, numerous clinical problems pertaining to it must be solved independently. The application of an appropriate orthotic system will affect the foot primarily and the remainder of the lower limb secondarily. Success of the foot device, however, may enhance the overall functional capabilities of the lower limb.

The integrity of the skin, especially the plantar surface, is mandatory for optimal function of the foot. Individuals with peripheral neuropathy complicated by rigidity or deformity of the foot are very vulnerable to the development of trophic ulcers. Should these lesions become compounded by infection, restoration of the involved foot may be seriously jeopardized. Management of patients should

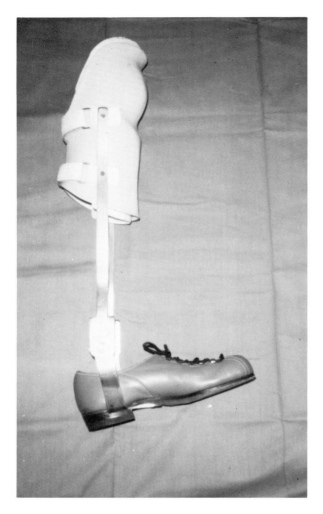

Fig. 9-12. Multipurpose ankle-foot orthosis with the capacity of controlling genu recurvatum, unloading the ankle partially, and providing mediolateral stability to the ankle joint.

include diagnostic evaluation, implementation of proper systemic care (e.g., diabetic control, removal of toxic substances, elimination of factors adversely influencing peripheral vascular problems, antibiotic therapy for control of infection), and vigorous treatment of the local soft-tissue lesion.

The initial goal in treating such ulcers should be the attainment of a clean, granulating wound base.[24] This is best achieved by a combination of techniques such as Betadine soaks, whirlpool baths, applications of effective topical agents, systemic antibiotics, and local debridement. Once satisfactory wound control is achieved, the application of a total contact short-leg cast (Fig. 9-13) aids in the elimination of significant barriers to wound healing, while allowing walking with or without external support.

The efficacy of this type of cast has been clearly demonstrated in the treatment of trophic ulcers in leprosy and diabetes mellitus.[15,21,23,24] It is thought to work by providing an effective means of controlling the limb edema that obstructs

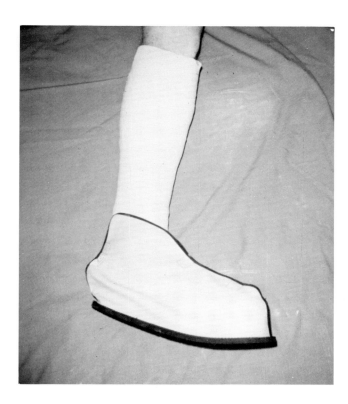

Fig. 9-13. Total-contact short leg cast applied over a healing trophic ulcer. Patient is allowed to walk as tolerated in 48 hours with the foot portion of the cast protected by a cast boot.

the diffusion of oxygen from the capillary loop to the cellular components involved in wound repair. In addition, the cast protects against further wound trauma and applies a compression force to the wound that reduces hypertrophic scar formation and probably improves the alignment of collagen fibers.

Following wound closure, the plaster cast is discontinued and the foot is immediately protected with properly designed footwear. The complexity of the system may vary from the simple selection of a structurally sound shoe (Fig. 9-14) with a proper accommodation to the shape of the patient's foot to the fabrication of a totally customized shoe with possible incorporation of a plastic ankle-foot orthosis (Fig. 9-15).

With any footwear system, the following objectives should be kept in mind: satisfactory contact of the shoe upper with the surface of the foot that is not bearing weight to create control of the foot without evidence of skin pressure (redness) over bony prominences; equalization of compression forces over all segments of the weight-bearing surface throughout the stance phase of gait; maintenance of a heel-toe gait pattern through shoe design or modification; and substitution of loss of joint motion by specific shoe modifications.

Successful achievement of the first objective is aided by selection of shoes with combination lasts, firm heel counters, low heels, and moderately thick leather or composition soles with a sturdy welt, a strong shank, and a high toe box or extra depth configuration. Shoes with a surgical opening (laced to the toe) facilitate donning of the footwear when marked joint rigidity or fixed structural

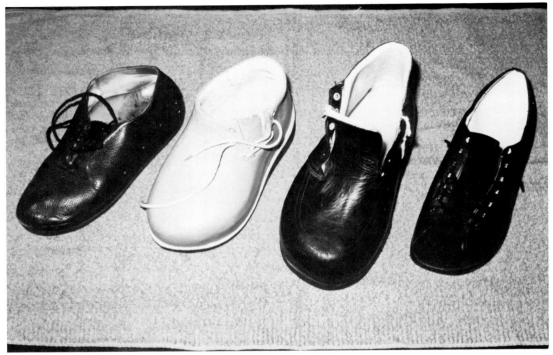

Fig. 9-14. Specific types of footwear for deformed and/or denervated feet. Left to right, custom-molded "space" shoe, custom-made Plastazote oxford with side lacing, custom-made Plastazote low boot, and extra-depth oxford with removable 0.938-cm inlay.

deformity is present. A removable depth inlay of .938–1.25 cm allows insertion of an interior shoe device without compromising the shoe fit.

Equalization of compression forces over the plantar surface of the foot may be maximized in several ways. A .938–1.25 cm sheet of Plastazote, a closed-cell polyethylene foam, can be heated to 140°F and molded against the plantar surface of the foot in a weight-bearing position.[20] The material cools in 3 minutes and retains its new shape. The plastic is cut to fit the interior of the shoe and is shaped by an emery wheel to reduce the thickness of the insert in areas where alterations of foot conformation require the relief of skin pressure and discomfort. Effectiveness of this total contact insert is gradually lost, due to the propensity of Plastazote to creep and compress under constant loads. Thus it loses its resiliency and unequal pressures will occur in localized areas of the foot. This characteristic necessitates periodic replacement of the Plastazote insert, the frequency depending on the body weight and level of activity of the patient. In some instances, backing the Plastazote with other materials will retard its "bottoming out." Latex, cork, acrylic, polypropylene, neoprene, Spenco, Pelite, and firmer grades of Plastazote have been used for this purpose. Spenco may also be used as a skin shear-reducing material on top of a Plastazote insole.

In patients with metatarsalgia, minor forefoot deformities secondary to rheumatoid arthritis, callosities under metatarsal heads, hammer toes, claw toes with prominent metatarsal heads, and similar conditions, the use of Plastazote foot

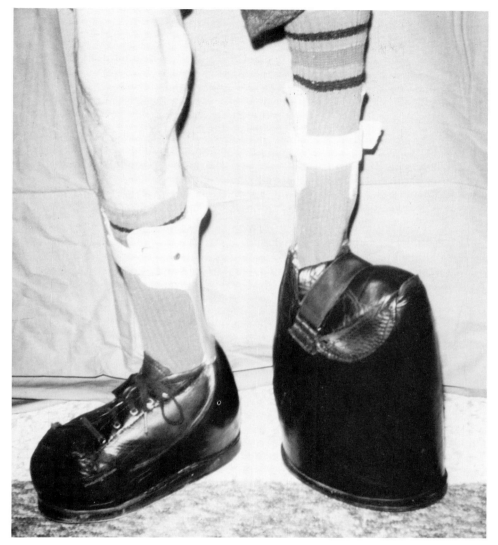

Fig. 9-15. Myelodysplastic patient fitted with custom-made footwear incorporating polypropylene ankle-foot orthoses.

inserts alone may be sufficient. In other patients, skin pressure and discomfort of the forefoot may be relieved only if further shoe modifications are undertaken. Metatarsal bars or metatarsal pads have long been used to transfer weight proximal to the metatarsal heads. To be efficacious the bar should be applied to a sole with enough flexibility to allow, as with a metatarsal pad, proximal weight transfer. The bar should also be .625–.938 cm higher than the proximal portion of the sole of the shoe and broad enough to provide a stable weight-bearing surface during mid-stance.

The rocker sole system is very effective in reducing painful motion at the metatarsophalangeal joints, as is found in hallux rigidus. The apex of the rocker must be located well proximal to the metatarsal heads and provide a satisfactory area for weight-bearing in mid-stance. The rake of the sole should be acute from the apex of the rocker to the toe of the shoe, allowing rapid dissipation of the compression loads applied to the forefoot from heel-off through toe-off. Usually the combination of Plastazote inserts and rocker soles will relieve most foot pressure and discomfort in the metatarsal and toe areas.

Historically, longitudinal arch strain has been managed quite successfully with classical arch supports constructed of a variety of materials. Frequently this condition is associated with problems in other areas of the foot. In this situation a full-foot Plastazote insert may be built up in the arch region by cementing together several layers of Plastazote and adjusting the arch height to conform to the longitudinal arch in the standing position.

Heel pain secondary to inflammation at the insertion of the Achilles tendon or at the origin of the flexor digitorum brevis on the anterior surface of the os calcis, pain associated with degenerative arthritis of the subtalar joint, or mild posterior tibial tendinitis are substantially relieved by a 1.25-cm Plastazote heel and arch device ending just proximal to the metatarsal heads. In order to relieve the compression loads applied to the heel in early stance phase, a SACH heel or 1.25-cm piece of neoprene may be inserted to take up the load at heel-strike. The combination of the SACH wedge heel with the interior Plastazote heel pad will alleviate considerable pain in the majority of hindfoot problems.

The Upper Limb

The Shoulder. The most common orthosis for the shoulder is a sling. It is useful in providing temporary support to an injured or paralyzed limb, but the limb is held in adduction and internal rotation which in turn may lead to shoulder tightness, particularly if spasticity is present. Daily range of motion activities in the absence of a fracture must be carried out to avoid joint stiffness.

Functional orthoses for shoulder abduction and flexion are nearly nonexistent.[18] Balanced forearm orthoses and spring-suspended arm slings that attach to a wheelchair have occasional application in aiding hand placement. They often are not very well accepted by patients because of problems in adjusting equipment, passage through doorways, and cosmesis. Static abduction orthoses of the shoulder are generally inferior to plaster casts.

The Elbow. Elbow orthoses are designed to meet one or more of three criteria: correction of deformity, joint stability, and motion control.

Corrective elbow orthoses may be subdivided further into static and dynamic systems. It must be understood that any static correction orthosis works by the application of an inelastic force. The soft tissues about the joint react to this applied force by an immediate elastic response, which is followed by a time-related plastic response due to the viscoelastic properties of the soft tissues. Any force system applied to a tight joint should be fitted to the point of producing a firm, stretching sensation, not pain. As the joint gradually loosens, the orthosis is adjusted again to the same end-point. Thus, through a series of corrective casts or repetitive adjustments of a static orthosis,[18] deformity of the elbow can be gently corrected without incurring intra-articular damage or periarticular ectopic

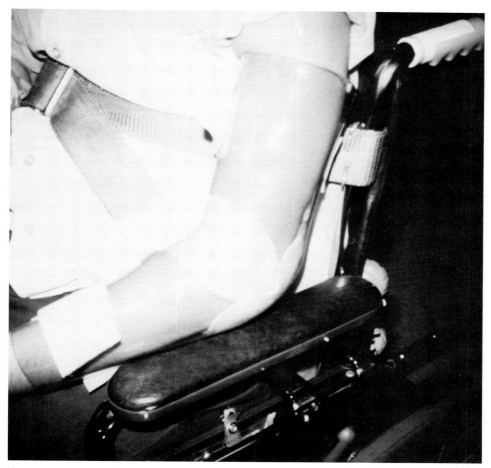

Fig. 9-16. A static elbow orthosis of molded plastic used to maintain correction of a flexion contracture. It has a medial opening with Velcro closures and a polyethylene foam pad to relieve pressure over the olecranon.

ossification. Once maximum correction has been achieved, the static orthosis (Fig. 9-16) may be used on a part-time basis to aid in the maintenance of joint correction. Both joint correction and maintenance of correction are best attained in conjunction with a vigorous program of active exercises and functional upper limb activities.

Nearly all dynamic corrective elbow orthoses are rubber-band or spring-wire devices applying a variable force over a period of time. More recently, plastic polymers, which have inherent viscoelastic properties, have been used to provide an intrinsic dynamic force within the orthotic system. Whether the dynamic force is created by the properties of the orthotic materials themselves or by means of rubber-bands or spring-wires, the orthosis must be articulated at the elbow axis to allow joint motion. The forearm and arm cuffs are designed to pivot during this process in order to prevent displacement and equalize soft-tissue forces. Carefully molded plastic forearm and arm components joined by single-axis or multicentric hinges usually fulfill these requirements. The dynamic force component can be designed in a variety of ways to meet the needs of the specific corrective orthosis. Stability in the elbow joint and control of joint motion can be provided by an unarticulated, molded plastic orthosis fabricated in a preselected position of function, an articulated single-axis elbow orthosis with molded plastic forearm and arm cuff (Fig. 9-17), or a body-powered, outside elbow-locking orthosis (Fig. 9-18).

The Wrist. Wrist control is very often incorporated into static or dynamic hand orthoses. When used independently, however, wrist orthoses are primarily directed toward the provision of joint stability or elimination of unwanted motion.

Properly designed wrist devices should hold the hand in a position between 5 degrees of volar flexion and 15 degrees of dorsiflexion, because that is the range of motion in which the majority of hand functions are best performed.

The device must be easily donned and removed, particularly in patients with associated hand impairment and deformity. For example, an acrylic, laminated wrist gauntlet (Fig. 9-19) can be fabricated with rigidity on the volar surface and flexibility on the dorsal surface by varying the lamination technique. Thus the entrance into the device is dorsal with closure secured by straps with Velcro, snaps, hooks, or buckles. Plastics make possible a light, durable, non-allergenic orthosis that is easily cleaned and relatively hygienic. Cosmesis is quite good.

In C5 quadriplegics, the action of the biceps muscle produces flexion at the elbow and supination of the forearm. Gravity alone acts to pronate the forearm if there is no opposing supination contracture. If some brachioradialis muscle function is present, it may initiate a ballistic pronation which is then completed by

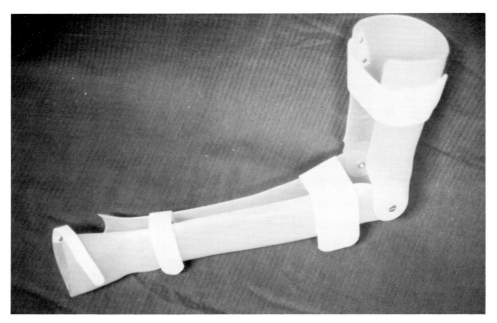

Fig. 9-17. An articulated single-axis elbow orthosis with a molded plastic forearm and arm cuffs.

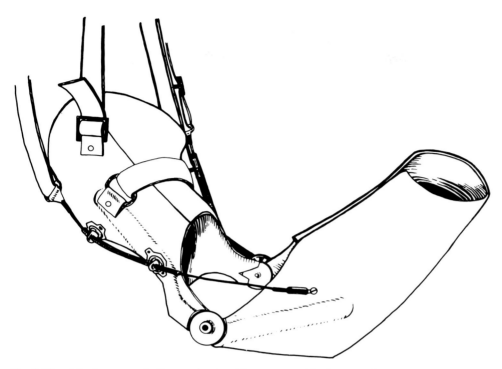

Fig. 9-18. A body-powered elbow orthosis with an external locking mechanism.

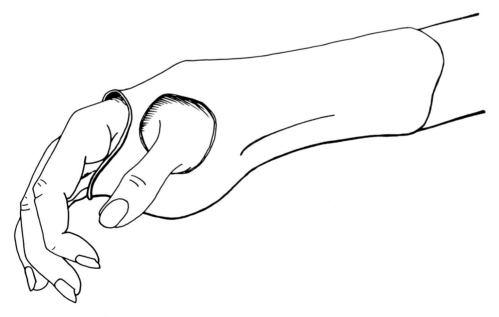

Fig. 9-19. An acrylic wrist-hand orthosis used to stabilize the wrist. The device is fabricated with dorsal flexibility for ease of application. The volar surface is rigid to secure joint control.

gravity.[1] For patients who are devoid of all brachioradialis action and are developing a supination contracture of the forearm, the fitting of a plastic pronatory forearm orthosis (Fig. 9-20) is beneficial. The proximal portion of this device is modeled after a Munster socket; the distal portion is designed to maintain the forearm in pronation without interfering with mobility of the hand. The entire orthosis can be attached to the arm rest of a wheelchair or a balanced forearm orthosis.

The Hand. Hand orthoses can be conveniently divided into two broad categories: splints and functional orthoses. Splints are devices usually intended for the short term. They may be used to prevent deformities in joints or soft tissue, as in hemiplegia, spinal cord injury, or burns. They also serve to hold injured tissue in position for optimal healing following surgical procedures, fractures, peripheral nerve injuries, or lacerations. Functional orthoses are expected to

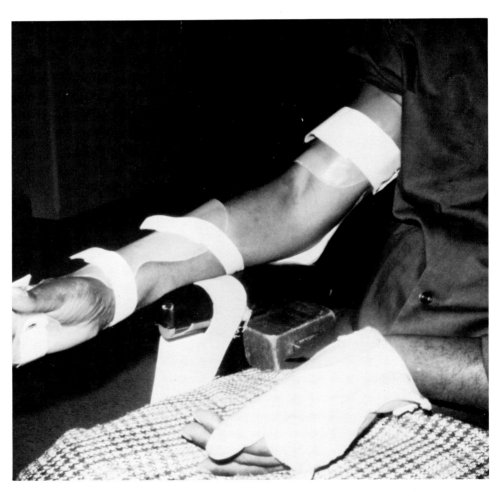

Fig. 9-20. An example of a thermoplastic elbow-wrist-hand orthosis used to compensate for the supination of the forearm due to an unopposed biceps brachii in a C5 quadriplegic.

provide improved hand function in patients who are left with residual impairment as a result of permanent injury or chronic disease. Devices in this group are often more complex, more precisely designed and are used for greater lengths of time. Unlike the splint, a functional orthosis frequently requires precise fitting and extensive training.

Treatment goals determine the design of the applied splint. In acute injuries, a static splint is selected to immobilize the hand in a functional position for optimal tissue healing. This device is used until sufficient tissue reconstitution has occurred. Then active range of motion is needed to regain joint mobility and tissue suppleness. These goals are best accomplished by exercise orthoses in conjunction with proper physical and occupational therapy programs.

As the name implies, dynamic splints are articulated devices with elastic or spring-resistance to augment weakened muscles or apply passive stretching.[1] They are indicated for exercise purposes rather than in activities of daily living. They are intended for limited use, determined by the patient's recovery of voluntary hand function. Although dynamic splints are commercially available, an experienced occupational therapist can rapidly fabricate a more comfortable device. Whether commercial or custom, care must be taken to avoid pain and skin pressure problems, both of which will interfere appreciably with the effectiveness of the exercise orthosis.

The rate and degree of recovery of diseases and injuries affecting the neuro-muscular or skeletal status of the upper limb are variable and often incomplete. In conditions such as hemiplegia, quadriplegia, brachial plexus lesions, peripheral nerve abnormalities, and rheumatic diseases, functional orthoses are often indicated to improve the capacities of a partially impaired upper limb. Despite possible subsequent recovery of voluntary upper limb control, these orthoses are valuable training devices during the period of marked impairment before functional recovery has been reached. Clinicians must realize that all orthoses are mechanical systems which are, at best, only partial replacements for functional losses. Moreover, patients will not use any orthosis providing a restoration of function that can be achieved by any other means.

The range of functional hand orthoses varies from adaptive cuffs to complex, externally powered devices. None of these replace all hand functions, so each should be viewed as a tool selected for specific tasks.[1] The more activities the patient can perform with the device, the more useful it will prove to be.

The most important functional goal for the patient and therapist to attain is effective use of the hand orthosis in activities of daily living. Success with a functional orthosis requires both training and experience. Assuming that the device is properly designed and fitted, skill in using the orthosis results from careful education of the patient under the supervision of an experienced therapist. Extensive efforts should be made to demonstrate multiple ways to use the orthosis; donning and removing the system should be made as easy as possible.[1] The lack of the therapist's involvement will only increase the probability of the patient's disappointment and resultant failure of the orthotic treatment.

Adaptive devices for greater independence in activities of daily living—such as shaving, grooming, bathing, feeding, dressing, and writing—are available commercially or may be fabricated by therapists and/or orthotists. One of the more frequently selected devices is the utensil-cuff, which is strapped onto the hand of severely paralyzed patients. Various instruments (fork, spoon, razor, toothbrush, page-turner, typing-stick) can be attached to the cuff and are easily interchanged for each task. Even these devices require some training and assistance from another person in order to be successful. Although these devices provide no active grasp or release of the hand, they do avoid the mechanical and fitting problems of functional orthoses. The basic functional hand orthosis is composed of a self-suspending palmar component that maintains the palmar arch and serves as the foundation for a positional upper-limb orthosis.[5] Either padded metal or plastics may be used to fabricate the device. The basic component is secured by a flange that rests against the radial side of the second metacarpal and by the recurved bar extending around the ulnar side of the hand.[1,5] The device continues on to the midline of the dorsal surface. The entire unit is prevented from distal slippage by a wrist strap. The unit does not interfere with any regular activity of the hand or wrist. Depending on the functional impairment of the upper limb, a wide variety of attachments may be added to deal with almost any dysfunction.[1]

Hyperextension of the metacarpophalangeal joint secondary to intrinsic muscle dysfunction can be prevented by the addition of a removable metacarpal bar to the basic hand orthosis. An opponens bar can control unopposed extension of the first metacarpal. The bar contacts the first metacarpal just proximal to the metacarpophalangeal joint of the thumb. When added to the basic hand unit, the entire device is called a short-opponens hand orthosis.[5] A C-bar can be added to the short-opponens orthosis to prevent web-space contracture and provide abduction of the thumb in opposition to the index and middle fingers. The C-bar is designed to avoid interference of flexion of the metacarpophalangeal joint of the index finger.

Ulnar deviation of the index finger can be controlled by the addition of a spring-resistant finger clasp, a device that substitutes for the first dorsal interosseus muscle. A similar aid can be applied to the long finger as well.

The long opponens wrist-hand orthosis provides wrist stabilization combined with the basic hand orthosis. This device increases grip strength when the extrinsic extensors are absent because it places the finger flexors at a more optimal length. Yet it may keep the fingers from opening by tenodesis action. Better assistance to opening the hand is more easily achievable with a "spider" splint or the attachment of an outrigger to the long opponens splint. This treatment would supply extension (via rubber bands) to the metacarpophalangeal joints of the fingers and thumb.

The flaccid hand should be splinted at the earliest opportunity to prevent rigid nonfunctional deformities. The use of a wrist-hand orthosis or a hand splint that holds the thumb abducted is indicated. Either a thumb post or short opponens hand splint may be selected. Joint stiffness can be prevented by passive ranging. Swelling of the hand while the patient is in a wheelchair is avoidable with an overhead outrigger having a spring-suspension of the forearm and hand or, more easily, with a trough attached to the wheelchair's arm rest. When the patient is in bed, the hand can be elevated on pillows to ensure dependent drainage. Preventing contractures of the metacarpophalangeal joints and tightening the first web space is mandatory to functional bracing of the severely paralyzed hand.

In high-level neurological deficits (C4 and C5), the hand has no intact motor control or useful sensation. Orthotic fitting for function can be approached by means of adaptive cuff devices or externally powered orthoses. If the patient lacks elbow and shoulder control, both a mobile arm unit and external power unit for the hand are needed. External power can be applied to reciprocal orthoses of the Rancho Los Amigos or Engen types via electric motors or carbon dioxide gas. Although harnessing shoulder elevation to a prosthetic-type cable is appealing, its use as an alternative external power source is limited by the requirement of satisfactory lateral trunk stability and the very high power : function ratio (15 : 1) necessary for activation of the orthosis. Usually the strongest or dominant side is selected for fitting. Bilateral fittings are poorly tolerated because of the complexity of the two control systems.

Complex, motor-driven, upper-limb orthoses have been developed and fitted to high-level neurological lesions. Experience has shown that patients with severe muscular paralysis whose sensory functions have remained intact are the most suitable candidates for fitting of this type of device. Conversely, the usual high cervical spinal cord patient with both motor and sensory deficits lacks the essential feedback for effective operation of the orthosis. Such devices are plagued by multiple maintenance and control problems without the compensation of consistent versatility in activities of daily living. Patient rejection due to "gadget intolerance" and orthotic inefficiency has virtually eliminated long-term use of these systems. Nevertheless, they remain important experimental aids.

In the presence of intact shoulder control and elbow control plus active radial wrist extension (C6), there is increased power for hand placement and sensation on the radial side of the hand. Wrist extension is provided by the extensor carpi radialis longus and brevis. Unfortunately, a portion of their power is lost in producing radial deviation along with wrist extension.[2,18]

To improve hand function any of the tenodesis orthoses—such as the Rancho, Engen, and Rehabilitation Institute of Chicago varieties—may be selected. These orthoses are based on the principles of reciprocal wrist and finger motions characteristic of a hand with a fixation of the finger flexors. Since three-jaw chuck prehension is the most useful configuration of the hand in activities of daily living and self-care,[16] reciprocal wrist orthoses furnish this type of prehension by stabilizing the thumb, immobilizing and positioning the interphalangeal joints of the index and middle fingers, and providing a mechanical linkage to the forearm. The Rancho and Engen orthoses (Fig. 9-21) have a mechanical parallelogram linkage, whereas the RIC splint has a volar cable from the forearm cuff to the finger component. All three orthoses have been called "wrist-driven finger orthoses" because the power of wrist dorsiflexion is transferred to the fingertips.[1]

In patients with an intact C7 neurological level (elbow extension, wrist dorsiflexion, forearm pronation, and radial wrist flexion), natural tenodesis usually develops and therapists must guard against vigorous stretching of the finger flexors and extensors. When a light grasp is required, the patient is encouraged to perform the task without the aid of an orthosis. If the tasks are more demanding, a reciprocal wrist orthosis is advantageous. Definitive surgical treatment may be seriously considered to provide active thumb abduction-opposition and finger flexion by suitable tendon transfers.[1,4,13]

C8 and T1 level patients rarely need any orthoses except to help in wrist positioning and thumb-web stretching during the acute phase of treatment. Ultimately these patients show adequate hand function spontaneously. Some may benefit from carefully planned tendon transfers.

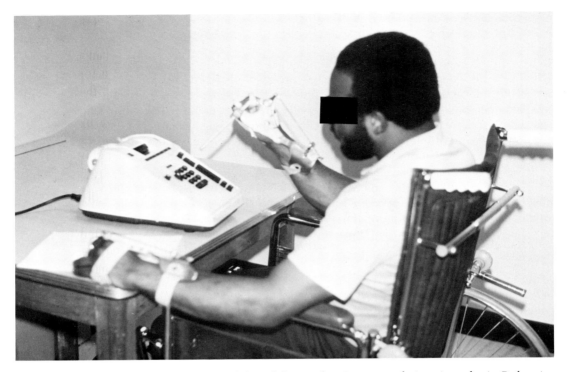

Fig. 9-21. A demonstration of bilateral fitting of an Engen tenodesis wrist orthosis. Prehension produced by the orthosis allows the patient to operate the calculator by depressing the buttons with a wooden rod.

Patients with primary rheumatic joint disease are aided by positional splints in the acute inflammatory stage, but bracing should be gradually withdrawn as the inflammatory response diminishes. It is far more important to regain joint mobility with active and passive exercises than to risk joint stiffness secondary to prolonged static splinting.

Mobile deformities of the interphalangeal, metacarpophalangeal, carpometacarpal, and wrist joints can result from destructive rheumatic joint disease. No currently available orthosis has been shown to prevent such conditions. It is much better to maintain maximum joint motion and teach the patient protective techniques that avoid deleterious forces being applied to the wrist and finger joints during performance of daily activities.

REPLACING ORTHOSES

Preventive maintenance is the basis of reliability, longevity, and performance of an orthosis. No orthosis is indestructible, but careful intermittent examination will identify minor maintenance problems before they result in serious malfunction of the device. Worn or defective components may produce alignment changes, increased resistance in joint motion control, alteration in the distribution of soft-tissue pressure, loss of motion control, or reduction in assistive forces. Many maintenance problems are easily correctable with minor adjustment of these components. Yet long-term wear eventually makes it mandatory to replace various materials and/or components. If a large number of parts of the orthosis must be changed, it may be more economical to fabricate a new brace.

Recent advances in materials, fabrication techniques, and orthotic design may also motivate members of the rehabilitation team to consider a new orthosis for selected patients. Although this option might seem attractive, one must keep in mind that many patients develop a high degree of reliance on their old devices. Some patients become insecure when threatened by any impending orthotic alteration. Even if the functional gain is considered beneficial by the treatment team, the patient may be reluctant to accept the change. Well planned counselling should precede any decision to prescribe a new device. If indicated, appropriate training with the new orthosis by the physical or occupational therapist should follow its fitting. Above all, patience, understanding, and encouragement must be demonstrated by rehabilitation team members during the entire conversion process.

Changes in the functional status of a patient may also create a need for an orthotic change. The patient should be carefully examined to determine if a modification of the current orthosis will suffice or a new one should be prescribed. In instances of progressive functional improvement, the decision is the relatively easy one of reducing the magnitude of the orthotic device versus elimination of the system altogether. Unfortunately, in circumstances of deteriorating neuromuscular function, the choice is more difficult because of the need to weigh the desire for preservation of function against such factors as more extensive orthotic design, higher expenditure of the patient's energy, increasing orthotic costs, and impact on the patient's psychological and emotional status.

Whatever the reasons for orthotic adjustment or replacement, the decision is usually best made during on-site consultation between the orthotist and health professionals involved in the care of the patient. The better the interdisciplinary communication, the more likely the process will be performed expeditiously.

PSYCHOLOGICAL ASPECTS OF ORTHOSES

Seldom does anyone desire to wear an orthosis unless it provides an important function that cannot otherwise be attained. Comfort, appearance, simplicity, efficiency, reliability, and ease of application and removal are all integral factors influencing a patient's acceptance of an orthosis. Failure to recognize the importance of these factors often results in frustration and eventual rejection of the device. Every effort should be expended to promote a favorable attitude on the part of the patient toward wearing the orthosis. In fact, team reassurance and encouragement are essential to the ultimate successful utilization of the orthotic system.

In situations in which the patient is incapable of applying and removing the orthosis, assistance must be given by family members, friends, or employed attendants. They must, of necessity, have a thorough knowledge of the orthosis and its objectives. Any lack of cooperation or failure of communication frequently results in complications or decreased efficiency of the device. Furthermore, any negative attitude of others toward the benefits of the orthosis is likely to influence the orthotic wearer adversely.

Identification of financial support, be it personal or third-party, for payment of the orthotic services is an endless source of frustration for the patient as well as the members of the rehabilitation team. Far too often, the orthosis is viewed by all parties as a minor adjunct to the patient's treatment program. No wonder third-party payers are reluctant to purchase devices of such alleged low priority in the face of today's enormous medical costs. Thus if the patient is unable to pay the cost of fabrication of the orthosis, the benefits of bracing are lost. It is imperative that health professionals educate governmental health agencies, insurance carriers, and private health foundations as to the importance of underwriting the cost of orthotic devices for improved care of disabled persons.

FUTURE DIRECTIONS IN ORTHOTICS

Where is the field of orthotics headed? For years it has lagged behind related bodies of knowledge in the development of technical skills, performance of fundamental research, and delivery of sophisticated patient services. Despite these weaknesses, the scope of orthotics has steadily expanded to meet new challenges, such as environmental control devices, orthotic implants, robot technology, and new concepts in mobility aids. How will orthotics accomplish the strengthening of its scientific foundation in order to fulfill increasing clinical and academic demands?

Advancement of the field may be achieved only through a simultaneous, multi-track approach: first, continued upgrading of educational and training standards of professional and technical personnel; second, further research in biomechanical analysis, new materials and fabrication techniques, functional electrical stimulation, biofeedback, human tissue properties, orthotic implants, and computerized orthotic systems; third, modernization of the delivery of services to consumers; fourth, encouragement of better utilization of orthotic technology by related health professionals; and finally, more effective interaction among health providers, medical engineers, and orthotists as they work to resolve the complex functional problems of the disabled.

REFERENCES

1. Bunch, W. H., and Keagy, R. D.: *Principles of Orthotic Treatment*. C. V. Mosby, St. Louis, 1976.
2. Cary, J. M., Lusskin, R., and Thompson, R. G.: Prescription principles. In American Academy of Orthopaedic Surgeons, Ed.: *Atlas of Orthotics*, pp. 235–244. C. V. Mosby, St. Louis, 1975.
3. Fisher, S. V., Bowar, J. F., Awad, E. A., and Gullickson, G., Jr.: Cervical orthoses' effect on cervical spine motion: Roentgenographic and goniometric method of study. Arch. Phys. Med. Rehabil. 58:109–115, 1977.
4. Freehafer, A. A., Van Haam, E. J., and Allen, V.: Tendon transfers to improve grasp after injuries of the cervical spinal cord. J. Bone Joint Surg. 56A:951–959, 1974.

5. Guilford, A. W., and Perry, J.: Orthotic components and systems. In American Academy of Orthopaedic Surgeons, Ed.: *Atlas of Orthotics,* pp. 81–104. C. V. Mosby, St. Louis, 1975.

6. Hartman, J. T., Palumbo, F., and Hill, H. B.: Cineradiography of the braced normal cervical spine: Comparative study of five commonly used cervical orthoses. Clin. Orthop. 109:97–102, 1975.

7. Johnson, R. M., Hart, D. L., Simmons, E. F., et al.: Cervical orthoses: A study comparing their effectiveness in restricting cervical motion in normal subjects. J. Bone Joint Surg. 59A:332–339, 1977.

8. Lehmann, J. F.: Lower limb orthotics. In Redford, J. B., Ed.: *Orthotics Etcetera,* pp. 283–335. Williams & Wilkins, Baltimore, 1980.

9. Lehmann, J. F., Delateur, B. J., Warren, C. G., et al.: Biomechanical evaluation of braces for paraplegics. Arch. Phys. Med. Rehabil. 50:179–188, 1969.

10. McCollough, N. C., III: Orthopedic evaluation and treatment of the stroke patient: Lower extremity orthotic management. In *Instructional Course Lectures,* vol. 24, pp. 29–40. American Academy of Orthopaedic Surgeons. C. V. Mosby, St. Louis, 1975.

11. McCollough, N. C., III: Orthopedic evaluation and the treatment of the stroke patient: Upper extremity evaluation and management. In *Instructional Course Lectures,* vol. 24, pp. 45–51. American Academy of Orthopaedic Surgeons. C. V. Mosby, St. Louis, 1975.

12. McCollough, N. C., III: The role of the orthopedic surgeon in the treatment of stroke. In Bowker, J. H., Ed.: Symposium on special problems in orthopedic rehabilitation. Orthop. Clin. North Am. 9:305–324, 1978.

13. Moberg, E.: Surgical treatment for absent single-hand grip and elbow extension in quadriplegia. J. Bone Joint Surg. 57A:196–206, 1975.

14. Mooney, V., and Cairns, D.: Management in the patient with chronic low back pain. In Bowker, J. H., Ed.: Symposium on special problems in orthopedic rehabilitation. Orthop. Clin. North Am. 9:543–557, 1978.

15. Mooney, V., and Wagner, F. W., Jr.: Neurocirculatory disorders of the foot. Clin. Orthop. 122:53–61, 1977.

16. Nickel, V. L., Perry, J., and Garrett, A. L.: Development of useful function in the severely paralyzed hand. J. Bone Joint Surg. 45A:933–952, 1963.

17. Perry, J.: Pathologic gait. In American Academy of Orthopaedic Surgeons, Ed.: *Atlas of Orthotics,* pp. 144–168. C. V. Mosby, St. Louis, 1975.

18. Perry, J.: Prescription principles. In American Academy of Orthopaedic Surgeons, Ed.: *Atlas of Orthotics,* pp. 105–129. C. V. Mosby, St. Louis, 1975.

19. Perry, J., and Waters, R. L.: Orthopedic evaluation and treatment of the stroke patient: Lower extremity surgery. In *Instructional Course Lectures,* vol. 24, pp. 40–44. American Academy of Orthopaedic Surgeons. C. V. Mosby, St. Louis, 1975.

20. Redford, J. B., and Licht, S.: Materials for orthotics. In Redford, J. B., Ed.: *Orthotics Etcetera,* pp. 53–79. Williams & Wilkins, Baltimore, 1980.

21. Soderberg, G.: Follow-up of application of plaster-of-Paris casts for noninfected plantar ulcers in field conditions. Leprosy Rev. 41:184–190, 1970.

22. Staros, A., and LeBlanc, M.: Orthotic components and systems. In American Academy of Orthopaedic Surgeons, Ed.: *Atlas of Orthotics,* pp. 184–234. C. V. Mosby, St. Louis, 1975.

23. Van Hanswyk, E. P.: The diabetic patient: Orthotic considerations. Orthop. Prosthet. 33(3):32–39, 1979.

24. Wagner, F. W. Jr.: Rehabilitation of the dysvascular lower limbs. In Bowker, J. H., Ed.: Symposium on special problems in orthopedic rehabilitation. Orthop. Clin. North Am. 9:325–350, 1978.

10

The Social Worker

Honora K. Wilson, M.S.W.
Ruth Cox Brunings, M.S.W.

The social worker diagnoses and treats any of the patient's social and emotional problems that affect his health and ability to benefit from medical care. The social worker by professional training is a specialist with expertise in helping individuals and families deal with personal problems that arise when they are faced with illness and disability. The psychosocial aspects of illness and disability are as profound as their physical symptoms.[11] The social worker's dual responsibility is to resolve the individual patient's psychosocial problems and at the same time to make changes in the health care delivery system to ensure that the psychosocial needs of all patients are met.[2]

HISTORY AND EMERGENCE OF THE PROFESSION

The specialty of medical social work in the profession of social work was inaugurated by a distinguished physician, Dr. Richard C. Cabot, Chief of Staff of the Massachusetts General Hospital in Boston. As the director of the Boston Children's Aid Society, he had observed social workers in action, sat in on case discussions, and studied case records. Later, when he saw some of the same children in the clinic, he realized how much better he understood them and their diseases through his knowledge of their psychosocial histories. For a complete diagnosis, he felt it was necessary to have information about a patient's home, diet, work, family, and personal problems.[7]

It was the realization of the close dependence of a person's physical well-being on his mental and socioeconomic condition that resulted in the formation of the first social work department in the Massachusetts General Hospital in 1905. Ida Cannon was appointed by Dr. Cabot as the first medical social worker in the United States.

From the beginning of this century, social work in hospitals expanded from settings in public hospitals to university hospitals to nonprofit and sectarian hospitals to proprietary hospitals to independent practice in the community. The expansion of social work in medical settings has occurred for the following reasons:

> Increased knowledge in the behavioral sciences with respect to the significance of social and emotional factors on physical health.
> Increased concern for medical care in the field of public welfare.
> Development of public health programs on local, state, federal, and international levels.
> Development of special rehabilitation programs.

Today more than 2000 United States hospitals have departments of social work. Moreover, the provision of social work services to patients is a standard for accreditation by the Joint Commission on Accreditation of Hospitals[9] and for licensure through Title 22. The health care field employs the majority of all social workers in this country.

SPECIAL QUALIFICATIONS

Formal professional education for social work was available in 1898.[6] Today the educational requirement for the professional social worker is a master's degree from an accredited school of social work. The degree takes two years to earn, and approximately 73 accredited colleges and universities in the United States and four in Canada award it. Two-thirds to one-half of each semester's hours must be spent in clinical practice with supervision by a social worker with a master's degree. Education for the master's degree covers five major areas: human behavior and the social environment, social welfare policy and services, social work treatment modalities, research, and clinical practice. The social worker in a medical setting takes specialized courses in the medical aspects of social work practice and has a clinical internship in a health care program. The social worker with a master's degree is the primary agent in the delivery of social work and carries responsibility for the provision of direct services to patients and families.

In California, as well as in approximately one-half of the other states, a social worker can secure a license as a licensed clinical social worker after two years of supervised practice followed by successful completion of written and oral examinations. These standards assure patients and the community that the clinical social worker has met professional educational requirements and has demonstrated clinical competence. Licensed clinical social workers can be expected to provide highly skilled, independent practice in psychosocial treatment of patients and families.

Twenty-three accredited colleges and universities in the United States and two in Canada now grant a doctoral degree in social work. Persons with such degrees are usually found in teaching, research, and administration. Numerous hospitals with large departments of social work have administrators with doctoral degrees.

Two hundred colleges and universities in the United States and two in Canada offer a bachelor's degree in social welfare. To meet accreditation standards, persons with such degrees must be supervised by social workers with master's degrees. They are found more frequently in large departments of social work and their duties are largely confined to performing specific tasks for patients—tasks that require concern for patients and awareness of community resources, but not professional knowledge and skills. Sometimes small hospitals employ social workers with bachelor's degrees, and contract for supervision by social workers with master's degrees. After a year or two of work experience, a social worker with a bachelor's degree tends to return to college or university to obtain a master's degree in social work.

In addition to the professional social work staff, social work assistants are trained on the job to perform concrete, specific tasks delegated by and under the supervision of the social worker. Increasingly, persons with a bachelor's degree in social welfare are being employed as social work assistants.

THE SOCIAL WORKER'S CONTRIBUTIONS AND FUNCTIONS IN REHABILITATION

The patient confronted by serious illness, particularly chronic illness, has a variety of tasks to be undertaken in order to negotiate the process of rehabilitation. These have been described as illness-related and general adaptive tasks. Activities related to illness involve facing pain and incapacitation, dealing with the hospital environment and special treatment procedures, and developing adequate relationships with the professional health care staff. The general adaptations a patient must make center on preserving a reasonable emotional balance, preserving a satisfactory self-image, preserving relationships with family and friends, and preparing for an uncertain future.[8]

Social work services are directly involved with the general adaptive tasks. Sometimes the medical staff requests the social worker's participation in the illness-related tasks. The social worker intervenes with both the patient and the family to assist in difficulties or adjustments having to do with work, finances, living arrangements, social life, marriage, child care, and emotional life. The social worker recognizes that acquired or congenital disability may affect the individual's self-esteem, as well as relationships with other people, including the family. Chronic illnesses may also produce emotional, financial, and sexual problems that may retard recovery.

The social worker's primary role is to make a psychosocial assessment,[3] that is, an evaluation of the patient as a person and the impact of the illness upon his ability to cope with medical treatment and rehabilitation. In this role, social workers are in the position of functioning in three areas of the treatment system. First, they use their knowledge and skill to assess the patients and their capacity to cope with illness. Second, in assessing the impact of the patient's illness on the family, they determine where the family fits into the treatment system, particularly as part of the patient's support system (Fig. 10-1). Third, social workers share and interpret their assessments with the rest of the health care team. These assessments influence all questions of management and treatment procedures for the patient.

Studies in the field of chronic illness have suggested that there are specific and predictable phases of adjustment through which most patients must pass to achieve resolution of emotional trauma and successful rehabilitation. For most illnesses and disabilities, the phases seem to be as follows.

First come confusion, doubt, and uncertainty. These emotions are frequently followed by denial resulting in aggressive behavior, euphoria, and inappropriate defense mechanisms. This stage is followed by depression as the patient perceives reality. After the depression is worked through, the patient is able to reassess the situation and move to restitution and adjustment.[5]

The family has its own experience similar to that of the patient. Just as the patient must go through several phases of adjustment until there is a restitution of self, so does the family experience the same. For the family there is loss and grief,

THE PATIENT'S SOCIAL SUPPORT SYSTEMS

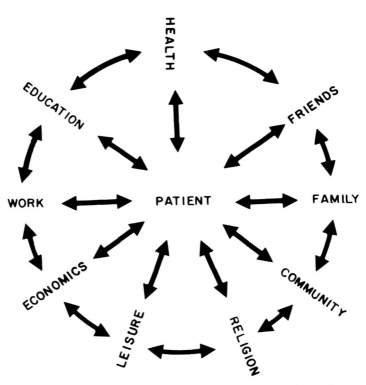

Fig. 10-1. Nine basic social systems interact with each other, influence a patient's social functioning, and together constitute a total social support system.

new roles, and change of status, followed by realignment of individuals, social systems, and finally an adjustment to a new style of living.

Family members also have pain over the guilt that they experience. The guilt comes from unresolved anger, ambivalence, fears, and a desire to escape from the patient and the whole problem. When guilt is recognized, accepted, and worked through, then the family is able to move to problem-solving, to making necessary decisions, to participating with the health care team, and to remaining involved with the patient.

In rehabilitation facilities, all patients and their families are interviewed at the time of admission by the social worker. The social assessment made then consists of the following factors:[4]

1. Any adjustment problems prior to illness.
2. Social, emotional, and economic problems created or intensified by the illness.
3. The patient's goals in life and how they may need to be redirected.
4. People important to the patient.
5. The nature of interpersonal relationships.
6. Usual social roles and present role changes.
7. Emotional reactions to impaired physical condition and the hospital environment.
8. The nature of coping mechanisms.
9. Expectations of the rehabilitation program.
10. Social resources and personal strengths.
11. Specific behaviors and attitudes that suggest mental illness, such as severe anxiety, depression, excessive grief, or suicidal ideation.

With this outline as a guide, and with information from interviews with the patient, family, involved friends, and other team members, the social worker makes a psychosocial diagnosis and treatment plan. This assessment is the basis for the information the social worker shares with the rest of the treatment team in order to contribute to their understanding of the significant social and emotional factors related to each individual's health problem and assist in their total evaluation and individualized treatment of each patient.

This psychosocial diagnosis is important to all team members, but it is of highest priority for the physician and the nurse. It is this knowledge that enables the physician to understand the patient's reaction to the medical environment, to the illness, and especially to surgical intervention. Knowledge of the patient's emotional status enables the surgeon to discuss an operation with an understanding of what it means to the patient. Thus the surgeon can realistically explain the intervention to the patient in terms of who is giving support to the patient, what the surgery threatens in relation to economic survival, how the patient's family views disability, what the patient's fears are, and what the prospect of surgery stirs up in the patient's unconscious. Orthopedic surgeons in particular, but perhaps all surgeons, need to understand with pride their own great skill in restoration, but also to not be disappointed when the patient is less than enthusiastic or responsive to the proposed surgery. The literature is full of references to the repressed anger of patients at the operation that removes a limb or modifies it. This anger is only indirectly aimed at the surgeon. It primarily is the way in which many patients express their psychic pain of illness and disability. When the social worker shares with the surgeon some of the pain, some of the disappointment, some of the failures in the patient's life, the surgeon is better able to hear and understand the repressed anger when he explains surgery. Some patients can be identified as poor surgical risks because of acute or chronic psychosocial problems.

The same knowledge of the family, the major factor in the patient's support system, can reinforce the surgeon's ability to interpret to the family what can be expected from the operation. The family support system is the major force upon which the health team can rely for successful rehabilitation. With knowledge of the family's hopes, fears, and disappointments, the physician can better deal with their expectations for treatment and rehabilitation.

The psychosocial assessment becomes important knowledge for the nurse in her daily care of the patient. Information from the social worker can help the nurse to understand the patient better, to know what approach to use for maximum cooperation, and to maintain nonjudgmental attitudes.

The main vehicle through which the social worker shares the data from the psychosocial assessment is the team conference. As these data are shared, all members of the team look at their own specific assessment with new insights as to how the patient and family will go through the medical treatment system. The psychosocial diagnosis is discussed and interpreted in the team conference. The plan of medical care as a comprehensive plan now includes a humanistic assessment of the patient's needs for psychosocial treatment.

As the psychosocial diagnosis and assessment continue with the patient, the social worker offers treatment in the areas of identified need. The treatment modalities of social work include individual psychotherapy, environmental therapy, advocacy therapy, group therapy, conjoint and family therapy, sexual counseling, and play therapy.

The psychosocial treatment given in individual one-to-one interviews can be advice, information, counseling, or psychotherapy.[1] The social worker listens to the patient's fears about his body, himself, his changes in role, and the unknowns of medical treatment. The social worker helps the patient to express his fears and anxieties and find emotional support for this experience.

As the patient begins to feel relief from emotional tensions, the social worker intervenes in each area of need. If he is concerned about money, help in securing financial assistance is given; if he is concerned about living arrangements, various housing alternatives are reviewed; if he is concerned about returning to work or change of work, referrals are made to vocational counselors. As the patient begins to deal with the physical and social limitations attendant upon his illness, the social worker helps if he is not able to do this himself. Environmental therapy may include assistance with negotiating the bureaucratic requirements of the public financial assistance system, securing vocational counseling, appropriate housing, homemaker, and home health aide assistance, home nursing services, and transportation. The above-mentioned services are also offered to the family, so as to ensure this resource as a part of the patient's support system.

Advocacy for the patient is a traditional role of the social worker and has high priority in the social worker's arena of function. Advocacy becomes imperative as more and more social services are available and as the social systems become more complicated and more difficult to negotiate. The social worker is also an advocate for the patient in the medical system. As medicine becomes more complex and as the medical system adds more team members, the distance between the patient and the physician becomes broader and the risk of dehumanization becomes greater. Here the social worker continually intervenes to assist the individual patient and to effect changes in the health care delivery system on behalf of human dignity.

Group treatment is a major tool in the social worker's armamentarium and it can be offered at any time in the course of the patient's medical experience. The social worker offers a variety of group experiences and uses different group techniques. Group treatment can be educational or therapeutic or a combination of both. Group treatment can be given for patients, families, or patients and families.

Peer groups are an important part of sharing experiences in chronic illness. The patient can be brought into a group at any time when the social worker ascertains his need and readiness. Groups meet on a regular basis for 60 to 90 minutes. They are primarily for support, sharing of physical and psychic pain, problem-solving, and expression of feelings. The social worker shares with the rest of the treatment team any significant feelings expressed during the group sessions but the content is kept confidential.

Other groups that perform some of the above functions and more are patient education groups. Usually the social worker organizes and plans these groups with all members of the team or individual team members throughout a series of meetings.

Social workers increasingly are offering group treatments for the families and significant others in the patient's life. They usually are planned for a certain number of meetings, primarily at night, when it is more convenient for those who work during the day. Family groups are for support, acquaintance with the medical team, sharing of information and knowledge, expression of feelings, and problem-solving. Such groups are particularly successful in helping parents of disabled children. More recently, groups for adults with elderly parents are being conducted.

The social worker frequently schedules family groups with the patient and the entire family to verbalize conflicts and misunderstandings and to solve problems. On other occasions, the social worker has conjoint family therapy sessions with a husband and wife. Again, these groups focus on expression of feelings, clarification of misunderstandings, planning, and problem-solving.

Family conferences with staff to discuss the patient's condition, medical treatment, and discharge plans are frequently led by the social worker. Many hospitals schedule weekly meetings to which different families are invited.

Sexual counseling is a well-established modality of treatment for the physically disabled. This treatment takes the form of individual counseling with the patient, conjoint counseling with the patient and sexual partner, and educational or therapeutic groups. The social worker, together with the physician, determines the area of sexual dysfunction and provides the appropriate treatment, which may include education, information, or therapy to resolve discomfort with body image, fear of rejection, or emotional problems that interfere with sexual functioning. The disabled patient and partner frequently develop sexual dysfunction as a symptom of other problems inherent in the relationship. Sexual problems are not isolated and therefore can best be treated in the context of the total therapeutic experience with the social worker or other primary therapist.

Play therapy is traditionally used with children as a medium of communication for the expression of problems, conflicts, and feelings. In working with physically disabled children with impaired speech, this modality of treatment can assume added importance.

These psychosocial treatments are continuously evaluated and shared with the health care team for interaction with medical management.

The social worker's involvement in discharge planning varies with individual patients and families, depending on the personal strengths and weaknesses of both the patient and the family and their willingness to utilize assistance in working through their problems. Discharge planning is a total process that involves all aspects of the patient's medical problem and rehabilitation. From the time of admission, much of the social worker's activity has been directed toward helping the patient come to a recognition, if not a resolution, of limited goals—that he has reached a maximum level of physical functioning and he now must begin the phase of living with the new self. This step includes awareness of physical limitations, of dependence on others for some part of his care, of a new identity, of a new role, and, one hopes, a series of achievements and new abilities.

There are four major factors that must be considered in assisting a person to make plans for discharge.[10] The first factor is the degree of physical function that the patient will attain. If the patient is fairly independent in activities of daily living and requires little or no help with personal care, he may be able to live alone with a minimum amount of help from family, friends, or a part-time housekeeper. If he requires considerable personal care and it is not feasible for him to live alone, he will need either a devoted family member or a live-in attendant to assist him.

A second consideration is the nature of a person's relationships with his family. The social worker assists the patient and the family in deciding if the patient will be cared for in the family home or in another living arrangement. This requires assessment of reality factors and the feelings the patient and the family. In order to assist the patient and family with the question of returning home or living elsewhere, weekend passes are encouraged to try out the plan for living. If the family can no longer care for the patient at home, then efforts must begin early in the hospital stay to work through the family's guilt, the patient's anger, disappointment, and feelings of rejection, and plans for other care.

A third factor to be considered is the emotional need of the patient for independence. If the family cannot allow the patient to dress or feed himself or to struggle with this kind of physical independence at his own pace, conflicts arise. The social worker must work to reconcile the patient's emotional need for independence with his actual physical dependence. He must be helped to assert realistic independence even if he is physically different than before.

The fourth factor is the financial and social resources available in the community for the physically disabled. The financial resources include public assistance programs, social security disability insurance programs, the Veterans Administration, and Crippled Children's Services, to name a few major ones.

Various agencies provide such specific services as vocational counseling, recreation, transportation, housing, child care, family counseling, and psychiatric care. As part of discharge planning, the social worker coordinates referrals to community agencies or arranges to provide continued direct services on an outpatient basis. In the last ten years the physically disabled have developed their own national and local support organizations, furnishing a wide range of services. These organizations, such as the Association of the Physically Handicapped, make the able-bodied community aware of the needs of the physically disabled and have been increasingly effective in lobbying for legislative changes, removing architectural barriers, and bringing about changes in attitudes toward the physically disabled. Other organizations, such as the Centers for Independent Living, are self-help programs. They are primarily staffed by volunteers with some paid professional staff (usually disabled). These centers have become a major resource for socialization, offer all kinds of services, group programs, and are continually available to prevent people from retreating from the mainstream of living.

Finally, the patient must be helped emotionally to leave the total support system of the hospital. This process is eased somewhat by follow-up care as an outpatient provided by the same inpatient rehabilitation team whom the patient has come to know and trust.

RELATIONSHIP OF THE SOCIAL WORKER TO REHABILITATION TEAM MEMBERS

Understanding of the interrelationships of the physical, social, and emotional factors that pertain in illness and disability has become a cornerstone of contemporary medical practice. Increasingly, the orthopedic surgeon who brings such skill in late 20th-century medicine to the treatment of some of the most disabling illnesses and disabilities finds himself unable any longer to limit his involvement to the patient's skeletal structure. Just as he increasingly becomes a team partner and relies upon the knowledge of his internist collaborator, so does he in turn heed the counsel and expertise of the nurse, physical therapist, occupational therapist, vocational counselor, and social worker. The primary medium of communication is the team conference, in which information is shared by all professional disciplines. At this conference the social worker may take the lead in encouraging the team to include the psychosocial aspects in the formulation of the total medical treatment plan.

RELATIONSHIP TO THE COMMUNITY

In recent years the hospital setting has come to be seen as a community. This philosophy is related to the concept of preventive medicine and to the hospital in the broadest sense as part of health services. This health service, of which prevention is a major part, demands that the medical caretakers move to share their knowledge and expertise with the total community. Social workers play a part in this design. Social workers participate in medical symposia for doctors, nurses, and all allied health professionals to share their knowledge of psychosocial factors in health care and the humanity of the patient. They are on faculties of medical schools and allied health schools. Social workers are on boards of the major voluntary health agencies across the country, such as those for heart disease, cancer, lung disease, and crippled children.

FUTURE DIRECTIONS

The practice of social work in health services is predicted to show continued expansion and improvement. More and more hospitals will comply with the standards of social work services for accreditation and licensing. As social workers demonstrate competence and effectiveness in more and more facilities, the demand for their services from both patients and hospital staff will increase.

Social work services can be billed on a fee-for-service basis, as insurance companies make direct payment for psychotherapy given by social workers. Now that social work services are revenue-producing, there is an opportunity for further expansion in health care facilities and in independent practice, with social workers accepting referrals from community physicians.

In addition to this predicted quantitative change, the quality of social work services in health care should improve as well, as more and more social workers with master's degrees and training in medical settings are employed to provide direct services. This increased use of professional social workers will occur as the standards for social work services are upgraded by the Joint Commission for the Accreditation of Hospitals and as licensing laws become effective in more states for licensed clinical social workers.

Another change in the future will concern access to social work services. The revisions in the welfare system in this country away from social work services and toward concentration on financial assistance have occurred at the same time as the expansion of social work services in the health care system. A person needing comprehensive social work services will increasingly obtain them in relation to health care rather than in relation to financial assistance. As health care facilities become the primary social system providing social work services to the community, the population served will increase to include all socioeconomic classes.

SUMMARY

The goal of social work is to maintain or restore each patient to his highest level of personal, social, and economic functioning. The factor determining whether or not a person has been successfully rehabilitated is the degree to which he adapts to his environment or his environment can be adapted to him. Social work with patients is directed toward the difficult transition between functioning in a hospital setting and returning home to assume responsibilities in the community. To achieve this readjustment and return to the community, social workers assist patients and their families in resolving personal and social problems. Social workers also use and develop community resources and serve as the liaison with community social agencies.[4]

REFERENCES

1. About Hospital Social Work Services, p. 6. Channing L. Bete, Greenfield, Mass., 1978 (pamphlet).

2. Bartlett, H. M.: *Social Work Practice in the Health Field*, p. 51. National Association of Social Workers, New York, 1966.

3. Bartlett, H. M.: *The Common Base of Social Work Practice*, pp. 139–160. National Association of Social Workers, New York, 1970.

4. Brunings, R. C.: *Social Work Policy and Procedure Manual*. Section II, Part 1: Rancho Los Amigos Hospital, Downey, Calif., 1979.

5. Dunham, O. C.: Phases of adjustment of the rehabilitation patient. Presented at the Institute on Rehabilitation and Chronic Disease for Faculty of Schools of Social Work, Rancho Los Amigos Hospital, Downey, Calif., February 1966.

6. Kahn, E.: The dynamic social work department, p. 3. American Hospital Association, Chicago, 1972.

7. Lurie, H. L.: *Encyclopedia of Social Work*, pp. 114–115. National Association of Social Workers, New York, 1965.

8. Moos, R. H.: *Coping with Physical Illness*, p. 9. Plenum Press, New York, 1977.

9. National Association of Social Workers and the American Hospital Association: Standards for hospital social services. Health Soc. Work 3(2):3–12, 1978.

10. Nickel, V. L., Stauffer, E. S., Wilcox, N. E., and Erickson, E.R.: *Final Report, Regional Spinal Cord Injury Rehabilitation Center SRS Grant 13-P-55279/9*, pp. 217–220. Attending Staff Association of the Rancho Los Amigos Hospital, Downey, Calif., May 1972.

11. The Hospital's Responsibility for the Psychosocial Aspects of Health Care. American Hospital Association, Chicago, 1970 (pamphlet).

11

The Clinical Psychologist

Douglas Cairns, Ph.D.

We place considerable limitations on understanding the role of the clinical psychologist, by using such a title as a description of who the psychologist is and what he does. About all that is to be inferred from this title is that the individual has participated in four years of graduate training devoted to the study of human behavior and two years of internship, possesses a doctoral degree, and assists people in achieving or maintaining a healthy adjustment. The manner in which he approaches the patient and applies his skills varies tremendously. This variability is generally a function of the differing philosophies of graduate programs around the country. Some are strongly oriented to the behaviorist viewpoint, in which the focus is on understanding factors that influence directly observable behavior. Others place more emphasis on internal events, such as thoughts and feelings, as the key to understanding and ministering to the patient's difficulties in adjustment. Although most programs require developing an expertise in areas of psychological testing, research design, statistics, neurophysiology, psychotherapy techniques, and psychopharmacology, the degree to which these are emphasized differs.

Considering the wide range of theoretical biases, training backgrounds, and available skills possessed by the clinical psychologist, it is understandable that problems can arise if he is asked to perform specific functions, such as ''I would like you to give this patient an MMPI,'' or ''Place this patient on a behavior modification program for weight loss.'' Whereas the psychologist may be fully qualified to perform these services, he may not feel they are appropriate. Instead of requesting specific functions of the psychologist, members of the rehabilitation team generally specify what information is needed or what changes they would like to see in the patient's emotional status. The psychologist then determines the best method of responding to the staff's request.

This chapter is certainly not free from theoretical biases. It should be considered representative of a behavioral approach to rehabilitation, except for the sections dealing with the psychologist's relationship to the treatment staff. I believe these sections transcend any particular theoretical positions in that most of my colleagues would agree that the clinical psychologist should be vigorously involved as a member of the rehabilitation team and have a firm understanding of each patient's treatment program.

DISABILITY

The Behavioral Viewpoint

Understanding factors governing human behavior and attempting to promote behavior change are the primary tasks of the clinical psychologist. Considering the complex nature of human behavior and the many forces exerting influence on it, these tasks appear quite formidable indeed. In an attempt to establish some rational framework within which human behavior might be examined, psychologists have always sought a model suitable to objective study.

For many years the clinical psychologist practiced within the medical model, in which abnormal behavior was seen to represent underlying emotional pathology. Pathology was viewed in terms of unconscious desires, unresolved childhood conflicts, weak egos, strong superegos, and other hypothetical constructs that, unless treated, would not permit return to "normal" behavior. For psychology, the medical model has not proved to be satisfactory. Numerous difficulties have been encountered attempting to measure the hypothetical constructs assumed to cause symptomatology. Moreover, symptomatology can be directly altered without treating the assumed underlying pathology. If symptomatic abnormal behavior can be eliminated without treating the underlying pathology, the medical model has questionable application at best. The past 20 years have been devoted to a large extent to developing and testing alternate models.

One such model evolved from behavioral science laboratories has been the "operant learning model." Assumptions of this model, stated simply, are that human behavior is dependent upon consequences it produces in the environment. That is, if a particular behavior leads to a reinforcement, the likelihood that the behavior will occur again under similar circumstances is increased.

The learning model does not assume that behavior is the function of an underlying unitary personality structure and its dynamics. Instead of seeking to explain behavior by theorizing about assumed intrapsychic causes, environmental consequences for expressing behaviors become the focus for examination. Understanding why one does or does not behave in a particular way requires knowledge of reinforcers specific to the individual. The process of ascertaining what is and what is not reinforcing for a given person is termed a "behavioral analysis."

Reinforcement is defined as anything that strengthens a behavior. Common examples of reinforcers are food and water, money, attention or approval from others, power, and prestige (it would be interesting to see how many books and articles would be written if the author's name were routinely omitted). Behavior is also strengthened if it produces an avoidance of punishment. Avoidance of unpleasant situations or people is an extremely powerful reinforcer, exerting influence over our behavior on a daily basis. Speed limits and traffic signals are obeyed to avoid traffic fines. We say "yes" when we would rather say "no" to avoid rejection and interpersonal difficulties.

Developing a Disability

Tissue pathology resulting in chronic illness significantly alters individual behavior. Changes in behavior that occur when the *person* becomes a *patient* range from taking medication, requesting help from others, and using assistive devices to total dependence devoid of self-responsibility.

Changes also occur in the patient's environment. Family and friends minister to him, expecting little in terms of independent function and offering much sympathy and support. If he enters the hospital, illness behavior is the norm. Typically, the hospital staff interacts with patients only if there is a problem. When the doctor makes bedside rounds, patients are asked to report their status. Often, the doctor responds to expressions of problems with a reassuring lengthy discussion. Statements of improvements usually result in less reinforcement—an inattentive smile and a perfunctory "that's good" as the doctor moves on to the next bed.

Consequences for expressions of illness behavior can produce a disability beyond what would be expected from the degree of tissue pathology. For example, continued expressions of disability may remove patients from intolerable work situations; provide them excuses for avoiding responsibility ("don't be upset by the fact that he slapped the child; after all, he *is* in a lot of pain," or, "not tonight, dear; I have a headache . . . backache . . . chest pain . . . an asthma attack"); offer the opportunity to avoid unpleasant social situations ("as soon as I get well my mother-in-law will move in with us—I am not fond of my mother-in-law"); or provide much needed attention and support ("so long as I'm unable to care for myself, my daughter will stay with me—after that I'll be alone again"). Under such circumstances, expressions of illness instead of well behavior are strongly reinforced.

The major concern related to reinforcement factors in chronic illness is that of time. The more time required for tissue healing, the more opportunity there is for illness behavior to be reinforced. If such a situation develops, treatment of tissue pathology alone may have little or no impact on altering the level of disability. It is therefore necessary for the clinical psychologist to determine if reinforcement factors are relevant. If they are, they must be dealt with in the rehabilitation process.

PREREQUISITES TO REHABILITATION: DETERMINING NEEDS

Prior to treatment, the psychologist determines the needs of the patient and staff. The most common need expressed by staff members is that patients cooperate with the treatment regimen. They are expected to arrive promptly at the treatment area and participate fully in therapy activities. They are expected to perform these activities often without understanding the rationale and without seeing progress for weeks or even months.

On the ward, medication is to be taken as prescribed without questions as to content and side effects. During bedside rounds, patients are expected to listen attentively and agree to "doctor's orders." They are expected to understand explanations of the disease process even when they involve such complex statements as "you have a defect in the pars interarticularis—you were born with it," or more simple-minded statements as "you have rusty pipes," or "you've slipped a disc." Much nodding of the head occurs on the part of the patient during these lectures and everyone assumes all is understood. Experience suggests that head-nodding is highly correlated with a complete lack of understanding. Furthermore, it can be assumed with some degree of validity that patients remember only about 20 percent of what is said to them at any given time.

Very often when the patient's response to treatment does not satisfy the needs and expectations of the staff, he receives various labels. "Unmotivated," "uncooperative," "combative," "manipulative," "a crank," and "flaky" are typical. In a few cases these may be apt descriptions. For the most part, however, they reflect an inadequate understanding of the patient's needs.

Many patients experience difficulty with a lengthy rehabilitation process because they need to understand their disability more completely. Others may need more frequent reinforcement than is typically available in therapy. Usually the only reinforcement for participation in therapy activities is an increase in functional ability. If improvement is not likely for several weeks at best, patients may give up in frustration.

Some patients require firm direction in their treatment program, whereas others need a close supportive relationship with staff. There are those, however, with whom such a relationship may foster dependency or self-pity. Still others may require support during early stages of rehabilitation and a push toward independence later on, and there are patients for whom the opposite sequence is better. The psychologist is often the only member of the rehabilitation team fully aware of the needs of patients *and* staff. Being aware of these needs serves to avoid misunderstandings and maintain communication. Once these needs are established, the rehabilitation program begins.

THE REHABILITATION PROCESS

Psychological Factors Affecting Rehabilitation

Rehabilitation is a most complex and comprehensive process requiring coordinated efforts of surgical and allied health specialists as well as those of the patient. Each individual enters this process with his own expectations and goals for the treatment's results. In general, the overall goals are to restore function or maintain existing function and improve the quality of life. If these aims are to be accomplished, the goals of each rehabilitation team member must not conflict and they must be consistent with those of the patient.

Having evaluated the patient, the psychologist gains an understanding of the emotional aspects of the disability, readiness for the program, and goals for treatment results. Emotional aspects of the disability can dramatically affect rehabilitation. Patients involved in orthopedic rehabilitation who have lost significant function or have lost an extremity from trauma or disease often progress through the stages of emotion usually seen with the terminally ill. Basically, these stages are denial, anger, bargaining, depression, and acceptance. This sequence of emotions is associated primarily with *loss* and is quite natural and in fact, according to some, necessary for eventual healthy adjustment.[6]

Patients who are depressed, that is, do not have access to reinforcement, may have no goals for treatment, appear passive, and receive a label of "unmotivated." Those who are angry or are attempting to fix blame for their condition may present as uncooperative, causing the staff to become impatient and request a discharge for disciplinary reasons. Patients in the denial phase might *appear* well-adjusted and accepting of the loss, but they may express unrealistic goals. For example, with one of the most devastating losses of all, the upper extremity amputation, the patient may wish to be fitted with a cosmetic hand to the exclusion of the more functional hook.

Careful discussion with the patient about his goals for treatment is conducted by each team member. The psychologist's advice regarding these goals usually is in response to requests from patients for a clear understanding of implications for future function and concerns about physical appearance. The psychological portion of rehabilitation, then, focuses on at least two major points: ensuring that patients have an adequate understanding of their disability and what they must *do* in the rehabilitation process; and assisting them to cope with demands of physical rehabilitation and, if necessary, adjustment to permanent loss of function or disfigurement and acceptance of assistive devices.

Since the patient's emotional status affects participation in all aspects of treatment on a day-to-day basis, the psychologist maintains daily contact with other members of the team. Close contact enables him to receive information about the patient's progress in therapy as well as apprise members of the rehabilitation team of relevant psychological information. For example, a patient might experience difficulty understanding and implementing self-care aspects of his therapy program for several interrelated reasons. He may wish to maintain a dependency relationship with family members; he may not adequately understand or may want to deny the permanent aspects of his disability and thus feel self-care is irrelevant; he may have difficulty paying attention because of worries or anxieties related to other matters; he may fear that too much progress will decrease the settlement of his pending litigation; or he may not like the therapist.

Often a great emphasis is placed on the need for understanding what implications disability has for the patient. This is certainly an appropriate and, in fact, a necessary part of rehabilitation. Also important is determining the implications for improving function. We assume that consequences for improved function can be nothing but positive. In some cases, however, improvement may have extremely negative consequences that far outweigh any gains made in rehabilitation. One patient, for example, had suffered separate injuries to his hand and lower back. Although he was progressing satisfactorily in his hand therapy program, he was resistant to low-back treatment. It was revealed that his low-back injury was work-related and compensable under worker's compensation. His hand injury was not work-related. If he were to progress with therapy for his low-back injury, he would eventually be rated as fit for work in regard to his back problem and compensation benefits would be discontinued. However, he would remain disabled from his job as a sheet-metal worker because of his hand disability, which was expected to require several additional months of rehabilitation. During this time, he could not receive adequate income. He saw as his only alternative, then, a continued low-back disability until his hand had regained enough function to permit return to work.

Another patient noted to have difficulty following through with his rehabilitation program indicated that once he recovered and was able to return to work, he would be required to resume alimony payments. So long as he remained on disability income, he was able to make more money than if he returned to work.

Careful monitoring of the patient's response to treatment places the psychologist in a position to deal with problems as they arise. To be effective, the psychologist's role must never be one of a consultant on the periphery to be called upon after problems have become unmanageable. If so, he enters the scene as a stranger, having little impact until he can develop a therapeutic relationship with the patient and a working relationship with the staff.

Techniques for Promoting Function

Having a thorough understanding of the patient's emotional reactions to disability and implications for improving, the psychologist is able to determine if certain behavioral techniques for promoting function would be worth including in the therapy programs. These techniques would involve application of the learning model defined earlier in the chapter. Behavioral techniques for promoting function have been well presented and documented elsewhere.[4] They will be referred to only briefly here.

The Therapist as a Behavioral Engineer. Viewing physical disability as a collection of behaviors subject to the influence of learning factors makes the distinction between physical and psychological disability less important than might be expected, provided the patient has the physical capacity for improved function. Virtually all rehabilitation can be seen as behavior modification even though it is performed by professionals in fields other than psychology. The power of social reinforcement in terms of the therapist's responses to the patient must never be underestimated. Often unknowingly, therapists produce significant change in the patient's level of disability simply by their reactions during treatment sessions. Since these reactions will occur regardless of a therapist's awareness of them, the psychologist assists therapists in recognizing their effect on the patient so as to assure change in the desired direction.

Biofeedback. A behavioral technique that has received considerable attention lately is biofeedback.[1] Advances in electrical instrumentation have made possible the manufacture of relatively inexpensive devices for measuring the physiological activity of body processes. Levels of activity are then displayed to the patient visually or auditorily. Feedback is then used by the patient to learn voluntary control over the system being monitored. For example, if it is felt that the patient is suffering from muscle tension headaches, surface electromyograph electrodes are placed over the frontalis muscles. Minute changes in muscle activity are measured and displayed on a meter. The patient then seeks to lower the meter reading, resulting in lower levels of muscle tension in hopes of decreasing headache pain. Although it is extremely difficult to reduce muscle activity when simply instructed to do so, appreciable decreases are achieved when feedback of small changes is made available to the patient.

Using a blood pressure cuff, the same principle has been employed to teach patients with essential hypertension to lower their blood pressure. Other disorders that appear to be treated successfully with biofeedback include migraine headaches, bruxism, epilepsy, insomnia, phobic reactions, and anxiety.

Biofeedback has been applied as well to muscle re-education. Stroke victims have been successsfully taught to strengthen muscles by a procedure opposite that of muscle relaxation. Instead of decreasing muscle activity, these patients learn to increase, in small increments, the activity of muscles affected by the stroke.

If it is possible to determine the underlying physiological process associated with a disorder and if small changes can be measured, it is then theoretically possible to treat the problem with biofeedback. Biofeedback, although currently finding wide applications, remains in the research stage. Any application of biofeedback requires a carefully planned protocol and evaluation of treatment results if it is to become a rational treatment procedure.

Contracts.   Behavioral contracts offer an additional technique for promoting function when the patient is not progressing sufficiently.[5] Staff concerns about his slow progress are presented to the patient and, with his cooperation, a contract is established whereby access to reinforcers is made dependent on specific amounts of improvement. The patient identifies the reinforcers and, by signing a contract, agrees that they are to be delivered only following specified behavior. For example, a 12-year-old boy with juvenile rheumatoid arthritis scheduled for bilateral total hip-joint replacement surgery was experiencing difficulty proning and ambulating because of pain. He refused to participate in physical therapy, spending most of his time in his room assembling model airplanes supplied by recreational therapy. With his cooperation, a contract was devised that required him to purchase model kits *and* gain access to them using tokens (poker chips) earned in physical therapy. The more progress he made, the more tokens he earned, and the more time he could spend working on his models in the evening. The result was improved participation and progress.

Progress in rehabilitation is typically quite gradual. Patients work for weeks and sometimes months before improvement is evident. Under these circumstances, reinforcement of participation by obvious signs of improvement is delayed. We know that if reinforcement is to strengthen behavior efficiently, it must occur as soon as possible following that behavior. In order to accomplish this more effectively, progress can be measured, recorded, and, in some cases, graphically displayed. Small gains can then be presented, thereby providing the patient with reinforcement to continue. These gains can also be recognized by staff in the form of attention and approval, providing additional reinforcement. All too often, attention from staff occurs only if the patient is not improving and serves to strengthen the wrong behavior—that is, lack of progress.

REHABILITATION OF CHRONIC SPINAL PAIN

Behavioral approaches to rehabilitation provide the basis for the Spinal Pain Service at Ranchos Los Amigos Hospital.[2,3,7] Over the past nine years, more than 4000 patients have been admitted to the program with encouraging results. The behavioral approach, embracing as it does the concept of operant conditioning, directs us to evaluate the consequences of pain behavior. Attention, sympathy, and support from significant others occur following complaints of pain—the patient's spouse exhibits concern, friends and relatives visit more frequently, and children become more helpful. Reinforcement continues so long as expressions of pain continue.

In most cases, family and friends eventually tire of this routine. If they stop providing reinforcement, however, pain behavior typically increases in strength and frequency. A normal gait becomes a limp. A limp now requires a cane or crutches. More time is spent in bed, and emergency room visits are more frequent. Under these conditions, it becomes increasingly difficult to withhold attention and sympathy.

As pain behavior increases, the resulting inactivity may cause joints to become stiff and muscles to weaken. Pain becomes the primary focus of attention and topic of conversation. Medication intake increases and aspirin is discarded in favor of narcotic analgesics. Behaviors associated with what was once an acute pain evolves into a disability strengthened by continued reinforcement.

Although social reinforcement in the form of attention and concern plays a role in the learning and maintenance of pain behavior, it is by no means the most important variable. Disability associated with low-back pain appears to develop more frequently under conditions in which expressions of pain remove unpleasant stimuli, provide time out from stress, and relieve the individual of responsibilities. Distasteful or dangerous work duties are avoided; and, if difficulties in self-assertion exist, expressions of pain provide greater control in social interactions.

Following the initial injury, activities that "aggravate" pain become less frequent. Close examination may reveal these to have a low reinforcing value or they may even be aversive. For example, riding in a car to and from an unpleasant job may be painful, or sitting long enough to perform the job may increase pain. Pain may be endured, however, while riding in a car to visit friends or sitting to watch a good movie. In a sense, the patient may be saying, "If I am going to hurt, I might as well hurt while I am doing something I like." Unfortunately, family members, employers, and insurance companies will rarely tolerate such an attitude. A husband may ask his wife why she is able to work in the garden, visit friends, and go shopping, but cannot wash clothes, clean the house, and prepare meals. The insurance company may wish to know why the patient can play golf and go fishing but cannot work. Not surprisingly, the inquisitions begin to acquire an aversive nature and to avoid them the patient becomes increasingly inactive. Under such circumstances, then, pain behavior originally associated with tissue pathology comes under the control of the patient's environment.

Evaluation

On admission to the Spinal Pain Service, the patient is routinely administered psychological tests, including the Minnesota Multiphasic Personality Inventory (MMPI). Testing is not designed to determine if pain is "real" or "imaginary," since this is an artificial distinction and is most always an unproductive pursuit. Instead, testing attempts to illustrate the degree to which pain complaints and perception may be influenced by reinforcing environmental factors and how the patient is likely to respond to treatment. A behavioral analysis is also conducted to determine further the role of environmental factors affecting expressions of pain by examining the consequences they produce in terms of attention, sympathy, and avoidance of unpleasant situations.

Results of the evaluation are then presented to rehabilitation team members for planning the treatment. Because the problem of chronic spinal pain cannot be treated medically alone or psychologically alone, yet does involve a considerable amount of psychological assessment, the psychologist serves as *coordinator* of the treatment program, consulting with patients and team members daily.

Target Activities

Target activities or goals take two forms: those identified by the treatment staff and those identified by the patient. Staff goals usually involve increasing muscle-strengthening exercises and functional ability, decreasing medication, returning the patient to work and recreational activity, and reducing his pain. Unless these too are the patient's goals, treatment will be unsuccessful. Patients are required to specify in behavioral terms activities they wish to perform. For example, "I would like to be able to stand 30 minutes for shopping and washing dishes, sit for 60 minutes, and walk for 15 minutes."

Almost any activity limited by pain may be objectively measured in time or frequency. Activity baselines may be obtained for walking distance and velocity, sitting time, time spent out of bed, standing time, exercise repetition, and time and distance on an exercycle.

Precise measures are essential, in some cases requiring counters or timers, so any initial slight change in the desired direction can be reinforced. For example, a switch similar to that which operates an automatic door may be placed beneath a chair and attached to an electric clock to measure sitting time. A similar apparatus, to be described, can be used to measure time out of bed. The physical therapist establishes the patient's tolerance for mat exercises, walking, exercycle, and quadriceps strengthening, and provides instruction in posture and basic spinal anatomy. The occupational therapist establishes tolerance for sitting and standing time, and provides instruction in relaxation, time management, body mechanics, and assertion skills to learn alternatives to using pain as an excuse for avoiding responsibility.

Medication Intake. Frequency, dosage, and type represent measures of medication intake. Since the patient is typically inaccurate when recording his own intake, the spouse may be recruited to make these recordings at home. Hospital baselines are obtained from the nurse when medication is initially prescribed on an "on-demand" basis.

Subjective Pain Level. Baseline pain levels are determined by asking the patient to rate his pain on a daily basis, using a scale of 0 = no pain to 100 = worst possible pain. The accuracy of this measure of pain is not a concern in the present setting, because pain ratings over time are more an indication of willingness to admit improvement than of actual intensity.

Up-time. Amount of time spent out of bed is most easily measured by an up-time recorder. This device consists of a pressure-activated switch placed under the mattress and connected to a clocklike apparatus mounted on the headboard. The clock only runs if the patient is out of bed, thereby measuring cumulative uptime.

Health Care Utilization. The number of doctor's visits, emergency room visits, hospitalizations, and the amounts of money spent for treatment and medication are measures of health care utilization. Baselines can be obtained prior to admission from the patient, spouse, or, in some cases, the insurance company. Continued recordings after discharge provide some indication of the effects of treatment.

Behavioral Treatment

Providing praise and attention for well behavior while remaining unresponsive to pain behavior appears to be an effective method of treatment for chronic low-back disability. At the outset, procedures are initiated to shift the focus of attention from pain sources and behavior to well behavior. Patients are informed that discussing their pain in daily conversation is counterproductive. Such talk does not reduce pain but instead provides a focus for attention. They are informed that staff members will avoid engaging in pain-related conversations. Instead, attempts are made to elicit other reinforceable conversation by responding to pain complaints with: "Let's not talk about your pain; let's talk about the progress you're making." Although this seldom eliminates all complaints, it does seem to reduce them appreciably.

Reluctance to stop *all* pain references probably reflects the caution with which most patients approach change. Treatment, for many, means a radical change in the way they conduct their lives. Most patients continue expressing pain simply in order to communicate: "I may be improving, but don't expect too much too soon. I'm not sure I'm ready to deal with what is expected of me when I get well."

Increasing amounts of each activity are prescribed daily by the therapists. The use of a publicly displayed performance graph is a particularly effective means of recording and reinforcing desired changes in target activities. A large graph (60 × 90 cm) is placed above the bed, and walking distance, sitting time, standing time, and other factors are plotted daily on it by staff making bedside rounds. If the plotted level represents an increase in activity, time is spent at the bedside praising the patient and engaging him in desirable conversation. If no improvement is noted, the graph is simply plotted and returned to its position over the bed.

Behavioral treatment also involves individual and group sessions in which techniques of pain management are presented and discussions about identifying sources of stress and reinforcers for pain behavior are held.

Medication. The frequency of narcotic usage found in treating chronic low-back pain is of such magnitude as to require a drug detoxification plan. First it is necessary to discontinue medication on a pain-dependent basis. Under these conditions, medication serves as a reinforcer for pain complaints. All narcotics, then, are mixed in a liquid masking agent and administered orally every four hours regardless of pain complaints. The amount of liquid is held constant at 15 ml while the active ingredients are gradually withdrawn. Eventually medication consists solely of the masking agent. The patient is informed that his medication will be decreased but will not be told when reduction occurs.

Family Education. If changes in target activities are to persist after discharge, the spouse or relatives must be willing and able to continue an atmosphere reinforcing these activities.

To accomplish this, the patient and principal relations meet with staff for instructions in reinforcement techniques. The staff emphasizes the importance of identifying and reinforcing well behavior. Videotaped examples of a patient expressing pain behavior and well behavior are presented. Instruction in the application of reinforcement techniques follows. Weekend passes are provided and then the patient and family attempt to apply these techniques in practice. Difficulties encountered are discussed with staff members during frequent contact with the spouse or relatives throughout treatment.

When patient and family become actively involved in the rehabilitation process, they assume a major portion of the responsibility for improvement. Accomplishing this step early in treatment makes the transition from hospital to home much smoother at discharge. For many patients, the rehabilitation process is lifelong, and only a small portion of this process occurs in the hospital. If progress is to continue, the family must be supportive in the proper direction.

SUMMARY

The role of the clinical psychologist is perhaps the most comprehensive compared with other members of the rehabilitation team. To understand the patient's emotional reaction to his disability, the psychologist must have a thorough understanding of both tissue pathology and the demands of physical rehabilitation. He must be able to monitor the patient's reaction to each aspect of the therapy program, maintaining close contact with both patient and staff. He also must know the patient's family so as to understand the interpersonal dynamics that may affect therapy and post-discharge follow-through.

Perhaps one of the most important functions of the clinical psychologist is to be able to communicate psychological information to the members of the rehabilitation team. Care must be taken to avoid useless esoteric terminology in written and verbal reports because psychological information is often used to alter the treatment approach or to understand patient reactions to particular aspects of therapy.

Examining the results of treatment by way of applied research represents the psychologist's contribution to the future of orthopedic rehabilitation. This future depends upon using rational treatment approaches of demonstrated effectiveness.

By virtue of his background and training, the clinical psychologist is often the member of the rehabilitation team called upon to design research and analyze data. In the rehabilitation setting where the goal of treatment is to improve the quality of life, the psychologist views all treatment as applied research to determine whether, in fact, this goal is accomplished. Research, then, does not necessarily take the form of testing hypotheses in carefully controlled laboratory settings. It involves careful evaluation of the patient's progress with various treatment approaches and an examination of follow-up results. These data, then, provide a rational basis for modifying the treatment furnished by all members of the rehabilitation team.

REFERENCES

1. Brown, B. B.: *Biofeedback—New Directions for the Mind.* Harper & Row, New York, 1974.
2. Cairns, D., and Pasino, J.: Comparison of verbal reinforcement and feedback in the operant treatment of disability due to chronic low back pain. Behav. Ther. 8:621–630, 1977.
3. Cairns, D., Thomas, L., Mooney, V., and Pace, J.: A comprehensive treatment approach to chronic low back pain. Pain 2:301–307, 1976.
4. Fordyce, W.: *Behavioral Methods for Chronic Pain and Illness.* C. V. Mosby, St. Louis, 1976.
5. Kanfer, F. J., and Phillips, J. S.: *Learning Foundations of Behavior Therapy,* pp. 437–438. John Wiley & Sons, New York, 1970.
6. Kubler-Ross, E.: *On Death and Dying.* Macmillan, New York, 1969.
7. Mooney, V., and Cairns, D.: Management in the patient with chronic low back pain. Orthop. Clin. North Am. 9:543–577, 1978.

12

Vocational Rehabilitation

Carolyn L. Vash, Ph.D.

THE IMPORTANCE OF WORK

For most human beings, work is just as important to psychological and social functioning as it is to economic survival. The activities and social status associated with work are as vital as earnings in avoiding the destructive effects of being powerless. The sense of powerlessness can cause immensely varied kinds of human suffering, including depression, suicide, failure to recover from illness and trauma, and failure to rebuild a life after even the best medical and rehabilitative care has been offered. In our society, the individual who is unable to work is deprived not only of the most effective survival tool that exists, but also of the major available path toward self-esteem and self-actualization.

Typically, work occupies nearly half of one's waking life, and considerably more than that for some people, including a fair proportion of physicians. You know how important your work as a health professional is to you. What would it mean in your life if you were suddenly unable to do it? Many if not most of your patients have similar attachments to their work. It gives structure to their time, it is the major determinant of their sense of identity, and frequently it constitutes their primary *raison d'être*—none of which can be relinquished lightly.

In a materialistically oriented society, to be without earnings is to be deprived of access to the vast array of material comforts and pleasures that one sees others enjoy. The barest necessities may be provided through a welfare system, but at enormous cost in terms of loss of privacy, loss of pride, and the devastating experience of what Erving Goffman[1] has termed "the mortification process." Thus, almost everyone needs to work, and for a wide spectrum of psychological, social, and economic reasons. The advent of a permanent orthopedic disability seldom changes any of those basic needs. What *does* change is the likelihood of being able to fulfill them. Ironically, the interference caused by the functional limitations of the disability itself may be minor compared to the additional and often unnecessary handicapping imposed upon the person by the external world.

BARRIERS TO EMPLOYMENT FOR WORKERS WITH DISABILITIES

To begin with, it is important to distinguish between the disability and any handicapping effects it may have. Residual anatomical, physiological, or psychological damage resulting from an illness, injury, or birth defect is the disability. Paralysis is an example. Whether or not a paralyzed person is also handicapped depends on what he or she is trying to do. For example, even a severely paralyzed person may not be particularly handicapped in delivering a lecture before a group. However, if a fire drill were suddenly ordered, that person might be seriously handicapped indeed. The extent of handicapping would depend on such external factors as the technology available to the lecturer, such as a wheelchair that can be independently operated, and whether or not the building is ramped or has fire emergency elevators. With these distinctions in mind, it is next necessary to look at the existing barriers to employment for many workers with orthopedic disabilities.

First, many employment sites have architectural barriers that make it difficult or impossible for workers with disabilities, especially wheelchair users, to work there. Unramped staircases, no elevators, inaccessible restrooms, narrow aisles, and cramped work stations are among the primary barriers to mobility within a work plant. In addition, even when a work plant is reasonably accessible, workers who are so severely disabled as to be unable to drive will not have access to public transportation to get to work. Fortunately, with the advent of federal and state legislation relating to mobility barrier abatement, the future looks more hopeful.

The second type of barrier to be circumvented is attitudinal. It is employer prejudice against disabled workers. Employers are better educated today than they were a decade ago about myths and realities concerning insurance risks. However, their fears that disabled workers will somehow be unable to deliver a high-quality product or service on time have proved more difficult to dislodge. Fortunately, again, recent federal and state legislation relating to equal employment opportunity, affirmative action, and fair employment practices is also making the prognosis for this matter more favorable.

A third type of barrier a worker with a disability may confront is procedural. This problem encompasses such diverse matters as labor contracts and job descriptions requiring job applicants to be able to perform certain duties, which, in fact, they may seldom or never be called on to do. Like mobility and attitudinal barriers, these procedural obstacles still persist to a significant degree, but they too are slowly being combatted by legislation.

However, one procedural barrier exists that has not been addressed by law and may never be. This involves procedures relating to medical and rehabilitative care. An important instance is the situation in which a disabled worker could return to work, or initiate work activity, if medical and rehabilitative appointment times were available outside of normal working hours—that is, evenings or weekends. The need to leave work for even one doctor's appointment or a session or two of physical therapy per week may seriously jeopardize the worker's relationship with his or her employer. Another frequently cited problem is the failure to take the disabled worker's job-related needs into account in the scheduling of surgery—considering only the demands on the surgeon's time and consequent operating room availability. However, there have been cases in which the actual surgical procedures have been altered as a result of the surgeon becoming aware of job-related functional demands on the patient.

The fourth and final type of barrier involved is that imposed by the disability itself—the loss of certain functions that would make job performance in certain areas possible or more accomplishable. This obstacle is listed last because, in view of the richness of feasible work areas for people with even severe orthopedic disabilities, it may actually cause less handicapping than the others with respect to obtaining *some* kind of employment. Yet it may be a significant barrier to getting and doing the specific type of job that individual has done in the past or wants to do in the future.

AVAILABLE SOLUTIONS

This section will proceed chronologically, to the extent such is possible, to illustrate the manner in which vocational rehabilitation progresses.

The vocational rehabilitation process generally begins with a contact with a *rehabilitation counselor,* who is primarily an expert in vocational counseling. These individuals typically have master's degrees in rehabilitation counseling and may be certified by the Council on Rehabilitation Education. The counselor helps clients identify interests, abilities, and skills that can be built upon to develop new or altered vocations. In so doing, the counselor also provides expert information on general occupational fields and specific labor markets to guide clients in making choices. Following initial counseling, if questions remain about what a client is able to do or would find satisfying on a relatively long-term basis, other vocational rehabilitation experts may be called upon. For example, *vocationally oriented psychologists* can administer and interpret standardized tests of interest, aptitudes, educational level, and skills and *work evaluators* can test the client on real or simulated work samples to discern strengths and weaknesses in performance. Work evaluators, like rehabilitation counselors, are striving for professional growth and the standard of the master's degree. Throughout these evaluative processes, the counselor and client use the information generated to move in successive approximations toward a suitable vocational choice.

At this point it is important to describe the types of agencies in which these and other vocational rehabilitation specialists work, because the policies of those agencies materially influence the types and extent of services to be provided. Nationwide, the state and federal vocational rehabilitation program is the major employer of rehabilitation counselors. This program was created by federal law in the 1930s and has continued to grow until the present. All American states and territories have a service-delivery arm of this state-federal partnership, and they employ rehabilitation counselors as their primary service providers. As such, they furnish the counseling and job placement services to clients directly, and they are responsible for procuring and coordinating all other specialized services their clients may need. Some of the small states employ less than 50 counselors for this purpose, whereas California, the most populous state, hires in excess of 700. The federal agency responsible for overseeing this program is the Rehabilitation Services Administration (RSA), housed within the United States Department of Education. RSA generates regulations governing who can be served, toward what ends, and to what extent by the state agencies—which are usually designated "Division," "Bureau," or "Department" of "Rehabilitation" or "Vocational Rehabilitation."

RSA has also assumed the responsibility for developing rehabilitation facilities in the private, nonprofit, and local government sectors that have the express purpose of vending the needed specialized services to the state agencies. They employ the full range of vocational rehabilitation specialists mentioned here. Like the state agencies, these facilities also have considerable history behind them.

Since the late 1970s, a third employer of significant numbers of vocational rehabilitation specialists has emerged, pursuant to legislation mandating rehabilitation for people who sustain industrial injuries. A private-practice market has appeared in the for-profit sector, and increasing numbers of rehabilitation counselors, work evaluators, and others can be found there.

In all three of these service delivery systems, sources of funds are available for persons who cannot afford to pay for the time-consuming and costly procedures necessary to obtain the help they need. The first two are supported by public funds and the third relies on insurance monies.

To return to the vocational rehabilitation process, once a tentative decision has been made, the client will begin a work preparation program if such is needed. Some persons who become disabled are fully able to continue their pre-disability training or work directions, either with or without adaptive equipment or services. Many more, however, must prepare to alter appreciably their career plans or methods of functioning in training or work.

For those who have not had a great deal of previous work experience, or who must radically change their vocational directions, *work adjustment specialists* may be called upon to plan and conduct programs for work habit training. Here, the client has an opportunity to experience realistic employer demands for such work habits as punctuality and acceptance of supervision, and to build up tolerance for a normal work day. Special settings—known colloquially as "sheltered workshops," but which actually attempt to minimize sheltering and maximize realistic work standards and expectations—may be used. When available, specially supervised work stations may be established in ordinary work settings for the same purposes.

Either simultaneously with or following the work adjustment process, the actual job skill training may take place. Just as the rehabilitation counselors coordinate the work evaluation and work adjustment services just described, they are also responsible for helping their clients secure vocational training in order to have saleable job skills to offer potential employers. The type of training will be selected on the basis of the evaluation results, the client's response to work adjustment, the length of training considered realistic given the client's needs and aptitudes, and costs. Training may range from as little as a few weeks for a circumscribed skill, to the seven or eight years required to obtain a graduate degree. If special equipment or services are required to permit the person to succeed in training, they are potentially available through both the publicly and insurance-funded programs. Specially equipped vans, motorized wheelchairs controllable by minute muscle action, and modified electric typewriters and tape recorders are among the more common devices secured to help severely orthopedically disabled students to function in training. *Vocationally oriented rehabilitation engineers* may be called upon to develop unique solutions to problems with equipment.

For the most part, ordinary resources for vocational education and training rather than programs designed solely for students with disabilities are employed. The reason is simple: future workers who have disabilities, even severe ones, need to be integrated into the mainstream as early as possible to avoid a heightened re-entry trauma later on. However, in some cases, specialized training programs have made it possible for severely disabled people to break into the world of work earlier and gradually. Their supports are rich at first, but they are reduced as independent means for solving day-to-day problems are found. Sometimes such training programs are located right on the grounds of a rehabilitation hospital.

After a patient completes his or her job skill training, the next steps are job search and development and job placement. *Job placement specialists* may be called upon to tutor the client in the fine arts of how to find and get a job. Methods of locating and understanding job market information are taught, as well as techniques for making a positive impression on potential employers. In addition to tutoring the client, the job placement specialist may personally assume responsibility for such activities as showing employers how they could benefit by redividing the labor in a way that could create a "do-able" job for a very severely disabled worker. Again, the rehabilitation engineer may be called upon to solve problems presented by the worker's physical limitations.

It is important at this juncture to make a distinction between "sheltered" versus "accommodated" employment for workers with disabilities. "Shelter" designates employment in which the worker is protected from the harsh necessity of meeting ordinary and usual performance expectations. The quantity or quality of production may be less than expected from the typical worker in an equivalent position without the usual sanctions being applied. "Accommodation," however, implies no such relaxation of standards. This term designates employment wherein needed adjustments and adaptations are made so the disabled worker *can* meet ordinary and usual performance expectations. The accommodations may be physical, as in the installation of ramps or machine modifications, or procedural, as in allowing a schedule with flexible hours or trade-offs in duties with another worker. A major aim within the entire, interdisciplinary, vocational rehabilitation field is to maximize the degree of accommodation that employers will offer disabled workers in order to minimize the degree of shelter they need.

After the client has been hired and the initial problems have been solved, the rehabilitation counselor will continue to maintain contact with the person (a minimum of three months is required by the state-federal program) to help solve problems that emerge as the job unfolds. Post-employment follow-up services may include anything from psychological counseling regarding anxieties about "making it" to additional fine tuning by the rehabilitation engineer.

For many, arriving at this moment closes the vocational rehabilitation process. Having been counseled, evaluated, adjusted, trained, placed, and checked out, they are through with vocational rehabilitation forever (unless, of course, they enter the field themselves, as quite a number of former clients are inclined to do). Others will find it necessary to go through at least part of the process again, which can only be expected in these days of accelerating job obsolescence. It is an important aspect of our society, and it touches everyone, including people with disabilities.

THE POLITICS OF VOCATIONAL REHABILITATION

This chapter began with a statement on the psychological, social, and economic importance of work to human beings. The fact is, however, that there are simply not enough jobs to go around. In recent years approximately 10 percent of the work force has always been unemployed. First the ethnic minorities, then women, and now disabled and older workers have coalesced into special interest groups fighting to ensure that they are not overrepresented among the inevitable unemployed. "The organized disabled" are now fighting hard and effectively to recapture their constitutional rights to equal protection under the law and, predictably, the central issue is jobs.

Lobbyists from a long roster of national and local "consumer" organizations address Congress, state legislatures, county boards of supervisors, city councils, and other public officials daily, demanding that their disabled constituents' needs be heard and responded to when decisions are made regarding such issues as job opportunity programs and welfare regulations, which, ironically, contain disincentives to gainful activity. The well-publicized suicide of an almost totally paralyzed young woman whose welfare grant was stopped because she earned a few dollars more than allowed, but who could not have survived outside of an institution without the grant, catalyzed a nationwide movement among disabled people to change the laws and regulations viewed as the proximal causes of such human tragedies.

As a result, ongoing job programs designed expressly for workers with disabilities have received added impetus. One of the best is nationwide and is known as "Projects with Industry," a partnership between the state-federal vocational rehabilitation program and industry. Here, special recruiting, selection, pre-job and on-the-job training procedures are established for getting workers with major disabilities integrated into the industry involved in the project.

Another important social trend in education is mainstreaming. Special segregated schools for youngsters with disabilities are being phased out and replaced with support systems allowing most of those children to be educated along with their non-disabled peers in local public schools. For children with orthopedic disabilities, the primary effort is the elimination of architectural barriers in the school plants. A few severely disabled children will also need special equipment and perhaps a little attendant care during the school day.

Mainstreaming is a drastic change currently causing all of the commotion change typically engenders. But when the new ways are familiar, they should contribute greatly to reducing the traditional attitudinal barriers toward people with disabilities. When employers think back on the fact that disabled children were not even allowed to go to the same schools they did, it is no wonder they have difficulty imagining that disabled grownups could fit into their work settings. Contact with people who have disabilities from childhood on should appreciably reduce the prejudices that develop about people we do not understand.

Through a combination of efforts, such as those described, plus the inclusion of disabled workers as a "protected population" under affirmative action, fair employment practice, and equal opportunity programs, the job picture for this group is gradually improving. The outlook should be a great comfort to orthopedists and other physicians who must sometimes wonder if all of the long, painstaking medical and rehabilitative care were worthwhile when they hear of their former patients sitting idle in nursing homes or choosing suicide over the kind of life they see in store for them.

REFERRAL BY THE PHYSICIAN

One of the questions physicians most frequently ask about vocational rehabilitation is, "How can I tell who is a good candidate to refer?" It is true that not everyone has the potential for becoming employed—the combination of the disability plus other factors may leave the person with too few resources to draw from in building saleable skills. Thus, it may be helpful to make a quick mental analysis of the patient's work-related resources when deciding whether to refer.

Most jobs can be seen as drawing from one or more of four basic types of worker resources: brawn, brain, hand, and personality. The meaning of "brawn" is as obvious as it seems. "Brain" includes the whole range of intellectual, creative, and aptitudinal capacities plus educational background. "Hand" means the dexterity and skill potential to manipulate, create, maintain, or use objects. "Personality" means strictly the ability to influence other people's behavior and attitudes. A fifth factor is not a worker resource per se, but it is an important backup variable—emotional stability. If a person has too little of it, no wealth of worker resources can guarantee employment.

The referring physician has only to imagine if the patient has some degree of usable strength in any one of the four worker resource areas, plus at least a moderate degree of emotional stability. Should the answer be an unequivocal "no," it would be better not to refer the person to an inevitable experience of failure. If the answer is "maybe" or "yes," the person should be referred to the state vocational rehabilitation office nearest his or her home. Every state has printed brochures about its program, and a supply should be available in the physician's office. In addition, there is a growing trend for the state vocational rehabilitation agencies to station one or more rehabilitation counselors in community hospitals. This simplifies and improves the quality of the communication between physicians and vocational rehabilitation specialists.

Well over a decade ago, the editor of this volume asked me to start a vocational services program at the hospital he then directed, saying, "It occurs to me that there is no point in all of this physical rehabilitation if we are just going to send them home to sit on the stoop and do nothing. We've got to help them get back into the mainstream of life and that means *work*." That is still the message.

REFERENCE

1. Goffman, E.: *Asylums*. Aldine, Chicago, 1961.

13

Sports Medicine and Rehabilitation

Michael J. Smith, M.D.
Marcus J. Stewart, M.D.

Sports medicine rehabilitation has been practiced for the last 3000 years. The ancient Greeks had athletic contests intermixed with their military drills. The need to recover from an injury or an illness was great, because the soldier-athlete was needed to defend his village from the surrounding towns' invasions. Herodicus, Hippocrates, and Galen were known to have treated athletes and worked in rehabilitation. By looking at classical art, we can find several advances in early sports medicine. Sculptures and paintings show that athletes began to gain weight as the value of good nutrition and developing muscles became appreciated. Some sculptures of the athletic participants are so naturalistic that in a boxer, for example, we can detect explicit athletic injuries, such as cauliflower ears and fractures of the nasal and maxilla bones.[7]

The object of treatment from the beginning of time has been the quick restoration of the injured or ill person to full functional capacity. Time, knowledge, and science have never altered this prime objective. Injury is too often equated with the musculoskeletal system and the plan of treatment is directed only toward restoration of the anatomy. We must appreciate that the injury may be not only to the body, but also to the athlete's mind and self-concept. Then it becomes evident that merely restoring the anatomy to normal may not restore the individual to his full capacity. In no place is this situation more evident than in the athlete.

With today's increased interest in physical fitness, sports medicine has become very popular as well. As athletes command higher and higher salaries, coaches and team owners have realized the necessity of returning professional athletes to action as quickly as possible. James Nicholas, the director of the Lenox Hill Institute for Sports Medicine and Trauma, told *The New York Times*, "You've got to recognize that in show business, if the star doesn't perform and the team doesn't sell tickets, you go bankrupt."[10] And coupled with the commitment to keeping professional athletes functioning is the general population's increasing devotion to physical culture and participation in sports. In the United States and in most other nations the professional and college athletes receive the most notice, publicity, and popularity. However, their injuries account for only about 10 percent of those among the athlete population. Therefore treatment and rehabilitation must be planned for the other 90 percent. That includes the young, the pre-college, and the recreational athlete of all ages. The principles of treatment and rehabilitation are the same for all athletes; only the speed and intensity of their application must be altered. The goal always remains the same: complete recovery and as rapid a return to normal activity as possible.

It is also important for the physicians, coaches, and trainers who are treating and taking care of the professional and recreational athlete to have a thorough understanding of the physiology of the injury and healing response. Knowledge of appropriate rehabilitation measures is imperative.

The physician and his allies who deal with athletes and sports injuries must also learn that their prime objective has to be to return the athlete to full, competitive capacity. Although proper and prompt treatment is imperative, merely treating the illness or injury will never suffice. The doctor must, from the day of his initial contact with the patient, have as the objective of his plan of treatment the complete restoration of *function*. The physician must gain the confidence and respect of the athlete, since the final result, regardless of the type and location of injury, will depend on the mental attitude of the patient and the rapport of the doctor with his patient. It is not sufficient to tell an athlete to rest until the injury no longer hurts. The physician must demonstrate to the athlete that he knows the sport itself and explain in terms of that sport why a certain treatment and rehabilitation program are needed. If the athlete doubts or distrusts the physician, he will not listen to his advice or follow the regimen.

The most neglected part of the musculoskeletal system in rehabilitation is the muscle itself. All too frequently attention is directed toward the bone or ligament injury and not enough understanding and time are spent on the muscle itself.

MUSCLE PHYSIOLOGY APPLIED TO SPORTS MEDICINE

After the injury, muscles atrophy. Lack of recognition of this diseased muscle motor unit leads to an inadequate rehabilitation. Not only must muscle strength be re-established, but the strength must be re-obtained in a functional capacity, which is always specific to the patient's performance.

Immobilization is detrimental to muscle function;[6] whenever possible, it should be avoided. Early active exercise is the key to prompt recovery. Activity decreases swelling and joint stiffness, and it is the swelling and joint stiffness that prolong the athlete's absence from competition.

Even though the athlete may have sustained only a partial injury, the total patient must be considered. Every attempt should be made to lessen the effects of decreased training, especially the loss of strength and cardiovascular fitness. An athlete with a broken hand can still run and participate in an exercise program for the lower extremities. A runner with shin splints should be allowed to swim or ride a bicycle to keep his overall conditioning at a peak level.

Muscles contract, and through the physiological lever system of bone and joints, cause the joint to move. A muscle may shorten when it contracts. This type of contraction is called a concentric contraction. The muscle contraction causes the joint to move and the muscle shortens as it contracts. Muscles also can contract eccentrically, meaning that the muscle actually lengthens as it contracts. An example of an eccentric contraction occurs when a person stands on his toes and then slowly lowers himself to the floor. The gastrocnemius and soleus muscle groups perform an eccentric contraction in preventing a quick flop back to the floor. Eccentric contractions produce more muscle soreness than concentric contractions.

There are two basic types of muscle fibers: slow-twitch muscle fibers and fast-twitch muscle fibers. They are named for the speed of their contraction. Actually there are two types of fast-twitch fibers, but for clarity and understanding of the rehabilitation concepts, only the primary slow- and fast-twitch fibers are described here.

The slow-twitch fibers contract at rates of 120 milliseconds. They are slow in contracting and relaxing. Their resistance to fatigue is very high, as are their mitochondria and capillary densities. They have a very low anaerobic potential and are often called "red fibers" because of their high capillary density. Slow-twitch fibers function well in postural support. For example, the soleus muscle has a high percentage of slow-twitch fibers.

Fast-twitch fibers contract at rates of approximately every 40 milliseconds. They are called white fibers because their capillary density is not as great as that of the slow-twitch fibers. Their mitochondrial density is low, yet they do have a high anaerobic potential. Fast-twitch fibers have a higher number of muscle fibers innervated by a single motor nerve. This allows larger tension development.[1] The biceps has a large population of fast-twitch fibers.

Fast-twitch fibers can be trained to build up some oxidative capacity. In endurance training, the adaptation of fast-twitch fibers to use aerobic pathways is of major importance.

After an injury, slow-twitch fibers atrophy first,[4,8,11] presumably due to the loss of normal proprioception to which the slow-twitch fibers respond. This fact is important to rehabilitation for two reasons. First, one must rehabilitate the slow-twitch and slow-speed work before the fast-speed work is started. (Slow-speed work allows muscles long periods of time to contract, as when a heavy weight is lifted through a range of motion of a joint. Fast-speed work requires that the muscle maximally exert its force over a short period of time, as during sprinting.) Secondly, proprioception must be retrained after all injuries. (Climbing stairs can be instituted for knees and figure-eight runs for ankles.)

Although slow fibers atrophy first, fast-twitch fibers also degenerate. Pain is one of the main inhibitors of fast-twitch function. Initially, the injured athlete cannot perform fast-speed exercise because of pain and swelling. As these subside, rehabilitation must also include work in the fast speeds. If this aspect is not included, the athlete will not be able to function competently in his sport, especially when quick acceleration movements are required. A muscle has a mixture of fast-twitch and slow-twitch fibers, as seen in Figure 13-1. The fibers respond differently to training.

Fast-twitch fibers respond to resistance training, such as weight lifting, better than slow-twitch fibers. This may account for the fact that some people do not hypertrophy as much as others with weight training.

With ageing, the preponderance of slow-twitch fibers increases. Fast-twitch fibers atrophy with age and slow-twitch fibers do not have the ability to hypertrophy. This explains why athletes tend to slow down with advancing age. The goals of rehabilitation must take this reality into account.

Despite the coexistence of fast-twitch and slow-twitch fibers, all muscle fibers are of the same type in a given motor unit. That is, a specific motor nerve innervates only one fiber type. When one performs a task calling for a low amount of force, such as drinking a glass of water, only about 20 percent of the maximal contraction capabilities of the arm are used. This fine tuning of motor control allows a person to perform specific tasks with the correct amount of force. If more force is needed in the event, more muscle fibers are recruited. Recruitment of motor units has a tremendous value in athletic training. For instance, intense concentration is needed to lift heavy weights. This concentration produces a high cortical output to recruit muscle fiber units that may not ordinarily be used.

Voluntary contraction cannot cause all of the muscle units to contract. This is actually a force deficit. However, an artificial impulse of electrical stimulation can theoretically cause contraction of every muscle fiber. This stimulation is being studied in the Soviet Union by Jakon Kots,[9] a neurophysiologist. By using the sine wave current (ac), less muscle pain is produced with stimulation. A frequency of 2500 Hz cycles is used to stimulate the muscle for 10 seconds with 50 seconds of rest; in total, stimulation is given for 100 seconds spread over ten minutes. Increases in strength of 40 percent have been recorded after 20 sessions. This gain in strength reportedly lasts for three months.

As the speed of contraction increases, production of force decreases (Fig. 13-

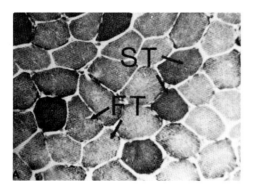

Fig. 13-1. Cross section of muscle demonstrating slow-twitch and fast-twitch muscle fibers. ST = slow-twitch fibers, FT = fast-twitch fibers. (From Armstrong, R. A.: Skeletal muscle physiology, pp. 29–48. In *Sports Medicine and Physiology,* edited by Richard H. Strauss. Copyright © 1979 by W. B. Saunders Company. Reprinted by permission of Holt, Rinehart and Winston.)

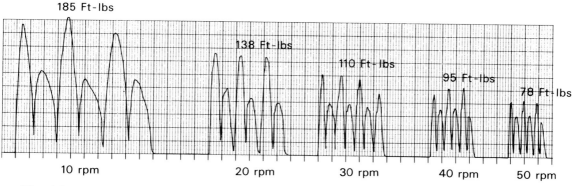

Fig. 13-2. Force production decreases as the speed of contraction increases. As the speed of the exercise increases from 10–50 rpm, the force production decreases.

2). No one is able to produce as much force at a high rate of speed as at a low rate. Why this happens is unknown. However, the most logical assumption is that the actin-myosin filaments are sliding past each other in a muscle contraction and do not have time to obtain the optimal tension needed for full-force production.

Sprinters, who only have about 40 milliseconds to develop their power as their feet push off the ground, tend to have a high percentage of fast-twitch fibers. Conversely, distance runners tend to have more slow-twitch fibers. The muscle biopsy studies of Costill et al.[3] in world class athletes have confirmed this difference. This research, however, looks at the athlete during one period of time. Did these athletes become world class performers because they genetically had the right type of muscle fibers or did they train their muscles to the fullest and possibly promote the right type of muscle activity? The correct answer probably involves both aspects.

Fast-twitch fibers can be trained to have good aerobic capacity and perform identically to slow-twitch fibers. But slow-twitch fibers cannot change. One cannot change the speed of contraction, which is a neurological event. Speed training calls for the athlete to command his motor recruitment more efficiently than he has done before. His efforts will produce a smoother flow, less internal resistance, and a greater potential for doing work.

Clearly it is advantageous not only to have, but also be able to train, the type of muscle fiber pertinent to one's athletic performance. This is the concept behind specific training. Not only must strength be increased in athletic training, but the muscle units must be overloaded at the limb speeds most similar to the athlete's endeavor or task.

The endogenous hormone (testosterone) level also affects the ability of the muscle fiber to respond to weight training and physical performances. There is no place in sports medicine rehabilitation and training for anabolic steroids. No study to date has shown that anabolic steroids clearly increase athletic performance. The improved performances from anabolic steroids reported by some researchers have been attributed to a placebo effect and to the fact that athletes who take anabolic steroids tend to be more aggressive than those who do not.[2] This aggressive athlete is usually on a conscientious nutrition and exercise regimen, which of itself produces a better result.[2]

MODES OF STRENGTH TRAINING

Orthopedists working in sports medicine are confronted with a baffling array of devices geared to improve an athlete's strength. It is crucial to understand the differences in modes of strength training in order to incorporate the equipment correctly into the rehabilitation program.

Isometric contractions (Fig. 13-3) are possible when the resistance is such that no motion is performed during the exercise. This allows a maximum loading of a muscle unit. However, the muscle is loaded solely at one point in the range of motion of the joint. Accordingly, isometric exercises have little effect on motor performance and have been found to be inadequate for prolonged strength training programs.

Isotonic contraction is an exercise done through a range of motion of the joint with a set resistance or weight (Fig. 13-4). A good example would be exercises performed with barbells or free weights. However, in isotonic exercises, because of the physiological skeletal lever system, neither the force on the system nor the resistance is constant through the arc of motion. Loading therefore occurs at the weakest point in the system, and the rest of the system is working at less than capacity. Another form of isotonics is a variable-resistance isotonic exercise. Nautilus exercise machines are an example of this (Fig. 13-5). To eliminate the disadvantage of the physiological skeletal lever, a cam (Fig. 13-6) is used. The cam

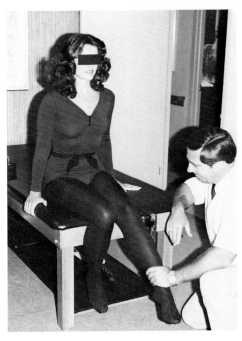

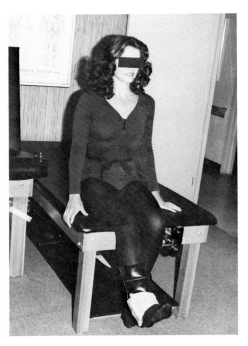

Fig. 13-3. An example of isometric exercise. The subject is maximally contracting her quadriceps muscle at one point in the range of motion of her knee. The resistance is applied by the assistant's hand.

Fig. 13-4. An example of isotonic exercise. The subject is contracting her quadriceps through a complete range of motion of the knee joint. The resistance is provided by the 2.25 kg sandbag attached to her leg.

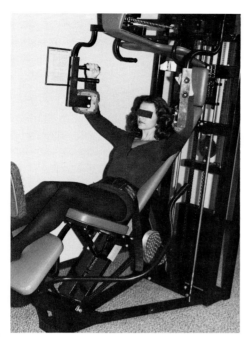

Fig. 13-5. An isotonic variable-resistance exercise. The individual is exercising on a Nautilus machine.

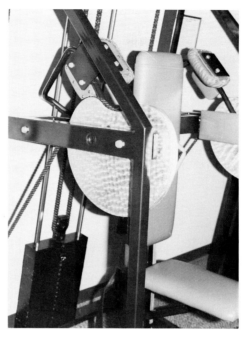

Fig. 13-6. A close-up view of the Nautilus cam.

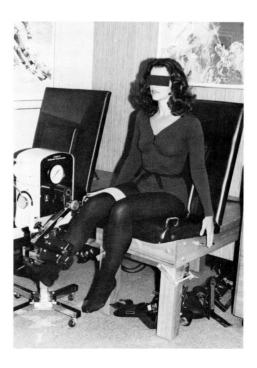

Fig. 13-7. An example of isokinetic exercise. The subject is exercising on a Cybex II isokinetic dynamometer.

adjusts the force produced by the particular joint lever system being used, allowing the patient to work the muscle harder throughout the total range of motion of the joint. Other machines use friction, hydraulics, or other forms of lever systems.

Isokinetic exercise is a modality in which the speed of the exercise is controlled and the resistance is varied. It can be done at fast and slow rates (Fig. 13-7). If a person moves less than the set speed, no resistance will be met. This type of variable resistance is totally accommodating to fatigue and pain. It loads the muscle at every point in the range of motion of the joint and enables one to do more work in the same period of time than is possible in the isotonic constant-resistance exercises. The basic kinds of isokinetic equipment are the Cybex and the Orthotron.

UNDERSTANDING THE CYBEX

One of the major advances in sports medicine rehabilitation in the past decade has been the development of the Cybex II isokinetic dynamometer. This machine gives a reproducible graphic representation of the force capabilities of the athletic patient (Fig. 13-8). The dual channel Cybex graph gives a reading of the force production in foot-pounds of torque. Torque is a twisting force measured in foot-pounds (force = weight × distance = foot-pounds). This torque can be measured at several speeds of limb movement, from 0–50 revolutions per minute (rpm). One rpm is the same motion velocity as an arc of motion of 6 degrees per second. Therefore, a setting of 5 rpm is the same as stating that the limb movement is 30 degrees per second. Likewise, 40 rpm is motion occurring at 240 degrees per second. Most day-to-day activities occur at 10–15 rpms (60–90 degrees per second), whereas accelerated levels of athletic performance require a limb movement of 40–50 rpm or more (240–300 degrees of motion a second).

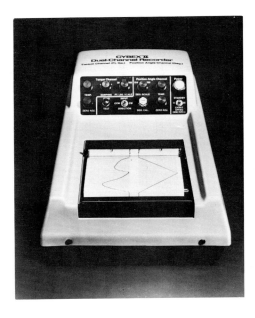

Fig. 13-8. The dual channel recorder on a Cybex II isokinetic dynamometer. The recorder on the left is giving a reading in foot-pounds of torque. The recording needle on the right is depicting the range of motion of the joint. (Courtesy of Cybex, a division of Lumex, Inc.)

   With this background, a patient's strength, power, endurance, and rate of tension development can be measured. By definition, the athlete's strength is measured at his peak torque at a slow speed, which by convenience is measured at 5 or 10 rpm (Fig. 13-9). The power of the patient is defined as the amount of peak torque produced at a fast rate of speed. This is usually measured at 30–40 rpm. It must be emphasized that this definition of power is different from the engineering definition of power, which is a calculation of the rate of doing work. Power as described in the athlete is concerned with the force produced at a fast rate of speed.

   The endurance of the patient is measured on the Cybex II at 30 rpm (Fig. 13-10). The endurance is counted by the number of repetitions necessary to reach the point when a patient can no longer make 50 percent of his original peak torque values.

   The rate of tension development is the amount of time it takes the individual to produce his peak torque (Fig. 13-11). Two individuals may have the same peak torque measured in foot-pounds. However, one may be able to produce that peak torque at 0.2 second, whereas the other might take 0.4 second. Obviously this has extreme implications for athletics and rehabilitation in that athletes who can

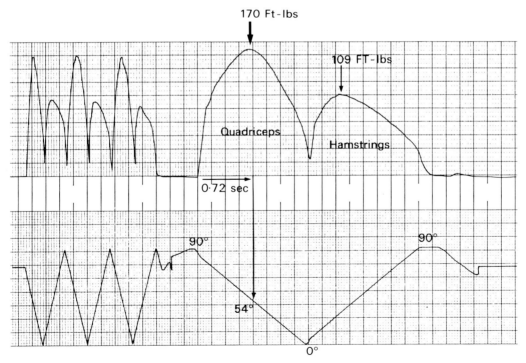

Fig. 13-9. A typical graph recording from a Cybex II taken at 10 rpm. The torque curves on the left are recorded at chart speeds of 5 mm per second. The labeled torque curves are produced with chart speed of 25 mm per second. This individual produced a maximum quadriceps contraction of 170 foot-pounds. The time that it took to produce this maximum quadriceps contraction was 0.72 seconds. This occurred at 54 degrees in the range of motion of the knee. The hamstrings produced 109 foot-pounds of torque. The total work performed is the area under each individual curve.

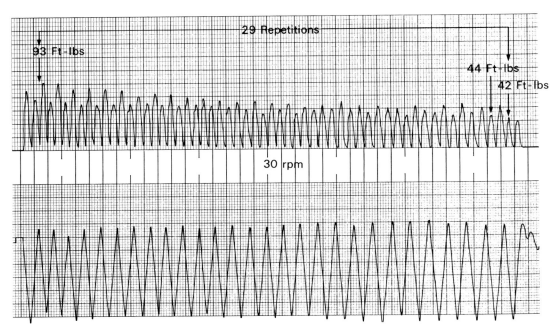

Fig. 13-10. Endurance calculation at 30 rpm. This patient initially produced 93 foot-pounds of torque. He was exercised until he produced two contractions that no longer make 50 percent of his original peak torque values. In this example it took 29 repetitions.

produce power at swifter rates will be able to compete better. Consider, for example, a baseball player hitting the t all. All else being equal, the faster the swing, the more energy delivered to the ball, and the farther the ball will go.

It used to be thought that a quadriceps : hamstring strength ratio should be 60 : 40. This is not necessarily true. Our tests of various athletic groups have shown that the ratio will depend on the development of the muscle groups as related to the specific sports. For instance, professional tennis players and basketball players have extraordinary high force capabilities in the hamstring muscles. This is not an abnormality; rather, it is an adaptation of the athlete's muscle to a specific performance demand.

All these measurements are compared with any produced with the uninvolved, uninjured extremity during the rehabilitation program. It is important to keep a record of the initial testing because these percentage values will change as the patient progresses. Usually both extremities are exercised in a rehabilitation program and therefore the percentage deficit will change accordingly. To facilitate and simplify data collection, we offer a method that organizes all the important information on one piece of paper (Fig. 13-12). A composite makes it easy to compare the patient's progress quickly because all figures and numbers are easily available.

If the patient has true pain, it is detectable on the graph by a reproducible ripple or abnormal mark that will be present on every range of motion that the joint performs, regardless of the speed at which the joint is tested (Fig. 13-13). This information is useful in prescribing a rehabilitation program. For instance, if the patient has chondromalacia and has pain at 30–40 degrees of knee flexion on

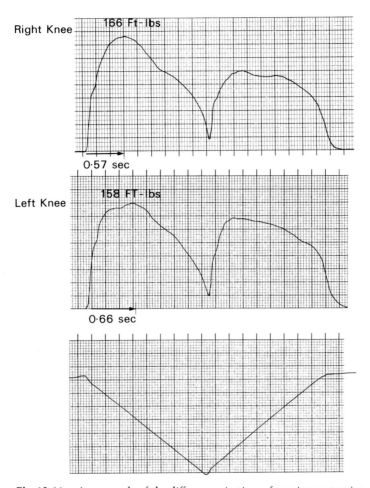

Fig. 13-11. An example of the differences in time of maximum tension development. This patient had an arthroscopic surgical procedure on his left knee two weeks before this graph was made. Although the peak torque values for his quadriceps muscle are relatively similar, it takes his left knee 0.09 seconds longer to develop the maximum tension in the muscle.

the Cybex, an exercise can be prescribed that blocks the joint from reaching 30–40 degrees of flexion (Fig. 13-14). This would eliminate the painful arc in the range of motion and allow the patient to exercise without injury. Towels or blankets can be placed under the knee to allow only 25 degrees of knee flexion. Then the patient can exercise the quadriceps in a short arc of motion.

KNEE REHABILITATION

Knee rehabilitation, like any other joint rehabilitation, requires the development of strength, power, and endurance. Failure to do this leads to an incompletely rehabilitated extremity and the likelihood of future injury is increased. A familiar

Text continues on p. 182

PATIENT NAME: _____   REFERRING PHYSICIAN: _____

SCALE: 180 ft–lbs/150 movt. _____   DIAGNOSIS: _____ Post op. arthroscopic rt,

_____ menisectomy   6/18/80 _____

	10 RPM		30 RPM	
Max. quadriceps (foot lbs. torque)	R 132	L 140	R 91	L
Max. hamstrings (foot lbs. torque)	R 99	L 102	R 56	L 56
% of unaffected quadriceps	R 94%	L	R 96%	L
% of unaffected hamstrings	R 97%	L	R 85%	L
Time rate of max. contraction (sec)	R 0.63 sec @ 53	L 0.65 sec @ 45	R	L
Endurance to 50% fatigue (reps)	R	L	R 26	L

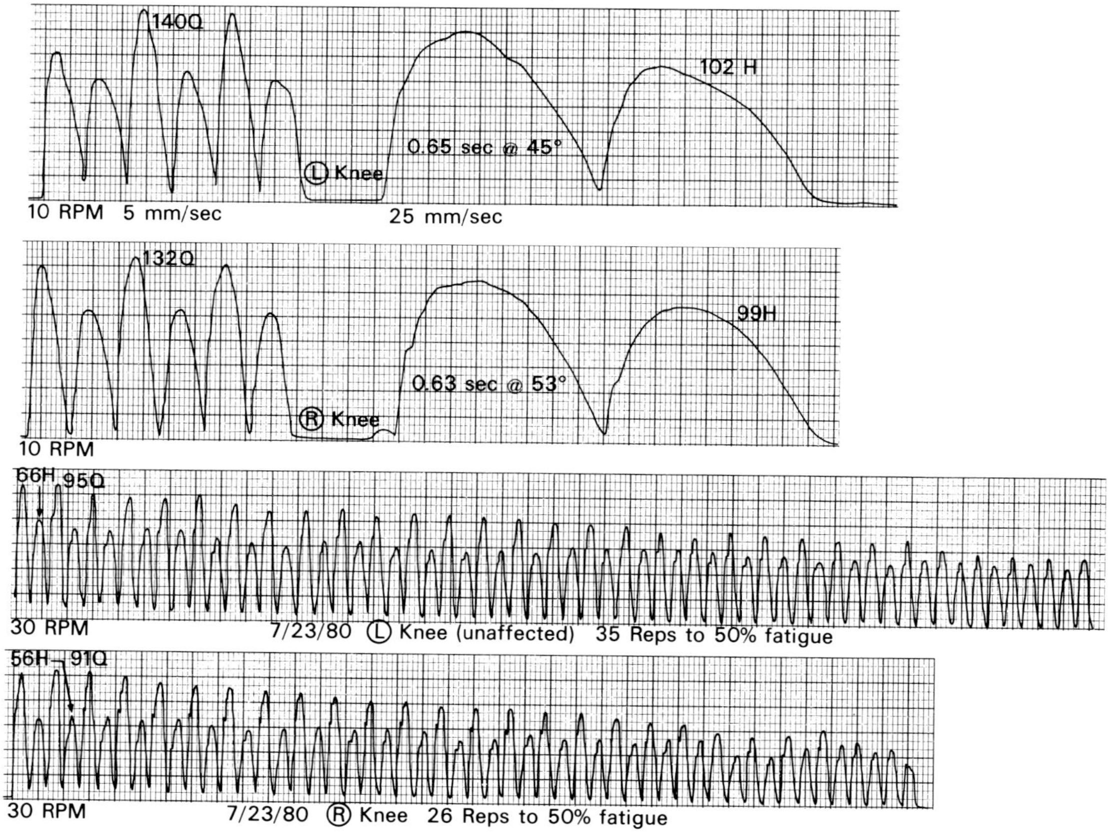

Fig. 13-12. A composite graph giving all pertinent information on one piece of paper. It allows quick and easy reference in comparing the athlete's progress.

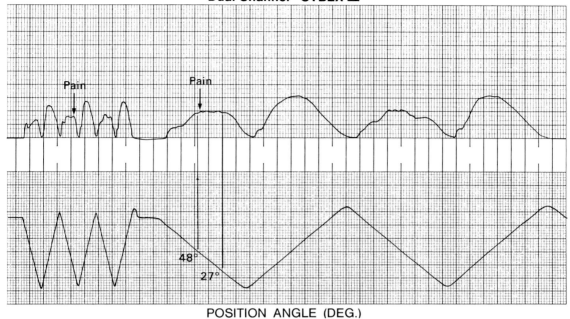

Dual Channel CYBEX II

POSITION ANGLE (DEG.)

Fig. 13-13. Example of a pain ripple. This torque curve was produced at 10 rpm. The torque speed on the left was done at 5 mm per second and chart speed on the right was produced at 25 mm per second. In this patient's range of motion, the pain ripple began at 48 degrees and lasted to 27 degrees.

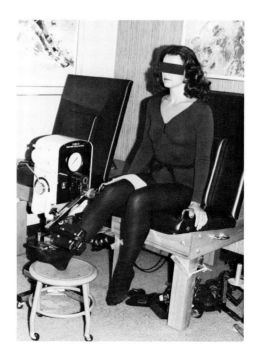

Fig. 13-14. A stool placed under the subject's right leg blocks her knee flexion past 30 degrees. She can now exercise on the isokinetic machine in a range of motion that does not proceed beyond 30 degrees of flexion. This is especially advantageous in patients with chondromalacia.

sight in any training room is an athlete who has had a meniscectomy followed by a postoperative program of vigorous progressive-resistance exercise. He may be able to lift 22.5 kg with his knee extensors, yet he is unable to return to full activity. There is nothing in the patient's athletic performance that requires him to lift one heavy weight, through one range of motion, given an indefinite amount of time, unless the patient is a weight lifter. Most athletes' limb speeds exceed 240 degrees per second, with some approaching 400–600 degrees per second. Therefore, if the rehabilitation program is concentrated only on strength, then the patient has not rehabilitated his knee fully and has no power and endurance. Also, because of the concept of specificity of training in exercise, it is prudent to train the patient in the manner most similar to his performance specifics and capabilities.[12] For an athlete who works basically in a fast speed, the anaerobic mechanism needs to be rehabilitated and exercised more. That exercise needs to be at 40–50 rpm. An athlete who performs at a slower speed needs speed and aerobic conditioning to fit that performance level.

The most important consideration in knee rehabilitation is education and exercise *before* the operation. All patients with knee injuries should be started on quadriceps-setting and straight-leg raising exercises. A muscle that has been exercised and trained preoperatively to function will regain that ability much sooner postoperatively than one that has not been trained. The patient is restarted on his quadriceps-setting exercises and straight-leg raising exercises immediately after surgery.

Pain is the initial limiting factor postoperatively, and every attempt should be made to reduce its intensity. A recent boon in this area has been the introduction of transcutaneous neural stimulation (TNS; Fig. 13-15). Sterile electrodes are placed on the patient at the operating table and the unit is hooked up in the recovery room. All patients who may have an arthrotomy are carefully educated

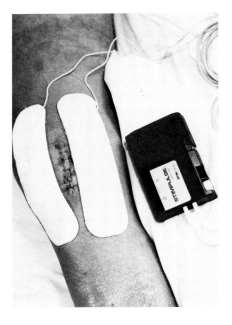

Fig. 13-15. An example of transcutaneous neural stimulation. Sterile electrodes have been placed next to the arthrotomy incision of the knee. The stimulator is shown to the right of the knee.

about TNS beforehand. Knowledge of the device and the education in its use will prevent problems and misunderstandings in using the TNS unit postoperatively. Frequently, patients will be able to do straight-leg raising exercises on the same day as their surgery.

Although the exact physiological reason for the TNS unit's efficacy is not known, it is thought that it works on the gate-threshold theory of pain. It may also raise the total body level of endorphins. The only known contraindication for its use is a cardiac pacemaker of the synchronous type.[5]

TNS units are used on all arthrotomies of the knee. TNS units are not used on arthroscopic procedures, since the patient's pain does not seem to warrant them. Usually the TNS unit is left on the patient for four to five days and then removed prior to discharge. Occasionally, patients will ask to take a TNS unit home with them, but this is usually not necessary.

Another method for inhibiting postoperative pain is to inject 10–20 cc of 0.5 percent Marcaine without epinephrine into subcutaneous tissues prior to skin closure. Marcaine can be administered in arthroscopic surgery as well, especially when the patient is only hospitalized for a day. In arthroscopic lateral retinacular releases, this anesthetic is most beneficial.

Stimulating muscles with a faradic current has been most beneficial for patients who are slow in regaining muscle tone. Eriksson and Haggmark[4] have shown that quadriceps treated with electrical stimulation at a frequency of 200 Hz had better muscle function and less muscle enzyme degradation than a control group did. Faradic stimulation causes a tetanic contraction of the whole quadriceps muscle. It is different than TNS, which is also given via alternating current. The amplitude on a TNS can be increased and, if placed near a motor point, it will produce a contraction. Triggering muscle contractions is not the basic application of the TNS, because it is primarily a pain suppressant. The muscle contraction produced by direct current has no practical benefit to sports medicine.

On the second or third day after the operation, a patient begins range of motion exercises. It was once thought that starting range of motion exercises before suture removal would be detrimental to skin healing. With the stronger synthetic suture material now available, this is no longer true. Patients can safely be started on a range of motion exercise three to four days after surgery. Most patients will show 90 degrees of flexion when the skin sutures are removed about two weeks later. There should not be any skin necrosis or healing problems with this early motion.

While in the hospital, the patient must try to obtain active terminal extension of the knee. He can work on this by exercising the quadriceps in short arcs. A towel or a blanket is placed under the knee and the patient starts exercising the vastus medialis in the last 20 degrees of terminal extension. The sooner terminal extension is obtained, the faster the rehabilitation program will progress and the more functional the knee will be.

At two weeks, the sutures are removed. Then, the patient, if not in a cast, is sent to physical therapy for whirlpool treatments and more range of motion exercises. If the patient is in cast, he waits for therapy until it is removed, about six weeks later. If the physical therapy facilities have a Kinetron (an isokinetic machine used for terminal extension exercises of the knee and for ambulation training after hip or knee surgery), the patient is placed on the machine and work on terminal extension is resumed. The patient is placed on the Cybex as soon as possible. To use the Cybex effectively, at least 70–90 degrees of knee motion are needed. If, for instance, the patient only has 70 degrees of knee motion, then the Cybex can be blocked with a stool or other device so that the range of motion exercised is comfortable to the patient, not injurious. What the rehabilitation program must guard against is the increase of any swelling in the joint. If the joint swells, the rehabilitation program is greatly prolonged. It is better to start with isometrics rather than a progressive resistance exercise program if the progressive resistance program is going to hurt and cause swelling.

Initially, the patient is exercised on the Cybex and seen in physical therapy five times a week for seven to ten days and then placed on a triweekly exercise program. The Orthotron is also an isokinetic machine. Although the Orthotron is a good exercise machine, it is not as accommodating as the Cybex. The patient must be able to lift at least 3.15 kg in a progressive-resistance fashion before he can be placed on the Orthotron, because the Orthotron's lever arm weighs 3.15–3.38 kg. The patient must be able to lift 3.38 kg easily, or the weight of the arm might be painful to lift.

We have not found any distinct isokinetic exercise protocols. We exercise our patients until they are 50 percent fatigued at a specific rpm. For three sets of exercises, the patient should be exercised both at slow (5, 10, and 15 rpm) and fast speeds (30, 40, and 50 rpm), with additional work prescribed depending on his specific athletic performance.

When a patient has 110 degrees of motion, he is ready to exercise with a standard bicycle. If the patient has some chondromalacia, it is advisable to have the bicycle seat very high, which will decrease the range of motion and avoid extensive knee flexion. Therefore riding the bicycle will not cause painful patellofemoral compression. If the patient has had a cruciate repair and should not gain full extension too quickly, then the bicycle seat is kept low. The knee will remain in a more flexed position during the pedalling. After three to six weeks, depending on the individual and the surgical procedure, the patient is started on a program at home. Treatment can include a Nautilus training or a free weight, depending upon the availability in the physician's area.

Some controversy ranges over the advisability of gaining terminal extension too quickly in patients who have had anterior cruciate repairs and reconstruction. Clearly, the substituted anterior cruciate ligament and the cruciate ligament repair do not have sufficient strength until 12–18 months after the repair, and some physicians leave the cruciate repairs in casts longer than the traditional six weeks. A flexion contracture can be far more disabling than the instability the athlete had prior to the operation. An athlete with a flexion contracture of 15 degrees has a severe handicap in running sports, particularly if he is a defensive back in football. He can no longer run backward and for all practical purposes cannot return to his sport. There is no real solution to the problem, but continued bracing after cast removal is the wisest therapy. The patient can exercise in his brace and the brace can be used later when the athlete returns to athletic participation. We are presently using a metal hinge, reinforced knee cage as well as the Lenox Hill derotation brace, depending upon the severity of the ligamentous injury and instability.

When the patient has regained 70 percent of his strength, as measured on the

Cybex, compared to the uninjured leg, he is started on walking fast. He is started on a running program when he reaches 80 percent. Then sharp running and cutting (at 45-degree angles) are permitted. If they are performed without pain or swelling, the patient progresses to 90-degree cuts and figure-eight runs.

The old adage that athletes can return to participation when they can perform a progressive-resistance exercise with 11.25–22.5 kg a certain number of times is unsound. By using the Cybex graphs, a more accurate measurement of the athlete's strength and performance can be made. The athlete is not allowed to return to his athletic event until he obtains at least 90 percent strength as compared to the uninjured leg. Preferably, he will obtain 95–100 percent. What must be remembered is that the 90 percent determination should not be made only for strength but for power and endurance as well.

Hamstrings (knee flexors) improve in function more quickly than the quadriceps if there has not been an anterior cruciate ligament repair on reconstruction. If there has been an anterior cruciate injury, then the hamstrings should be extensively worked upon, since by their mechanism of action they prevent forward translation of the tibia on the femur.

After a knee injury, the quadriceps and hamstrings are not the only muscle groups that need rehabilitation. The hip flexors, extensors, abductors, and adductors will also atrophy and become weak. Vigorous rehabilitation of the gastrocsoleus muscles will be necessary.

A stretching program for the hamstrings, quadriceps, groin muscles, and gastrocsoleus muscles is not only a vital part of a rehabilitation program, but also an integral part of a preseason injury prevention program. Proprioceptive neuromuscular facilitation (PNF) is a popular addition to the stretching exercise program. PNF is a form of steady, passive stretching of muscles. When the point of maximum stretch is reached, the antagonist muscle is contracted. Through the neuromuscular pathway (Golgi tendon apparatus), the stretched muscle is relaxed even more (Figs. 13-16A, B). PNF is effective in stretching out tight hamstrings. The subject maximally, slowly, passively stretches his hamstrings and then at the maximum point of stretch contracts his quadriceps. By contracting his quadriceps, he relaxes the hamstring even further, allowing more stretch to be obtained.

Chondromalacia

Chondromalacia is a softening of the patella's articular cartilage at the patella femoral joint. It is also known as "patella compression syndrome." Causative factors may be direct trauma, a deficiency of the vastus medialis, or a mechanical malalignment of the legs or feet. Pronated feet are a common cause of knee pain from chondromalacia in runners. This condition may require a foot orthosis to correct the abnormal foot mechanics. Chondromalacia may also be associated with patella subluxations and dislocations.

Patients usually complain of peripatellar pain associated with activity and prolonged knee flexion. Characteristically this is worse in descending stairs and inclines, or when sitting in theatres. Subpatella crepitus and tenderness are noted, especially when the patella is compressed against the femur. A plica may be associated with this condition and may accentuate roughness and pain in the cartilage.

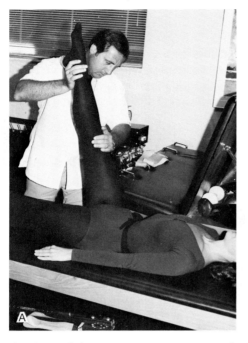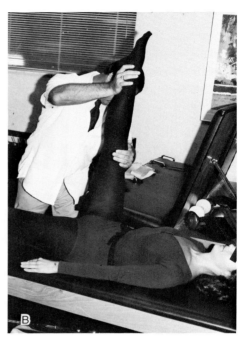

Fig. 13-16. (A) A proprioceptive neuromuscular facilitation. The subject has slowly, steadily, and passively stretched her right hamstrings to the maximum point. (B) The quadriceps muscles are then contracted, reflexively allowing more stretching to be accomplished in the hamstrings.

Initially, the rehabilitation of an injured knee with chondromalacia involves resting the joint and protecting it from irritation. This will reduce the initial pain and swelling. Aspirin is given at a dosage of 625 mg, four times a day, for two to four weeks. Other anti-inflammatory agents (ibuprofen or indomethacin) may be of benefit. Ice compresses are also used to decrease the initial pain and swelling.

At this point it is important to institute a strong program of patient education. The athlete needs to understand the anatomical aspect of the patella with regard to exercise and function, and how it relates to his specific sport. If this is not explained, the athlete will attempt to do various exercises and training programs on his own that most likely will accentuate his chondromalacia symptoms and therefore hinder his return to full participation.

After the initial pain and swelling have subsided, exercises are instituted to strengthen the vastus medialis. Proper quadriceps-setting exercises, straight-leg raising exercises, isometric exercises, and terminal extension exercises are initiated. It is important that the athlete exercise the vastus medialis, since strength in the vastus medialis will determine the ultimate outcome of the chondromalacia symptoms. The vastus medialis can be worked extensively by dorsiflexing the foot on the involved side, internally rotating the thigh at the hip, and performing a straight-leg raising exercise. At first, the knee is exercised only in 10–20 degrees of flexion to full extension. As muscular strength increases, more knee flexion can be exercised. An effective way of determining the specific joint angle responsible for the discomfort is to use the Cybex II. If a patient has a "pain ripple'' in his Cybex readout, the specific range of motion in the involved joint can be found and an exercise program to block knee flexion past the painful area can be tailored.

At this point in the rehabilitation program, flexibility exercises are instituted. Tight hamstrings, triceps surae, and tensor fascia lata all place abnormal force vectors on the knee and accentuate chondromalacia symptoms. A proprioceptive neuromuscular facilitation program for stretching tight hamstrings is very beneficial.

As the patient regains his strength, motion, and flexibility, more strenuous exercises are undertaken. Isokinetic exercise at fast speeds (40–50 rpm) is effective in alleviating chondromalacia symptoms. At this rate of limb movement, the patella does not have enough time to develop a detrimental compressive load as it articulates with the femur.[14] This means the muscles are exercised in ranges of motion that would not be acceptable using a slower rate of limb speed, as in traditional progressive-resistance exercises based on weights. If the patient feels some minor discomfort with the high-speed isokinetic work, ice can be applied during the training program. Ice not only reduces the discomfort, but also prevents swelling from occurring. Exercise should be done on a bicycle with the seat elevated to decrease knee flexion, for that decreases patella femoral compression. Bicycle exercises can be done at a fast rpm, which works on muscle strengthening and endurance.

Exercise programs for the gastrocnemius and soleus muscles, the hamstrings, and the hip muscles are also instituted, as in any knee injury.

Chondromalacia may occur in conjunction with other knee injuries as well. Therefore it is important to understand the rehabilitation program for chondromalacia, so that other rehabilitation programs can be adjusted if chondromalacia is present. Often muscle atrophy secondary to another injury may precipitate chondromalacia pain that perhaps was not evident before the injury. For instance, a patient with a torn meniscus may be found to have moderate retropatellar crepitus, which then becomes symptomatic due to the muscle atrophy, which resulted from the injury. Therefore if the traditional exercise and rehabilitation program is instigated without knowledge of the fact that chrondromalacia is present, the patient will suffer marked pain and swelling in the knee because of the roughening of the patella. Such discomfort will greatly hinder the rehabilitation program.

REHABILITATING ANKLE INJURIES

Ankle sprains are the most common injury in sports medicine. This discussion does not deal with operative and cast immobilization in Grade III ankle ligamentous tears because Grade I tears of the anterior talofibular ligament, which may or may not be combined with the tear of the calcaneofibular ligament, are most frequently seen. Yet they tend to be an injury singularly neglected during rehabilitation.

The most important rehabilitative treatment of this type of injury is the prevention of swelling. The more the ankle joint becomes swollen, the less range of motion is available in the joint, and the more prolonged the recovery rate.

Ankle injuries should immediately be treated with ice, compression, and elevation. Crushed ice is the cheapest and the best form of initial treatment. The commercially available blue ice tends to be quite stiff and does not conform as well as crushed ice to bony areas, such as the ankle and knee. In addition, the commercially available products tend to be colder than the zero-degree centigrade temperature of crushed ice, and the extreme frigidity can cause thermal injury to the skin. Ethyl chloride coats the skin and acts as an analgesic, but it does not cool the injury effectively. The ankle should be wrapped with an elastic wrap and completely surrounded by the crushed ice for a minimum of 20 minutes. Active exercise can be started before weight bearing by the application of ice. The ice works both as an anesthetic and as a suppressant to swelling.

Besides the ice, compression, and elevation, the athlete is given crutches. The ice is kept on the extremity until the swelling stops (24–48 hours). The athlete uses the crutches until he has full, painless weight-bearing. Then range of motion exercises for the ankle are instituted. (One easy way to instruct the patient in performing range of motion exercises is to tell him to pretend to write the alphabet with his toes.) Contrast baths can be used to encourage range of motion. At first the ankle is immersed into a whirlpool or bucket of warm water (100 F) for five minutes, followed by range of motion exercises and limbering up. Then the ankle is taken out of the warm water and placed in cold water (a slush of ice water) for one minute. Immersion in the cold water helps prevent swelling. The ankle is returned to the warm water for four minutes and cold water for one minute; this regimen continues as the warm water time is decreased by one-minute intervals. Again, rehabilitation is working to prevent an increase in swelling. If swelling is occurring with the contrast baths, then more ice and less heat should be applied. The worst problem in ankle rehabilitation is the application of heat too soon and too frequently. Therefore, adequate supervision is imperative.

Once range of motion exercises are started, so too can manual resistance exercises and isotonic exercises begin. Exercises must work on not only the gastrocsoleus, but on the peroneal muscles. Isokinetic equipment has useful ankle adaptation that works on the foot invertors, everters, and dorsiflexion and plantar flexors (Fig. 13-17). When the athlete reaches 70 percent of the range of motion in his ankle, and 70–80 percent of his strength, he can progress from walking to jogging to running full speed. Protective ankle taping has been beneficial in this stage of rehabilitation. A Louisiana heel lock is best used in the taping program,

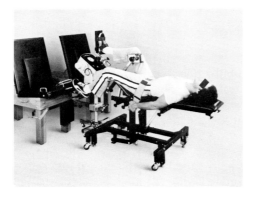

Fig. 13-17. An ankle exercise adaptation that fits on a Cybex II. It works on ankle inversion and eversion. (Courtesy of Cybex, a division of Lumex, Inc.)

because it prevents abnormal subtalar motion. Taping also has a positive psychological function in that it can give an athlete a sense of security.

All patients with ankle injuries should do stretching exercises. Athletes who repeatedly suffer inversion-type ankle sprains are found to have a very tight heel cord. A special box designed to stretch a heel cord is effective in alleviating the problem.

When the patient's complete range of motion returns to his ankle, he is started on 45 degrees running and cutting and progresses to 90-degree cuts and figure-eight runs. He can return to his sport when he has recovered his strength and has 100 percent range of motion and feels no pain or swelling during the exercise program.

SHOULDER REHABILITATION

Shoulder rehabilitation depends largely on the underlying pathology involved. For recurrent anterior dislocations of the shoulder, strengthening the internal rotators is crucial. That in itself, however, will not prevent recurrent dislocations of the shoulder. If the patient has already undergone a surgical procedure, then the previous operation will dictate the speed of his return to performance. It has been our experience that patients receiving the Bristow surgical procedures for their dislocated shoulder require the longest time to return to athletic competition because it takes time for the coracoid process and the glenoid neck to heal. A capsulorrhaphy by a DuToit staple allows the patient to return much sooner to his athletic endeavor. The DuToit staple allows much less external rotation to be lost, a real benefit to the throwing athlete.

Rehabilitation after acromioclavicular separation depends upon the severity of the injury and the type of medical or surgical treatment given to it. Complete acromioclavicular separations that are treated with an open reduction and a resection of the distal end of the clavicle,[13] combined with a ligament reconstruction using a Meadox dacron prosthesis, allow the athlete to return to sports in as little as four weeks. This recovery rate is almost as fast as nonoperative treatment. With the ligament prosthesis, overhead presses are allowed at three weeks and resumption of the patient's sport gradually follows.

Rehabilitation of the shoulder must include all components of the shoulder girdle musculature. Not only should shoulder flexors be exercised but also shoulder abductors, internal rotators, and external rotators. The shoulder rotators provide most of the important functional movements. Failure to recognize their importance will seriously hinder the athlete's recovery.

Shoulder rehabilitation can be done isokinetically or isotonically. There are adaptation devices for the upper body that hook onto most isokinetic equipment (Figs. 13-18, 13-19). These exercises are very beneficial to the athlete who has a rotator cuff tear, be it acute and not complete or old and degenerative. The key to shoulder rehabilitation when there are rotator cuff tears is to start with a light weight and perform 15 to 20 repetitions of the exercises. Too heavy a weight will only increase the pain.

A Nautilus program consisting of light weights and several repetitions is extremely beneficial for these rotator cuff problems. Baseball pitchers, tennis

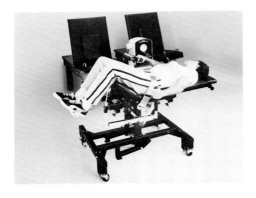

Fig. 13-18. Adaptation for Cybex II that allows the shoulder to be exercised in internal and external rotation in 90 degrees of abduction. (Courtesy of Cybex, a division of Lumex, Inc.)

players, and older weight lifters are most likely to have rotator cuff injuries and impingement syndromes. Work on the shoulder's internal and external rotation should not be neglected.

THE REHABILITATION TEAM

The interest of the physician should extend beyond the physical rehabilitation of the patient and should include social, vocational, and psychological restoration. This goal requires a team effort and, thus, allied health personnel who specialize in the various aspects of rehabilitation. The team should include the physician, and, if available, a senior orthopedic resident; physical and occupational therapists;

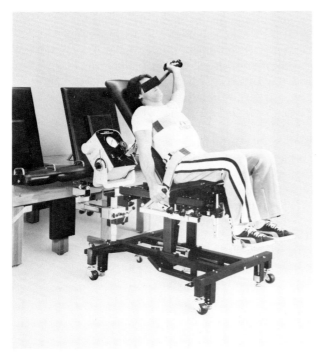

Fig. 13-19. An adaptation that allows patients to exercise the shoulder in abduction and adduction. (Courtesy of Cybex, a division of Lumex, Inc.)

representatives from the nursing staff; a prosthetist; an orthotist; a vocational rehabilitation representative; and medical consultants. We would add to the team a physical training instructor, for in dealing with athletes of all ages, this person is indispensable. The good trainer is often much closer to the athlete than the doctor or the coach. This comradeship and confidence are extremely helpful in rehabilitation and in returning the athlete to competition. Although most athletes are already well-motivated for work and exercise, the psychology of group therapy can play an important role in the individual desire for achievement. However, in the long run, it is the responsibility of the doctor in charge, because of his training and his understanding of the pathophysiology that has caused the difficulty, to direct the program of therapy to be used for each patient.

Helping the Professional Athlete

Most patients in sports medicine are highly paid professional athletes who are continually subjected to injury and athletic trauma and who must, for economic as well as medical reasons, remain in action as much as possible.

Treatment and rehabilitation are essential in professional and collegiate sports of all kinds, so much so that one famous football coach said, "Without prompt medical and surgical treatment followed by efficient rehabilitation, I could not field a team next year." It is the restoration of function that is so vital to the athlete and, thus, to his team. Because no operation will help an athlete regain function unless it is immediately followed by a sophisticated rehabilitation program, rehabilitation must begin on the day of injury. That is, the doctor, the trainer, and the coach must plan from the first day of injury the physical, mental, and psychological treatment that will return the athlete to his sport as soon and as completely as possible. If a part of the body (like a knee, leg, or arm) is so injured that it must be immobilized, then continual muscle rehabilitation must be instituted for the rest of the body. This activity must be carried out in a scheduled, systematic, progressive program. Once the injured part can be activated, a definite program must be outlined for it, too, and followed vigorously and routinely.

FUTURE RESEARCH

The future of sports rehabilitation in sports medicine is exciting. With the work of the biomechanical engineers and the adaptations of computers to sports technology, major advances are being made.[15] By translating athletic actions to stick figures and then programming the actions into a computer, diverse analyses can be made of the athlete's performance. These investigations should lead to recommendations for the optimal way of training injured athletes.

SUMMARY

The key to sports medicine rehabilitation is sports injury prevention. Everyone concerned with sports medicine should cooperate in making participation in sports safer. An intensive preseason training program to build up strength, coupled with aerobic conditioning and flexibility exercises, will keep the athlete "fine tuned" and in the best possible shape to perform his sport and reduce the potential for injury.

REFERENCES

1. Armstrong, R. A.: Skeletal muscle physiology. In Strauss, R. H., Ed.: *Sports Medicine and Physiology,* pp. 29–48. W. B. Saunders, Philadelphia, 1979.
2. Brooks, R. V.: Anabolic steroids and athletes. Phys. Sports Med. 8:161–163, 1980.
3. Costill, D. L., Coyle, E. F., and Fink, W. F.: Adaptations in skeletal muscle following strength training. J. Appl. Physiol. 46:96–99, 1979.
4. Eriksson, E., and Haggmark, T.: Comparison of isometric muscle training and electrical stimulation supplementing isometric muscle training in the recovery after major knee ligament surgery. Am. J. Sports Med. 7:169–171, 1979.
5. Eriksson, M., Schuller, H., and Sjoiund, B.: Hazard from TNS in patients with pacemakers. Lancet 1:1319, 1978.
6. Haggmark, T., and Erikkson, E.: Cylinder or mobile cast brace after knee ligament surgery. Am. J. Sports Med. 7:48–56, 1979.
7. Howell, M. L., and Howell, R.: Training and medicine in the ancient Olympic games. Phys. Sports Med. 4:61–67, 1976.
8. Karpati, G., and Enyel, W. K.: Correlative histochemical study of skeletal muscle after suprasegmental denervation, peripheral nerve section, and skeletal fixation. Neurology 18:681–692, 1968.
9. Kots, J.: Electromuscular stimulation. Unpublished research.
10. Leavy, J.: Doctors practice so the athletes can play. New York Times, V, pp. 1, 22, July 22, 1979.
11. Patel, A. N., Razzak, Z. A., and Dustur, D. K.: Diffuse atrophy of human skeletal muscles. Arch. Neurol. 20:413–421, 1969.
12. Smith, M. J., and Melton, P.: Isokinetic vs. isotonic variable resistance training. Am. J. Sports Med. 9:275–279, 1981.
13. Smith, M. J., and Stewart, M. J.: Acute acromioclavicular separations. Am. J. Sports Med. 7:62–71, 1979.
14. Steadman, J. R.: Rehabilitation of athletic injuries. Am. J. Sports Med. 7:147–149, 1979.
15. Whieldon, D.: Biomechanics: Space-age sports medicine. Phys. Sports Med. 7:106–117, 1979.

Rehabilitation of the Hand

Sidney J. Blair, M.D.

This chapter discusses rehabilitation of the hand following injury or disease. The goal of rehabilitation is to return the patient to as close to normal activities of daily living as early as possible. Hand rehabilitation is in reality the rehabilitation of the entire upper extremity.

Not every patient with an upper extremity disability will require formal rehabilitative efforts. Most patients with hand problems, when given instructions for further care, carry out the instructions with minimal difficulty. Our purpose here is to focus on those problems that cause prolonged disability. Such patients need further treatment and guidance to make their final recovery; thus, they require trained personnel, such as can be found in an organized hand rehabilitation center.

HAND REHABILITATION CENTERS

Access to a hand rehabilitation center is vital to a patient's rehabilitation, as Wynn-Parry[23] has written: "If patients with severe injuries to the hand are to regain maximum function as quickly as possible, intensive treatment for several hours a day is required from a highly skilled therapeutic staff under the direction of a doctor with specialized knowledge of all aspects of the problem."

There has been a marked proliferation of hand rehabilitation centers in the United States. Some of the early centers were under the direction of Earl Peacock of the University of North Carolina and John Madden of the University of Arizona. Occupational therapists, such as Lois Barber of Downey Community Hospital in Downey, California, and Janet Waylett of Loma Linda, California, also helped to organize hand rehabilitation centers. In 1976, the first symposium on rehabilitation of the hand took place under Dr. James Hunter.[10] In the same year the organization of the Society of Hand Therapists was founded, indicating the tremendous interest in hand rehabilitation over the past few years.

The benefit of the center is the intensive therapy concept. A wide range of facilities for occupational and physical therapy exists. One of the greatest benefits is the atmosphere of confidence and optimism in such a center. Regular assessment of the patient's progress is possible.[17] Patients attend the center daily for either full or half-day sessions. A single flat fee is charged, which includes treatment, supplies, and the construction of simple orthoses. The hand rehabilitation center's goals are to correct as far as possible the problems frequently encountered in diseases and trauma to the upper extremity and to achieve a *painless, strong, and supple extremity* capable of carrying out the multitudinous tasks and activities of daily living.

PHASES OF FUNCTION IN THE HAND AND UPPER EXTREMITY

Functional activities require the hand to reach a distant object or area.[1] The hand must be placed forward at the level of a work surface, forward being in relation to the mouth and face. There must be at least 10–15 degrees of flexion at the glenohumeral joint to bring the hand to the mouth. There must be adequate, painless, functional range of motion in all proximal joints of the upper extremity. Sufficient stabilization should be present in the shoulder as well as the elbow. Hand function can be divided into three categories: nonprehensile function, prehensile function, and hand sensation.

Nonprehensile function encompasses the hook action of the fingers, which includes such acts as carrying a suitcase, and percussive activities, which include such skills as typing and playing the piano. Prehensile functions encompass the precision and power grips.

The various functions just discussed depend on hand sensation, the ability of the fingers to feel what they are holding, and to know how and with what strength they are holding it. The tremendous concentration of nerve endings gives notice of any thermal or mechanical factor that may cause injury to the hand. Moberg[14] has coined the term "tactile gnosis," which refers to the quality of sensation that makes a precision sensory grip possible. This sensitivity allows us to perform the fine tactics required in occupations and activities of daily living. Peripheral nerve repair and nerve re-education programs are attempts to restore this fine sensitivity in the injured or diseased hand. At times, one must settle for the lesser quality of cutaneous protective sensation.

Sensation itself needs to be distinguished from the concept of sensitivity. Whereas sensation is the acceptance and activation of impulses in the afferent nerves, sensibility refers to the interpretation and conscious appreciation of the stimulus that produced the sensation.

COMMON PROBLEMS IN REHABILITATING THE HAND

Frequently encountered problems in diseases and trauma to the upper extremity that tend to delay rehabilitation are acute and chronic edema, pain and hypersensitivity, loss of range of motion, loss of strength and endurance, and shoulder stiffness. Each of these disabilities can be minimized if the physician spends sufficient time on alleviating them and is aggressive in treating the early phases of the disease or trauma. Aggressive care requires careful, precise surgery, careful positioning of the hand, early reversal of pain patterns, frequent patient visits in order to assess progress scrupulously, and judicious advice to the patient regarding activities.

Acute and Chronic Edema

Edema is commonly associated with trauma, infections, and diseases of the hand. All the movable parts and compartments are bathed in a serofibrinous exudate. Affected areas include the subcutaneous tissue, fascial spaces, and fascia and paratendon between muscles and folds of the joint capsule. Visualize this exudate bathing all these vital structures, which swell and thicken and the exudate organizes so soon that these structures become strongly adherent to each other. Gliding ceases between tissue layers, between tendon and tendon sheaths, and between fascia and muscle. Severe stiffness ensues. The stiff structures become painful and motion ceases. Immobility increases stiffness and a vicious cycle may begin. This process is reversible and, if controlled, early deleterious effects can be kept to a minimum. Therefore in all postoperative and post-traumatic cases, for burns and infections, and in some arthritic patients, the extremity is elevated with the hand positioned above the heart. This technique is usually accomplished with a commercial elevator hooked to an intravenous pole. The elbow can rest on the bed, just so the hand remains above the heart.

All cases are fitted with a volar plastic or plaster splint to maintain wrist support. The splint does not immobilize the metacarpophalangeal (MCP) joints unless there is reason to do so. Therefore all fingers fall into flexion, and finger motion can continue. Compression dressings are not used, nor is any dressing placed between the fingers except one layer of fine mesh gauze. No circular dressings are used on fingers. No heat or soaks are used, nor are whirlpools icepacks, or massage—only active motion of the uninjured parts. Dressings must be inspected frequently for tightness. No circular casts are used early in surgical or injury cases. No slings are prescribed; patients are encouraged to place their hand over their head several times a day. Therefore *elevation, both day and night, plus motion of the joints of the upper extremity, are essential in preventing edema.*

Once edema becomes established or chronic and the scar phase ensues, techniques of occupational therapy, physical therapy, and therapeutic devices are needed. Initial treatment of chronic edema includes elevation, active motion, careful splinting, Jobst elastic garments worn intermittently, and various types of viscoelastic foam wraps.

Pain and Hypersensitivity

Pain is normally associated with hand diseases and injuries because of the hand's concentration of nerve endings, the superficial position of the sensory nerves, especially the radial sensory and the ulnar sensory, and the relatively tight carpal canal. The presence of nerve endings in the many synovial, tenosynovial, and periosteal structures can account for this symptom. Most patients respond with simple medication and appropriate treatment, with the pain gradually subsiding.

We have come to recognize a syndrome of pain with varied characteristics. These features are severe pain out of proportion to the injury, vasomotor instability, sweat disturbance, osteoporosis, and atrophy of muscles. These characteristics are grouped under the syndrome of reflex sympathetic dystrophy (RSD) and can be further divided into the following conditions:[11]

> *Causalgia major* is most commonly seen in wartime. It is usually caused by gunshot wounds, and there is injury to major mixed nerves.
> *Causalgia minor* is burning pain associated with sensory nerves, such as the digital, radial, and ulnar nerves at the wrists.
> *Sudeck's atrophy* is usually associated with wrist injuries. It is characterized by severe osteoporosis.
> *Shoulder-hand syndrome* usually starts in the shoulder. It is seen with myocardial infarctions and strokes.
> *Minor traumatic dystrophy* is associated with minor crush injuries to the hand and fingers.
> *Major traumatic dystrophy* is associated with major crush or mutilating injuries to the entire extremity.

There are three stages of the RSD syndrome. The first stage, lasting from a day to several weeks, is characterized by increased superficial blood flow, erythema, warmth, edema of the hand, increased hair and nail growth, hyperhidrosis, muscle wasting, pain aggravated by motion, and osteoporosis. The second stage, starting about three months after onset, is characterized by cool, pale skin (perhaps becoming cyanotic), brawny edema, loss of hair, brittle nails, and limitation of joint motion. The third stage generally shows atrophy of the skin, atrophy of the digital soft tissues, proximal and intractable pain, rigid joints, and severe osteoporosis. Traumas that bring on the RSD syndrome include crush injuries, which are the most common cause; fractures and sprains, especially about the wrist and ankle; elective operations, in particular the carpal tunnel release and Dupuytren's contracture release; gunshot wounds; and burns.

Prevention and recognition before three months are important. Once pain patterns become fixed, the prognosis becomes poor. Sixty percent of all patients with this condition will make a spontaneous recovery, leaving 40 percent who will require further treatment.

In summary:

1. Early recognition is important.
2. Always splint injured parts.
3. Elevate all injuries to control edema.

4. Exercise uninjured parts.
5. Prescribe pain medication.
6. Hospitalize and examine frequently.
7. Let motion occur by not applying constricting dressings.
8. Prescribe tranquilizers, trifluoperazine (Stelazine) twice a day. For younger persons, chlordiazepoxide hydrochloride (Librium) or diazepam (Valium) are more suitable.
9. Refer early to a hand rehabilitation center, where activities can be supervised.
10. Look for nerve compression syndrome after injury, particularly median nerve compression at the wrist.
11. Consider the use of transcutaneous electrical nerve stimulation (TENS), which has been recommended for chronic and acute pain syndromes.[9] TENS has been found to decrease pain in some patients enough so that they can participate in a rehabilitation program. Essentially this device attempts to control pain by selectively stimulating certain nerve fibers (large myelin sensory fibers) in order to eliminate or block other fibers that carry pain (small unmyelinated C axons). The direct current stimulator delivers a modified square-wave pulse with controllable frequency, pulse width, and voltage.
12. Use stellate ganglion blocks early on to decrease pain. They are given as a series of three to five on consecutive days if there is marked temporary relief after sympathetic block. With continued symptoms, dorsal sympathectomy is indicated. These will have a 90–95 percent good result.

To repeat: *Early recognition is important!*

Loss of Range of Motion of Joints

The origin of joint contracture from edema and subsequent immobilization from it have been previously discussed. When ligaments are relaxed and then become edematous with subsequent fibrin deposition, contracture and shortening ensue. For example, the two most difficult problems seen are hyperextension of the MCP joints with loss of flexion, and contracture of the proximal interphalangeal (PIP) joints in flexion with loss of extension. Again, prevention and early recognition are the key factors in controlling the range of motion loss. When an injury occurs, the wrist is usually hyperextended and the MCP joints are markedly flexed, applying maximum length to the collateral ligaments. The PIP joints are extended or slightly flexed 10–15 degrees and the hand is held in the so-called "clam-digger" position. Early motion and control of edema are necessary once the stiffness begins.

The two methods of treatment are nonoperative and operative mobilization. In nonoperative mobilization, application of stress to the offending scar tissue is the only accepted method we have of remodeling the tissues. As is well known, deliberate tearing of the tissues usually causes hemorrhage, pain, more edema, and then more scar. The three basic methods of nonoperative mobilization follow.[22]

Activation of the Musculotendinous Unit by the Patient. This method is excellent for most minor contractures but inadequate for moderate or major contractures.

Dynamic Orthoses. These aids are commercially available but they also can be made in the occupational therapy department of the hand rehabilitation center.

Progressive Casting. The orthosis is placed on the part under tension and every day, or every other day, the orthosis is changed.

The average person can tolerate well up to 6 ounces of force up to four hours. It is important to keep accurate records of the progress of the patient. When a plateau is reached, a decision must be made whether to accept the limitation or apply surgical methods. An operation is indicated if a patient exhibits a lack of 65 degrees of MCP motion or 75 degrees of PIP motion.

Various techniques have been described for operative or surgical mobilization of the joints, and readers are referred to the work of Curtis[5] and Weeks and Wray[22] for more detailed discussions.

Loss of Strength and Endurance

Most activities of daily living require a combination of endurance and strength. Therefore rehabilitation programs are aimed at not only building up strength, but also toward increasing hand endurance and decreasing body fatigue.[8] The use of progressive-resistance exercises is indicated to increase strength, but it is important that exercises dependent upon high repetition for their effect be included to improve cardiovascular function and musculature.

Shoulder Stiffness*

The shoulders have a lax capsule to allow marked mobility of that joint. Frequently with upper extremity injury, the bursal structures quickly develop capsular contracture and adhesions. Because of the numerous pain endings in the bursa, pain ensues, causing further restriction of motion, with the hand becoming dependent. Edema and pain increase in the hands. Sleep is interfered with, because the patient is awakened by pain. To prevent shoulder stiffness, the patient's shoulders must be moved through a full range of motion over the head 25 to 50 times per day. Cortisone injections can be used if a chronic state exists; slings are not advised.

---

* See also Chapter 21.

MAJOR DISEASES AND INJURIES OF THE HAND

Trauma

Crush Injuries. Most industrial hand injuries involve varying degrees of crush to the fingers or to the hand, characterized by severe edema and great pain. The pain is usually the result of crushed nerve and periosteum. When these patients are first seen, they are elevated with volar orthoses to allow MCP flexion and observed for circulatory and vascular impairment. Frequently surgical decompression in the operating room is performed, namely, dorsal decompression of skin and interosseous spaces and volar decompression of the forearm anterior compartment. The operation is followed by continued elevation without tight dressing, stellate blocks to decrease pain, and encouragement of early motion. Persistent edema problems can be handled with Jobst garments, exercises, and activities above the heart. Exercises aimed at increasing range of motion, strength, and endurance will need to be instituted later. The patients must be prepared for a long period of rehabilitation and given psychological support when the weeks and months wear on. The therapist and physician must continue to be optimistic in order not to discourage the patient.

Fractures and Dislocations of the Upper Extremity. After the fracture is reduced by open or closed methods, elevation must be instituted. Elevation is advised for injuries from the phalanges to the elbow. (It would not be possible in cases of humeral fracture.) The patient should be encouraged to place his hand above his head at least 25 to 50 times a day, and to move those joints that are not immobilized. Casts that do not need to immobilize the MCP joints should be carefully trimmed in the palm, so full MCP joint motion, as well as thenar motion, is possible. Regarding hand fractures and dislocations, it is important that reduction be accurate and attention paid to alignment of the fingers. Use of Kirschner wire inserted by open means or by the percutaneous method will allow early mobilization of the joints. With shaft fractures, one should begin early protected motion to prevent joint stiffness. Edema, decreased range of motion, pain, and decreased strength and endurance are commonly seen. An early carpal tunnel decompression for median compression in Colle's fracture will prevent further problems of RSD and stiffness.

Tendon Injuries. With the advent of atraumatic tendon repair as advocated by Koch, Mason, Allen, and Bunnell and the early motion techniques of Kleinert and Verdan,[22] some of the tendon-gliding problems have diminished. However, joint motion limitation, tendon rupture, and adherence still must be faced. Following repair of a flexor tendon, the patient will be in plaster with a rubber band attached to the fingernail. The patient is encouraged to extend the finger while the rubber band pulls the finger (or fingers) into flexion. The band is removed in three weeks and the fingers protected for an additional week. Active range of motion exercises then begin. Progressive-resistive exercises begin six weeks after the operation. Frequently there will be contracture at the PIP joint, which can be treated with a dynamic orthosis worn to decrease the original contracture. Repetitive exercises can be given later to increase endurance. In treating extensor tendon injuries when the injury is at the distal interphalangeal (DIP) joint, immobilization in extension must be undergone for four to six weeks, allowing motion at the PIP joint. With injuries at the PIP joint, again, four to six weeks of immobilization in extension are needed, allowing motion of the MCP and DIP joints. In injuries more proximal to the MCP joint and dorsum of the hand, immobilization should take place for four weeks, allowing 20 degrees flexion at the MCP joint and motion at the DIP and PIP joints. After immobilization is removed, the patient begins the active range of motion exercises. Progressive-resistance exercises can be prescribed if muscle weakness is noted.

If after three months the patient has not attained the motion needed through an adequate therapy program, surgical tenolysis should be discussed with the patient. If it is planned that tenolysis will be performed, it should be done in a program outlined by Schneider and Mackin[18] using a combination of a local anesthetic and fentanyl citrate-droperidol (Innovar). If during the procedure it is found that too much scar has formed, then a staged tendon reconstruction should be undertaken.[16]

Peripheral Nerve Injuries.* Nerve injuries can be caused by thermal or mechanical agents. Among the thermal is electricity. The most common mechanical agents are sharp objects like knives and glass, and missiles (gunshot wounds) and crushing injuries account for the others. Since the advent of careful nerve repair and the use of magnification, much improvement has been seen in the return of motor function and sensory function. With actual nerve loss of approximately 1–2 cm or more at the hand, and 4 or more cm at the elbow, some surgeons advocate nerve grafting rather than immobilizing the wrist and elbow in marked flexed positions. The following paragraphs discuss the rehabilitation of radial, ulnar, and median nerve injuries.

High radial nerve injuries must be fitted with dynamic wrist-finger-thumb orthoses to prevent stretching of the extensor and to allow the use of the hand during the opening and release phases.[4]

Ulnar nerve injuries cause paralysis and weakness of the ulnar lumbrical, thumb adductor, and dorsal and palmar interossei. Because the interossei are primary flexors of the MCP joints, an imbalance will occur with common extension and a "claw deformity" will ensue with hyperextension of the MCP joint. The proximal phalanges will assume a flexed attitude on attempts at finger extension. The power grip will weaken and a secondary contracture of the PIP joint will be observed. At that time a dynamic orthosis must be fitted, which would include a wrist and hand orthosis that has a MCP stop with an extension assist for the PIP joint. Active exercise, later moving to progressive resistance exercise, will help maintain strength while the nerve motor function returns.

In all median nerve injuries, the loss of sensation of the volar thumb, index, middle, and part of the ring finger make it mandatory that the patient be aware of the possibility of thermal or mechanical injury, and that precautions must be taken

---

* See also Chapter 19.

for protection of those sensations. In the low median nerve injury, the overactive long extensor of the thumb with the first dorsal interossei and adductor pull the thumb into extension and adduction, which produces adduction contracture. This disability can be treated with an orthosis, such as a splint with a rubber band encircling the base of the thumb attached to a leather cuff around the wrist to bring the thumb into palmar abduction. With higher injuries, the flexor pronator group of muscles is involved; therefore a program to protect weak muscles is necessary. Active exercises are begun once motor function returns, eventually followed by graded repeated exercises to reinforce prehension.

A vital aspect in treating median nerve injury is sensory re-education. Dellon and associates[6,12] have demonstrated that improvement in sensory function is possible even several years after nerve injury. Essentially the program reeducates the patient to interpret correctly the changed impulses that occur after nerve injury by application of specific sensory exercises at different times in the recovery process. Early-phase sensory education starts when the patient can perceive moving touch and vibration at 30 cps. Constant touch starts when the patient can perceive 256 cps. In late-phase sensory education, which begins after the patient can identify moving and constant touch, two-point discrimination is allowed. Various coins, hexagonal nuts, and washers are given to the patient; the objects are first felt with the uninjured hand, then with the injured hand. This exercise is first done with the eyes open, and then with the eyes closed for about 15 to 30 minutes each day.

Traumatic Amputations.* From wrist disarticulation to above-elbow amputation, treatment of the injury has the following objectives: shrinking and toughening the stump, training the patient in the use of a prosthesis in daily living activity, and increasing the motion of the involved joints. Strengthening the endurance of the shoulder and the remaining musculature must also be considered as necessary goals. Traumatic amputations about the hand, especially the digits, will need desensitization of the stumps. Pain is a common problem associated with amputation and it is therefore important that stellate blocks be applied early. Range of motion exercises and elevation for prevention of edema in the hand and fingers are prescribed early, too. Often strength and endurance will be lost in the remainder of the hand, and a program to improve these modalities must be instituted. It is of vital importance that the physician be optimistic about further function, not only with the patient, but with the patient's family. Discussion with the family should begin the day of injury to ensure their optimism at all times while talking with the patient.

Burns of the Upper Extremity.† Preservation of function is one of the three main problems facing the severely burned patient, the other two being survival and appearance.[21] In burns, loss of function is equated with a loss of active joint motion. The main cause of loss of motion is contracture, influenced by two factors: the contractive nature of the scar and the position of the extremity. In the

---

* See also Chapter 24.
† See also Chapter 23.

first instance, the physician and the team should obtain skin coverage as soon as possible so that joints can be moved freely and easily. The second factor is positioning of the joints. The contractures occur in joints in positions of comfort, that is, flexion of the extremities, which are drawn toward the trunk—shoulders are adducted, elbows are flexed and pronated, hands and wrist are flexed, the MCP joints are extended, the PIP joints are flexed, and often, too, the dorsum of the hand is edematous.

When multiple burns occur, early proper positioning should place the shoulder in abduction, elevate the hand, and support the wrist in extension with an orthosis so that the MCP joints fall into flexion. Motion of the fingers should be encouraged. The little and ring finger MCP joints often hyperextend late. Therefore it is important that the orthosis not interfere with the flexion of the ulnar side of the hand. The orthosis should be easily removable. Its materials should be lightweight and flexible to permit the patient to lift the extremity and to allow for the orthosis to be remolded easily for prevention of deformity. The orthosis should be removed several times a day and joints gently moved through a full range of motion. This would, of course, be modified during skin grafting. Many of the motion exercises can be performed while the patient is in the tub. The shoulders must be put through a full range of motion every day to prevent stiffness.

After the patient leaves the burn unit and the extremities have been grafted, the patient should attend the hand rehabilitation center for daily living instruction and treatment for increased range of motion of joints and improved strength and endurance. The constant changes necessary in the orthosis can be made in the center, including the application of dynamic orthoses for established scar. The most frequent hand deformity is that of the claw deformity position, with loss of the first web space. To prevent this, all rehabilitative efforts must be aggressive and constant.

Rehabilitating the Hand in Cerebral Palsy*

It is of primary importance to have an accurate evaluative record of the functional and cosmetic potential of rehabilitation efforts when dealing with cerebral palsy patients.[20] The complete patient must be considered first, then the upper extremity, and lastly the hand.

The functional evaluation of the hand must include coordination, strength, reach, hand placement, as well as close observation of grasp and release patterns and voluntary control. Sensibility must be determined. The pattern of common deformities seen include thumb-in-palm deformities, swan-neck deformities, flexion of the wrist, pronation of the forearm, flexion of the elbow, and internal rotation of the shoulder. Many patients are unable to open their hand for grasp. Many have unstable PIP joints, leading to hyperextension deformities of those joints. Some patients are helped by selective surgical procedures. The goals of such operations include good grasp and release, good hand placement, extension of the fingers with wrist extension, and supination with good sensibility. In 10–20 percent of the cases, operative procedures may assist in rehabilitation.

---

* See also Chapter 28.

Conservative methods and orthoses should precede any operations. However, when the patient presents with a contracture or moderate spasticity, it is then that a release sometimes should be undertaken prior to beginning further care.

Early care involves the use of orthoses to prevent fixed contractures of the joints and muscles. The position of the hand in the device should be that of wrist extension, finger extension, and the thumb held out from the palm. After long-term conservative care, the patients who are cooperative and well motivated, and who have some function of the hand regarding grasp and release, as well as some sensation, can be considered for operative procedures.

Rehabilitation of the Hand in Rheumatoid Arthritis*

The aim of rehabilitation of the arthritis patient is to restore maximum function to all the extremities, although this discussion emphasizes the upper extremity.[7] The main goal is to enable patients to continue the activities they engaged in before the onset of the illness. Resumption of daily tasks is made difficult by pain, remission, exacerbation, and deformity.

Before initiating rehabilitation, the patient's function and mobility must be assessed. Such an evaluation includes current status of function, pain, range of motion, strength, endurance, activities normally undertaken, and psychological status. The rehabilitation program would include medical and surgical treatment, physical and occupational therapy, and social service guidance.

Physical therapy decreases pain and stiffness, restores range of motion to involved joints, and increases muscle strength and endurance. Heat therapy can be used prior to exercise, preferably moist heat in the form of hot towels, mud packs, paraffin, wax, or infrared devices. Initially, active assistive, static, or active independent exercises would be prescribed, followed by active resistive exercises. After restoration of muscle strength and joint motion, the patient must be trained to use his hand in such a way that deformities will not develop. Repeated exercises are prescribed for endurance but they should show some end product. The patient could engage in wood or metalworking, basket weaving, or loom weaving.

The patient should be provided with the various self-help devices that assist in daily living activities, such as opening jars, opening house and car doors, and dressing. Various orthoses can be prescribed to rest acutely inflamed joints. Serial orthoses can be prescribed to correct existing deformities.

Millender and Nalebuff[13] have divided rheumatoid disease of the hands into four stages: early tenosynovitis and synovitis, persistent synovitis (synovitis continuing more than six months), specific rheumatoid deformity, and severely crippled and destroyed hands. The first stage of treatment includes steroid injection, resting orthoses, and making sure the patient understands the importance of rest and exercise. Resting orthoses decrease muscle spasm, relieve pain, and decrease inflammation. They can be worn day and night, but most patients will wear them only part of the day because they tend to interfere with activities.

_____

* See also Chapter 33.

A balance between rest and exercise is important. Active exercise with little resistance is recommended. Frequent short periods of exercise with rest breaks are better than any prolonged exercise. Orthoses can be constructed for immobilizing inflamed joints; resting shells can be made for each joint and can be easily removed for gentle exercise. During postoperative care, the elbows and shoulders are moved for ten minutes three times a day.

For patients in the second stage, in which a dorsal tenosynovectomy would be performed, the therapy prescribed to regain extension of the MCP joints would initially be instruction in active assisted exercises, whereby the patient extends the MCP joints and then uses the other hand to bring the finger to full extension. If full extension is not achieved, dynamic orthoses are used. Where the extensor tendon has been repaired, immobilization of the MCP joint in 20 degrees of flexion is necessary for three to four weeks while the PIP joint is allowed to move freely.

In the third stage, in which specific deformities are present, the most common are volar and ulnar subluxation and dislocation of the MCP joints. To re-establish the phalangeal relationships while still allowing motion, silicone spacers can be applied. The metacarpal heads are resected and the remaining soft tissues about the joint are retained and sutured to resist the strong volar and ulnar dislocating forces. The various orthoses have been designed to remodel the collagen about the joint. Problems that occur following implant arthroplasty include edema, which is controlled by elevation, and decreased range of motion, which is treated in a program of finger flexion and extension exercises in dynamic orthoses, such as the Swanson splint made by the Pope Company of Kankakee, Illinois.[19] This splint allows flexion and extension of the fingers, yet ulnar deviation is controlled. The splinting allows individual control of the degree of MCP motion obtained. Since the patient will frequently be unable to obtain full flexion and extension—this being the ultimate goal—emphasis may be switched to flexion in the ulnar two fingers and to extension on the radial two fingers at the MCP joints. For decreased strength, light manual resistive exercises can be prescribed, followed by repetitive prehension exercises. To increase hand dexterity, repetitive functional activities and prehension activities can be prescribed. These postoperative activities can start as early as five days following surgery.

For patients having fourth-stage deformities, that is, deformities in which salvage procedures are used, orthoses are designed and exercises prescribed as in the third stage.

Rehabilitation of the Upper Extremity in Stroke Patients*

Because the recovery of normal upper extremity function is so poor in the stroke patient, rehabilitative efforts focus on training the patient to accomplish the activities of daily living as a single-limbed individual.[3] Training for assistive functions occurs when there has been some recovery in the limb. As with many other areas in rehabilitation, the early care is the most important.

As with the RSD syndrome and burns, a vicious cycle of pain, swelling, and

_____

* See also Chapter 18.

stiffness transpires; so, also, in the stroke patient in whom spasticity leads to contracture, contracture leads to pain, which leads to more spasticity. Therefore early treatment must be aggressive and constant. The physician must pay careful attention to positioning in order to prevent deformity. Abduction of the shoulder to prevent the vicious internal rotation and abduction contracture, and extension of the wrist to prevent flexion contracture, is most important.

In addition to proper positioning, range of motion exercises and the application of a temporary orthosis to prevent flexion contracture are indicated. A sling to prevent glenohumeral subluxation is sometimes prescribed. Besides treatment for preventing contracture of the upper extremity on the afflicted side, attention must be directed to the normal side of the body, to which strengthening exercises should be given. On the involved side, splinting should be continued at night for the wrist if necessary.

When shoulder contracture becomes established, pain may accompany abduction. The pain is usually severe, interfering with sleep. Steroid injections into the shoulder to relieve a subdeltoid bursitis or a bicipital tendinitis are in order. Continued gentle manipulation by the patient with the good arm, or by a system of pulleys, should be instituted. Release of the adduction-internal rotation contracture can be accomplished by severing the subcapularis, pectoralis major, and latissimus tendons.

In cases of major sensory loss, the patient should be trained as a single-limbed individual. Major rehabilitation efforts should not be attempted, nor should the patients be kept in the hospital for prolonged periods to try to increase use of the hemiplegic limb when it has been shown such efforts are useless. In addition to releases at the shoulder, release of flexion contracture at the elbow as well as pronation-flexion release of the forearm and hand can be accomplished. Where there is marked flexion contracture of the wrist, the surgeon can undertake sublimis-to-profundus transfer, as described by Braun et al.[2] for cosmesis and hygiene.

Rehabilitating Children with Congenitally Deficient Upper Limbs

Treatment of recurrent limb and prosthetic problems is a long-term process, and it is important that care should be undertaken by a pediatric amputee team consisting of a pediatric orthopedist, pediatrician, occupational and physical therapists, social worker, psychologist, and prosthetist. One of the major problems facing the team is that of the emotional impact on the family. The family should be counseled regarding their feelings of pity, guilt, and rejection to avoid imparting these feelings to the child.

The prosthetic device should be fitted as early in life as possible and should be consistent with motor development. The rehabilitation of a child who has a congenital or acquired limb loss is essentially directed toward prehension. Grasp and release develop in a normal manner, and grasp always precedes release. From birth to the age of 9 months, infants grasp by means of bimanual palmar prehension. Later, they grasp by means of thumb, index, middle, and ring fingers.

At 18–24 months, children have controlled release, along with adequate stereoscopic vision, which allows release to occur in proper location. At ages 2–4, a well-coordinated release pattern plus arm coordination are seen when the child can throw overhanded.

Based on these patterns, a small child would be fitted with a nonfunctional mitten-type upper extremity, which could be used as an assistive device against a normal hand. The child could then graduate to a functional device. Activation of the hook terminal device with cable and harnessing could occur between the ages of 12 and 16 months.

Rehabilitating the Upper Limb in Complete Traumatic Quadriplegia

Restoration of function of the hands is one of the main goals in rehabilitating the quadriplegic patient. The patient who is young is restricted to wheelchair existence, and hence it becomes his instrument of mobility. He must see the partially paralyzed limbs for this activity as well as for transfer activities. Add all the other normal upper extremity functions, and it becomes evident that maximum rehabilitative efforts must be made to gain as much function as possible. An initial program of splinting and evaluation should be followed by surgical restoration of maximum hand function.

There must be a good initial program of occupational and physical therapies. Because there is sometimes a delay in the recovery of muscles and improvement in their strength, stiff, contracted hands may develop. Therefore orthoses are made to maintain the hands in a functional position, and the devices are coupled with a program of sensory re-education. Later, tendon transfers can improve the remaining function.

Bunch and Keagy[4] have recommended a functional analysis in the selection of the proper devices for rehabilitation. Major factors in this analysis are spinal stability, hand placement, and grasp and release pattern.

Spinal Stability. Frequently the patient must use his upper extremities to support his trunk, and thus cannot use them for routine activities of daily living. Providing support for the trunk becomes important to the extremities.

Hand Placement. The hands must be placed accurately in a space where the tasks are. Therefore assistive devices for the shoulder and elbow are frequently needed.

Grasp and Release Pattern. The pattern of open, grasp, and release is basic to hand function and forms the basis for the many functional orthoses and operative procedures that have been devised and used for rehabilitation purposes.

Zancolli[24] has divided quadriplegic patients into clinical groups. These divisions are based on the lowest functioning cord segment: Group 1: flexor of the elbow, C5; Group 2: extension of the wrist, C6; Group 3: extension of the finger, C7; and Group 4: common extensors and flexors of the fingers, C8.

In Group 1, the biceps and brachials are functioning, as are the scapulohumeral joints, letting hand placement occur. The rehabilitation program consists of an orthosis for wrist support with additional self-help devices to assist in feeding. The brachioradial muscles can be used if present, as a transfer to the extensor carpi radialis brevis, if present. Sometimes, externally powered finger-driven orthoses are prescribed for the patient.

For Group 2, Moberg[15] has pointed out that through injury or congenital defects, the extent of function diminishes in the movable sensory parts of the hand. The functions of the hand that are normally performed with the jaw-chuck pinch or grip decreases, and key or pinch grip increases. Normally, the pulp pinch is used for 50 percent of the daily activities, and the key pinch for the remaining 50 percent. His efforts to rehabilitate quadriplegic patients have been directed at obtaining key pinch, especially in the Group 1 and 2 (C5 and C6 injuries, respectively) patients. (The key pinch works so well because sensation remains on the radial side of the hand—it is possible for a patient to attain position sense, motor sense, and grip at the same time.) With extension of the wrist, the surgeon can perform a tenodesis of the flexor pollicis longus, stabilize the interphalangeal joint of the thumb, and obtain a useful hand for various tasks.

For Group 3 patients, who have good finger as well as good thumb extension, rehabilitation is aimed toward restoring opposition to the thumb, intrinsic function to the fingers, and finger flexion.

For Group 4, rehabilitation is directed toward restoring active instrinsic function to the fingers.

SUMMARY

The importance of aggressive, early care in the prevention of deformity and disability cannot be overstated. Good early care devoted to reducing pain, minimizing edema, and establishing early joint motion is mandatory. Those involved in the care of these diseases and injuries of the upper extremity must be much more than aggressive. They must be patient, kind, and optimistic, too.

REFERENCES

1. American Academy of Orthopaedic Surgeons: *Atlas of Orthotics, Biomechanical Principles, and Application.* C. V. Mosby, St. Louis, 1975.
2. Braun, R. M., Vise, G. T., and Rober, B.: Preliminary experience with superficialis to posfundus tendon transfer in the hemiplegic upper extremity. J. Bone Joint Surg. 56A:466–472, 1974.
3. Braun, R. M., West, E., Mooney, V., et al.: Surgical treatment of the painful shoulder contracture in the stroke patient. J. Bone Joint Surg. 53A:1307–1312, 1971.
4. Bunch, W. H., and Keagy, R. D.: *Principles of Orthotic Treatment.* C. V. Mosby, St. Louis, 1976.
5. Curtis, R. M.: Joints of the hand in hand surgery. In Flynn, J. E., Ed.: *Hand Surgery,* 2d ed., pp. 222–239. Williams & Wilkins, Baltimore, 1975.
6. Dellon, A. L., Curtis, R. M., and Edgerton, M. T.: Re-education of sensation in the hand following nerve injury. Johns Hopkins Med. J. 130:235–243, 1972.
7. Hall, A. P.: The decision to operate in rheumatoid arthritis. Orthop. Clin. North Am. 6(3): 675–684, 1975.
8. Herbison, G. J.: Finger motion related to rehabilitation. In Littler, J. W., Cramer, L. M., and Smith, J. W., Eds.: *Symposium in Reconstructive Hand Surgery,* pp. 246–260. C. V. Mosby, St. Louis, 1974.

9. Holdeman, V. A., and Wilson, R. L.: Transcutaneous nerve stimulator. In Hunter, J. M., Schneider, L. H., Mackin, E. J., and Bell, J. A., Eds.: *Rehabilitation of the Hand*, pp. 369–375. C. V. Mosby, St. Louis, 1978.

10. Hunter, J. M., Schneider, L. H., Mackin, E. J., and Bell, J. A., Eds.: *Rehabilitation of the Hand*. C. V. Mosby, St. Louis, 1978.

11. Lankford, L. L., and Thompson, J. E.: Reflex sympathetic dystrophy. In *Instructional Course Lectures*, pp. 163–178. American Academy of Orthopaedic Surgeons. C. V. Mosby, St. Louis, 1977.

12. Maynard, C. J.: Sensory re-education following peripheral nerve injury. In Hunter, J. M., Schneider, L. H., Mackin, E. J., and Bell, J. A., Eds.: *Rehabilitation of the Hand*, pp. 318–323. C. V. Mosby, St. Louis, 1978.

13. Millender, L. H., and Nalebuff, E. A.: Early rheumatoid hand involvement. Orthop. Clin. North Am. 6(3):697–708, 1975.

14. Moberg, E.: Method for examining sensibility of the hand. In Flynn, J. E., Ed.: *Hand Surgery*, 2nd ed., pp. 435–449. Williams & Wilkins, Baltimore, 1975.

15. Moberg, E.: Surgical treatment for absent single hand grip and elbow extension in quadriplegia. J. Bone Joint Surg. 57A:196–206, 1975.

16. Mackin, E.: Physical therapy and the staged tendon graft, preoperative and postoperative management. In *Symposium on Tendon Surgery in the Hand*, pp. 283–291. American Academy of Orthopaedic Surgeons. C. V. Mosby, St. Louis, 1975.

17. Nickel, V. L.: The model of a hand rehabilitation center. In Hunter, J. M., Schneider, L. H., Mackin, E. J., and Bell, J. A., Eds.: *Rehabilitation of the Hand*, pp. 655–659. C. V. Mosby, St. Louis, 1978.

18. Schneider, L. H., and Mackin, E. J.: Tenolysis. In Hunter, J. M., Schneider, L. H., Mackin, E. J., and Bell, J. A., Eds.: *Rehabilitation of the Hand*, pp. 229–234. C. V. Mosby, St. Louis, 1978.

19. Swanson, A. B.: *Flexible Implant Resection Arthroplasty in the Hand and Extremities*. C. V. Mosby, St. Louis, 1973.

20. Swanson, A. B.: Surgery of the hand in cerebral palsy. In Flynn, J. E., Ed.: *Hand Surgery*, pp. 328–337. Williams & Wilkins, Baltimore, 1975.

21. Reardon, J. C.: Occupational therapy treatment of the patient with thermally injured upper extremity. Burns of the upper extremity. In Salisbury, R. E. J., and Pruitt, B. A., Eds.: *Major Problems in Clinical Surgery*, vol. 19, pp. 127–147. W. B. Saunders, Philadelphia, 1976.

22. Weeks, C. M., and Wray, R. C.: *Management of Acute Hand Injuries*. C. V. Mosby, St. Louis, 1978.

23. Wynn-Parry, C. B.: *Rehabilitation of the Hand*. Butterworth, London, 1973.

24. Zancolli, E.: *Structural and Dynamic Bases of Hand Surgery*. J. B. Lippincott, Philadelphia, 1968.

15

Spinal Cord Injuries

Robert W. Hussey, M.D.

Spinal cord injury is the most disabling consistently survivable injury that occurs to man. It can be defined as a traumatically induced dysfunction of the spinal cord that results in a nonprogressive loss of sensory and motor function distal to the point of injury. There is usually an associated injury to the spine impairing its structural stability; it is this impaired stability that is the most common factor leading to the spinal cord injury. Effective management of the injury to the spine and spinal cord in the initial phases must recognize this interrelationship. This definition excludes paralysis due to diseases of the central nervous system, such as degenerative diseases, primary or metastatic neoplasms, or vascular diseases, because these conditions are most often progressive. However, certain patients with a vascular anomaly, such as arteriovenous malformation, or with vascular accidents, such as a ruptured aorta or degenerative disk disease, may experience a sudden onset of nonprogressive paralysis as the result of the process or its treatment. It can be treated like a traumatic lesion.

There are two broad categories of spinal cord injury: complete and incomplete. A complete spinal cord injury is one in which there is no detectable sensory or voluntary motor function below the level of injury. The most significant feature of complete injury is that there is little or no chance of functional recovery if that situation persists for more than a few hours. An incomplete injury is one with preservation to some degree of sensory or motor function below the level of injury. Incomplete injuries are capable of further functional recovery.

Injury to the spinal cord from the first cervical segment to and including the first thoracic segment produces sensory and motor deficits in all four limbs and is referred to as quadriplegia or tetraplegia. Injuries from the second thoracic segment and below spare the upper extremities and result in paraplegia.

PREVALENCE, INCIDENCE, AND CAUSES

Accurate prevalence and incidence figures are difficult to obtain, and there are few published reports. The prevalence rate for persons with complete or partial paralysis as the result of injury is 0.8 per 1000 population or 145 to 170,000 persons in 1971 in the United States.[20]

The annual incidence of spinal cord injury is estimated at 25 to 35 injuries per million population.[20] In a recent study of northern California countries, incidence was 52.4 per million. If those admitted dead on arrival or who died immediately after admission to the hospital were excluded, the incidence rate was 32 per million per year.[10] In the same study, the case fatality rate was 48.3 percent, of which 79 percent died prior to hospital admission. The case fatality rate for persons admitted to the hospital was 17 percent. In a survival study conducted on Veterans Administration patients, the 10-year survival for patients who survived the first three months was 86 percent for paraplegics and 80 percent for quadriplegics.[11]

The leading cause of spinal cord injury is motor vehicle accidents. Falls, sports injuries, particularly diving, and gunshot wounds are the other common causes.[20]

HISTORICAL PERSPECTIVE

Until World War II, little effective rehabilitation was even considered for victims of spinal cord injury, and most persons so injured died within a short time of injury. Dr. Donald Munro, who set up a unit at Boston City Hospital, reported in 1954 on results of 445 patients treated since 1930. He emphasized that comprehensive rehabilitation could return the spinal cord injured patient to a productive life in the community. During World War II, more patients survived spinal cord injury, and Sir Ludwig Guttmann founded the National Spinal Cord Injury Center at Stoke-Mandeville, England. In large measure based on Guttmann's results, the concept of a comprehensive spinal cord injury center gained worldwide acceptance. In the United States, the Veterans Administration set up similar centers for American spinal cord injured veterans. This system now has grown to 18 centers. With the support of the industrial accident insurance carriers, and more recently the U.S. Department of Health, Education, and Welfare and the National Institutes of Health, regional spinal cord injury centers have been established throughout the country. They all follow the principles established by Munro and Guttmann: that the care and rehabilitation of spinal cord injured patients are best provided in spinal cord injury centers to which the patients are admitted for comprehensive treatment as soon as possible after injury.

GENERAL PHILOSOPHY OF TREATMENT

The basic philosophy of treatment is to minimize functional deficits, prevent complications, and use all remaining function, both voluntary and reflex, to the maximum extent in order to return the patient in as short a time as reasonable to a productive life in society. One must bear in mind that with modern care the spinal cord injured person has a nearly normal life expectancy, and this potential should not be compromised in order to achieve short-term objectives.

The first treatment priority is survival of the patient. Associated life-threatening injuries and conditions take precedence over the spinal cord injury in the treatment plan. The second priority is reduction and stabilization of the injured spine. The third priority is to reverse, if possible, the effects of the injury to the spinal cord. It might be argued that this should be the first priority. However, it is sad but true that there is at present no generally accepted surgical or pharmacological treatment that has been shown to be efficacious in reversing the neurological deficit. Rehabilitation starts at the moment of injury. At first, the goals are to preserve normal range of motion in all joints, maintain the strength of existing muscles, and prevent deformity.

The care of the spinal cord injured person is complex and requires the skill of diverse professions. This care is best delivered by the team headed by a single responsible physician who has knowledge of all aspects of the care and rehabilitation of the spinal cord injured patient. This essential body of knowledge is of a multidisciplinary nature and no single specialty can legitimately claim primacy for the direction of the care. The leader of the team must appreciate and understand the role of all the medical and paramedical specialties involved and treat them as professionals with needed expertise. There is no ideal team, but at least representatives from general medicine, general surgery, plastic surgery, urology, neurology, neurosurgery, orthopedics, physical and occupational therapy, social work, psychology, and, most importantly, nursing should be included.

As soon as the extent and nature of the spinal cord, spine, and injuries to other parts of the body are determined, it should be possible to determine the prognosis for survival and neurological recovery. Based on this knowledge, therapeutic and rehabilitation goals can be established, and an estimate made of the time required to meet those goals. It is important to set this timetable as early as possible so that both the patient and family know what to expect and can begin planning and preparing. These goals may be difficult for the patient and the family to accept initially and may require modification and change based on the patient's progress.

EVALUATION OF THE PATIENT

General Care

The general examination with a complete history and physical is as important in the spinal cord injured person as any other patient. A point to be remembered is that the neurological injury may eliminate important findings usually relied upon, such as pain, tenderness, and muscle spasm. The laboratory examination includes complete blood count, blood urea nitrogen, sodium, potassium, chloride, calcium, phosphorus, alkaline phosphatase, and determination of the pH, oxygen partial pressure, and carbon dioxide partial pressure of arterial blood. The basic roentgenographic examination should include lateral x-rays of the entire spine, chest x-ray, and anterioposterior views of the injured area of the spine. Additional spinal x-rays are determined by the level involved. In the cervical area in particular, oblique x-rays and an open-mouth anterioposterior view of C1 are important for a complete examination of the cervical spine. X-rays should be taken of any extremity with external evidence of trauma, abnormal or false motion in any of the long bones, or abnormal motion of any joint.

A complete and accurately recorded neurological examination is the single most important procedure in establishing treatment for the injured spinal cord. It serves as the basis for determining further diagnostic evaluation, treatment, prognosis, and planning of rehabilitation. The sensory examination is best recorded on an outline drawing or, in the emergency phase, on the patient himself.

Figure 15-1 shows the major sensory and motor tracks and blood supply to the spinal cord. The anterior spinal artery supplies the anterior two-thirds of the central gray matter and the white matter anterior to the posterior horn. The paired posterior spinal arteries supply the posterior one-third, and the interconnecting circumferential arteries, the narrow band in the periphery of the cord. Of particular importance is the fact that the lateral cortical spinal motor tract and the lateral spinal thalamic tract are not only in close anatomical relationship, but have a common blood supply. Therefore sparing of pain and temperature sensation carries not only a favorable prognosis for further recovery of these modalities, but for motor function as well.

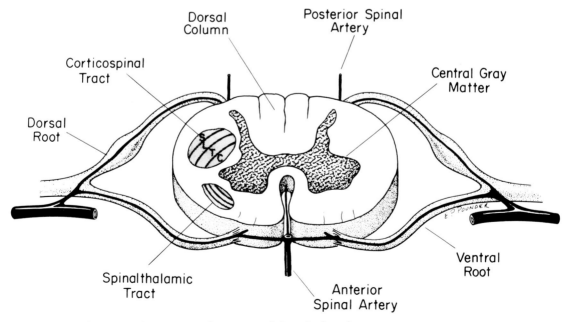

Fig. 15-1. Cross-sectional anatomy of the spinal cord.

In experimental spinal cord injury, the first effects are seen in the gray matter, with decreased blood flow, decreased oxygen content, intra- and extracellular edema, and petechial hemorrhage. This process then evolves, with enlarging and coalescence of the hemorrhagic areas and cellular necrosis. The process then extends out into the white matter. In complete injuries, the process extends to the periphery of the cord, and all neural elements in this area are destroyed. In incomplete injuries, the same processes are seen but are less intense and do not extend to the periphery of the cord. The fibers in the long tracts going to and from the sacral segments are located peripherally, which is felt to be the basis for the finding of sacral sparing in incomplete injuries as possibly the only sign of incompleteness. The entire process of hemorrhagic necrosis in experimental models evolves over a four to eight hour period. However, the neurological deficit is usually instantaneous. The process in the experimental model can be modified and ameliorated by a variety of physical and pharmacological manipulations, such as cooling, myelotomy, steroids, and sympatholytic drugs. To date, however, none of these manipulations have proved to work consistently for human beings.[18]

The first element of the neurological examination relevant to the spinal cord injury is the determination of the sensory and motor level. In determining the neurological level, it is important to remember that the segments C5 through T1 are not represented on the anterior portion of the trunk but are found only on the arms. If the level is determined only by testing the trunk in any cervical injury, the level will be found at the junction of C4 and T2 dermatomes 4 to 5 cm below the clavicle. When doing this part of the examination, it is most convenient to place the patient's arms away from the side of the body in the palm-up position. One then does the testing in the mid-axillary line moving across the axilla and then down the postaxial border of the arm across the palm and up the preaxial border of the arm to the shoulder. In this way, each dermatome from T2 to C4 is crossed in succession. The accurate determination of the neurological level, particularly in the zone between C7 and T3, is especially important because the corresponding segments of the spine are difficult to demonstrate by standard radiographic technique. In order to diagnose the spine injury in this area, it is often necessary to use special radiographic techniques, such as swimmers' views, oblique views, tomography, and even fluoroscopic examination. The author has seen on several occasions major dislocations in the C7, T1, and T2 areas missed because the neurological level was not accurately defined and therefore the radiographic examination was not properly pursued. On one occasion in an incomplete injury with major motor and sensory sparing, the patient was ordered to begin strenuous transfer activities on the assumption that there was no spine injury. Fortunately, before the patient began these activities an accurate neurological level was determined at T1-T2. An x-ray examination revealed a complete dislocation of T1 on T2. Activity was immediately restricted until the spine was properly stabilized and the patient suffered no additional neurological damage.

The next step is to determine if the injury is complete or incomplete. This may be obvious and already determined along with the level, but particularly in extremely acute injuries preserved function may be confined to sacral segments, or the so-called "sacral sparing." Only after careful examination of the perianal, perineal, and genital regions, and checks for motion of the toe muscles and sphincter reveal no sparing can the patient be considered to have a complete injury. This examination should be repeated after satisfactory spine alignment has been obtained. On a number of occasions, I have seen initially complete patients become incomplete after reduction of the dislocation or displacement.

Table 15-1 lists the incomplete syndromes, their major features, and their prognosis for recovery.[3] Several generalizations can be made. The earlier and more rapidly the recovery occurs, the better the end result. Motor sparing carries the best prognosis for major functional improvement followed by preservation to pain. It is common for a definitely incomplete patient to go as long as three weeks before the first signs of motor recovery are seen. E. S. Stauffer, in discussing prognosis based on neurological examination, states that in the presence of complete spinal shock as evidenced by a complete state of areflexia the absence of sacral sparing may not indicate a complete lesion. The bulbocavernosus reflex (reflex contraction of the anal sphincter on the squeezing of the glans penis or clitoris or tugging on the catheter) is usually the first reflex to return, often so quickly after injury that one can question if it were ever lost. Stauffer uses the return of this reflex to indicate the end of the spinal shock phase and that at this point, if there is no sacral sparing, the injury can be truly considered to be complete. The experience at our center does not support this hypothesis and we do not feel that the absence of the bulbocavernosus reflex invalidates the finding of no sacral sparing in determining that the patient is complete. We have found, however, that some patients are spastic with hyperactive deep-tendon reflexes

Table 15-1.   Incomplete Spinal Cord Injuries and their Prognoses for Recovery

SYNDROME	SALIENT FEATURES	PROGNOSIS
Brown-Sequard (functional hemi-section)	Motor loss one side, pain and temperature loss opposite side	Good
Central cord syndrome	Usually cervical; all sensory motor functions involved; involvement greatest at level of lesion; greater sparing distally	Variable; spasticity and poor hand function
Anterior cord syndrome	Complete or partial loss of pain, temperature and motor function; touch and position sense spared	Poor for motor recovery unless pain sensation spared
Posterior cord syndrome	Normal pain; temperature and motor loss; absent touch and position sense	Extremely rare
Concussion	Complete or partial loss momentary with rapid recovery	Normal within 48 hours

immediately after injury and that these patients become incomplete, as evidenced by the appearance of sensory sparing even though initially they had none. Therefore while we consider testing for the bulbocavernosus reflex an integral part of the initial complete neurological examination, we have not been able to relate its presence or absence to final neurological outcome.[15,16]

Standard Radiology

The standard radiographic examination of the spine includes anterior, posterior, and lateral views of all segments of the spine. All should be obtained without moving the patient. In the cervical spine in addition, oblique views that can be obtained without moving the patient through angling the x-ray tube 50 degrees are vital to determine the presence of unilateral facet dislocations, dislocations in the lower cervical and upper thoracic spine, and fractures of pedicles, facets, and laminae. Oblique views are of little value in thoracic spine due to superimposed rib shadow, but they may help to define some injuries in the lumbar spine. The open-mouth view for the odontoid fracture should be included in patients with head trauma or cervical spine injury. Tomography, in particular polytomography, aids in defining the skeletal injury, particularly if the standard radiographs are equivocal or if the spine is obscured by superimposed structures. Lateral views in flexion and extension should be obtained when static films fail to show an injury in patients with spine pain or neurological deficit. These views, however, should be performed carefully and only by individuals experienced in obtaining such studies in spine-injured persons, and usually under fluoroscopic control.

Neuroradiological Examination

The most commonly performed neuroradiological examination is myelography. The oil-based contrast materials yield little information of value because their density obscures the spinal cord, and their viscosity results in a completely obstructed flow of contrast material if there is any compromise in the diameter of the spinal canal from cord edema or bone or soft tissue. Gas myelography combined with polytomography gives a negative contrast image that demonstrates the spinal cord and any soft tissues or bone in the canal,[13] showing the relationship of these materials to the spinal cord. Similarly, water-soluble contrast materials, such as metrizamide, can demonstrate many of the same structures.

The most exciting development is computerized axial tomography (CAT scanning) of the spine, with or without the addition of water-soluble contrast material. The enhanced imagery of the new equipment shows both the spine and spinal cord and demonstrates fractures and other pathology that cannot be picked up by the previously mentioned techniques. The experience with this technique in spinal cord injury is limited to date, and its proper role in the evaluation of spinal cord injury has not been fully defined. Quite possibly CAT scanning could replace all the other forms of neuroradiological assessment of the spinal cord injured person.

Other tests that may be used are electromyography and evoked cortical potentials. In general, a careful neurological examination will yield as much useful clinical information as these electrodiagnostic tests. They may, however, distinguish between spinal cord and plexus or peripheral nerve injuries. They also have value in the evaluation of patients with altered states of consciousness when the usual neurological examination gives unreliable information.

ACUTE MANAGEMENT

General Care

The general care of the acutely injured patient is first directed toward survival of the patient. The standard treatment programs applicable to any victim of trauma are followed: frequent monitoring of vital signs, urinary output, arterial blood gases, serial hemoglobin and hematocrit, white blood count, and serum electrolytes.

Steroids, either dexamethasone or methylprednisolone, are given in the acute phase. The program followed in our center is to give 10–20 mg of dexamethasone intravenously as soon as the newly injured patient is admitted. This injection is followed by 4–6 mg intravenously or intramuscularly every six hours for one to two days. Over the next five days, the schedule is tapered off. This program tends to be used more often with incomplete and cervical spine lesions. Complete thoracic and thoracolumbar lesions are given only a three-day course of steroids. If the patient has responses indicating neurological improvement, steroid dosage may be continued for up to ten days and then tapered over three to five days. All patients are started on 300 mg of cimetidine intravenously every six hours until they begin taking oral fluids and then are given 300 mg by mouth three times a day for the first three weeks as prophylaxis for stress ulceration.

The patient must be turned every two hours to avoid pressure sores. This can be accomplished in a regular hospital bed, even with the patient in traction, by log rolling from side to back to side. Specialized beds and frames may make this safer and simpler with less personnel, but no single such device is universally applicable. Patients with cervical levels of C4 and above do not tolerate the prone position because of their decreased ventilation, and fatal hypoxia can result. The circoelectric bed in particular is not thought to be appropriate for acutely injured patients. These patients may have severe postural hypotension during turning; the gravitational loading of the spine during turning can cause displacement, and the pressure placed on the heels during rapid turning results in pressure sores of the plantar surface of the heels.

The leading cause of early morbidity and mortality is pulmonary dysfunction. Close monitoring of the pulmonary status by auscultation of the chest, by chest x-rays, and by arterial blood gas determinations will enable one to anticipate problems. Chest physical therapy should be instituted at once, with deep breathing exercises, assisted coughing exercises, and mechanical aids, such as the incentive respirometer or intermittent positive-pressure breathing machine. In patients unable to mobilize their secretions, nasotracheal suctioning or therapeutic bronchoscopy may be needed. If it is necessary to use a mechanical respirator, endotracheal intubation by the oral or nasal route is preferable to immediate tracheostomy. If one anticipates the need for long ventilatory support, then elective tracheostomy can be performed five to ten days following injury.

The prompt restoration of normal spine alignment and mobilization of the injured segments of the spine are the next priorities. For cervical spine injuries, these are best accomplished by skeletal traction, using either calvarial tongs or the halo ring. The halo ring has the advantage of being able to be incorporated into an orthotic device or cast. It provides rigid immobilization of the spine and early mobilization of the patient. Reduction of cervical dislocation should ideally be accomplished within four to eight hours by increasing weights and close x-ray monitoring. Closed manipulation is not routinely practiced or advocated in this country, in contrast to Australia and South Africa. If done, it should only be carried out by someone experienced in the technique. If reduction cannot be obtained by closed means, then emergency open reduction should be performed unless contraindicated by the condition of the patient. If open reduction is performed, it should be accompanied by internal fixation and fusion. There is less unanimity of opinion as to the handling of thoracic and thoracolumbar fracture dislocations. The postural reduction techniques advocated by Guttmann[7] have the greatest worldwide acceptance. In this country, the use of open reduction internal fixation using the Harrington instrumentation system is rapidly gaining popularity. An alternative has recently been advocated, the use of traction reduction via the pelvic band or the halo femoral traction.[5,19] Our personal preference is pelvic band traction, and with this method we have been able to obtain realignment of the injured spine rapidly without the need for emergency surgery.

The other injuries, in particular life-threatening thoracic and abdominal injuries, take preference in the treatment plan, even over emergency spinal surgery. The treatment of associated extremity fractures utilizes the same general therapeutic principles applied to comparable injuries in the patient whose spinal cord is not injured, with two exceptions. Solid circular casts should never be applied below the level of injury, and traction is difficult to handle, particularly with regard to the need for routinely turning the patient. Whenever possible, taking into consideration the type of fracture and condition of the patient, early open reduction and internal fixation will significantly simplify the care of the patient and the fracture. External skeletal fixation may be ideal for the spinal cord injured patients in that the method eliminates the need for casts and immobilization of adjacent joints. Therefore it allows continual skin inspection and early range of motion to adjacent joints without the necessity of major surgical procedures.

The initial rehabilitation efforts begin on the day of injury. These include accurate recording of muscle strength and joint range of motion, range of motion exercises several times per day of all paralyzed joints, and active exercises for the unparalyzed muscles. Resting splints should be fabricated for the hands of all quadriplegics and they must be worn continuously except during exercise periods and inspection. The patient should be positioned to prevent the development of deformities, in particular, equinus deformity of the feet and ankles, adduction and internal rotation deformity of the shoulders, and flexion deformity at the elbows. Whenever and as soon as possible, the patient should begin self-feeding and doing light hygiene activities, even though on bed rest and in traction.

Deep venous thrombosis and thromboembolic disease pose a real hazard to the spinal cord injured patient. The reported incidence varies widely, in large measure related to the criteria for diagnosis, but it has been reported to be as high as 80 percent. There is no standard accepted means for prevention in the spinal cord injured patient, as in the rest of orthopedic practice. The preventive means advocated as beneficial range from frequent range of motion exercises through stocking and intermittent compression boots to anticoagulation with heparin or warfarin. The lethal potential of this complication is such that some measure should be taken for prevention and early recognition in order to prevent a massive, fatal, pulmonary embolus.

Early Urological and Bowel Care. The accepted standard in most spinal cord injury units for bladder management is intermittent catheterization. This means emptying the bladder at regular four- to eight-hour intervals using an aseptic technique of catherization. The intervals of catheterization and the fluid intake must be adjusted so that no more than 500 cc of urine are allowed to accumulate in the bladder between catheterizations. If it is necessary to monitor urinary output closely, or give large amounts of fluids, such as blood or plasma, it is best to put the patient on constant catheter drainage until these needs are past.

Reflex ileus occurs following most spine fractures and spinal cord injury. The patient should not be given liquids or food orally until coordinated intestinal activity returns, as evidenced by passage of flatus and feces. If there is any tendency to abdominal distention, gastric dilatation, or vomiting, a nasogastric tube should be passed to decompress the stomach until coordinated intestinal function resumes. The patient is started on a daily program of suppository with a small enema every three days if there is no result from the suppository, until a pattern of regular fecal elimination is established. This program is usually modified in a few weeks to one bowel movement every other day both for the patient's and the staff's convenience. This establishes a pattern that the patient should retain the rest of his life, with minimal risk of "accidents" between periods of bowel evacuation.

SPINE STABILIZATION

The mechanical function of the spine is to provide a flexible axial support for the body in the upright position, and the goal of treatment is to restore this function. Support is provided by the combined effect of the vertebrae, ligaments, and spinal musculature. The keys are the osseous integrity of the vertebra and the continuity of its ligaments. The structural stability anteriorly is provided by the vertebral bodies, the intervertebral disk, and the anterior and posterior longitudinal ligaments. Posteriorly the facet joints, their capsular ligaments, the interspinous ligaments, the interlamina ligamentum flavum, and the attached muscles provide the stability. The posterior complex is the key to alignment of the spine, since it is composed of the arthroidal or gliding joints that limit motion by their structure.

The spine when injured heals by three means: healing of the fractured bones, healing of the disrupted ligaments, and spontaneous fusion between injured vertebrae. The healing of the fractured bone occurs through the normal processes of fracture healing and results in solid bony union. The spontaneous fusion between vertebrae occurs most commonly through the formation of new bone anteriorly between injured vertebra or across the disk spaces at the point of dislocation. These two forms of healing bring about the most stable form of union.

The healing of torn ligaments is accomplished, however, by the formation of fibrous scar tissue. This fibrous scar is often not as strong as the original ligament and does not prevent abnormal mobility in the area of injury. When the healing process consists of only this type of healing, abnormal mobility or instability is frequently the result.

Late instability following spine injury can take two forms. The first and most common is the result of a failure of the healing process, leading to persisting abnormal mobility in the area of injury. This is usually the result of inadequate immobilization during the healing phase or inadequate length of time of immobilization to allow adequate healing. The second form of late instability is progressive deformity in the area of injury. This results from healing in a markedly deformed position so that normal gravitational and muscular stresses produce a progressive deformity. Most spine injuries will heal if the patient is immobilized by bed rest with careful turning and positioning and, when the injury is in the cervical region, with traction. This process is usually completed within three months and only rarely is the degree of damage and deformity so great as to prevent it. As mentioned, the only major exception is the purely ligamentous injury, as is seen in cervical spine dislocations in which the resulting ligamentous scar is insufficient to prevent abnormal mobility.

The methods of treatment available are bed rest alone, bed rest with traction, orthotic support, and surgical stabilization that is usually accompanied by some form of internal fixation. Bed rest with or without traction results in stable healing in the majority of instances. This, of course, eliminates the risk of surgery but, particularly in units not accustomed to dealing with acute injuries, increases the risk of such complications as pneumonia, atelectasis, pressure sores, deep venous thrombosis, and restriction of joint motion. Orthotic support alone is usually insufficient to provide immobilization of the injured spine. The halo cast or brace combinations will immobilize the cervical spine sufficiently to allow healing without confining the patient to bed. When the skin underneath the orthotic device is anesthetic, there is a risk of pressure necrosis, but in incompletely injured patients halo brace immobilization is an ideal, nonoperative means of stabilization that allows early mobilization of the patient. Operative stabilization in properly selected patients will allow early mobilization of the patient, but these procedures should be performed only by surgeons experienced in these operations in spinal cord injured patients.

Cervical spine stabilization is classically obtained by the use of skull traction and bed rest. Turning frames help in maintaining spine alignment, but they are not essential. The traction device most widely used today is the Gardner-Wells tongs, which are easily applied and need no additional equipment beyond the tongs themselves. The halo can be used as a traction device in the same way as the tongs; later they can be attached to an orthotic device if indicated. The traction, in addition to immobilizing the spine, is used to reduce the displacement and deformity. Surgical stabilization can be obtained by anterior or posterior fusion, depending on the nature of the skeletal injury. The anterior approach is best for burst and comminuted fractures of the vertebral body. It usually combines resection of the fractured body and replacement with a fibula or iliac strut graft. If present, facet joint dislocations should be reduced prior to anterior fusion, because it is difficult to reduce facet dislocations indirectly from the anterior approach.[14] The interbody types of fusions, such as the Cloward procedure used for cervical disk disease, are not appropriate for this class of injury, since they do not restore the instability created by the fractured vertebral body. Posterior fusion is used in cases of facet dislocations, either as part of open reduction of locked facet dislocations or as a stabilizing measure for a previously reduced facet dislocation.

For purposes of this discussion, the thoracic spine is limited to the segments of thoracic vertebrae 1–10. These segments' articulation with ribs attached to the sternum provides stabilization of vertebral segments themselves in addition to the intrinsic spinal structures. Of the three areas of the spine, this is least frequently associated with spinal cord injury. When injured, it is usually by extreme and often direct force and associated with injuries to the thorax and intrathoracic structures. The spinal cord injury in this region is usually complete and has an extremely rare indication for surgical intervention. The bony injury is often complex: typically, it is one of multiple fragments, that despite a tendency toward gross displacement, go on to solid bone union. Therefore injuries in this region of the spine stabilized by the ribs can be mobilized more quickly and rarely require surgical stabilization. If it is necessary, posterior fusion fixation with Harrington rods is the method of choice.

Injuries to the thoracolumbar spine, that is, the eleventh thoracic through second lumbar vertebrae, initially are the most unstable encountered. Most are caused by a combination of flexion, rotation, and compression forces, resulting in the slice fracture dislocation or burst fracture.[8] Either of these conditions can seriously disrupt the anterior and posterior bony and ligamentous structures. Prompt closed reduction similar to that used in cervical spine injury is more difficult, but recent experience with traction methods is encouraging.[5,19] The accepted closed method has been ''postural'' reduction, in which pads or pillows slowly correct the anterior-posterior deformity, but not the rotary or lateral deformity. Due to the instability and difficulty in reduction, operative reduction through internal fixation has been advocated by a number of authorities.[2,4,7,16] Currently, the most popular technique is correction and internal fixation using Harrington distraction rods.[6] These rods should extend at least two segments above and below the injured segments, and autogenous bone grafts should be added for fusion. Compression rods or springs are used for those injuries with primary forward or flexion deformity and intact posterior structures.

In considering surgical versus nonsurgical stabilization, several points must be considered. Fractured vertebrae, like any other bone, will heal if the fragments are in reasonable approximation and adequately immobilized for a sufficient time. Purely ligamentous injuries heal less well, but in most instances there is sufficient injury to the bone or periosteal tissue to stimulate spontaneous intersegmental fusion. Therefore at least 80–90 percent of spine injuries will heal within 12 weeks on a program of recumbent immobilization. Most spine fractures and dislocations can be satisfactorily realigned by closed traction or postural means. The neurological outcome has not been improved by surgical stabilization. The only clear difference is a shortening of the period of bed rest in the surgically stabilized group and a slightly shortened initial hospital stay.[6] In each instance therefore one must weigh the risk of surgery, the type of operation required, and the benefit expected from the reduction of the period of bed rest. Certainly, there is no clear advantage that would enable one to say that surgical stabilization is the preferred method of treatment.

PHYSICAL REHABILITATION

The Rehabilitation Team

The rehabilitation team is really only a subset of the basic treatment team. Classically, it is composed of physical and occupational therapists under the direction of a physician familiar with rehabilitation techniques. Ideally, this is the same physician who has primary responsibility for overall treatment of the patient so that all aspects of rehabilitation and treatment remain coordinated. Other members of the team are orthotists, driver training instructors, and other specialized types of therapists. The exact composition is determined in large measure by the institution and its traditions.

The remainder of the treatment team contributes and should be considered part of the rehabilitation team. In particular, nursing personnel play a pivotal role, for they have the closest and most frequent contact with the patient and must reinforce the newly learned skills, provide supervision, and, most important, insist that the patient utilize the new skills. Social workers, psychologists, and vocational counselors must be up to date as to the patient's potential and inform the team of specific therapy needs of which they may become aware.

The working relationships between the members of the team depend upon the establishment of responsibility for the various aspects of rehabilitation. As in any team, all members must know their responsibility and assignments. Usually this means assigning specific aspects to specific therapy groups or therapists, such as dressing to occupational therapy and transferring to physical therapy. There can, however, be no hard and fast rules in this regard, and much of it depends on institutional organization, training, and tradition. It matters little who does what so long as everyone does his or her job, and the entire program is accomplished. Regular team meetings are essential to keep the patient's program coordinated and give everyone the opportunity to contribute expertise.

Rehabilitation Methods and Techniques

The first rehabilitation treatment goal is to maintain a normal range of motion in all joints. This is accomplished by proper positioning and regular range of motion exercises—active assistance for those portions with functioning muscles and passive for paralyzed joints. Therapy is started as soon as the patient is injured. Formal range of motion exercises by a therapist should be carried out at least daily, and more frequently if the patient has restricted motion or is developing restriction of motion. This problem is most apt to appear in joints with an unopposed major muscle, such as at the elbow when the biceps is of normal strength yet the triceps is absent. Range of motion exercises are supplemented by static positioning orthoses or other devices, such as blocks or pillows. These aids prevent deformity, particularly of the hands and wrists in the quadriplegic and equinus deformity of the foot and ankle to all patients with paralysis of the legs. The patient should be instructed as soon as possible in self-ranging and exercising.

The nursing team participates informally in ranging by positioning the patient properly to prevent loss of motion and deformity. The patient in the side-back-side turning program should have the lower leg positioned in full extension at the hip and knee, and the upper leg positioned in full flexion at the hip and knee. This means that every time the patient is turned, these joints are carried through a full range of motion. A common deformity, especially in patients in turning frames, is internal rotation and adduction deformity of the shoulder. It can be prevented by positioning the arms in abduction and external rotation through part of the day.

The modalities of heat, cold, ultrasound, and diathermy play a small role in rehabilitating the spinal cord injured patient. Extreme care must be exercised when these modalities are used in areas of reduced sensation so as not to injure the patient. The primary value of these modalities is to relieve pain and spasm and to gain the patient's cooperation in the range of motion program. No one modality is clearly superior to the others, and different modalities may be effective in different patients with the same problem.

Prescribing appropriate orthotic devices and equipment is one of the most important aspects in rehabilitation of the spinal cord injured person. The proper equipment can make the patient more independent, make employment possible, and improve the quality of life.

The single most important item for most patients is the wheelchair. The basic objective must be to keep the chair as light and narrow as possible. The back height should be adjusted so that it comes just below the point of the scapula so as not to interfere with pushing. The seat depth is measured to make the front edge 5 cm proximal to the popliteal crease, and the foot rest adjusted so that the knees are slightly lower than the hips. This increases the weight carried by the thighs, takes weight off the ischial region, and distributes the weight over the greatest possible surface, all of which help decrease the risk of ischial pressure sores. Manual propulsion is feasible for most patients with functional levels below C6, although modifications of the rims may be needed for the quadriplegic patient. High backs and reclining backs are rarely needed, and then only for patients with levels at C4 and above.

Motorized wheelchairs are needed for most patients with functional levels of C5 and higher. The best controller is the proportional hand or joy stick control. Nonproportional control may be needed in patients with poor arm control, spasticity, or involuntary movements. Chin control would be adequate for the majority of patients unable to use hand controls, but some patients may require other means, such as the tongue switch, puff and sip, or more sophisticated control mechanisms.

A proper cushion is equally vital. No cushion exists that completely prevents pressure sores. The patient or whoever is responsible for his care must periodically relieve the weight on the sitting surfaces or pressure sores will develop. The most satisfactory cushion remains the 7.5–10 cm thick, latex, pin core, foam rubber variety. Other cushions of special materials, construction, or configuration may be needed in special circumstances, in particular, for those patients with scars from previous pressure sores or fixed deformities.

Patients with functional levels between C5 and C7 may benefit from a functional hand orthosis. The two most useful are the wrist-driven, flexor-hinge hand splint for those with functioning wrist extensors, and the ratchet hand splint for patients without wrist extensors. The ratchet splint is a modification of the wrist-driven splint, giving passive prehension by means of a one-way ratchet.

Paraplegics with functional levels below L1 and L2 may achieve functional ambulation with the use of lower limb orthoses. For limbs without knee, ankle, and foot control, the long leg brace or a knee-ankle-foot orthosis (KAFO) will be needed. Essential features of this brace are the rigid foot-ankle unit and either a drop lock or bail lock knee unit. The Scott Craig orthosis is one of the most satisfactory forms of KAFO. It is rare that a patient who requires bilateral KAFO will become functionally ambulatory. For a limb with knee control, but with little or no foot or ankle control, a short leg brace or ankle-foot orthosis (AFO) is needed. The molded plastic insert orthoses are very satisfactory in these instances. Patients who require a KAFO on one side and AFO on the other or a bilateral AFO will frequently become functionally ambulatory.

Patient and family teaching is an essential part of the rehabilitation. The patient should become the expert in his own care. Even if he is unable to do it, he should be able to instruct others in his care. Family members should also be instructed in the care, particularly for the more dependent patient. Typical complications, such as pressure sores, contractures, and bowel and bladder problems, can be prevented by a knowledgeable patient and family.

Table 15-2 lists the goals for the average spinal cord injured patient at each functional level, and the equipment that helps the patient meet and sustain those functional expectations. As soon as the patient's functional level has become stable, the goal should be set, explained to the patient, and a timetable established to meet the goals. Everybody is an individual and these are average expectations. Age-associated problems, body size, and development may modify these goals for given patients. The goals are based on the functional level at the time the rehabilitation program is instituted, not on some vague expectation of future recovery. If the functional level improves, then the goals can be changed to meet the new conditions.[9]

Table 15-2. Functional Goals of Spinal Cord Damaged Patients by Level of Injury

FUNCTIONAL SPINAL CORD LEVEL	MUSCLE FUNCTION	FUNCTIONAL GOALS
C4	Neck control Scapular elevators	Manipulate electric wheel-chair with devices Mouth stick (communication) Use environmental controls
C5	Partial shoulder control Partial elbow flexion	Independent in light hygiene and feeding activities with devices Propel wheelchair with assistive devices or electric wheelchair Swivel bar transfer Adapted sports: swimming, archery, bowling

Continued on next page

Table 15-2. Functional Goals of Spinal Cord Damaged Patients by Level of Injury (*continued*)

FUNCTIONAL SPINAL CORD LEVEL	MUSCLE FUNCTION	FUNCTIONAL GOALS
C6	Shoulder control Elbow flexion Wrist extension Supinators	Independent in dressing activities Independent in transfer activities, car and bed Driving with adapted equipment Adapted sports: track and field, table tennis
C7 and C8	Shoulder depression Elbow extension Some hand function	Independent in eating without adapted devices Independent in application of condom drainage Independent transfers—car, bed, commode chair, or tub stool Assisted bowel care
T1–T5	Normal upper extremity muscle function	Total wheelchair independence Independent transfers—wheelchair to tub Move from wheelchair to floor and back Assisted standing activities All wheelchair sports
T6–T10	Partial trunk stability	Exercise ambulation with bilateral long leg brace and crutches
T11–L1	Trunk stability	Possible household ambulation
L2	Hip flexors	Household ambulation
L3–L4	Adductors, quadriceps	Community ambulation
L5–S2	Hip extensors, abductors Knee flexors Ankle control	Community ambulation

Bladder Rehabilitation

The goals of bladder rehabilitation are achieving adequate bladder emptying, either reflexly or by external pressure, and avoiding chronic urinary tract infection. The technique that best meets these objectives is bladder retraining by intermittent catheterization. This is started in the acute phase at four- to six-hour intervals. When the patient begins to void, the intervals between catheterizations can be increased and the fluid restrictions relaxed. The bladder is considered balanced when the post-voiding residuals are less than 100–150 cc and the emptying is achieved without high intravesicle pressure. A urologist experienced in the care of the neurogenic bladder is a vital member of the team.

Bowel rehabilitation is started immediately after the injury to establish the regular pattern of bowel evacuation. Suppositories or rectal stimulation are the usual means of achieving evacuation. The best schedule to strive for is bowel evacuation every day or every other day at the same time (usually following a meal) to take advantage of normal gastrocolic reflexes. A stool softener or lubricator, such as dioctyl sodium sulfosuccinate (Colace), helps maintain proper consistency, and on occasion a mild laxative, such as milk of magnesia or concentrated prune juice, will help facilitate regular evacuation. There is significant individual variation, but once an effective program is established it should be strictly adhered to.

PSYCHOSOCIAL AND VOCATIONAL REHABILITATION

Effective psychosocial rehabilitation is as essential as aggressive physical rehabilitation for the spinal cord injured patient to retain and maintain the maximum potential. A patient who cannot accept injury and disability and cannot see himself as a valuable member of society and who will not cooperate in the rehabilitation process or take care of himself will present with a never-ending series of complications. Psychosocial rehabilitation involves close interaction among the patient and all members of the rehabilitation team. Of special importance in this regard are the social workers and psychologists working with the patient and family. At one time it was popular to categorize stages of readjustment to the injury, but with increasing experience psychologists and psychiatrists working with spinal cord injured patients are discarding such theories. Unquestionably, most if not all patients initially deny the seriousness and permanency of the injury and its functional consequences, but with time the majority come to terms with themselves and their disability sufficiently to work toward effective rehabilitation.

Community placement is one of the major goals. Ideally, this means returning the patient to his home. Such structural alterations as ramps, wide doors, and adapted bathrooms may be required. Planning should begin as soon as the patient is admitted. When required, the provision for an attendant must be planned with identification and training, whether it be a family member, friend, or paid attendant. If appropriate living arrangements cannot be identified, then some alternative must be found, such as congregate or communal facilities. Institutional placement should be considered as a last resort for the spinal cord injured patient.

Vocational and educational counseling and training are frequently needed.

The average patient is in his early 20s, and has not made a career choice or completed his education. If his reintegration into society is to be truly complete, he must be trained in an appropriate skill or occupation. With a proper attitude and education, there is no degree of disability that precludes the patient from finding a meaningful vocation. Obviously, the choices and opportunities are more limited for the more severely disabled.

SPECIAL PROBLEMS

Heterotopic Ossification

This is a condition of unknown etiology in which heterotopic new bone begins forming in the soft tissues near major joints below the level of injury. In its most severe form, it can lead to bony ankylosis of the joint. Ossification occurs most frequently in hip joints. Especially when complete ankylosis occurs, the patient will be unable to reach the expected rehabilitation goals and become completely dependent. In those instances, surgical resection of the ankylosing bar will restore functional range of motion and the functional capability of the patient.[12]

Surgery must not be performed until the process has fully matured or massive recurrence is inevitable. The signs of maturity are smooth cortical outline in the new bone mass, a normal serum alkaline phosphatase, and, most important, a stable, low uptake ratio on bone scan for at least three consecutive months. This is determined by serial bone scan in which the activity in the highest uptake area of the new bone is compared to the activity in a normal reference bone by using computerized counting. The uptake ratio will reach a maximum when the process is most active and then decrease to a stable lower level. At this point, resection of the ankylosing bar can be performed and major recurrence will not occur.[17] It frequently takes two years from the time the process first appears to reach sufficient maturity for a safe surgical resection.

Pressure Sores

Pressure sores are the most common avoidable complication of spinal cord injury. They are formed when sustained pressure exceeds capillary filling pressures, which then leads to necrosis of skin and underlying soft tissue. Pressure sores most commonly occur in two distinctly different settings with typical sores unique to each.

The first setting is in the newly injured patient with sacral or heel sores. These are due to inadequate turning and positioning during the period of vascular instability in the immediate postinjury period. Prevention requires turning every two to three hours, plus protecting bony prominences with pillows; in particular, the heels must be kept off the bed. Most heel sores are allowed to heal by granulation and re-epithelialization, because it is a difficult area to treat surgically. The sacral sores, if small, can be healed similarly, but large ones may require skin grafting or flaps. What is most distressing about these sores is that they may delay rehabilitation by at least three to four months and leave the patient with permanently scarred skin before he even gets started.

The second setting is the "sitting sore" of the rehabilitated patient. These are most common in the ischial and trochanteric regions. The most common cause is lack of proper care by the patient. They can be prevented by a properly fitted wheelchair and having the patient regularly relieve pressure by raising himself off the cushion. These sores frequently require surgical closure.

The *sine qua non* of pressure sore treatment is to keep the sore free of pressure at all times. As R. Vilan, a French plastic surgeon, said, "You can put anything but the patient on the sore and it will heal." It is a mistake to get the patient up with a sore even if for only a short time, if your objective is to heal the sore.

The High Quadriplegic

In the past ten years, improved emergency treatment and pulmonary therapy have made possible the appearance of the "high quadriplegic," that is, someone with a neurological level of C4 or higher. They have no functional limb musculature, and their diaphragmatic function is compromised or absent.

In the initial phases, artificial ventilation and intensive pulmonary care are the keys to survival. If the patient is complete (having a level of C3, C4, or higher), elective tracheostomy will improve care and make the patient more comfortable. This decision should be made within the first ten days. When diaphragm function is compromised, weaning is easier with a tracheostomy, and if the diaphragm is completely paralyzed, tracheostomy is essential. If the zone of injury includes the region of the third and fourth cervical segments, then the anterior horn motor neurons have been destroyed, meaning that permanent, artificial ventilation by means of a ventilator is required. If the zone of injury is above this level, resulting in diaphragmatic paralysis of the upper motor neurons, then ventilation by electrical stimulation of the phrenic nerves is possible through the use of an implanted electrophrenic pacemaker.

High quadriplegics can utilize breath-activated environmental control units. These units operate a number of electrical appliances and components, such as radios, televisions, telephones, tape recorders, alarms, and door openers. Typewriters and wheelchairs can also be operated by the same control mechanism. These units are commercially available. Their use gives the patient a form of independence and in some cases can make possible some type of income-producing occupation.

Reconstructive Hand Surgery

In certain carefully selected quadriplegics' hands, surgery can bestow improved function. The total patient and his function must be taken into consideration, particularly transfer capability and wheelchair propulsion. There are a few basic points to keep in mind. Never compromise active wrist extension. Do not utilize spastic muscles for transfer. The results are always better in hands with good sensation, specifically, those with two-point discrimination.

FUTURE DIRECTIONS

Spinal Cord Regeneration

There is an increasing amount of basic research into the problem of regeneration. We must gain an understanding of the factors that influence axon growth, myelination, and glial growth within the central nervous system. Peripheral axons attempt to grow into the central nervous system and will grow into connecting tissue scar, but they do not seem to be able to grow into regions where glial cells produce myelin and support the axon. If we could understand the processes of axonal growth within glial support structures, we might be able to accomplish regeneration.

Acute Care and Reversal of Cord Damage

Since the first experiment by Allen,[1] a wide variety of physical and pharmacological treatments of the experimentally injured spinal cord in laboratory animals have resulted in reversal or lessening the effect of injury. To date none of these treatments has been shown to produce a similar effect in a clinical series of spinal cord injured patients. A number of explanations can account for this: species differences, mode of injury, and the time from injury to start of treatment. Emergency medical services are improving rapidly and now treatment of a variety of conditions is started at the scene of the accident by paramedics. Perhaps other specific therapies can be started within minutes of injury to minimize the extent of cord damage. Newer techniques of diagnosis, in particular, CAT scanning, can supply better information more rapidly and further point to specific therapies. Prevention and early reversal are more likely to be effected before restoration of function through regeneration.

Rehabilitation Engineering

The gains in engineering technology in the past two decades have been phenomenal. We can control complex machines at the edge of the solar system and purchase at the corner drug store a pocket computer with a greater capability than that first computer which filled a room. Some of these advances have been used to improve capabilities and life of the spinal cord injured. Much of this current knowledge and technology has not as yet been applied to rehabilitation. Increasingly, engineers and rehabilitation professionals are working together, and in most every instance this collaboration has been beneficial to the disabled person. This trend will continue and increase in magnitude, and, if past experience is an indicator, the rewards will be great. Functional electrical stimulation has the possibility of providing useful function in muscles without central nervous system control. Electrophrenic pacemakers can now successfully give a patient diaphragmmatic function over prolonged periods of time. The problems of fatigue, synchronization, and recruitment are the obstacles that still must be overcome to make functional electrical stimulation practical.

Space-age technology is being applied to mobility aids. There are now vans that can be safely operated by quadriplegics who less than five years ago were considered practically or legally incapable of driving a vehicle. This technology will be applied to other mobility aids, such as the wheelchair, which has not had a major design modification since it was introduced.

Since the end of World War II, great strides have been made in the care and rehabilitation of the spinal cord injured patient. The value of specialized spinal cord injury units has now become well accepted, and nationwide systems of spinal cord injury centers are being established. These centers are now functioning within regional trauma systems so that persons with a spinal cord injury are rapidly transferred there for treatment. However, considering the number of patients sustaining spinal cord injury, and the number of centers available, it is obvious that most patients in this country still are not receiving this type of care. It is hoped that this chapter will provide some guidelines and indications as to the type of care needed by spinal cord injured patients and emphasize not only the need for skilled and coordinated care, but also the challenges and rewards from dealing with the rehabilitation of the spinal cord injured patient.

REFERENCES

1. Allen, A. R.: Surgery of experimental lesion of spinal cord equivalent to crush injury of fracture dislocation of spinal column. J.A.M.A. 57:878–880, 1911.
2. Bedbrook, G. M.: Spinal injuries with tetraplegia and paraplegia. J. Bone Joint Surg. 61B:267–284, 1979.
3. Bosch, A., Stauffer, E. S., and Nickel, V. L.: Incomplete traumatic quadriplegia, ten year review. J.A.M.A. 216:473–478, 1971.
4. Burke, D. C., and Murray, D. D.: The management of thoracic and thoracolumbar injuries of the spine with neurological involvement. J. Bone Joint Surg. 56B:72–78, 1974.
5. Cahal, A. S.: Care of spinal cord injuries in the armed forces of India. Paraplegia 13:25–28, 1975.
6. Dickson, J., Harrington, P., and Erwin, W.: Results of reduction and stabilization of the severely fractured thoracic and lumbar spine. J. Bone Joint Surg. 60A:799–805, 1978.
7. Guttman, L.: *Spinal Cord Injuries: Comprehensive Management and Research.* Blackwell Scientific Publications, Oxford, 1973.
8. Holdsworth, F. W.: Fractures, dislocations and fracture-dislocations. J. Bone Joint Surg. 52A:1534–1551, 1970.
9. Hussey, R. W., and Stauffer, E. S.: Spinal cord injury: Requirements for ambulation. Arch. Phys. Med. Rehabil. 54:544–547, 1973.
10. Kraus, J. F., Franti, C. E., Riggins, R. S., et al.: Incidence of traumatic spinal cord lesions. J. Chronic Dis. 28:471–492, 1975.
11. Messard, L., Carmody, A., Mannarino, E., and Ruge, D.: Survival after spinal cord trauma. Arch. Neurol. 35:78–83, 1978.
12. Rossier, A. B., et al.: Current facts on para-osteo-arthropathy. Paraplegia 11:36–78, 1973.
13. Rossier, A. B., Berney, J., Rosenbaum, A. E., and Hachen, J.: Value of gas myelography in early management of acute spinal cord injuries. J. Neurosurg. 42:330–337, 1975.
14. Rossier, A. B., Hussey, R. W., and Kenzora, J. E.: Anterior fibular interbody fusion in the treatment of cervical spinal cord injuries. Surg. Neurol. 7:55–60, 1977.
15. Rossier, A. B., Fam, B. A., di Benedetto, M., and Sarakarati, M.: Urethro-vesical function during spinal shock. Urol. Res. 8:53–65, 1980.
16. Stauffer, E. S., and Kaufer, H.: Fractures and dislocations of the spine. In Rockwood, C. A., and Green, D. P., Eds.: *Fractures,* pp. 817–903. J. B. Lippincott, Philadelphia, 1975.

17. Tanaka, T., Rossier, A. B., Hussey, R. W., et al.: Quantitative assessment of para-osteo-arthropathy and its maturation on serial radionuclide bone images. Radiology 123:217–221, 1977.

18. Tator, C. H.: Acute spinal cord injury: A review of recent studies of treatment and pathophysiology. Can. Med. Assoc. J. 107:143–150, 1972.

19. Wang, F. J., Whitehill, R., Stamp, W. G., and Rosenberger, R.: The treatment of fracture dislocations of the thoraco lumbar spine with halo-femoral traction and Harrington rod instrumentation. Clin. Orthop. 142:168–175, 1979.

20. Young, J. S., and Northrup, N. E.: Statistical information pertaining to some of the most commonly asked questions about SCI, part I. SCI Dig 1:11–31, 1979.

16

The Dysvascular Lower Limb

F. William Wagner, Jr., M.D.

Obstructive vascular disease of the heart and brain is the leading cause of death in modern western society. The same pathological processes are involved in the arterial tree of the lower extremities and produce the condition known as the dysvascular limb. The usual early symptoms or disabilities secondary to vascular dysfunction that lead a patient to seek the services of a physician are pain and a nonhealing lesion of the leg or foot (Fig. 16-1). Gross decrease in the flow of blood leads to the characteristic pain of intermittent claudication, one of the earliest and quite specific complaints. Discomfort in the muscle mass of back, buttocks, thigh, calf, or foot will cause the patient to stop walking after a given distance. This is frequently so specific that it can be graded as one-block or two-block claudication. Relief is rapid when activity is stopped. Walking can usually be continued after a short rest.

With progression of atherogenic deposits, the patient will begin to experience pain at rest. As ischemia advances, the pain shifts to the area farthest from the heart. Rather than in the calf or thigh, the pain will now be in the forefoot or arch of the foot. One of the most distressing complaints is that of pain or cramp after falling asleep. With recumbancy and sleep, the heart rate and output are slowed and blood supply is even smaller than during daytime activities. Patients experiment with different positions and report increased pain with elevation. Conversely, they may obtain relief with sleeping semi-upright in a chair or with the painful leg hanging over the side of the bed. Pain of this degree while at rest indicates severe arterial insufficiency and a pregangrenous state.

If diabetes mellitus is present, the patient may also suffer from microangiopathy as well as neuropathy. The microangiopathy of diabetes is characterized by an exaggeration of the capillary basement membrane thickening that is present with normal aging. Our work at Rancho Los Amigos Hospital with Doppler ultrasound has shown that diabetics need a higher ischemic index to heal a specific lesion than do nondiabetics.[20-24] The lower limit for healing in diabetics is 0.45, and 0.35 for nondiabetics. We feel that this 0.10 difference may be due to diabetic microangiopathy. It is further postulated that the thickening interferes both with nutrient and oxygen transfer to cells and with pick-up of metabolites and other waste products by the capillary and venular systems.

On occasion the presenting complaint may be that of a nonhealing lesion of the foot or leg. It may have started with minor trauma or from pressure of a shoe. Dysfunction of the vascular system must be suspected if the lesion does not heal in the expected time. If the lesion is painless or relatively so, diabetes mellitus must be ruled out.

Other divisions of the vascular system may be involved as well as the arterial tree. Venous and lymphatic dysfunctions must be considered and treated as indicated. Included would be hypertension, cardiovascular disease, previous vascular surgery, previous stroke or heart attack, Raynaud's syndrome or disease, Buerger's disease, post-phlebitic syndromes, lymphangitis, and other similar diseases.

PREVALENCE AND CAUSES

In the western world, obstructive vascular disease of the heart and brain continue to lead or be high on the lists of causes of death. Many studies have been performed on plasma and serum components in the past 100 years. In 1885 Liebermann[12] introduced a method of measuring cholesterol, which was improved by Burchard[5] in 1890. Tswett[19] described chromatography in 1906. Despite continued refinements of laboratory analysis and the accumulation of vast amounts of data, marked controversies still exist as to the exact nature of the causes and treatment of atherosclerosis. The list of associated factors grows with each year of study. In 1897, William Osler listed the factors contributing to "angeiosclerosis" as food, drink, tobacco, and personal and occupational stresses. In addition, genetic factors, softened drinking water, increased sucrose ingestion, increased saturated fat ingestion, autoimmune reactions, arterial hypertension, obesity, and lack of exercise have all been implicated.

The exact mechanism of atheroma formation is still under continuing study and there are several tenable theories. Intimal infiltration of lipids from plasma overly rich in lipoproteins, mural thrombosis, and actual cholesterol synthesis in the intima due to impaired mitochondrial function have all been proposed.[18,26,27] The most plausible theory at present appears to be that of infiltration.[2] Sucrose intake appears to enhance this infiltration.[27] Tobacco smoking is also apparently related to intimal damage. After grafting procedures, those who stop smoking have a statistically better chance of graft success.

In rabbits, hypercholesterolemia is a prerequisite for the deposition of cholesterol and subsequent atherosclerotic plaque formation. Quantitative dietary

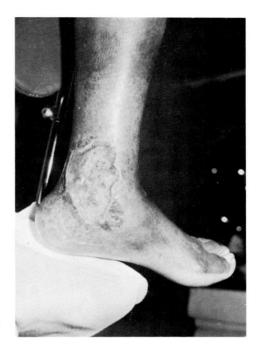

Fig. 16-1. Typical vascular lesion over the medial malleolus. (Courtesy of Rancho Los Amigos Hospital.)

experiments in both healthy volunteers and in known atherosclerotic patients have shown that saturated fat enhances and polyunsaturated fat depresses serum cholesterol levels.[14,16,18] Unfortunately, experiments with human beings have not been performed in large enough numbers and over long enough periods to make unequivocal statements that a reduced risk for atherogenic cardiovascular disease follows dietary changes. Thus, rehabilitation in the preventive stage would probably include a program of regular exercise, discontinuance of smoking, regular rest and relaxation, and multiple small feedings of a balanced diet with minimum sucrose, minimum saturated fats, and moderate polyunsaturated fats.

VASCULAR SURGERY

Modern vascular surgery has made most of its major advances in the past three decades. Diagnostic methods, new surgical techniques, and artificial graft materials have all contributed to the spectacular achievements that are occurring. The number of operations appears to be increasing each year, reflected in the fact that in the United States at least 73,000 reconstructive procedures are performed on major arteries each year.

Historically, the first anastamosis and grafting of vessels began with the work of Von Eck in 1879. Alexis Carrel made notable contributions in techniques of anastamosis soon after the turn of the century. Traumatic vascular surgery really did not come into its own until 1952 during the Korean War, when the recent advances in civilian blood vessel surgery were applied to wartime vascular surgery. Refinement of techniques, antibiotics, and synthetic materials allowed the development of the modern era of vascular surgery following the 1940s. Diagnostic techniques, such as angiography, had their beginning in 1923 when Sicard and Forestiere opacified parts of the arterial system with iodized poppy seed oil. In 1953 Seldinger[17] reported the percutaneous arterial catheterization technique that allowed more precise and selective visualization of the vessels. Anticoagulants, which became clinically available in 1936, have decreased the complication of clotting.

Replacement and bypass of diseased arterial segments have become major reconstructive procedures.[1,13] Shortcomings associated with homologous tissue grafts, such as inadequate procurement of homotransplants, inadequate veins in certain vascular areas, and long-term morphological alterations observed in both types of transplants, pushed the search for artificial replacement materials. In 1952 the first successful arterial replacement with synthetic fabric was reported. However, the concept was not completely new, since blood vessel replacements had been attempted with plastic tubes, glass, aluminum tubes, paraffin-coated silver tubes, and many other inert materials, such as Vitallium, polyethylene, siliconized rubber, steel mesh, and Ivalon.

Intra-arterial surgery was first attempted in 1880 and again in 1909. Early thrombectomies were unsuccessful and were not tried again until 1947 when J. Cid dos Santos described the procedure known as thromboendarterectomy. This appeared to be revolutionary because it actually injured the intima surgically, which was thought to lead inevitably to vascular thrombosis. Improved surgical techniques and anticoagulants have made thrombectomies and endarterectomies successful procedures.

Arterial embolectomy is also one of the earliest known direct arterial procedures. It was first successfully performed in 1911; however, the introduction of the Fogarty balloon catheter in 1963 gave it its greatest impetus.

Microsurgical techniques have been made possible because of two advances. One is the operating microscope or magnifying loop; the other is the development of the small instruments and sutures needed to work under higher magnification. Arteries as small as 1 mm or less in diameter can be reconstructed.[8]

Even more complicated procedures are now accomplished. The first reconstructions were done by surgeons with no vascular training. Thus, their helpers became the first trainees. Now success in extensive and difficult-of-access arterial lesions is due to better anesthesia, better special equipment for surgery and postoperative care, and, perhaps most important, better vascular surgeons.

DIAGNOSIS

Physical Examination

Visual inspection of the lower limb in a good light may reveal the presence of vascular disease. Atrophy of muscle and subcutaneous tissues may result from chronic ischemia. The hair may start to disappear distal to the lesion. The skin becomes shiny, pale, and waxy. The nails may grow at a decreased rate and become thick and bizarre in shape, or they may stop growing. The skin may be dry and crack between the toes. Ulcers or patches of gangrenous skin may form over such pressure points as the malleoli, metatarsal heads, and interphalangeal joints of the toes. These ulcers are frequently exquisitely painful and tender (Fig. 16-1). However, they may be relatively painless in the diabetic except for those whose neuropathy is in the hyperesthetic stage. In the hypoesthetic phase, the patient may be so unaware of pain or discomfort that severe infection or gangrene may develop before medical aid is sought.

The foundation of all vascular examination is palpation for the presence of arterial pulses. Presence of normal pulsations in the dorsum of the foot and below the medial malleolus implies that there is little or no peripheral arterial disease. The popliteal and femoral pulses must be evaluated if foot and ankle pulses are diminished or absent.

Diagnostic Methods

When pulses are abnormal, the symptoms are severe enough, and arterial disease appears to be causative, further tests must be performed. Contrary to popular belief, the arteriogram is the last test to be performed. It is technically a "roadmap" to indicate the area of blockage and aid in planning the type of revascularization to be performed. It is ordered by the vascular surgeon.

Clinical assessment by noninvasive techniques can be carried out by transcutaneous Doppler ultrasound (Fig. 16-2).[3,21,22,24] This instrument emits a beam that is pulsed between 5 and 10 MHz in frequency. The beam is transmitted through a coupling gel and the skin to the blood vessel that is being examined. The beam is reflected back to the probe by each surface that it strikes and is then analyzed by the electronic circuitry. The moving bloodstream reflects a signal that is increased in frequency compared to the speed of flow of the cells. The difference in frequency between the transmitted and received signals is the Doppler shift. This difference is converted to an audible or electric signal that can be heard through a stethoscope or loud speaker, can be seen on an oscilloscope as a wave form, or printed on a tape. The instrument can be used as a sensitive stethoscope to map the arterial tree and measure systolic pressures at the toes, midfoot, ankle, calf, knee, thigh, and groin. Systolic pressure is also taken in the brachial artery at the elbow. The brachial artery pressure is considered to be normal for each person unless upper extremity vascular problems are present. At all of the levels measured, the width of the sphygmomanometer cuff should be 120 percent of the diameter of the extremity being measured.

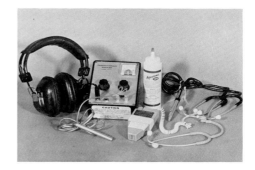

Fig. 16-2. Portable Doppler ultrasound instruments, three examples. Left: Parks Electronics, Beaverton, Oregon. Model 802, pencil probe 9.1 MHz. Center: Medsonic, Inc., Mountain View, California. Model 874A, 5.3 MHz. Right: Physio Control, Redmond, Washington. Doplett 10, pocket size, 10 MHz. (Courtesy of Rancho Los Amigos Hospital.)

Each leg systolic pressure is divided by the brachial artery systolic pressure. This gives a percentage of flow at each level and is referred to as the ischemic index (Fig. 16-3). As atheromatous blockage increases, the systolic pressure decreases at that level, and the ischemic index decreases.

At Rancho Los Amigos Hospital, a high correlation has been found between healing rates and the ischemic index. If a diabetic patient's index is greater than 0.45, there is more than a 90 percent chance of healing an ulcer or a surgical procedure at that level. For a patient who is not diabetic, the ratio should be 0.35 for a similar healing rate. It is felt that the 0.10 difference represents the microvascular defect referred to as the basement membrane thickening. If the ischemic index is below 0.35 or 0.45, respectively, the patient is referred to the hospital's vascular service for further work-up and treatment. If the foot pain appears to be due to other than arterial insufficiency, consultation with other services is indicated. Musculoskeletal lesions as well as nerve compression can produce symptoms similar to claudication. Most of these may be differentiated by the history and usually there is no direct relation to the distance walked.

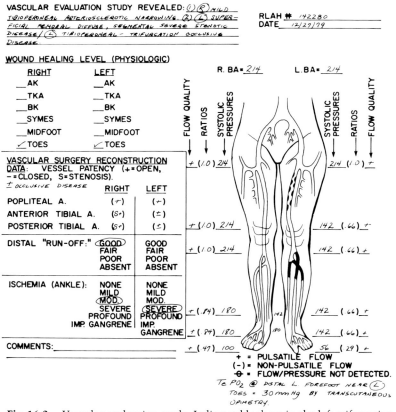

Fig. 16-3. Vascular evaluation study. Indicates blockage in the left trifurcation. Collateral flow is sufficient to permit toe amputation (coupled with transcutaneous oxygen measurement). The ischemic index is indicated in parentheses; wound healing is predicted at the toe level. (Courtesy of Rancho Los Amigos Hospital.)

Table 16-1. Dysvascular Surgical Cases with Ischemic Index Greater Than 0.45 in Diabetic and 0.35 in Nondiabetic Patients*

| | | HEALING RATES, % | | |
LEVEL OF SURGERY	CASES	Diabetic	Nondiabetic	Combined Average
Above knee	29	88	100	94
Through knee	25	100	100	100
Below knee	49	95	88	92
Syme's	79	82	95	91
Transmetatarsal	21	100	100	100
Ray and partial ray	33	81	100	90
Toe	30	100	100	100
Incision and drainage	11	100	100	100
Total	277	93	98	96

* Courtesy of Rancho Los Amigos Hospital.

Ulceration may be also due to venous stasis. These lesions will usually have surrounding edema, stasic dermatitis, and pigmentation. Nonvascular conditions also may cause ulcerated areas. If the pulses and noninvasive tests are normal, a dermatological consultation is indicated.

Additional Diagnostic Tests

Oscillometry, fluorescein dye tests, histamine wheals, thermography, ergometry, plethysmography, and radioactive tests[9,11] of skin circulation have all had their vehement adherents as well as detractors. Success rates in prediction of healing with the Doppler ischemic index have been so successful that this test alone, coupled with clinical examination, is now being used in the preoperative evaluation of patients at Rancho Los Amigos Hospital. Table 16-1 indicates the results for 277 consecutive surgical cases in which the healing level was determined by Doppler ultrasound.

GRADING DYSVASCULAR FOOT LESIONS

To aid further in selecting treatment for the dysvascular foot, lesions have been graded in severity to enable a better matching of treatment with the disease process. Analysis of foot lesions from potential breakdown through beginning ulceration to final complete breakdown has led to a classification in six grades.[15] This classification was designed by the staff of the ortho-diabetes service at Rancho Los Amigos Hospital with the assistance of Dr. Bernard Meggitt.

In Grade 0, the skin is intact. There may be multiple foot deformities and hyperkeratotic areas that may break down with poor care. In Grade 1, the skin is broken and the ulcer is in the superficial layers only. This lesion may be overlying a bony prominence or may be due to a penetrating injury. In Grade 2, the ulcer is deeper and penetrates to tendon, ligament, joint, or bone. The Grade 3 lesion represents progression of a Grade 2 lesion to formation of a deep abscess or osteomyelitis. A Grade 4 lesion shows gangrenous changes in a toe, toes, or some portion of the forefoot. In Grade 5, the whole foot or greatest percentage is gangrenous and no local foot procedures are possible. Amputations are performed at the level indicated by the Doppler study and the patient's general condition.

TREATMENT AND DIAGNOSIS

Matching of various tests and treatment methods with the graded lesions has enabled us to achieve a high percentage of healed foot lesions and a high success rate in surgical procedures. Each of the following is indicated in the flow charts (Figs. 16-4, 16-5, 16-8, 16-9, 16-12, 16-15) or in the discussion.

Medical Treatment ①*

Close cooperation between the surgical and medical teams is essential. A hopeless-looking foot often may be transformed into one that is salvageable when bed rest, intravenous antibiotics determined by appropriate cultures, and vigorous control of diabetes and other underlying diseases are instituted. In general, surgery should be delayed until the white blood count has dropped below 10,000/ml³ and the temperature is decreasing. On occasion, a fluctuant abscess may require urgent surgical drainage.

Doppler Evaluation ②

This test is performed on each patient. If the ischemic index is sufficient to allow healing, treatment is begun as indicated in Figure 16-4. If the index is below the healing level, the patient is then referred to the vascular service.

Vascular Service ③

Arteriography and other diagnostic tests as indicated are carried out on the vascular service. Endarterectomy, profundaplasty, and bypass procedures are the most frequently recommended. Revascularization has allowed lesions to heal without surgical intervention, toe and Syme's amputations to be carried out in the foot, and below-knee amputations to be substituted for above-knee levels in limbs that otherwise would have undergone an above-knee amputation. A series of femoral-popliteal vein grafts for limb salvage recently reported had a five-year patency of 72 percent and an increase of ischemic index at the ankle from 0.33 to 0.75.[13]

---

* Encircled numbers correspond with stages of diagnosis and treatment presented in the flow charts.

Irrigation and Drainage Tubes

Kritter[10] has described a method of irrigating smaller foot wounds through a small plastic tube led into the depths of the wound through a separate stab incision. An antibiotic solution perfuses the wound and exits between the sutures, carrying with it debris, hematoma, and bacteria. This system has allowed closure of virtually all wounds with a resulting higher primary healing rate.

The Shirley abdominal sump drain has been modified to irrigate larger cavities (as in Syme's or through-knee disarticulations) and allow drainage through the second lumen.[20-23] This system has been used for ten years with excellent results. Virtually no tubes have clogged, as the suction drainage systems once did. An antibiotic solution is fed into the tube normally used for air. Drainage fluids exit by gravity through the perforated tube. The drain tube is clamped for about five minutes every few hours. This distends the cavity slightly and aids in irrigation of debris. The tube is then unclamped for regular drainage.

Shoe Wear: Healing Shoes (5) (10)

Claw toes and depressed metatarsal heads are deformities frequently found in the dysvascular foot. At first, self-procured treatment usually consists of a metatarsal pad. This will frequently push the clawed proximal interphalangeal joint against the top of the shoe with a resultant callus and finally an ulcer. An important shoe modification has been the extra high toe box now available (Fig. 16-7). Every patient should be directed to a shoe store with a pedorthist (a member of the Prescription Footwear Association) where such shoes are available.

Plastazote, Pelite, Aliplast, and other foamed polyethylene materials make excellent insoles for such shoes. They distribute the pressure evenly and help in the reduction of keratoses.

Following surgery, walking casts are frequently necessary. In the stage between the cast and the regular shoe, a healing shoe is prescribed. This is formed of a foam polyethylene plastic, such as Plastazote, over an enlarged shoe last. This shoe allows dressings to be worn and virtually no areas can cause pressure.

Biological Materials (6)

Various enzymes have been used for nonsurgical debridement of ulcers. Streptokinase, streptodornase, pancreatic enzymes, sutilains (Travase), fibrinolysin and desoxyribonuclease combined (Elase), and many others have been tried with varying degrees of success. Most enzymes split material in the ulcers. The breakdown products must be irrigated away or they will reconstitute. Thus, there is daily attention and dressing of the wound. We have performed daily dressings on a wet-to-dry basis with Ringer's solution or saline solution and found the results similar to enzymatic treatment.

Temporary sealing of ulcers with heterografts, or xenografts, may aid in creating a near-sterile wound. Porcine grafts have been used with some early success. Epigard, a manufactured plastic synthetic skin, has much of the same properties of aiding in sealing the wound. It may also be used as a dressing over homografts.

Surgical Treatment: Prophylactic, Excisional, Minor Amputations ⑦

Prophylactic surgery is an important part of the rehabilitation plan for the dysvascular foot. Claw toes, bunions, depressed metatarsal heads, deformed nails or other bony prominences can all be corrected by standard orthopedic procedures. Neuropathic joints can be fused in the diabetic patient to prevent further breakdown. Doppler ultrasound testing gives an assessment of the vascular supply and the operation is performed when the index is high enough to indicate that the foot will heal.

Excision of infected tissue, especially tendons, fascia, and bone, is an absolute must in the surgical treatment. The dysvascular foot does not have the ability to rid itself of necrotic and diseased tissue. Treatment of large plantar ulcers frequently requires a wedge resection of toe and metatarsal head and a portion of the shaft. If the area must be packed open, it may be secondarily closed, may fill in with time, or may be skin-grafted.

Foot Amputations[20,23]

Toes. To amputate a toe, the incision may be of any design so long as the base is wide enough for the length of the flap. The bone may be removed through disarticulation or through osteotomy.

Metatarsal. This level provides a functional residual foot. Rounding or beveling of the under surface of the distal metatarsal prevents later pressure points in the sole of the foot when the patient is wearing a shoe.

Lisfranc and Chopart Procedures. These levels require lengthening or division of the Achilles tendon and resuturing of the dorsiflexors to prevent equinus of the residual foot. A polypropylene ankle-foot orthosis aids in ambulation. This level is infrequently performed in most centers.

Major Amputation Levels and Techniques

There are no longer sites of election as once practiced. Except for the leg below the calf, as much length is saved as possible in each amputation.

Syme's Amputation.[20-23] The ankle disarticulation of James Syme is the most functional of the major lower extremity amputations. When the forefoot is infected, a two-stage procedure has been effective in preventing the spread of infection proximally. Newer materials aid in construction of a functional prosthesis. Gait studies show a virtually normal walking pattern except for toe dorsiflexion. Ankle motion is simulated by the SACH (solid ankle cushion heel) foot. In our clinic, the amputation has withstood the test of time.

Below the Knee. The long posterior flap produces a well-rounded residual limb. Pressure sores over the anterior tibial crest have been virtually eliminated with this procedure. The fascial myodesis probably results in slightly less secure muscle stabilization than with direct myodesis. However, the drill holes needed for direct myodesis frequently heal with bony excrescences that become painful under a prosthesis.

The patellar tendon bearing and supramalleolar brims are just about the standard for all below-knee prostheses. Construction techniques with plastics permit better contouring of the sockets. Modular components decrease the amount of hand work in each prosthesis and frequently lead to a lighter prosthesis.

Through the Knee. This level has had varied acceptance in amputation centers. Its two major advantages are that it is a disarticulation and relatively few muscles and no bones are cut through·and that it is an end-bearing stump. Lesser advantages are the long lever arm, better muscle stabilization in closure, and the virtual lack of hip flexion contractures resulting.

A polypropylene socket with anterior opening and Velcro closures allow donning in a sitting position. This is far easier for elderly amputees. Newer knee joints and linkages have added to the function and cosmetic appearance. The flare of the condyles aids suspension.

Above the Knee. Most amputations at this level are in patients whose vascularity is insufficient to support healing at a lower level. They are also performed when infection or gangrene in the calf area will not allow a below-knee amputation.

Lighter materials have reduced the weight of the prosthesis, but, unfortunately, control and safety mechanisms have added weight. Relatively few above-knee amputees over the age of 55 are community ambulators. Most of those for whom a prosthesis is constructed abandon it within six months and resort to wheelchair and crutches. Gait and oxygen consumption studies show that above-knee amputees can perform better with crutches than with prostheses.

Hip Disarticulation. This amputation is indicated when infection and gangrene are so high that above-knee techniques are not possible. Revascularization is usually not indicated in a case of this sort. The prosthesis requires excellent muscular control and endurance and is usually not suitable for elderly patients.

Immediate Prosthetic Fitting

In the early 1960s, Weiss[25] of Poland popularized surgical myodesis, fitting of a plaster pylon, and immediate weight-bearing for below-knee amputees. A wave of enthusiasm spread across the world and the procedure was widely tested. It is obvious that the increased attention paid to the amputee was of value. However, it soon became apparent that stress on the just-operated residual limb had a deleterious effect on the dysvascular amputee. Most centers now wait 10–14 days before allowing weight bearing.

The rigid plaster dressing is of benefit in the control of edema and pain and in the prevention of contractures. This concept is not new. In World War I amputees were casted for easier transportation and it was noted that those casted healed better than those uncasted.

Iodine-Containing Materials ⑨

Iodine is one of the more effective broad-spectrum antimicrobial surface agents. In the tincture form, it is painful and can harm healing tissues. Organic iodine complexes, such as povidone-iodine, do not sting or irritate skin and mucous membranes. They can be used as a wash, an irrigant, a pack in soaked sponges, and in a viscous cream or foam. As far as can be told, strains resistant to iodine have not developed. These products are available over the counter.

An iodine solution with more rapid and deeper penetrating powers has been developed by Collens et al.[6] It also is water-soluble and relatively nonirritating. It must be prepared by the pharmacist. It has been of great help in cleansing both superficial and deep wounds. It has been injected into moist gangrenous tissues with resultant cessation of putrefaction. The article by Collens and associates should be read for a description of preparation of the material and its use.

Iodoform gauze is still a standard treatment for packing infected wounds and it is used for small cavities.

Walking Casts ⑩

Grade 1 and 2 lesions are frequently treated with a walking cast as soon as Doppler evaluation and bacteriological tests are completed. If there has been much swelling, it will go down quickly and a new cast must be applied to prevent motion in the cast and possible new pressure sores. These casts are also used after partial foot and Syme's amputations. Weight bearing is allowed after 10–12 days. Wounds from wedge resections of a toe and metatarsals are sometimes left open if the skin is not sufficient to close. Walking casts can sometimes heal these lesions without secondary surgery. Neuropathic joints in patients with diabetic neuropathy are treated with walking casts until clinical signs of redness, swelling, and pain are gone. A cast or ankle-foot orthosis is then used until x-ray evidence of healing is complete.

Patient Education ⑤

Prevention, prophylaxis, and patient education are important facets of the treatment program. Without the patient's cooperation, much of the treatment can fail and amputation result. Liaison nurses assigned to both diabetic and foot clinics carry on a constant teaching program to supplement the information given to the patient when admitted to the hospital. Many of the following therapeutic necessities are well known to everyone but need frequent re-emphasis.

1. The feet must be inspected daily for cracks, cuts, blisters, bruises, and skin breakdown, especially between the toes.
2. The shoes must be inspected inside each day for foreign objects, bunching of lining, nail points, hardened accumulation of foot powder, and any other pressure points.
3. Feet should be washed daily with mild soap and tepid water. They should be dried carefully. Vaseline or lanolin should be applied to the skin to keep in the moisture obtained with washing.

Medicated powders should be used carefully and only at the direction of the physician.

4. Avoid extremes of temperature in all bathing. Water temperature should be tested before bathing. If the patient is insensitive to heat or cold, a member of the family should perform the testing.

5. Do not use external sources of heat for cold feet. Use down boots or wool socks to conserve body heat. Heating pads, floor furnaces, hot water bottles, and similar devices are dangerous. In cold climates, do not sit with the feet next to the car heater.

6. Wear properly fitted hose. Avoid thick seams or irregular mends. Change to clean socks at least daily.

7. Do not wear circular garters or twist the tops of the stockings. If support is necessary, use a garter belt.

8. Do not use chemical agents to remove corns or calluses. Do not perform "bathroom surgery." See a physician for recommended care.

9. Wear properly fitted shoes. Find a pedorthist who has been specially trained in the fitting of shoes for dysvascular feet. When the toes are clawed, a higher toe box is necessary. Break in shoes gradually. Never wear a new pair of shoes for more than an hour or so without taking them off and inspecting for reddened areas. If the patient's eyesight is poor, a member of the family should check.

10. Do not walk barefooted. This includes going to the bathroom at night. One cut from a small sharp object may lead to infection and subsequent amputation.

11. Cut toenails straight across. Do not dig into the corners. If the nails are too thick for scissors, use clippers. If the nails are too severely thickened or deformed, see a physician for cutting.

12. The patient's feet should be examined by the physician at each visit.

TREATMENT FLOW CHARTS: ALGORITHMS

To aid in decision-making, treatment flow charts (algorithms) have been developed for each grade of lesion. The oval represents a starting or finishing condition. The rectangle indicates a procedure or treatment to be performed, usually as a result of some previous test or set of conditions. The diamond represents a question that can be answered with "yes" or "no" and directs further treatment based on that answer.

Grade 0

The typical Grade 0 foot (no open lesion) in a dysvascular patient has claw toes, depressed metatarsal heads, dry skin, toenail problems, and calluses over bony prominences (Fig. 16-4). If vascular or neuropathic symptoms are present, the patient is referred to the vascular or medical services. If there are no deformities, the patient is given education and advice and shoe wear is prescribed.

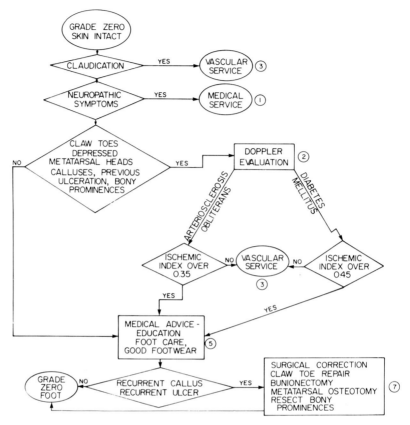

Fig. 16-4. Algorithm for Grade 0 foot. (Courtesy of Rancho Los Amigos Hospital.)

If calluses become severe or an ulcer should recur, surgical correction is considered.

Grade 1

Localized superficial ulcers usually occur over a bony prominence (Fig. 16-5). Medical and vascular evaluations and treatment are carried out. Iodine solutions are used for surface treatment. Walking casts may aid in epithelialization. On occasion, surgical treatment may be necessary. Large surface losses require skin grafting (Fig. 16-6). With healing of the wound, patient education and proper shoes are emphasized. Polypropylene orthoses and rocker-bottom shoes may be required for accompanying joint deformities (Fig. 16-7).

Grade 2

Lesions that go to the tendon, ligament, bone, or joint are usually infected enough to require vigorous antibiotic treatment (Fig. 16-8). An occasional lesion

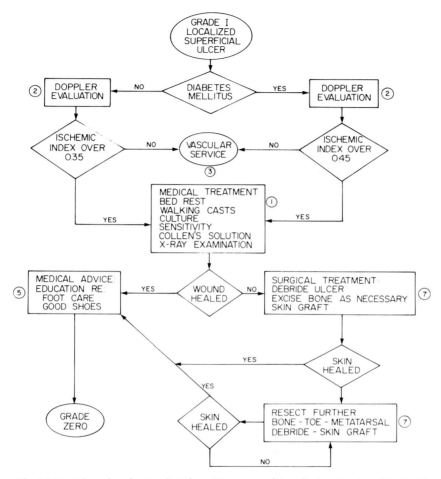

Fig. 16-5. Algorithm for Grade 1 foot. (Courtesy of Rancho Los Amigos Hospital.)

may heal with local iodine packing and walking cast treatment. Most require a surgical procedure. Very few go to amputation. Patient education starts in the hospital and is reinforced in the clinic by all members of the team.

Grade 3

Deep abscesses and osteomyelitis must be removed surgically (Fig. 16-9). Patients with decreased vascularity are not able to discharge pus, infected connective tissue, and bone. The most common reason for continued infection after a debriding procedure is the failure to remove all infected tissue. Closed wounds appear to heal better than those left open to granulate. If possible, primary skin grafting is performed (Figs. 16-10, 16-11). Drainage tubes have aided in healing these closed wounds. Occasionally, wounds are left open when the skin is insufficient to close them. Secondary closure with grafts is usually successful.

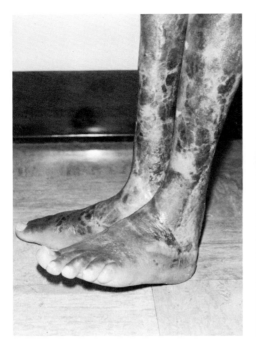

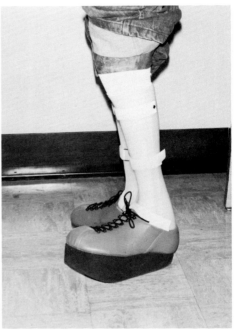

Fig. 16-6. Moderate arteriosclerotic. Grade 2 lesions over feet and both shins; grafted. Left ankle contracture from immobilization. (Courtesy of Rancho Los Amigos Hospital.)

Fig. 16-7. Polypropylene ankle-foot orthosis with anterior tongue for edema control. Extra depth shoes to allow Plastazote inserts. Rocker-bottom left shoe to simulate ankle motion; gait is virtually normal. (Courtesy of Rancho Los Amigos Hospital.)

Grade 4

Gangrene of the toes or forefoot indicates that some tissue must be removed (Fig. 16-12). This can range from a single toe to a Syme's amputation. Wet gangrene represents one of the few types of emergency surgery performed. Gas gangrene is most often nonclostridial. Dry gangrene of a single toe or of several toe tips may self-amputate if kept dry (Figs. 16-13, 16-14). Iodine may aid in control of local infection.

After healing of the surgical wound, the patient is fitted for shoes or prosthesis as indicated. Education is reinforced at each clinic visit.

Grade 5

Gangrene of the whole foot requires amputation at the lowest level, indicated by Doppler evaluation when the patient is under good medical control (Fig. 16-15). Revascularization may allow performance of a below-knee rather than an above-knee amputation. Education and care of the remaining foot are of major importance because bilateral amputees have markedly decreased function.

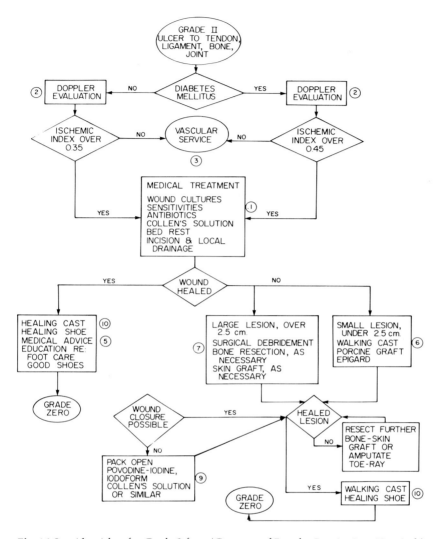

Fig. 16-8. Algorithm for Grade 2 foot. (Courtesy of Rancho Los Amigos Hospital.)

THE TEAM APPROACH

Much of the discussion to this point has revolved around the immediate medical or surgical care. However, medical and surgical corrections of a disability do not by themselves solve the problem of disabled persons. The medical or surgical procedures are only links in the long chain of related steps that finally leads to useful function. With good support, the patient can aid in the selection of the treatment plan.

The team will vary at each institution, depending on the size of the hospital and the special departments available. The team approach allows larger numbers

Text continues on p. 250

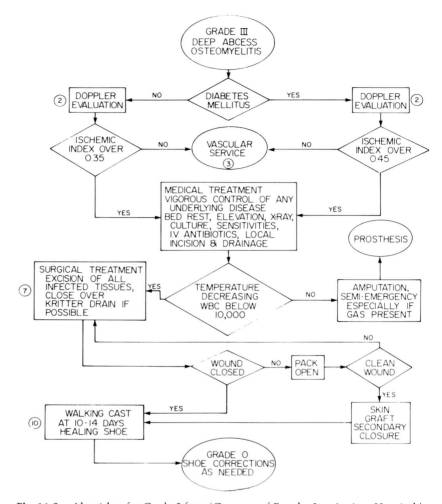

Fig. 16-9. Algorithm for Grade 3 foot. (Courtesy of Rancho Los Amigos Hospital.)

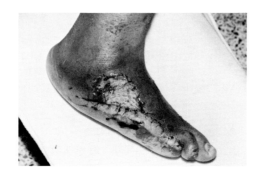

Fig. 16-10. Healing Grade 3 foot after resection of 3, 4, 5 toes and partial metatarsal shafts. Skin graft to ulcerated area. Foot had deep abscess and ulcer. (Courtesy of Rancho Los Amigos Hospital.)

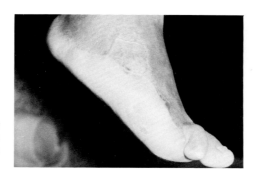

Fig. 16-11. Healed foot of Figure 10. Now wearing extra depth shoes with Plastazote filler and sole insert. (Courtesy of Rancho Los Amigos Hospital.)

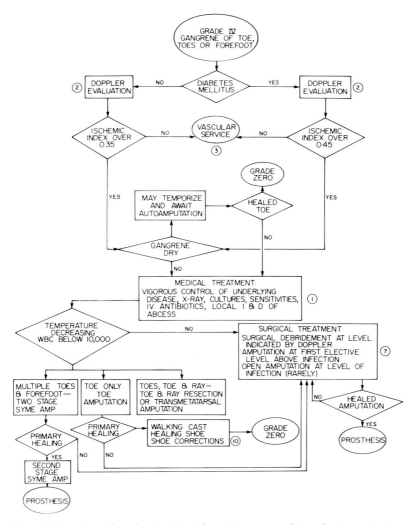

Fig. 16-12. Algorithm for Grade 4 foot. (Courtesy of Rancho Los Amigos Hospital.)

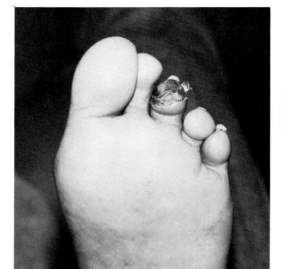

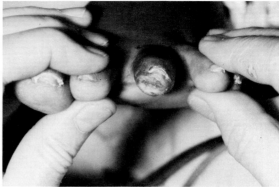

Fig. 16-14. Toe shown in Figure 16-13 after removal of dry gangrene. (Courtesy of Rancho Los Amigos Hospital.)

Fig. 16-13. Grade 4, gangrene of tip of toe, allowed to self-amputate. (Courtesy of Rancho Los Amigos Hospital.)

of patients to come together. Talking with other patients frequently aids the patient in solving problems and allaying fears. An environment is also provided that is specially suited to the training of additional personnel to treat this ever-growing number of patients.

Although the patient may, on occasion, form a close bond with a particular member of the team, each team must have a leader. This person will usually be the surgeon responsible for the final surgical decision and performance of the surgical procedure. Medical care should be directed by a co-chief. The team and consultants at Rancho Los Amigos Hospital represent a typical team and are as follows.

Team Leader

Orthopedic surgeon. The orthopedic surgeon is assisted by an orthopedic fellow, residents, and occasionally an intern on elective rotation. Medical students may also rotate on electives. Patients are seen with other team members for decisions on continuing medical care, surgical care, postoperative care, prosthetic care, discharge planning, and clinic care.

Co-leader

Internist, diabetologist, or endocrinologist. The co-leader is assisted by medical fellows, residents, interns, and on occasion by medical students. Pre- and

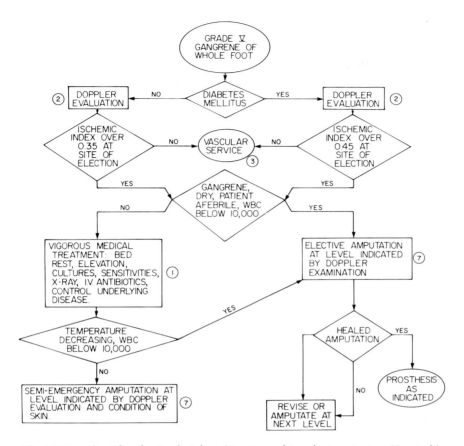

Fig. 16-15. Algorithm for Grade 5 foot. (Courtesy of Rancho Los Amigos Hospital.)

postoperative care is carefully watched, especially for diabetic and hypertensive patients and those with cardiovascular problems. Antibiotic coverage is coordinated between the medical and surgical departments.

Medical Consultants

Family Physician. Before the patient is discharged, the outside treating doctor is contacted to assure follow-up care. If none is available, the patient is followed in the outpatient clinic.

Cardiologist. Cardiovascular function may be compromised when the stress of using a prosthesis is added. Preoperative consultation may reveal that the patient cannot use a prosthesis, which will influence the level of amputation. In the case of debilitated patients, involved procedures, staged procedures, and other complex surgical treatments are not indicated; the simplest one-stage procedure is performed.

Anesthesiologist. Preoperative consultation is obtained and anesthesia planned. Many regional and local procedures are done for patients for whom general anesthesia is too risky. Excluding above-knee amputations in very ill patients, our death rates are at or below 1 percent.

The anesthesiologist also supervises the administration of anesthesia by nurse anesthetists.

Radiologist. Invasive diagnostic vascular procedures are indicated before revascularization surgery is performed. Radioactive studies are used to detect infected areas and possible new growths.

Psychiatrist. Body image is markedly altered following major amputations. Serious questions arise as to sexual performance. These problems are best handled early by consultation with a psychiatrist or psychologist.

Plastic Surgeon. On occasion, it may be necessary to rotate a flap or perform a cross-leg flap. If the orthopedic and vascular surgeon are not sure of the techniques, a plastic surgeon's consultation is obtained.

Vascular Surgeon. When Doppler assessment reveals an index too low for local healing, additional tests are ordered by the vascular surgeon. Revascularization procedures are effective in aiding healing at local levels or permitting lower amputation levels.

Allied Health Professionals

Ward Nurse. The surgeon's and patient's staunchest allies have been the nurses. Care of the ill patient preoperatively is frequently difficult when diabetic control is added to infection and cardiac and kidney problems. In addition, the daily wound care given is one of the major factors in recovery of the patient who heals without surgical ablation.

Nurse Anesthetist. A team of nurse anesthetists is supervised by an anesthesiologist. Their care has been excellent. If the patient is too ill for inhalation anesthesia, regional intravenous lidocaine, regional nerve block, or local anesthesia is given by the surgeon or anesthetist.

Intensive Care Nurse. Postoperative care of difficult cases is started on an intensive care ward for 24 hours when necessary. These nurses are well trained in the special care of the postoperative patient. They are well versed in reading electrocardiograms and can give intravenous medication for cardiac problems.

Nurse Practitioner. Each outpatient is assigned to a nurse practitioner. The patient may call if problems arise outside the regular clinic hours. The nurses also make house calls to check on home health problems.

Liaison Nurse (Coordinator). Medical and surgical clinics meet at different hours and on different days. These nurses attend each clinic and can aid in diabetic treatment at the surgical clinic and arrange needed surgical clinic visits through the medical clinic. They have been taught foot and nail care and aid in such treatment.

Physical Therapist. Physical therapists perform pre- and postoperative evaluations to aid in the determination of potential prosthetic use. Gait training and strengthening exercises are used after application of a pylon or temporary prosthesis and after delivery of the final prosthesis. The patient is instructed in doffing and donning as a reinforcement to the instruction started by the prosthetist. House calls are made to assess the need for such equipment as ramps and rails.

Occupational Therapist. The occupational therapist supervises strengthening and training of the upper extremities. Instruction is given in household tasks. Special care is taken in training in the kitchen.

Medical Social Worker. A hospitalized patient frequently needs a go-between to aid in solving problems with insurance, housing, transportation, finances, government agencies, and even other family members. The amputee will, on occasion, not be able to return to the same environment. This is frequently apparent preoperatively and allows time for resettling to be arranged before discharge.

Psychologist. Not all patients suffer enough mental anguish or personality changes to require aid. However, it is well recognized that major loss of limb can be accompanied by severe depression, distortion of body image, or even complete personality decompensation. Ward personnel are aware of such changes and are quick to ask for consultation.

Pedorthist. The Prescription Footwear Association has been formed in response to a need for trained professionals in the dispensing of prescription shoes. Its members, pedorthists, are trained in the fabrication, modification, and repair of footwear prescribed for the disabled foot. They must pass an examination before certification is granted.

The Association distributes literature describing shoe modification and the materials used. A list of trained pedorthists is available from the Prescription Footwear Association, 200 Madison Avenue, New York, New York 10016.

Orthotist. In some centers the orthotist is now providing all therapeutic shoe corrections in addition to manufacturing braces. Toe blocks, sole stiffeners, rocker bottoms, and ankle-foot orthoses are all fabricated to prescription for the dysvascular foot patient.

Prosthetist. The input of the whole team aids in selecting an amputation level and then, in turn, deciding if a prosthesis should be prescribed. The prosthetist advises as to availability of types of prostheses and their suitability for a particular patient. He fabricates the prosthesis and initiates much of the care that is taken over by the physical therapist. In addition, he maintains or devises new prostheses and makes another in cases in which the prosthesis finally wears out.

Vascular Technician. Transcutaneous Doppler analyses as to wave forms and pressure, transcutaneous oxygen measurements, and similar tests are performed in the vascular laboratory. The ischemic index is calculated by the technician and a prediction is made as to healing level. In addition, the technician consults with the vascular surgeon and performs additional tests as required.

Vocational Counselor. After lower extremity amputation, certain more vigorous occupations are no longer possible. Working within the medical limits set for the patient, a counselor works with physical and occupational therapists to arrive at a line of training. A sheltered workshop provides work experience. The final happy day is the return of the amputee to gainful occupation.

FUTURE DIRECTIONS FOR REHABILITATION OF DYSVASCULAR DISEASED PATIENTS

The major portion of this chapter has been taken in describing treatment of a disease entity well along its downward course by the time the patient is symptomatic enough to seek medical help. It suddenly becomes crystal clear that the most efficient form of treatment would be prevention.

A cursory review of the voluminous literature on generalized and coronary artery atherosclerosis reveals many controversies and questions. Is cholesterol of major importance? What are the genetic and environmental factors? Has increased sucrose become a causative factor?[27] Has the electron microscope finally provided direct evidence of lipid infiltration of arterial walls?[2] Can atherosclerosis be prevented by dietary control of hyperlipidemia; is a national fat-control diet possible or indicated?[14,16,18] Are animal studies directly applicable to human beings? At the present state of knowledge, is intestinal bypass surgery indicated in the control of hyperlipidemia?[4,7]

From the foregoing, it is apparent that causation is polyvalent. Many scientists are searching for answers. No program of prevention is at present accepted by all investigators.

For surgical treatment in the vascular field, there are many promising advancements being studied. In the search for the "ideal vascular graft," many new plastic and biological materials are being tested. Umbilical veins appear to be a reliable source, and glutaraldehyde-stabilized, alcohol-stored grafts have been used in sufficient numbers to indicate their usefulness.

Advancement in surgical correction of the defects will probably be in refinements of present techniques and instruments. Endoscopic evaluation of intimal disorders is being perfected. Assessment of surgical anastamoses and removal of thrombi and debris are additional functions of the endoscope.

Diagnostic techniques for assessment of healing potential and surgical levels are becoming more accurate. Noninvasive transcutaneous oxygen tension probes are being miniaturized and made more stable. Laser-beam Doppler analysis may provide direct prediction of healing along the proposed suture line.

The orthopedist and other amputation surgeons are looking for additional techniques to stabilize the limb-prosthesis contact. The ultimate solution would be attaching the prosthesis to the skeleton, which in turn would be a combined mechanical-electrical device that could mimic normal gait exactly.

The immediate goal is an activity and dietary program that will achieve an atheroma-free vascular system without major disruption of daily life. Treatment at any stage must be decided between the patient and his treating physician with sufficient consultation to satisfy both.

REFERENCES

1. Baier, R. E., Akers, C. K., and Perlmutter, S.: Processed human umbilical cord veins for vascular reconstruction surgery. Trans. Am. Soc. Artif. Organs 22:514–526, 1976.

2. Balis, J. V., Haust, M. D., and More, R. H.: Electron-microscopic studies in human atherosclerosis. Cellular elements in aorta fatty streaks. Exp. Mol. Pathol. 3:511–525, 1964.

3. Barnes, R. W., Shanick, G. D., and Slaymaker, E. E.: An index of healing in below-knee amputation: Leg blood pressure by Doppler ultrasound. Surgery 79:13–20, 1976.

4. Buchwald, H.: A surgical operation to lower circulatory cholesterol. Circulation 28(2):649–650, 1963.

5. Burchard, H.: Beiträge zur Kenntnis des Cholesterins. Chem 261 61:1–25, 1890.

6. Collens, W. D., Vlahos, E., Dobkin, G. B., et al.: Conservative management of gangrene in the diabetic patient. J.A.M.A. 181:692–698, 1962.

7. Fritz, S. H., and Walker, W. J.: Ileal bypass in the control of intractable hypercholesterolemia. Am. Surg. 32:691–694, 1966.

8. Jacobson, J. H., and Suarez, E. L.: Microsurgery in anastamosis of small vessels. Surg. Forum 11: 243–248, 1960.

9. Kety, S. A.: Measurement of regional circulation by the local clearance of radioactive sodium. Am. Heart J. 38:321–328, 1949.

10. Kritter, A. E.: A technique for salvage of the infected diabetic gangrenous foot. Orthop. Clin. North Am. 4:21–30, 1973.

11. Lassen, N. A., and Holstein, P.: Use of radio isotopes in assessment of distal blood flow and distal blood pressure in arterial insufficiency. Surg. Clin. North Am. 54:39–55, 1974.

12. Liebermann, C.: Über das Oxychinoterten. Ber Dtsch Chemges 18:1803, 1885.

13. Lo Gerfo, F. W., Corson, J. D., and Mannick, J. A.: Improved results with femoropopliteal vein grafts in limb salvage. Arch. Surg. 112:567–570, 1977.

14. Malmros, H., and Wigand, G.: The effect on serum cholesterol of diets containing different fats. Lancet 2:1–8, 1957.

15. Meggit, B. F.: Orthopedic management of foot breakdown in the diabetic patient. J. Bone Joint Surg. 55B:882–883, 1973.

16. Miettinen, M., Turpeinen, O., Karvonen, M. J., et al.: Effect of cholesterol-lowering diet on mortality from coronary heart disease and other causes. Lancet 2:835–838, 1972.

17. Seldinger, S.: Catheter replacement of the needle in percutaneous arteriography. Acta Radiol. 39:368–376, 1953.

18. Spritz, N., and Mishkel, M. A.: Effects of dietary fats on plasma lipids and lipoproteins. J. Clin. Invest. 48:78–86, 1969.

19. Tswett, M: Adsorptions Analyse und Chromatographische Methode. Anwendung auf die Chemie des Chlorophylls. Ber. Dtsch. Bot. Ges. 24:384–392, 1906.

20. Wagner, F. W., Jr.: Amputations of the foot and ankle: Current status. Clin. Orthop. 122:62–69, 1977.

21. Wagner, F. W., Jr.: Orthopedic rehabilitation of the dysvascular lower limb. Orthop. Clin. North Am. 9:325–350, 1978.

22. Wagner, F. W., Jr.: Syme's amputation for ischemia of the toes and forefoot. In Bergan, J. J., and Yao, J. S. T., Eds.: *Gangrene and Severe Ischemia of the Lower Extremities,* pp. 419–434. Grune & Stratton, New York, 1978.

23. Wagner, F. W., Jr.: The diabetic foot and amputations of the foot. In Mann, R. A., Ed.: *Du Vries' Surgery of the Foot,* pp. 341–380. C. V. Mosby, St. Louis, 1978.

24. Wagner, F. W., Jr.: Use of Doppler ultrasound in determining healing levels in diabetic dysvascular lower extremity problems. In Bergan, J. J., and Yao, J. S. T., Eds.: *Gangrene and Severe Ischemia of the Lower Extremities,* pp. 131–138. Grune & Stratton, New York, 1978.

25. Weiss, M.: The prosthesis on the operating table from the neurophysical point of view. Report of Workshop Panel on Lower Prosthesis Fitting. National Academy of Sciences, Washington, D.C., 1966.

26. Whereat, A. F.: Is atherosclerosis a disease of intramitochondrial respiration? Ann. Intern. Med. 73:125–127, 1970.

27. Yudkin, J.: Dietary fat and dietary sugar in relation to ischaemic heart disease and diabetes. Lancet 2:4–5, 1964.

17

Head Injuries in Adults

Douglas E. Garland, M.D.

Three million head injuries occur each year. This figure includes minor injuries, such as simple lacerations. Automobile accidents account for 500,000 head injuries yearly. Head trauma is found in 70 percent of the injured occupants and multiple injuries are common. Every year 30,000 persons, primarily young men aged 15 to 24, are hospitalized for severe head injuries.

PREDICTION AND RECOVERY

Although prediction of neurological recovery is not in the orthopedic realm, an understanding of the neurosurgeon's prediction techniques will help the orthopedist in providing the best acute fracture care and rehabilitation. Predicting the neurological recovery of head-injured adults is difficult, but reasonably accurate estimates of neurological and functional return in patients with cerebrovascular accidents are possible.[2] Isolated lesions, such as occlusion of the middle cerebral artery or one of its tributaries, are common; in these cases, clinical syndromes, recovery patterns, and functional outcome can be readily defined. However, closed head injuries frequently involve more than one area of the cerebrum, the brain stem, and the cerebellum, and their clinical patterns may also vary, depending on the magnitude and type of injury. Coma, confusion, agitation, and decreased cognition also make evaluation and consequent prognostication of neurological return much more difficult than in the stroke patient.

Prediction

Teasdale and Jennett[11] have attempted to predict in the first few days after severe head injury the patient's final neurological results. The responsiveness scale developed was based on various aspects of coma routinely observed clinically (Table 17-1). A hierarchy of responses was recognized for each of the components and given numerical values, which were then compared to the neurological results at one year. By defining the initial and final results, they were able to calculate a mathematical relationship between the two. Prospective studies have now verified the usefulness and accuracy of the coma scale and neurological results can now be confidently foreseen early after injury.[8]

Recovery

Outcome as defined by Teasdale and Jennett was divided into five groups: good recovery, meaning near normal to normal recovery; moderate disability, or independence in activities of daily living with residual neurological problems; severe disability, or total dependence because of cognitive or physical problems; persistent vegetative state or unresponsiveness to external stimuli; and death.[11] Their classification is practical for predicting early general prognoses and it is an aid for appropriate orthopedic intervention in acute care and in the rehabilitation setting.

The Neurosurgical Service at the University of Southern California, Los Angeles County, recently participated in a multi-university effort to determine

Table 17-1. The Glasgow Coma Scale*

RESPONSE	QUALITY	NUMERICAL VALUE†
Eye opening	Spontaneous	4
	Speech	3
	Pain	2
	None	1
Motor response	Obeys	6
	Localize	5
	Withdrawal	4
	Abnormal flexion	3
	Extension	2
	None	1
Verbal response	Oriented	5
	Confused conversation	4
	Inappropriate	3
	Incomprehensible	2
	None	1

* From Teasdale, G., and Jennett, B.: Assessment of coma and impaired consciousness. A practical scale. Lancet 2:81–84, 1974.
† Responsiveness or coma sum equals 3–15 points.

Table 17-2. Condition of 184 Head-Injured Adults One Year after Injury*

CONDITION	1 MONTH, %	6 MONTHS, %	12 MONTHS, %
Dead	41	48	53
Persistent vegetative state	15	5	2
Severe disability	32	14	10
Moderate disability	8	19	16
Good recovery	4	14	19

* Modified from Heiden, J., Small, R., Caton, W., et al.: Severe injury and outcome (a prospective study). In Popp, A. J., Bourke, R. S., Nelson, L. R., and Kimelberg, H. K., Eds.: *Neural Trauma*, p. 190. Raven Press, New York, 1979.

neurological results of severe head injuries by using Jennett and Teasdale's initial concepts.[6-8] The study, based on data from 184 consecutive head-injured adults followed at least one year, concludes that most patients who survive their head injury will become rehabilitation candidates (Table 17-2). Age has a significant effect on prognosis (Table 17-3). Patients younger than 19 years of age showed the best results, although few children younger than 10 years were represented in the study. The level of recovery from diffuse cerebral injury as compared with surgical hematomas is comparable. Ninety percent of the patients obtained optimal level of recovery within six months. No patients severely involved at six months improved to a good recovery at one year. Permanent mental rather than physical sequelae were more frequently the primary cause of debility in patients with a moderate or severe disability (Table 17-4).

An independent retrospective review of patients from the Head Trauma Service at Rancho Los Amigos Hospital also demonstrated that age was an extremely important factor in a good recovery.[10] The authors also noted that the

Table 17-3. Age and Condition of 184 Head-Injured Adults One Year after Injury*

		CONDITION	
AGE	NO. PATIENTS	Dead or Persistent Vegetative State, %	Moderate Disability or Good Recovery, %
0–19	39	26	62
20–29	56	41	46
30–39	25	56	32
40–49	21	81	19
50–59	19	68	11
60	24	100	0

* Modified from Heiden, J., Small, R., Caton, W., et al.: Severe injury and outcome (a prospective study). In Popp, A. J., Bourke, R. S., Nelson, L. R., and Kimelberg, H. K., Eds.: *Neural Trauma*, p. 185. Raven Press, New York, 1979.

Table 17-4. Contribution of Mental and Physical Factors to Residual Disability*

DISABILITY	MODERATE, %	SEVERE, %
Mental > physical	67	53
Physical = mental	12	47
Mental < physical	21	0

* Modified from Heiden, J., Small, R., Caton, W., et al.: Severe injury and outcome (a prospective study). In Popp, A. J., Bourke, R. S., Nelson, L. R., and Kimelberg, H. K., Eds.: *Neural Trauma*, p. 190. Raven Press, New York, 1979.

longer the duration of coma, the poorer the prognosis. Finally, approximately two-thirds of the patients became ambulatory and independent in self-care activities. This latter finding would undoubtedly be similar to the University of Southern California study if those survivors were further evaluated and the neurological outcome more specifically defined.

MENTAL DISABILITIES

As demonstrated in the previous discussion, mental sequelae may be a greater disability than the physical residual. Cognitive rehabilitation is paramount in obtaining a good recovery and may be the only impairment. Mental residual problems include personality and behavioral changes, apathy, impaired selective attention and retention, and decreased capacity for judgment, thought organization, and new learning.

The following levels of cognitive functioning observed in patients with head injuries have been defined by the Communication Disorders Service at Rancho Los Amigos Hospital:

1. No response: the patient is completely unresponsive to stimuli.
2. Generalized response: the patient reacts inconsistently and unpurposefully to stimuli in a general manner.
3. Localized response: the patient reacts specifically but inconsistently to stimuli, as in instances of withdrawing an extremity to a painful stimulus.
4. Confused, agitated: the patient is in a heightened state of activity and exhibits severely decreased ability to process information.
5. Confused, inappropriate, unagitated: the patient appears alert and is able to respond to simple commands fairly consistently.
6. Confused, appropriate: the patient shows goal-directed behavior, but is dependent on external help for direction.

7. Automatic, appropriate: the patient appears appropriately oriented within hospital and home settings with minimal-to-absent confusion but has shallow recall of what he has been doing.
8. Purposeful, appropriate: the patient is alert, oriented, and able to recall and integrate past and recent events.

Although this classification is not absolute, it is practical. An individual patient's level can be identified and each discipline may implement complementary techniques suitable for that level. Furthermore, the patient's progress can be charted systematically. In general, programs for the first three levels are directed toward stimulation of the patient. At level 4, treatment attempts to control agitation and begins to help the patient restructure the environment and its events and activities. Therapies for levels 5 and 6 work to provide further structure. By this stage the patient usually demonstrates difficulty in processing information relative to the amount, complexity, duration, and rate at which information is given. By simplifying the task sufficiently, the patient will begin to respond appropriately. The higher cognitive skills of reasoning, judgment, and problem-solving may eventually be attained by increasing one task at a time. Treatment at levels 7 and 8 is directed toward the care of one's self and return to the community.

The exact usefulness and role of speech and language therapy for the patient with impaired communication is difficult to ascertain due to the number of variables among patients. Hagen's study[5] of hemiplegic stroke patients has demonstrated the most accelerated rate of recovery occurs during the first six months. Whereas the control group spontaneously recovered functional visual and auditory abilities, only those receiving communication therapy acquired functional reading comprehension, language formulation, speech production, spelling, and arithmetic abilities. In general, attempts at making cognitive gains with a patient who has not had treatment within six months after injury are less than rewarding.

PHYSICAL DISABILITIES: THE ORTHOPEDIC PROGRAM

Physical rehabilitation is complicated by the patient's inability to cooperate. Intellectual and physical disabilities are managed through complementary techniques. Team members stimulate the patient frequently, briefly, meaningfully through intelligent explanations and in an organized multisensory manner. This is illustrated, for example, in teaching activities of daily living. By daily repetition of correct steps for transfers to and from the bed, wheelchair, and toilet, the patient not only gains motor control but his learning ability and memory are stimulated.

The orthopedic surgeon's role has been well-defined in the care of the head-injured adult.[1] In the acute period, fracture care that may include open reduction and internal fixation must be undertaken. In the recovery phase, which persists for approximately a year, the orthopedist must prevent spastic deformities and decubitus ulcerations and identify and initiate management of heterotopic ossification. Finally, when return of neurological function has stabilized, reconstructive surgery may be undertaken and heterotopic bone may be resected.

FRACTURE TREATMENT

Acute fracture care for the head-injured patient is often difficult because of priorities that must be accorded to the multiple injuries. Life-saving resuscitation may detract from complete recognition and treatment of musculoskeletal injuries. In some instances, an injury may be diagnosed but an uncertainty regarding proper treatment often prevails because of a poor understanding of the extent of the head injury and the prognosis. In 1978, 91 brain-injured patients who sustained 99 skeletal injuries were reviewed two years after their injury.[1] An attempt was made to identify the etiology of unsatisfactory fracture results. From this review, five rules were formulated for the treatment of fractures:

1. *Establish the diagnosis completely.* These patients are comatose and cannot direct the physician's attention to the area of pain or injury. At least one of ten patients arriving at a head trauma unit has a missed musculoskeletal injury. The first review showed that 10 of 91 patients had 12 missed injuries. These injuries were of significant magnitude—five were spine injuries and three were about the hip. The prospective review over a two-year period has recently demonstrated a changing pattern of missed injuries. Ten skeletal injuries were identified; however, no hip injuries and only one unrecognized spine injury were found. There were 29 peripheral nerve injuries that were often associated with a fracture. Initial roentgenograms should include anteroposterior (AP) and lateral views of the cervical spine, an AP of the pelvis, including both hips, and an AP of both knees, especially if the victim has been struck by an automobile.[4] Repeated examinations are essential to diagnose peripheral nerve injuries, since they frequently are not manifest until the patient can cooperate or physical signs are evident.

2. *Base the treatment on the assumption that the patient who survives a head injury will make a good neurological recovery.* According to Jennett et al.,[8] approximately 50 percent of patients who sustain severe head injuries succumb. Fewer than 10 percent of the survivors remain totally dependent. The largest group of survivors, more than 20 percent, make a good neurological recovery. Furthermore, neurologically compromised patients require excellent fracture care, because they may not be able to compensate for skeletal deformities as well as the normal person.

3. *Anticipate uncontrolled limb motion.* Slings, splints, and braces should be secure because these patients are frequently confused, agitated, and lack judgment. Tenuous open reduction and internal fixations should be protected by external devices.

4. *Do not cast joints in a flexed position.* Flexion attitude is frequently the position many joints assume after a head injury. Joints cast in a flexed position may result in aligned fractures but joint contractures. If reduction cannot be maintained because of flexor tone, open reduction and internal fixation should be entertained. In the upper extremity, the elbow should be immobilized at 135 degrees, the wrist at neutral, the metacarpophalangeal joints at 45–60 degrees, the interphalangeal joints extended, and the thumb extended and abducted. In the lower extremity, the hip, knee, and ankle should be immobilized in neutral positions.

5. *Do not impose traction methods as a matter of course.* Traction methods, especially when they involve skin, often prove unsatisfactory for prolonged fracture management. Furthermore, traction in the confused and agitated patient adds to nursing problems, and pulmonary care and feedings become extremely difficult. Mobilization of the patient in traction for diagnostic tests and surgery is difficult. Therefore an aggressive surgical approach may be required to facilitate overall care.

Anesthesia

Except in life-saving situations, neurosurgeons are reluctant to authorize anesthesia in comatose patients, since they are unable to monitor neurological status. Moreover, an already elevated intracranial pressure can be increased during intubation secondary to hypercapnia, since carbon dioxide is a potent vasodilator. Lastly, most anesthetic agents are cerebral vasodilators. Increasing cerebral blood flow and cerebral blood volume can increase intracranial pressure and decrease cerebral perfusion, thus increasing the possibility of cortical damage from ischemia.

If general anesthesia is required, certain guidelines should be followed:

The patient should be neurologically stable. Neurosurgeons frequently request that general anesthesia be delayed until there is no worsening in neurological status over a 24-hour period.

Any patient with evidence of post-traumatic encephalopathy or altered state of consciousness should have computerized axial tomography to rule out intracerebral hemorrhage. However, approximately 25 percent of head-injured adults have increased intracranial pressure without mass effect and are still at risk.

The anesthesiologist must be familiar with basic principles of neuroanesthesia. Controlled hyperventilation should be used to prevent hypercapnia and the anesthetic agent selected should have the least effect on cerebral blood flow. Blood should be replaced with blood and dextrose and water must be avoided.

Approximately half the head-injured patients who eventually succumb die within two weeks of their accident (Table 17-5).[7] Those dying in the third or fourth weeks usually have declared their fate by significant medical complications, such

Table 17-5. Deaths and Day of Expiration after Injury in 123 Consecutive Patients*

DAYS AFTER INJURY	NO. DEATHS
1	1
2–3	10
4–7	9
8–14	12
15–28	19
>30	9
	60

* Modified from Heiden, J., Small, R., Caton, W., et al.: Personal communication—unpublished data.

as pneumonia, stress ulcers, and metabolic abnormalities. Cerebral edema appears by 24 hours. The maximal edema is reached by three to five days and resolves by seven to ten days. The risks of anesthesia are minimal after this time. Therefore, since anesthesia is safe after ten days, half of the potential deaths have already occurred, and many patients have declared their fate, most elective orthopedic procedures may be safely undertaken at or about ten days. This assumption was recently verified when 122 head-injured patients underwent general anesthesia later than two weeks after their injury with no neurological deterioration.[3]

Upper Extremity Fractures

The incidence of upper extremity injuries associated with head injuries is less than lower extremity injuries, especially in cases of pedestrians struck by automobiles.[4] More than half of upper extremity injuries occur in the shoulder girdle area and can be diagnosed with routine chest roentgenograms.[1] Missed musculoskeletal injuries are infrequent although unobserved peripheral nerve injuries are common.

Shoulder Girdle. The most common area of injury in the upper extremity is the shoulder girdle. Fractures of the clavicle and acromioclavicular separations are common, whereas scapular and proximal humerus fractures occur less frequently. Most injuries can be treated symptomatically. The injury should alert the examiner to the potential underlying brachial plexus palsy. A flail upper extremity with a fracture around the shoulder girdle has a brachial plexus injury until proved otherwise, especially if the patient has been injured on a motorcycle.

Humerus. Fractures of the humerus are not common and routine methods of treatment may not be applicable. The principles of the hanging arm cast cannot be applied to the bedridden patient. Splints and Velpeau bandages may be difficult to keep in place. Further difficulties arise in middle and distal one-third shaft fractures in which the radial nerve may be injured. Traction through an olecranon pin is not desirable and may not prevent initial or subsequent injury to the radial nerve. Open reduction and internal fixation afford the opportunity to explore the radial nerve and protect it from further damage.

Elbow. Fortunately, fractures about the elbow are rare. Closed treatment with circular plaster may result in a flexion contracture. Heterotopic bone is often a complication of elbow fractures and may decrease motion. Further complications arise when the heterotopic bone obliterates the ulnar groove. External pressure from merely resting the elbow on the bed may lead to a tardy ulnar palsy. If open reduction and internal fixation are attempted, fixation should be secure and the ulnar nerve should be transferred anteriorly. Instituting therapy for range of motion soon after an operation is advantageous.

Forearm. This is the second most common fracture in the upper extremity. Unreduced fractures often heal in a short period of time. If open reduction and internal fixation are undertaken, excellent fixation should be obtained in order to initiate early a range of motion. Heterotopic bone frequently appears across the interosseous membrane. Surgical dissection should be minimal, precise, and gentle, and bone grafting should not be required even in delayed surgeries.

Distal Radius. Occasionally, initial reduction of this fracture is not maintained, yet re-manipulation is not performed because the neurological recovery is expected to be poor. When patients are young, an acceptable range of motion can still be achieved; however, median and ulnar palsies are common when the fracture is left unreduced.

Lower Extremity and Pelvic Fractures

The incidence and number of complications in lower extremity fractures are increased over upper extremity fractures. Diagnosis is more difficult due to overlying soft tissue and multiple fractures are frequent.

Pelvis. It is frequently of greater significance to identify a pelvic fracture early because of bleeding diathesis than treatment. These fractures heal rapidly even with minimal apposition. The sacroiliac joint and symphysis pubis often ossify if they have been injured. Pelvic fractures are the most frequent skeletal injury in the victim struck by an automobile.[4]

Injuries About the Hip. Hip dislocations and fractures and acetabular fractures always present potential difficulties. They have a tendency to remain undiagnosed, the potential for heterotopic bone formation is high, appreciable pain is frequent on attempted motion, and hip flexion contractures are common. Regardless of mode of treatment, aggressive physical therapy is often needed to ensure a good result.

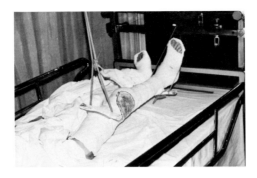

Fig. 17-1. Fractured femur in cast traction. A femoral pin was inserted. Note that the hip, knee, and ankle are in a neutral position. Removal of the rubber tubing from the dowels will mobilize the patient.

Femur.   Traction methods are frequently a hindrance to overall care. When traction is used, cast traction is often beneficial (Fig. 17-1). A tibial or femoral pin is inserted and a short leg cast is applied. While an attendant applies traction to the leg, an attempt is made to reduce the fracture and a tight thigh gaiter is applied. The gaiter and short leg cast are then connected with plaster. Wooden dowels are attached to the anterior thigh and posterior to the calf. Rubber tubing is applied distally with sufficient tension to elevate the cast off the bed. The proximal dowel can be suspended by rubber tubing if difficulty is encountered in aligning the fracture or stabilizing the leg. Advantages of this method are as follows: patients can be easily mobilized while the leg is still contained; traction set-up is minimal and can be handled easily on nonorthopedic wards; the hip, knee, and ankle are maintained in a neutral position; and the agitated patient's leg will not thrash around and will remain in a midline position because the rubber tubing offers resistance to movement in any other direction. Femoral fractures are best treated by internal fixation with an intramedullary nail. Care must be taken to use a nail of sufficient diameter to engage both fragments. Some patients demonstrate spastic internal or external rotators about the hip and it is common for one of the fragments to rotate on the nail. A one-and-one-half body cast spica is not desirable in the comatose, confused, or agitated patient.

Knee.   Knee ligament injuries are rare except in the patient struck by an automobile. It is not necessary to operate on these injuries early. If the knee injury is on the same side as the hemiplegia, a flexion contracture often persists after casting. Quadriceps exercises are difficult to learn postoperatively and, once again, full range of motion is difficult to achieve. If the involved knee is contralateral to the neurologically impaired extremity, surgical repair and casting will render ambulation impossible. Due to mental confusion, rehabilitation of the nonspastic surgical knee is also very difficult. Delayed surgical reconstruction should give a functional knee to most of these patients.

Tibia.   Tibial plateau fractures that meet routine surgical criteria should be repaired in head-injured patients. Tibial shaft fractures pose no significant problem and usually heal with standard plaster techniques.

Spine Fractures

Head injury and spine fracture combinations are frequently lethal. Consequently, severe cervical spinal cord and head injuries are clinically rare. Routine cervical spine roentgenograms should be obtained in all patients in whom coma is secondary to trauma.

Cervical Spine. Halo traction is the best skull traction in the agitated patient. The halo also is useful in patients with previous surgical skull decompression. However, these patients do not tolerate cervical traction. Unstable fractures should be stabilized internally and grafted early. Surgery during the first couple of days after injury has an extremely high mortality rate.

Thoracic Spine. As in the cervical spine injuries, unstable fractures even in the complete lesion should be stabilized internally. Mobility and rehabilitation are greatly enhanced and healing is rapid. External protection is still advised, since these patients fail to protect themselves and their spines.

MANAGEMENT OF SPASTIC DEFORMITIES

Muscles, even when fully relaxed, still possess small amounts of tension. When the muscle is stretched, as in moving a joint, a certain unconscious resistance is encountered. This is known as muscle tone. Tonus can be abolished by severing the ventral roots, which contain the motor nerve fibers, or the dorsal roots, which contain sensory fibers from muscle. Tonus is maintained and regulated in muscles by reflex activity in the nervous system, specifically the stretch reflex system with its supraspinal inhibitor-facilitatory modulation. Spasticity indicates that the muscle-stretch reflex has become isolated from the latter and is mediated through the γ-efferent system.

Physiology: The Stretch Reflex System

The stretch reflex system consists of muscle fibers (extrafusal), muscle spindles (intrafusal), and sensory afferent and motor efferent fibers (Fig. 17-2A). Muscle spindles are parallel to striated muscle fibers and consist of a sheath with a number of nuclei and small striated muscle fibers at each pole. Muscle spindles have packs of nuclei at the central portion (nuclear bag) or a single row of nuclei (nuclear chain). Annulospiral fibers give rise to Group I-A ($12–30\ \mu$ in diameter) fibers, which are the largest sensory afferents and thus transmit at the most rapid rate. Group II fibers ($4–12\ \mu$) arise from the flower spray organs. Group I-A fibers signal the rate of change in the muscle, whereas those in Group II reflect static muscle length.

The Golgi tendon organs arise at the muscle-tendon junction and are in series with the extrafusal fibers. Group I-B sensory fibers arise from these organs and signal increasing muscle tension. Sensory inhibition impulses decrease motor activity.

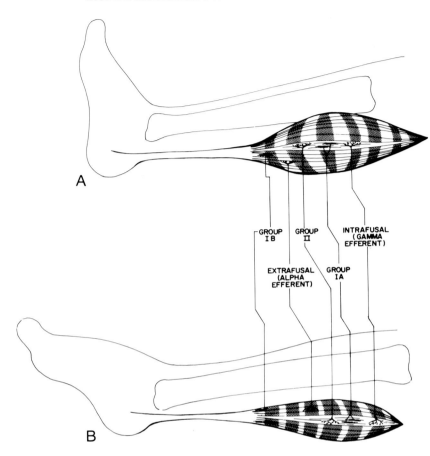

Fig. 17-2. (A) The stretch reflex system. (B) The foot has developed an equinus attitude with a myostatic contracture of the gastrocnemius-soleus muscle group. The muscle is now smaller and its fibers must lengthen to a greater extent for each dorsiflexion degree arc at the ankle than the muscle in (A). Because the muscle is smaller and must now lengthen more per degree of dorsiflexion arc, and because potential for spasticity should remain the same in both muscles, a greater volley of spastic activity will be seen in (B) over (A) in a stretch response. Consequently there is a relative increase in spasticity in (B).

The motor nerve fibers consist of α- and γ-efferents. The α-efferents are thick, high-velocity conduction fibers that terminate on the motor end-plates of extrafusal muscle fibers. The γ-efferent nerves innervate the intrafusal fibers and are thin and conduct slowly.

Treatment with Plaster of Paris Casts

Plaster of Paris casts are the mainstay of severe spastic deformity care. Flexed joints allow the formation of myostatic contractures that increase the spastic response to stretch (Fig. 17-2B). Plaster casts maintain the muscles at proper length and joints in an acceptable position (Figs. 17-3A, B). Casts also aid in stretching contracted tissue and decrease the stretch response (Figs. 17-4A, B).

Decorticate (lower extremity extended, upper extremity flexed) and decerebrate (extremities extended) rigidities require the most aggressive initial plaster treatment. These patients have severe tone and, if left untreated, develop early myostatic contractures. The spasticity of hemiplegia is usually not as intense as extensor rigidity, but at times it may also need aggressive plaster of Paris treatment.

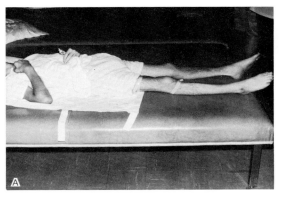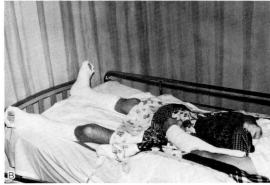

Fig. 17-3. (A) A patient with quadriparesis. Position of equinus at the ankles and the flexed elbows will lead to fixed deformities. (B) The same patient with his ankles positioned at neutral and elbow in near full extension. The opposite elbow could be fully extended with minimal difficulty. It may be necessary to treat all extremities with plaster.

Hip.   Adductor tone is uncommon and not usually a major problem except in the brain stem insult. If casts have already been applied to the lower extremities for plantar flexion tone, a spreader bar may be added to maintain abduction. Tone secondary to brain stem injury does not always respond to casting. An early percutaneous adductor tenotomy may be beneficial. Hip flexion deformities are infrequent and are generally secondary to knee contractures. They normally respond to proning.

Knee.   Knee flexion deformity is commonly seen in spastic hemiplegia. A circular long leg plaster is initially applied in maximum extension. This stretches the soft tissue contracture, avoids stimulation of the stretch reflex, and seems to make the stretch response less sensitive. Dropout casts are then used, to be changed as needed until the knee is neutral (Fig. 17-5). AP splints or posterior splints alone may be required at night to maintain a neutral position.

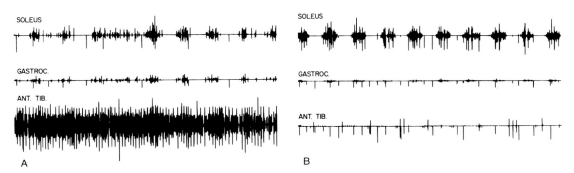

Fig. 17-4. (A) Graph of a spastic patient ambulating without a brace. Note the marked activity in all three muscles. (B) Graph of the same patient ambulating with a brace. Note the marked decrease in activity of all muscles. Plaster of Paris casting has the same effect and it can thus be used to decrease the stretch response.

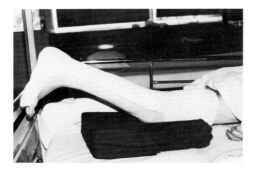

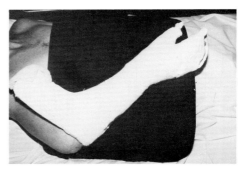

Fig. 17-5. The knee dropout cast. The patient is prone and the anterior portion of the tibial cast is removed. While proning to stretch out the hip, the weight of the leg stretches the knee contracture. A therapist may perform passive extension. As the contracture decreases, new casts may need to be applied. The posterior shell prevents further contracture.

Fig. 17-6. The elbow dropout cast. The posterior portion of the arm is removed and passive stretching can be undertaken. The anterior shell prevents further contracture. Serial casts will be required as the contracture decreases.

Ankle.   Short leg casts are required to prevent equinus (Fig. 17-3B). Serial casts may be needed if equinus is fixed, and they should be changed at intervals of seven to ten days. Once a neutral position is attained, AP splints are useful in maintaining it.

Elbow.   As with knee flexion contractures, a circular plaster is often initially used for elbow flexion contractures. Dropout casts are then used until full extension is gained (Fig. 17-6). Once again, AP splints may be required at night. The wrist and fingers can be incorporated into the dropout cast and treated simultaneously with the elbow if flexor tone is present (Figs. 17-3B, 17-6). It is rare to treat isolated finger and wrist flexion deformities early and then not to have elbow deformities. The elbow is often the most refractory to treatment. If neurological recovery does not occur and the upper extremity remains nonfunctional, the wrist and fingers will not respond to plaster treatment either.

Treatment with Anesthetic Nerve Blocks

Local anesthetics disturb the free transfer of ions across the axon membrane. When the inflow of sodium ions and the outflow of potassium ions are blocked, axon transmission ceases. The effectiveness is determined by agent concentration and the surface area:volume ratio of the nerve.[9] Thus, thinner fibers, such as the γ-efferents with greater relative surface areas, are the most readily blocked.

Local anesthetic nerve blocks are both diagnostic and therapeutic. Diagnostic nerve blocks aid in differentiating myostatic contracture from spasticity. They also aid in predicting the results of any surgical or chemical neurolysis. Nerves can be therapeutically blocked prior to cast application. By decreasing γ-efferent activity and thus spasticity, the maximal joint correction will be attained prior to cast application. At least 10 cc of a 0.5–2 percent procaine solution is used for each nerve block. Although the block may not be anesthetically complete, the γ-efferents will be the first involved because they have the largest surface area:volume ratio. In fact, it is at times possible to demonstrate voluntary muscle activity and sensation along with loss of deep tendon reflexes and clonus. Nerves commonly blocked are the musculocutaneous, median, ulnar, posterior tibial, and sciatic.

Anesthetic nerve blocks are also therapeutic in that, unpredictably, some blocks may last for days. This carry-over is best and most consistently demonstrated in the obturator nerve block for adductor tone. One of the long-lasting procaines should be used for its anesthetic effects.

Treatment with Phenol Nerve Blocks

Phenol destroys peripheral nerve conduction when injected directly into the nerve. Two actions of phenol on nerve tissue have been identified. First, it has an immediate local effect similar to other anesthetic agents and may selectively block the thinner nerve fibers. Secondly, it causes coagulation of protein. Thus, nerve destruction depends on diffusion and destruction of protein within the nerve. Consequently, phenol is not selective in this function.[9]

Phenol injection of nerves is an open technique. Three percent phenol is mixed with glycerine. Phenol blocks are usually used during the initial six months after injury when the spasticity is the most severe. Its effects are variable but they usually last three to six months. By the time nerve regeneration occurs, it is hoped that normal or maximal neurological recovery will have ensued. Traditionally phenol has been injected into most peripheral nerves. Today, however, the most common indications are the posterior tibial nerve for ankle-plantar flexion tone and the musculocutaneous nerve for elbow flexion tone.

Musculocutaneous Nerve. The main indication for phenol nerve block is the inability to gain elbow extension despite casting. The entire nerve is blocked under direct vision in the proximal arm. Sensory loss is not a problem. Dropout casts are required postoperatively. Roentgenograms of the elbow are required preoperatively to ensure that heterotopic bone is not present.

Posterior Tibial Nerve. Indications for posterior tibial block are: inability to bring the ankle to a neutral position despite serial casting; inability to prevent clonic gastrocnemius-soleus activity despite bracing on attempted ambulation; and inability to maintain the foot in an orthosis (pistoning) when ambulating despite a neutral ankle position at rest. The posterior tibial nerve is visualized at the popliteal fossa. With the aid of a nerve stimulator, the motor branches of the gastrocnemius, soleus, posterior tibialis, and toe flexors are identified and injected. The sensory branch is spared. Depending on preoperative indications, casting may be required postoperatively.[1]

DECUBITUS ULCERS

Soon after head injury, acute decubitus ulcers occur most commonly at the heel and over the malleoli. Later, especially in the severely involved patient who remains dependent and becomes malnourished, decubitus ulcers occur in their more common locations at the trochanters and sacrum.

Initially the malleoli and heel are subject to constant vertical force from the weight of the leg during coma and flaccidity. As spasticity ensues, shear forces and friction play an important role in blister and decubitus ulcer formation. Further, as agitation ensues (level 4), these same factors may become significant even in the normal extremity.

Plaster of Paris casts are an excellent mode of treatment for these ulcers. Casts may be used as a preventive or protective measure. During agitation it is desirable to use a cast for protection of the foot and ankle from trauma. Once an ulcer has formed, a cast can prevent additional trauma to the injured area, since these patients cannot always cooperate with a positioning program.

Casts distribute pressures over the entire enclosed leg more evenly, relieving localized pressure over the bony prominences. Edema, which is often associated with pressure ulcers, is better controlled by circular casts. Lastly, casting will decrease the stretch response of the gastrocnemius-soleus muscle across the ankle joint (Figs. 17-4A, B). Thus, shear and friction forces at the heel will be decreased.

Decubitus ulcers secondary to plaster of Paris are uncommon but do occasionally occur. This development may mean a poorly applied or padded cast or that limb synergies have allowed proximal joint motion and consequent motion within the cast. This ulcer should be treated by an appropriate reapplication of the short leg cast. A long leg cast is required if limb synergies are present.

MANAGEMENT OF HETEROTOPIC OSSIFICATION

It is common knowledge that heterotopic ossification occurs in head-injured adults. However, little information is available regarding its incidence, location, and treatment.

Clinically, heterotopic ossification differs from that observed in paraplegics. The incidence in paraplegia ranges from 10–50 percent, but it is 10–15 percent in head injuries. In paraplegia the location in decreasing order of frequency is hip, knee, elbow, and shoulder.[14] In head injury, occurrence of heterotopic bone is common at the hip but uncommon at the knee. Although ankylosis of the hip is common in both entities, ankylosis of the elbow is much more common in head-injured patients. Lastly, because head-injured patients have the potential for a near-normal neurological recovery, the stimulus for heterotopic ossification may disappear. Consequently, when resection of new bone is undertaken, the possibility of recurrence should be decreased, as opposed to the case of the spinal cord injured patient.

Diagnosis is made by tests for elevated alkaline phosphatase and bone scans, and later confirmed by roentgenograms. However, due to the frequent association of fractures, the alkaline phosphatase may be elevated during fracture healing.

Bone scans may be difficult to obtain in the agitated patient, so roentgenograms may be the best available method of diagnosis.

Once heterotopic bone has been identified, programs for vigorous range of motion and positioning should be instituted. Unfortunately, such regimens often produce pain, which exaggerates spasticity and makes range of motion even more difficult. The efficacy of diphosphonates during the early phase of heterotopic ossification is not known. The diphosphonates do not prevent formation but the calcification of collagen and osteoids. Whether calcium deposition will occur once the drug has been stopped remains to be seen.

Surgery should not be undertaken until at least 18 months have elapsed since injury. Serial bone scans are helpful in determining if a patient is ready, since resection should not be performed unless there is little or no uptake activity. Alkaline phosphatase levels should be normal. Good voluntary muscle control about the joint is also beneficial because maintenance of joint motion will not be dependent upon a therapist.

The Hip

Three basic types of heterotopic bone form at the hip. Combinations of these types can occur, especially if there is an injury about the hip. Occasionally range of motion during the acute phase is impossible even though ankylosis has not occurred. Anterior bone formation lies below the rectus femoris and sartorius and anterior to the hip capsule. These patients lie in external rotation and internal rotation is difficult. Hip flexion can frequently be maintained. Resection at the correct time may provide excellent hip motion.

Heterotopic bone associated with adductor tone is detected on the medial aspect of the proximal femur. Hip flexion can frequently be maintained. Early percutaneous or open adductor myotomy and obturator neurectomy frequently are useful in maintaining hip abduction.

Posterior heterotopic ossification about the hip is a serious problem. Although some degree of motion is maintained, a hip flexion contracture is almost always present. Resection of the bone may not be helpful, since the flexion contracture frequently persists. Extension osteotomy of the proximal femur to utilize present motion in a more favorable arc may be a more acceptable alternative.

When injury about the hip has occurred, considerable ectopic bone may form in all planes. An approach similar to that used in cases of posterior bone formation may yield the best results surgically.

The Elbow

Formation of extra bone at the elbow may pose considerable difficulties in range of motion. Bone formation tends to occur anteriorly or posteriorly but if the elbow has been traumatized, bone may form in any plane.

Posterior bone formation is generally seen with decerebrate rigidity (elbows extended). Frequently, the elbow will ankylose in extension. Preoperatively the bone consists of a shell between the humerus and triceps; resection frequently allows acceptable motion.

Anterior bone formation is a more difficult problem than posterior formation. It is commonly associated with spastic hemiplegia and decorticate (elbows flexed) rigidity. Phenol injection to the musculocutaneous nerve may preserve an acceptable range of motion during early ossification. By the time the bone matures, a flexion contracture has usually developed. Resection of the bone is technically difficult because of neurovascular structures and muscle involvement. Postoperatively, the flexion contracture usually persists and such complications as skin sloughs and wound complications are extremely common.

The Shoulder

Although small amounts of bone are common about the shoulder, significant functional disabilities are rare. Spasticity is present in the internal rotators but, with persistence by the therapist, acceptable motion can be achieved. Ankylosis is rare; occasionally it is seen with brain stem injuries resulting in vegetative or severe disability states.

The Knee

Heterotopic bone formation is not common and only small amounts of bone are detected, usually at the medial femoral condyle. Hamstring spasm can be primary or secondary to associated knee pain. Knee effusions are frequent. Loss of motion is rare if ranging can be instituted.

SURGERY

Reconstructive surgery should not be undertaken until 18 months after injury.[1] Reviews of operations for patients with head trauma have been published,[1-3] and surgical procedures developed for stroke patients* may be applied to the head-injured patient as well.[12,13]

REFERENCES

1. Garland, D. E., and Rhoades, M. E.: Orthopedic management of brain injured adults: Part II. Clin. Orthop. 131:111–123, 1978.
2. Garland, D. E., and Waters, R. L.: Orthopedic evaluation in hemiplegic stroke. Orthop. Clin. North Am. 9:291–305, 1978.
3. Garland, D. E., Capen, D., and Waters, R. L.: Surgical morbidity in patients with neurologic dysfunction. Clin. Orthop. 145:189–192, 1979.
4. Garland, D. E., Glogovac, S. V., and Waters, R. L.: Orthopedic aspects of pedestrian victims of automobile accidents. Orthopedics 2(3):242–244, 1979.
5. Hagen, C.: Communication abilities in hemiplegia: Effect of special therapy. Arch. Phys. Med. Rehabil. 54:454–463, 1973.

---

* See also Chapter 18.

6. Heiden, J., Small, R., Caton, W., et al.: Severe injury and outcome: A prospective study. In Popp, A. J., Bourke, R. S., Nelson, L. R., and Kimelberg, H. K., Eds.: *Neural Trauma,* pp. 181–193. Raven Press, New York, 1979.

7. Heiden, J., Small, R., Caton, W., et al.: Personal communication—unpublished data.

8. Jennett, B., Teasdale, G., Galbraith, S., et al.: Severe head injuries in three countries. J. Neurol. Neurosurg. Psychiatry 40:291–298, 1977.

9. Mooney, V., Frykman, G., and McLamb, J.: Current status of intraneural phenol injections. Clin. Orthop. 63:122–131, 1969.

10. Rhoades, M. E., and Garland, D. E.: Orthopedic prognosis of brain injured adults: Part I. Clin. Orthop. 131:104–110, 1978.

11. Teasdale, G., and Jennett, B.: Assessment of coma and impaired consciousness. A practical scale. Lancet 2:81–84, 1974.

12. Waters, R. L.: Upper extremity surgery in stroke patients. Clin. Orthop. 131:30–37, 1978.

13. Waters, R. L., Perry, J., and Garland, D. E.: Surgical correction of gait abnormalities following stroke. Clin. Orthop. 131:54–63, 1978.

14. Wharton, G. W., and Morgan, T. H.: Ankylosis in the paralyzed patient. J. Bone Joint Surg. 52A:105–112, 1970.

18

Stroke

Christopher Jordan, M.D.
Robert L. Waters, M.D.

Cerebrovascular accidents (CVAs) are one of the most common medical problems in the United States. They are the third leading cause of death, responsible for about 200,000 deaths per year. Table 18-1 summarizes the survival and functional prognosis of stroke patients and documents that they survive long enough and have enough residual function to justify aggressive rehabilitation.

The different clinical syndromes of stroke arise from insults to different areas of the cerebral cortex, as shown in Figure 18-1. The middle cerebral artery supplies the greatest area of the cortex and this area controls numerous different body functions. This artery is most commonly involved in strokes and a middle cerebral artery problem produces the typical hemiplegic picture, that is, greater involvement of the upper than the lower extremity. The anterior cerebral artery leaves the circle of Willis anteriorly but is in reality the midline cerebral artery, for its area of vascular supply extends far posterior. The anterior cerebral artery supplies the area of the cortex representing the leg, illustrated in Figure 18-2. This explains anatomically why following a middle cerebral artery stroke there is less leg than arm involvement.

CVAs in the vertebral-basilar system are less common, but when they occur rehabilitation is difficult because of the balance and coordination problems resulting from interruption of afferent and efferent pathways between the brain and spinal cord.

Table 18-1. Prognosis Following CVAs*

	TOTAL NUMBER OF CVAs, %	SURVIVAL RATE AFTER			FUNCTIONAL PROGNOSIS OF SURVIVORS, %	
		30 Days, %	5 Years, %	10 Years, %		
All CVAs		62			29	Normal
					33	Able to work
					3	Total care
Thrombosis	71	90	43	22	27	Normal
					34	Able to work
					2	Total care
Emboli	8	75	30	15	27	Normal
					34	Able to work
					2	Total care
Hemorrhage, overall	16				49	Normal
					14	Able to work
					49	Total care
Intracerebral bleeding		22	7	0		
Subarachnoid bleeding		55	37	30		

* Modified from Matsumoto, N., Whisnant, J. P., Kurland, L. T., et al.: Natural history of stroke in Rochester, Minnesota, 1955 to 1969. Stroke 4:20–29, 1973. By permission of the American Heart Association.

EVALUATION OF REHABILITATION POTENTIAL

An accurate assessment of a patient's remaining functional potential is essential before starting to treat the neurologically stable stroke patient.[1] Goals and benefits of rehabilitation, a patient's eventual placement, and a family teaching program should be defined before therapy starts.

Severe medical problems and severely decreased cognition usually are relative contraindications to rehabilitation. Physical problems should not be of such severity that they prevent the patient from participating in the rehabilitation program. The patient must tolerate the minimum activity level required by the rehabilitation program if the patient is to be considered a candidate. Cognitive impairment with decreased short-term memory and decreased learning ability also inhibits the potential for rehabilitation. Cognitive abilities are judged by the appropriateness of responses to questions, by the ability to follow commands, by psychological testing, and by testing learning ability in a rehabilitation setting. Cognitive impairment is pervasive, affects all aspects of rehabilitation, and must be carefully assessed. Table 18-2 lists major obstacles to successful rehabilitation.

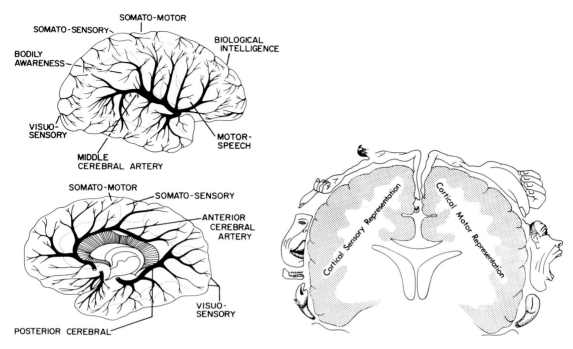

Fig. 18-1. Areas of cerebral cortex that control the various functions and their arterial supply.

Fig. 18-2. Areas of the motor and sensory cortex that control the extremities. The portion affecting the lower extremity is in the midline.

Other factors that limit rehabilitation potential are the perceptual problems of body neglect and sensory deficits. Body neglect becomes a major problem when a patient ignores his involved extremities and cannot be taught to use them until his self-image returns. They also may ignore safety factors on that side and thus stay at the supervised level of activity. Neglect, when more subtly present, can be

Table 18-2. Inhibitors of Rehabilitation Potential

Severe Inhibitors
    Severely impaired cognition and learning ability
    Decreased activity tolerance because of severe medical problems

Relative Inhibitors
    Bilateral cerebral damage
    Obesity
    Contralateral extremity problems
    Body neglect
    Impaired balance
    Marked sensory impairment
    Prolonged flaccidity
    Placement in a nursing home

documented by having the patient make body image drawings and noting the lack of symmetry of the two sides in the drawing. Other clues are the absence of spontaneous use of an extremity in the presence of functioning muscles unless verbal cues are given, neglect of safety factors on that side, and the failure to look across midline toward their affected side. Most patients eventually overcome this stage of neglect, and it does not remain a major isolated clinical problem. Some neglect, however, frequently remains as part of the total stroke picture.

In the normal course of recovery a patient will have flaccid extremities for about 48 hours following a CVA. Thereafter, the deep tendon reflexes become hyperactive and the patient becomes spastic. At this time, the patient's motor control becomes patterned and he can usually initiate a primitive flexor (withdrawal) or extensor pattern in an all-or-none fashion. Gradually, as the recovery continues, the patient is able to use his muscles selectively out of pattern; eventually full selective motor control may return. The usual course of motor return in a stroke patient is from proximal to distal. At any point along this course, an individual patient's progress may be halted. The longer flaccidity persists, the poorer the prognosis.[12] If a patient is flaccid for six weeks, then no functional return in that extremity can be expected. In the lower extremity the motor return rarely changes after three months and has plateaued fully by six months. The same is generally true in the upper extremity, but recent trials of long-term outpatient therapy have suggested that slow improvement in arm function may go on for as long as 18 months. The amount of selective control needed for functional use of the leg is much less than in the arm, so that the prognosis for functional return in the lower extremity is much better than in the upper extremity. A patient can walk with some pattern overlay in the lower extremity, but very little can be done with that same degree of control in the upper extremity.

Evaluation of Ambulation Potential

The common misconception that CVA patients never become functional is far from the truth. About 20–30 percent of the patients will walk fairly normally, and research has shown that roughly 75 percent of the patients return to some level of ambulation.[6–11] There are three basic requirements for ambulation. The first is balance, which in the stroke patient means the ability to lean over his unaffected leg and support himself with a cane held in his intact hand. This ability is critical, because the stroke patient with an impaired upper extremity is unable to use a walker. The patient must be able to stand before he can walk. Second, some method of limb advancement is required. Generally, this requires trunk control and functioning hip flexors. The third is stance stability of the hip, knee, and ankle on the affected side. This loss is the easiest to compensate for—the patient can do it, or an ankle orthosis and cane can be provided. Also, spasticity may offer some stance stability.

Evaluation of the patient's ambulation potential can then be fairly easily done on physical examination.[14–15] The examination must be done with the patient upright. When checking balance, sitting balance should be checked first, because standing balance will not be present if sitting balance is absent. If the patient has double limb balance, then limb advancement and stance stability are checked by assisting him to ambulate. If the patient does not demonstrate ambulation potential, then lower extremity rehabilitation goals consist of maintaining range of motion, transfer techniques, and wheelchair management.

Evaluation of Upper Extremity Potential

For the stroke patient and his family, regaining the use of the leg and the ability to walk are highly visible and very important goals. Equally important, if a patient is to become independent in normal activities of daily living, is functional return in the arm. Nearly two-thirds of the patients will get some return in their arm, but in only about 30 percent does it approach the functional control of the intact side.[12] Hand function is less automatic and is much more affected by perceptual and sensory problems than the leg. The normal requirements for hand use are proximal joint stability, the ability to place the hand in space, sensory feedback, and the ability to grasp and release.

Body neglect can be a significant problem and affects the arm more than the leg. Patients will not use what function they have if neglect persists—they will forget to use the arm unless given constant verbal cues. Sensory losses, especially of the higher-level functions of proprioception and two-point discrimination, will also prevent spontaneous hand use. Most stroke patients regain deep pain and light touch sensation, but these modalities alone are insufficient. The sensory tests that correlates best with spontaneous use are proprioception and two-point discrimination.

Motor control may vary from selective to pattern motion in an all-or-none fashion to no motion at all. Any voluntary hand function that elicits proximal patterning is of no functional benefit. Since flexor spasticity predominates in the arm, a patient's ability to extend his fingers must be checked. A hand with impaired release can be used only as a gross assist or as a paperweight. Also, problems in motor planning, such as difficulty in sequencing the steps of a complex task, will decrease hand use.

Evaluation of potential hand use then requires a careful physical examination. It is important to check for signs of neglect, for sensory losses of the more integrative functions, for the ability to use the hand without triggering pattern movements, for motor planning deficits, and for impaired hand release. Only the last of these is ever amenable to surgical treatment. Because hand function depends on so many uncontrollable factors, if the impairment is significant, the goal of upper extremity rehabilitation becomes teaching the patient to do things one-handedly and to prevent joint contractures on the affected side.*

Nonoperative Treatment of Extremity Problems

In the preceding section, the importance of cognitive abilities, sensory losses, balance problems, and motor planning problems was stressed. Unfortunately, these problems are not easily amenable to treatment. Using repetition, facilitory techniques, and functional electrical stimulation, progress can be made in those

---

* See also Chapter 14.

areas but it is often inconsistent and incomplete.[19] The bulk of the extremity conditions that are treated by an orthopedic surgeon are the results of two problems—spasticity and contractures. Spasticity, with its resultant abnormal joint positioning, may interfere with extremity function, cause pain, and lead to contractures. Currently available medications used to reduce spasticity are usually ineffective or sedate the patient, decreasing his cognitive awareness.

The cornerstone of nonoperative treatment of spasticity is maintaining a normal range of motion. The physical or occupational therapist, the patient, or a family member must range the spastic extremity. The ranging program must be aggressive and the importance of obtaining full joint range should be emphasized. A joint fully ranged twice a day will seldom become contracted. Myostatic contractures enhance spasticity, creating a vicious circle. In general, obstructive spasticity and contractures are frequently the results of early inadequate care. An occasional patient is so spastic that even conscientious efforts fail, but most contractures are preventable with range of motion exercises. An important adjunct to the ranging program is the use of night casts to maintain proper joint positioning while the patient sleeps.

A recent trend in managing spasticity is to apply electrical stimulation to the antagonist muscles via cutaneous electrodes.[20] Electrical stimulation helps maintain the strength of the antagonist muscles so that they can compete more successfully with the spastic muscles. It may speed sensorimotor re-education in the return of selective control of the muscles by making the patient more aware of the sensation of contraction in the muscles he is attempting to fire voluntarily. In addition, working through a spinal cord reflex, stimulation may decrease the spasticity of the offending muscles.

An important part of managing the functional problems resulting from spasticity is the use of orthoses.[12] The orthosis is used to hold the joint in a functional position. By decreasing motion, the spastic muscles will receive less stimulation of their stretch reflex and it may be possible to correct a spastic deformity. Some patients are so spastic that the deformity cannot be controlled with an orthosis and these patients may need surgery. Orthotic principles work equally well in the upper or lower extremities, but frequently an orthosis interferes with hand function or is too cumbersome to be of value in the upper extremity.

An adjunct to these techniques is the use of serial local anesthetic blocks, which temporarily eliminate spasticity and may have some long-lasting effects. Nerve blocks are also helpful in differentiating true contracture from spasticity as the cause of decreased joint range. The techniques of nerve blocks have been well documented.[13]

Contractures may occur separately from spasticity in stroke patients and cause problems with pain, positioning, pressure sores, skin maceration, and increased difficulty with transfers or ambulation. The nonoperative treatment of these problems is discussed in the chapter on head injuries. If nonoperative treatment fails, then surgery may be required.

Surgical Management of Disabled Extremities

Surgery is indicated when nonoperative methods have failed or when the goal is to make the patient braceable or brace-free.[4] Hygiene and pressure sore problems are the most absolute surgical indication, even in totally bedridden patients with functionless extremities. The procedure is most commonly indicated for hip adductor spasticity, which causes problems with perineal hygiene. It is sometimes indicated for shoulder, elbow, and wrist deformities. This type of surgery markedly eases the nursing care problems in these severely spastic patients.

Spasticity or contractures may cause pain by holding joints constantly in a fixed position; this is especially significant at the shoulder, but such fixedness also occurs at the wrist and occasionally at the knee. It, too, is an indication for surgical release. However, not all joint pain in stroke patients stems from contractures or spasticity, so other causes must be ruled out before performing releases.

Cosmesis is an uncommon surgical indication. It is limited to those patients with so much elbow and wrist flexor tone that the arm goes into a position of elbow and wrist flexion with walking, causing a noticeable cosmetic problem. A related problem is elbow and wrist flexor clonus with walking; it too is cosmetically unattractive. These arms are routinely nonfunctional, and a musculocutaneous neurectomy or a wrist flexor release will improve their appearance.

Functional improvement is the most frequent and most satisfying surgical indication. To operate with improved function as a goal presupposes that there is some reason to expect the patient has potential to improve. Because stroke patients spontaneously recover for at least six months following a CVA, surgery to improve function is not done before that period of spontaneous recovery is completed.

Finally, the type of surgery to be done should be emphasized. In the adult stroke patient, who presumably had normal bone structure prior to the CVA, the deformity is caused by abnormal muscle forces and not by bone deformity. Therefore any surgical correction should be directed at those muscles; in general, bone surgery is not indicated in the adult stroke patient. The deformity seen clinically can be corrected by performing the appropriate tendon lengthening or release. If the goal of surgery is to decrease but not eliminate the muscle's function, a lengthening and not a release should be done. This consideration is especially important in the potentially functional hand. If an operation is being performed on a functionless extremity, then a release is generally indicated, because it is easier to do and it lessens the chance of recurrent deformity.

Preoperative Evaluation

Surgical procedures performed to improve function in cerebral spastic patients have not enjoyed universal acclaim. Many patients developed recurrent deformities or the opposite deformity. Surgical intervention is complex. First it is necessary to identify all the muscles contributing to the deformity, then indicate what the antagonist muscle function is, and then predict what the result of the release or transfer will be. Careful preoperative evaluation then is the key to consistent surgical results and it consists of four steps. There must be a careful examination, and usually a physical therapy or occupational therapy evaluation that should document that the deformity seen clinically is, in fact, a functional problem. Next the patient must be fitted with a trial orthosis that reproduces the desired postoperative extremity position and allows the physician to observe if the new position is more functional. Then nerve blocks must be applied. By eliminating the spasticity in a defined group of muscles, the blocks reveal which muscles are causing a clinical deformity. They also allow testing of the muscle strength of the antagonists, temporarily not overpowered by the anesthetized muscles. This knowledge is especially useful if a transfer to augment the antagonist muscle power is being considered. Lastly, the dynamic electromyogram (EMG), an invaluable preoperative test, is administered. Figures 18-3 through 18-6 are examples of dynamic EMG.

The dynamic EMG is the newest and must useful part of the preoperative work-up.[3] This type of EMG does not assess nerve conduction velocities, abnormal wavelengths, or muscle strength. It demonstrates the phase in which a muscle is active during a functional activity, and this knowledge of timing is essential. Spastic muscles never change phase postoperatively, so out-of-phase tendon transfers cannot be expected to function except as a tenodesis. Conversely, if a muscle is continually spastic preoperatively and is transferred, it remains spastic postoperatively and may lead to the opposite deformity. Further, the EMG will identify all muscles contributing to the deformity seen clinically as well as those muscles that are electrically quiet so the correct muscles can be lengthened or released. The dynamic EMG then shows the surgeon what to cut, what to leave, and what can be transferred. Its predictive capabilities have led to improved surgical consistency in the spastic patient. Proper balance and activity of antagonist muscle forces are the keys to normal function. Careful preoperative evaluation makes these goals consistently attainable.

NORMAL

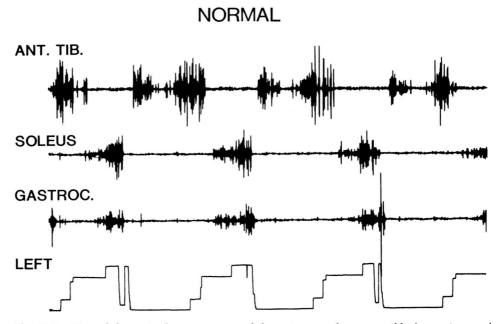

Fig. 18-3. Normal dynamic electromyogram of the major muscles responsible for equinus and varus. The lowest tracing is the foot switch, which records swing phase (baseline), heel strike (first level), metatarsal head contact (second level), and first toe contact at roll-off (highest level).

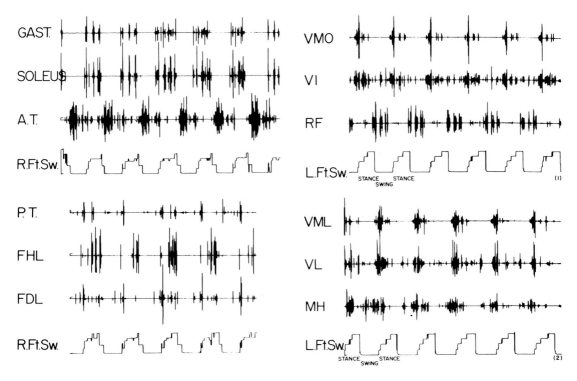

Fig. 18-4. Typical EMG of a stroke patient, showing gastrocnemius (GAST) and soleus firing inappropriately in late swing, the anterior tibialis (AT) firing continuously, the posterior tibialis (PT) with little activity, and the toe flexors firing inappropriately in late swing and early stance. (FHL = flexor hallicus longus, FDL = flexor digitorum longus, RFTSW = right foot switch.)

Fig. 18-5. Typical EMG of a patient with a stiff-legged gait that is surgically correctable. The vastus intermedius (VI) is continuously active and the rectus femoris is firing out of phase in late stance and early swing. If the vastus medialis (VML) and vastus medialis obliquus (VMO) or the vastus lateralis (VL) had shown marked activity during that period, the patient would not be a candidate for surgery. (LFTSW = left foot switch.)

SURGICAL MANAGEMENT OF SPECIFIC ABNORMALITIES

Lower Extremities

The Foot and Ankle. Equinovarus is the most common deformity of the lower extremity treated in the stroke patient; however, equinus and varus will be discussed as separate entities. The penalty of equinus is a decreased base of support, difficulty in clearing the toes in swing phase, and back knee deformity. It is caused by overactivity of the soleus and gastrocnemius. The other muscles crossing posterior to the ankle are smaller, have a short level arm, and are not primary causes of the equinus deformity. Nonoperative treatment of equinus consists of a locked ankle orthosis. The indications for Achilles tendon lengthening are brace-free ambulation or failure of the orthosis to control the equinus, as

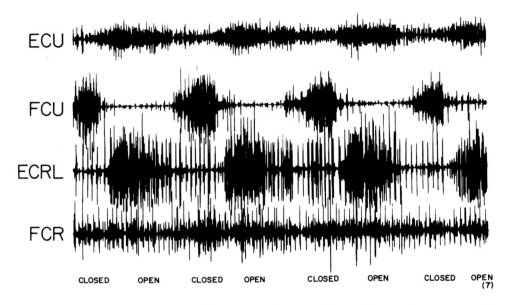

ECU

FCU

ECRL

FCR

CLOSED   OPEN   CLOSED   OPEN   CLOSED   OPEN   CLOSED   OPEN
(7)

Fig. 18-6. An upper extremity EMG of a patient with a wrist flexion deformity showing a spastic flexor carpi radialis (FCR) and a phasic flexor carpi ulnaris (FCU). The overactivity of the extensor carpi ulnaris (ECU) and extensor carpi radialis longus (ECRL) may be of central origin or the result of chronic stretching by the stronger flexors.

when the foot pistons up and down in the shoe during walking. We routinely use a percutaneous Hoke triple-hemisection tenotomy with the proximal and distal cuts medial and the middle hemisection laterally. Postoperative management consists of six weeks in a short leg walking cast with the ankle in neutral or 5 degrees of plantar flexion. Immediate ambulation is allowed. After cast removal, a locked ankle orthosis and night splints are used for another 4.5 months.

Varus is the second most common problem detected alone or in combination with equinus. Weight bearing, which may precipitate pressure sores and eventually cause pain, is confined to the lateral border of the foot. Treatment consists of a locked ankle orthosis. Again, surgical indications are failure to maintain correction in the brace or brace-free ambulation. Two groups of patients cannot become brace-free with surgery: those sustaining severe proprioceptive loss require the deep pressure sensation from the brace calf band for sensory feedback and patients with weak calf strength need the orthosis to stabilize the tibia during stance.

An EMG study made in 1978 of 34 stroke patients showed that the varus is almost always caused by the anterior tibial muscle.[18] In the 17 patients the posterior tibial muscle was totally inactive and in only a few was it normally active. Lengthening procedures described previously for correcting varus are only rarely prescribed. If indicated, the surgical treatment of varus is a split anterior tibial tendon transfer (SPLATT).[17–23] When performing a SPLATT procedure, some consideration should be given to a tendon transfer in order to augment dorsiflexion. If the EMG shows an available muscle firing in swing phase, then a posterior tibial nerve block should be administered to eliminate calf tone so that the patient's dorsiflexor power can be assessed accurately. If the patient still has a foot drop after calf paralysis is complete, then a transfer is indicated. Usually it is the flexor hallucis longus that is transferred.

Toe curling is the next most common problem seen. It frequently causes pain. Treatment is a long toe flexor tenotomy. This is performed in the midfoot through the medial incision if a SPLATT procedure is also being done.[23] Otherwise it is done at the metatarsal-phalangeal joints. A toe flexor release should always accompany an Achilles tendon lengthening (TAL) even if clawing was not observed preoperatively. Once the foot is dorsiflexed, the toes will curl from a tenodesis effect if they are not released. Occasionally a patient will also have an intrinsic plus-deformity of the toes, treatable by a release at the metatarsal-phalangeal joint.

Valgus of the foot is rare. It is seen only in those patients with a pes planus prior to their stroke. If it cannot be managed orthotically, it is treated with a lateral-based TAL. Evertor muscle releases or transfers are unusual.

A recent follow-up study surveying 35 patients 2.5 years after their SPLATT, TAL, or toe flexor release demonstrated that nine patients had some residual varus, four showed residual equinus, but none required further surgery. Three had a residual foot drop from inadequate dorsiflexion. Ninety percent of the patients improved, 60 percent improved their ambulation by at least one level, and 50 percent became brace-free.[2]

Knee Surgery. Two surgically correctable problems are seen at the knee. The first is flexion contractures. In the nonambulating patient, such contractures increase pressure on the heels when the patient lies supine, which can lead to pressure sores. In ambulation the contractures increase the demand on the quadriceps and hip extensors, which increases the energy cost of walking. Quadriceps demand rises rapidly when a contracture exceeds 15 degrees. If nonoperative measures fail, a hamstring tenotomy is indicated. For the potential ambulatory patient, a selective hamstring release is done based on the EMG. In the nonambulator all four tendons are released. A posterior capsulotomy is not performed. Any residual contracture is treated by serial casting.

The second problem is abnormal quadriceps activity in late stance and early swing. It prevents the normal 35 degrees of passive pre-swing knee flexion and leads to a stiff-legged gait causing the patients to hip-hike, circumduct, and decrease their velocity. There is no good nonoperative treatment. A walking EMG of all heads of the quadriceps is essential for selecting patients for the operation. Patients who will consistently show good results are those in whom the overactivity is limited to the rectus femoris and the vastus intermediate portions of the quadriceps. If all four heads are overactive, then releasing two is not sufficient. If the vastus medialis and vastus lateralis are firing improperly, their release may cause knee instability, and therefore the procedure is not indicated. If these EMG criteria of activity limited to the rectus and intermedius are adhered to, good results occur in 88 percent of the patients, and if they are not followed, good results will be seen in only 25 percent. The operation consists of an anterior midline incision from 4 cm above the patella going proximally, followed by identification and resection of 2 cm of the muscle. Postoperative ambulation with a soft dressing is allowed as soon as pain ceases sufficiently.

Hip Deformities. The major problems about the hip are flexion contractures and adductor tightness. Hip flexion contractures are initially treated by a ranging and proning program. If these measures fail and the contractures are severe enough to cause a flexed attitude during ambulation or render a sitter unable to prone, then a surgical release is indicated. The operation is usually performed via an anterior approach.

Adductor spasticity and tightness are not as serious problems in stroke patients as in other spastic diseases because they are usually unilateral. The intact leg presumably has a normal hip range, so hygiene is usually not troublesome. It may cause scissoring in the ambulating patient. The initial treatment is a series of anesthetic obturator nerve blocks, which have some long-lasting effect in approximately 50 percent of the patients. If this fails, then an adductor release is performed.

An uncommon problem in the hips of stroke patients is heterotopic ossification.* Also, uncommonly seen is an excessive flexor (withdrawal) pattern causing stroking when the patient is standing, which may require a muscle release.

Upper Extremities

The Shoulder. The major shoulder problems are contractures, subluxation, and pain. Contractures form quickly, the result of inadequate ranging and the early return of spasticity in the shoulder. The contracture is always one of adduction and internal rotation. The initial treatment is an aggressive ranging program. If this fails, indications for surgical release are poor hygiene, pain, and a functional impairment from decreased placement abilities. The insertions of the pectoralis major, subscapularis, latissimus dorsi, and teres major are transected. Postoperative management consists of an aggressive ranging program as soon as wound healing is secure.

Subluxation of the shoulder caused by flaccid musculature is also a common problem affecting many stroke patients. In most cases the arm is functionless because a stroke patient's motor return is from proximal to distal. The subluxation often leads to a decreased range of motion and pain. Therefore the treatment is a ranging program and a sling to hold the humerus in place. Several elective operations for subluxation are described by Saha in his monograph on the flaccid shoulder.[19]

Pain can be a persistent problem in the shoulder. The possible causes are contracture, subluxation, shoulder-hand syndrome, degenerative joint disease, and pain of central origin. This last is characterized by head, arm, and leg pain on the affected side. The treatment of shoulder pain consists of identifying and treating the underlying cause.

The Elbow. The elbow is almost as severely affected by the ravages of spasticity and contractures as the shoulder. Some loss of elbow range can be tolerated without functional impairment. In addition to decreased range of motion, elbow flexor spasticity may lead to biceps clonus or flexor patterning, which cause cosmetic difficulties. Severe tone also can impair hand placement abilities and, if the spasticity is severe, it may lead to poor hygiene in the antecubital fossa. The

---

* See Chapter 17.

initial treatment is ranging and positioning. If that fails, then treatment hinges on differentiating contracture from spasticity, which can be done during a physical examination augmented by a musculocutaneous Xylocaine nerve block. If contracture of more than 90 degrees is found, then an elbow release through a straight incision lateral to the midline is performed. Releases of the biceps, brachialis, and brachioradialis are frequently required. If spasticity is the cause, then treatment consists of a musculocutaneous neurectomy. This is done with an incision parallel and just posterior to the biceps, starting at the level of the pectoralis major insertion and proceeding distally. Of 19 patients who had musculocutaneous neurectomies for cosmesis and improvement in activities of daily living, 18 retained elbow flexion in the fair or better strength range from residual brachioradialis function. Operations on 11 other patients for other reasons were successful in all cases, with the average increased extension being 67 degrees.[5]

The Forearm and Hand. In stroke patients, the forearm and hand are the parts of the upper extremity most often operated upon. Preoperative evaluation often necessitates trial orthoses, nerve blocks, and dynamic EMG to avoid the inconsistent results that have plagued these procedures in the past. It is especially important to evaluate the residual extensor power, which usually requires a median nerve block, and identify the flexor muscles that are spastic, which requires an EMG. The most common deformity is wrist and finger flexor overactivity and the most common clinical problem is impaired hand opening or release. In 1963, in a study of 70 normal volunteers, Perry et al.[16] demonstrated that only 37 percent had EMG activity of the extensor digitorum communis during release and only 9 percent used the wrist extensors during release. Release is basically the absence of grasp. The most common way to improve release in spastic patients is to weaken their grasp spasticity. In the functional hand, hand opening is increased by fractional or Z-lengthening tendons, not releasing tendons.

The muscles most prone to spasticity in the forearm are the wrist flexors. When they show spasticity, usually the finger flexors do too, but a group of patients with selective finger control and wrist flexor spasticity can be identified. In such cases releases may be performed, since lengthenings, especially those of the flexor carpi ulnaris, have a high incidence of recurrent deformities. In addition, because the finger flexors can substitute for the wrist flexors, the wrist flexors are more expendable. If the finger flexors are tight with the wrist neutral or dorsiflexed, performing a concomitant muscle tendon junction slide may be indicated.

Finger flexor spasticity is the next common deformity. It may be present in the sublimis without profundis activity and vice versa. This state is best documented by EMG and points out the value of the test. If a patient has functional potential, a muscle-tendon slide lengthening is prescribed. It can be done at two levels of the same muscle if extra length is necessary. Three centimeters of length can be gained. Since it is not necessary to have full finger extension for good hand function, and since over-lengthening will cause excessive loss of grip strength, it is better to lengthen too little than too much. The Z-lengthening is usually not done, because a Z-plasty of multiple tendons may cause adhesions between the tendons.

Finger flexor lengthening in a nonfunctional hand is accomplished by a sublimis to profundis transfer if more than 3 or 4 cm is needed.[21] The sublimis is cut distally and sewn en masse to the profundis tendons, which are cut proximally. This procedure was originally described as having some functional potential but is now considered to be a salvage procedure in the nonfunctional hand. If there is any evidence of intrinsic spasticity, an ulnar nerve motor branch neurectomy is performed at the same time to prevent a secondary intrinsic deformity.

The Thumb. The thumb-in-palm deformity is the most frequently seen thumb deformity. It has three variations. The first is the thumb-in-palm from flexor pollicis longus spasticity, which is associated clinically with flexion of the interphalangeal joint and can be documented by EMG. Treatment is a tendon lengthening.

Next is thenar muscle tightness, characterized by metacarpophalangeal flexion, a relaxed interphalangeal joint, and a perpendicular abducted position of the thumb. Because 70 percent of normal persons have a dual innervation of the flexor pollicis brevis and opponens, both median and ulnar nerves have to be blocked to relax those muscles and differentiate this deformity from the first type.[7] An EMG delineates which of the thenar muscles is the offender. Treatment involves releasing the offending muscle and suturing it into the extensor brevis tendon proximal to the metacarpophalangeal joint. In some cases at surgery, the abductor brevis has been found to have migrated volarward and to be acting as a metacarpophalangeal flexor. Suturing these muscles into the extensor brevis preserves some of their thumb placement function and eliminates their metacarpophalangeal flexor function. An associated hyperextension deformity of the interphalangeal joint may cause a boutonniere deformity. If severe, treatment is an interphalangeal fusion.

The third type of thumb-in-palm deformity is the adducted thumb, characterized by tight first web space. It is caused by hyperactivity in the adductor or in that portion of the first dorsal interosseous originating from the first metacarpal. Since both are ulnar innervated, nerve blocks will not distinguish between them, but an EMG will identify which muscle is the main offender. Treatment is an adductor release or stripping of the first dorsal interosseous.

SUMMARY

Cerebrovascular accidents affect several body systems. Accordingly, certain accompanying disabilities have not been addressed because they are beyond the scope of this chapter. Most significant of these are the communication disorders, feeding difficulties for patients with bulbar involvement, and the social problems caused by stroke. The goal of this chapter has been to emphasize the rehabilitation potential of stroke patients, how to evaluate it, and how to maximize it surgically. Surgery is just one aspect of the total rehabilitation for stroke patients. Preoperative evaluation is the key to consistent functional improvement. The patient must demonstrate enough cognition, coordination, and sensation to make use of the increased motor skills that an operation can provide. The physical examination, nerve block, and EMG aid in identifying exactly which muscles are causing the clinical deformity. If careful examinations are made, operations can be performed with little risk and consistent results.

REFERENCES

1. Block, R., and Bayer, N.: Prognosis in stroke. Clin. Orthop. 131:10, 1978.

2. Eroche, W. J.: Correction of spastic equinovarus deformity by split anterior tibial tendon transfer: A long-term study. In *Orthopedic Seminars*. Rancho Los Amigos Hospital, Downey, Calif., 1978.

3. Frazier, J.: An electromyographic analysis of the ankle and foot in the hemiplegic patient. In *Orthopedic Seminars*. Rancho Los Amigos Hospital, Downey, Calif., 1979.

4. Garland, D. E., Capen, D., and Waters, R. L.: Surgical morbidity in patients with neurologic dysfunction. Clin. Orthop. 145:189–192, 1979.

5. Garland, D. E., Thompson, R., and Waters, R. L.: Musculocutaneous neurectomy for spastic elbow flexion in nonfunctional upper extremities in adults. J. Bone Joint Surg. 62A:108–112, 1980.

6. Gresham, G. E., Fitzpatrick, T. E., Wolf, P. A., et al.: Residual disability in survivors of stroke— the Framingham Study. N. Engl. J. Med. 293:954–956, 1975.

7. Harness, D., Sekeles, E., and Chaco, J.: The double motor innervation of the opponens pollicis muscles: An electromyographic report. J. Anat. 1172:329–331, 1974.

8. Kannel, W. B., Dawber, T. R., Cohen, M. E., et al.: Vascular disease of the brain—epidemiologic aspects: The Framingham Study. Am. J. Public Health 55:1355–1366, 1965.

9. Lehman, J. F., et al.: Stroke: Does rehabilitation affect outcome? Arch. Phys. Med. Rehabil. 56:375–382, 1975.

10. Levine, J., and Swanson, P. D.: Nonatherosclerotic causes of stroke. Ann. Intern. Med. 70:807–816, 1969.

11. Matsumoto, N., Whisnant, J. P., Kurland, L. T., et al.: Natural history of stroke in Rochester, Minnesota, 1955 to 1969. Stroke 4:20–29, 1973.

12. McCollough, N. S.: Orthopedic evaluation and treatment of the stroke patient. In American Academy of Orthopaedic Surgeons: *Instructional Course Lectures*, pp. 21, 24, 45. C. V. Mosby, St. Louis, 1975.

13. Moore, D.: *Regional Block*. Charles C Thomas, Springfield, Ill, 1957.

14. Perry, J.: Lower extremity management in stroke. Examination: A neurologic basis for treatment. In American Academy of Orthopaedic Surgeons: *Instructional Course Lectures*, p. 26. C. V. Mosby, St. Louis, 1975.

15. Perry, J., Giovan, P., Harris, L. J., et al.: The determinants of muscle action in the hemiparetic lower extremity. Clin. Orthop. 131: 71–89, 1978.

16. Perry, J., Dail, C., and Allen, J. R.: Phasic relations of hand muscles applied to tendon transplants. Final Project Report. NIH Grant AM-07192. Attending Staff Association of the Rancho Los Amigos Hospital. January 1, 1962–March 31, 1967.

17. Perry, J., and Waters, R. L.: Orthopedic evaluation and treatment of the stroke patient. In American Academy of Orthopaedic Surgeons: *Instructional Course Lectures*, p. 40. C. V. Mosby, St. Louis, 1975.

18. Perry, J., Waters, R. L., and Perrin, T.: Electromyographic analysis of equinovarus following stroke. Clin. Orthop. 131:47–53, 1978.

19. Saha, A. K.: Surgery of the paralyzed and flail shoulder. Acta Orthop. Scand., Suppl. 97, 1967.

20. Vodovnik, L., Kralj, A., Stanic U., et al.: Recent applications of functional electrical stimulation to stroke patients in Ljubljana. Clin. Orthop. 131:64–70, 1978.

21. Waters, R. L.: Upper extremity surgery in stroke patients. Clin. Orthop. 131:30–37, 1978.

22. Waters, R. L., Garland, D. E., Perry, J., et al.: Stiff-legged gait in hemiplegia: Surgical correction. J. Bone Joint Surg. 61A:927–933, 1979.

23. Waters, R. L., Perry, J., and Garland, D. E.: Surgical correction of gait abnormalities following stroke. Clin. Orthop. 131:54–63, 1978.

19

Peripheral Nerve Injuries

Gary K. Frykman, M.D., F.A.C.S.

Even when expertly repaired, peripheral nerve injuries are known to recover much more slowly and incompletely than other non-nervous tissue injury. However, the total scope of disability due to peripheral nerve injuries has never been precisely assessed. In 1977, 65,155 patients with median and ulnar nerve neuropathies were hospitalized in the United States, with an average hospital stay of 3.3 days.[9] If a $140 per day hospitalization charge is assumed, the cost of hospitalization alone was $30 million. Although no statistics are available, if we included hospitalization costs for all peripheral nerve injuries, we could easily double that figure. If this amount is added to the unknown value of physician fees, rehabilitation costs, lost work time, and temporary and permanent disability payments, it is easy to arrive at a cost of several hundred million dollars annually for treating these injuries.

The traditional attitude toward peripheral nerve injuries was that little could be done to rehabilitate the patient other than the performing of a technically good nerve repair. However, when a contracted, painful, useless extremity results from a peripheral nerve injury, it is obvious that some measures can and should be taken to prevent additional and unnecessary disability and to enhance the functional return of the nerve-injured extremity.

In this chapter, methods of evaluating peripheral nerve injuries, complications, patient education, and the roles of the therapist, physician, and patient in the rehabilitation setting will be reviewed. Some of the newer approaches to rehabilitating nerve injuries used at the Hand Rehabilitation Center of Loma

Linda University will be emphasized. Causalgia and sympathetic dystrophies will not be discussed.

ASSESSMENT

Accurate documentation of the extent and nature of a peripheral nerve injury deficit is extremely important to the physician and the therapist. In cases in which the nature, location, and extent of nerve injury are unknown, accurate documentation of motor and sensory loss is essential to localize the nerve injury. Where the extent of nerve injury is known, such as postoperatively following nerve repair, progressive reassessment is necessary to determine the extent of nerve regeneration.

Methods of Evaluation

Motor Evaluation. Muscle strength is tested and graded into one of six standard grades by the method of Daniels et al.[4] All the pertinent muscles in the extremity are examined. Other factors, such as independence of action, endurance, and speed of muscle action, may also be assessed but evaluative methods for these attributes are not yet standardized. Beware of trick movements[18] in muscle testing because some patients are adept at substituting muscle functions. It is always necessary to palpate over the belly of the muscle being tested, feel a contraction, and also watch and feel its tendon action before accepting the movement as being due to that particular muscle.

Sensibility Evaluation. Many tests for sensory modalities have been devised: touch, pressure, heat and cold, and sweating.[14] However, these are generally not too useful because the correlation between their presence and functional recovery is poor.[7,8,10] Seddon[11] has emphasized the distinction between academic, found by testing, and functional recovery of peripheral nerve lesions. Moberg[7] coined the term "tactile gnosis," which is that quality of sensation necessary for the fine precision function of the hand necessary for such activities as screwing a nut on a bolt, winding a watch, or buttoning clothes without visual clues. Testing for sensibility should not be burdensome or overly time-consuming, yet it should give practical information.[14]

The Von Frey hairs and their modern successor, the Semmes-Weinstein monofilaments for assessing light touch to deep pressure, have been well studied.[6,12,15,17] Moberg[7] found that Von Frey hairs have no correlation with degree of functional sensory loss. Levin et al.,[6] because of "variable and poorly understood results" with the Semmes-Weinstein esthesiometer, conducted an engineering analysis of these probes. They found that "gross errors arise from careless application" and variations in the temperature, humidity, and ends of the filaments could cause inconsistencies. The probes were noted to be "simple to use but easy to misinterpret."[6]

These probes have been extensively studied by others and are advocated as being the most reliable and consistent method of sensibility evaluation.[2,15] However, 13 variations in response patterns were described.[17] The probes as described are perhaps valuable as research tools but because they are laborious and tedious, they are not yet practical for general use.

The form used by the Hand Rehabilitation Center of Loma Linda University for making sensory evaluations is shown in Figure 19-1. We evaluate hyperesthesia first. If the patient overreacts or shows dysesthesias from the stimulus, no further testing of sensibility in that area is reliable. Skin atrophy, change in color, dry skin, and lack of callosities all indicate areas of impaired or absent sensibility and lack of use.

Six grades of sensibility are distinguished and each grade is assigned a color, which is then entered on the diagram of the hand shown in Figure 19-1 by the therapist for quick and easy visual identification. Usefulness of this method can be readily seen in Figure 19-2, which illustrates the sensory findings of a patient with injured median and ulnar nerves. The patient was tested six times during a six-month period until full recovery was imminent.

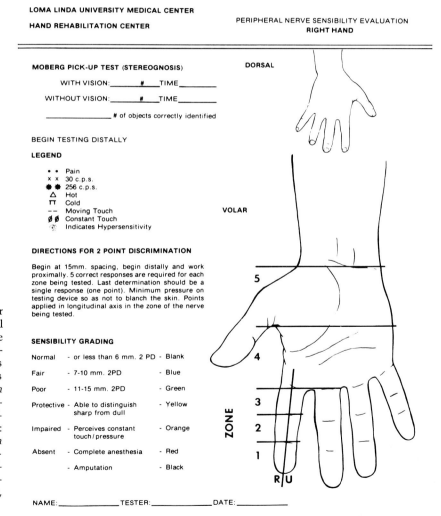

Fig. 19-1. This form for evaluating peripheral nerve sensibility in the right hand is also available for the left. It is discussed in Waylett's *Hand Rehabilitation Center Procedure Manual and Teaching Syllabus.* (Waylett, J. G.: *Hand Rehabilitation Center Procedure Manual and Teaching Syllabus,* 2nd ed., pp. 149–150. Fred Sammons, Brookfield, Il., 1979.)

LOMA LINDA UNIVERSITY MEDICAL CENTER

HAND REHABILITATION CENTER

PERIPHERAL NERVE SENSIBILITY EVALUATION
RIGHT HAND

MOBERG PICK-UP TEST (STEREOGNOSIS)

WITH VISION:_____#____TIME_____

WITHOUT VISION:_____#____TIME_____

_____ # of objects correctly identified

BEGIN TESTING DISTALLY

LEGEND

• •	Pain
x x	30 c.p.s.
✳ ✳	256 c.p.s.
△	Hot
⊓	Cold
– –	Moving Touch
∅ ∅	Constant Touch
⠿	Indicates Hypersensitivity

DIRECTIONS FOR 2 POINT DISCRIMINATION

Begin at 15mm. spacing, begin distally and work proximally. 5 correct responses are required for each zone being tested. Last determination should be a single response (one point). Minimum pressure on testing device so as not to blanch the skin. Points applied in longitudinal axis in the zone of the nerve being tested.

SENSIBILITY GRADING

Normal	- or less than 6 mm. 2 PD	- Blank
Fair	- 7-10 mm. 2PD	- Blue
Poor	- 11-15 mm. 2PD	- Green
Protective	- Able to distinguish sharp from dull	- Yellow
Impaired	- Perceives constant touch/pressure	- Orange
Absent	- Complete anesthesia	- Red
	- Amputation	- Black

DORSAL

VOLAR

ZONE

NAME:_____ TESTER:_____ DATE:_____

Weber's two-point discrimination (2PD) test, which uses two points made from a simple paper clip, has been found to be the most reliable and consistent method of sensibility evaluation that correlates with functional use.[2,8] Moberg has found that 2PD of greater than 10–12 mm does not show tactile gnosis.[8] Two PD of greater than 15 mm on the volar surface of the hand is not significant. If 2PD is greater than 15 mm, but the patient can distinguish the sharp from dull end of a safety pin and has no evidence of injury due to lack of sensation, that is, from ulcerations, burns, or lacerations, we consider him as having protective sensibility from sharp injury. However, he still may not have enough sensation to protect him from injury due to excessive pressure from splints, repetitive stresses of use, or thermal injury from hot packs.

Impaired sensation means that the patient can perceive such stimuli as a pin prick, a light touch, or pressure but is unable to identify the nature of the stimulus. Absent sensation indicates the inability to detect any of the stimuli used.

Functional Testing. We administer the Moberg picking-up test, first with vision and then without. When the patient is prevented from seeing, it is also useful to have him attempt to identify the objects while picking them up.

Such tests as the Purdue pegboard and O'Conner dexterity tests disclose specific functions and are particularly useful in vocational testing to assess the patient's ability to return to work.

Other Methods of Evaluation. Nerve conduction studies and electromyography are useful adjunctive methods for evaluating peripheral nerves for localization of a nerve lesion, determination of the degree of nerve injury, and detection of reinnervation prior to clinical evidence of motor return.[10]

Tinel's sign is of only moderate usefulness in ascertaining lesions or regeneration. The presence of a strong Tinel's sign at the site of a nerve injury or suture and the absence of one distally can indicate little or no regeneration. The presence of a Tinel's sign advancing with time along a nerve trunk does indicate that some nerves are regenerating. However, the strength of Tinel's sign is not quantitative and does not correlate with usefulness of nerve return.[11]

Hand edema can be measured objectively by using the hand volumeter, which is shown in Figure 19-3.

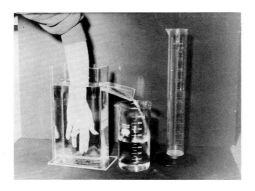

Fig. 19-3. The hand volumeter is adapted from the original design by Dr. Paul Brand of Carville, La. It is accurate to within 1 percent and is available from G. D. Creelman, P.O. Box 146, Idylwild, Calif. 92349.

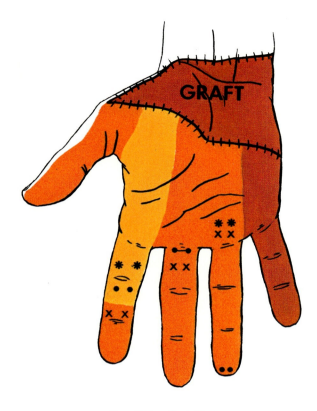

A. 12-2-77

Fig. 19-2. The sensibility of the right hand of a 30-year-old man who caught his right hand in a rolling machine sustaining a crush-avulsion injury to the wrist and palm. He avulsed a distally based flap volarly over the entire width of the palm, beginning at the wrist flexion crease. Both median and ulnar nerves were in anatomical continuity but sustained local crush. There was a complete loss of sensation in the ulnar nerve distribution and a partial loss of median nerve sensation. Because of subsequent skin loss, a split-thickness skin graft was applied to the wrist and proximal palm on November 18, 1978. This graphic color scheme and symbols are interpreted in Figure 19-1. Note that the sensory modalities tested do not always evenly progress distally with time. (A) Complete loss of sensation to little finger and skin graft area is shown. (B) One month later, sensation was protective in all of the hand except the grafted area, and some 2PD was found in the index finger.

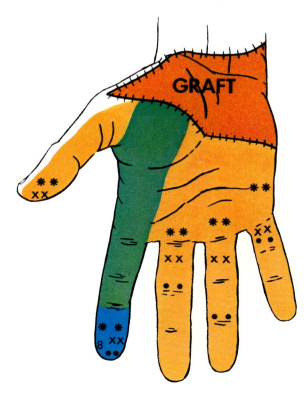

B. 1-3-78

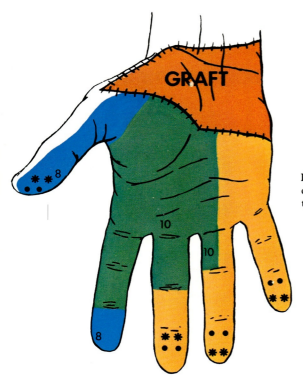

Fig. 19-2 (Continued). (C) 2PD was still impaired in nerve distribution (numbers indicate mm of 2PD). (D) The fingertip's 2PD had returned to normal in median distribution.

C. 1-20-78

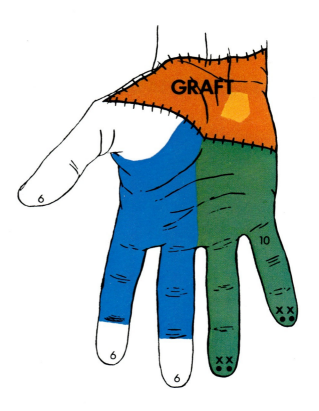

D 2-22-78

Fig. 19-2 (Continued). (E) Some 2PD had returned in ulnar nerve distribution. (F) Normal sensation had returned to almost all of hand. Note that the graft did not have even protective sensation throughout.

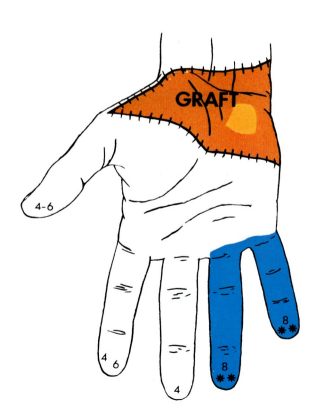

F. 5-23-78

E. 4-3-78

FACTORS ADVERSE TO FUNCTIONAL RECOVERY

Swelling and stiffness are two related problems that adversely affect recovery.

Swelling

Swelling from edema is a natural tissue reaction to trauma. All measures possible should be taken to minimize the tendency for edema because chronic edema fluid is protein-rich, which allows for the formation of collagen in the tissues. Collagen formation in the tissues leads to chronic and perhaps permanent joint contracture.

Elevation of the injured extremity higher than the heart level is used to encourage the downward flow of edema fluid. We use stockinette elevation to an intravenous pole with the elbow flexed 90 degrees when the patient is in bed to maintain the elevation. Tight casts, bandages, or dressings may become constricting and must always be loosened when detected. We do not use ice bags for cooling the upper extremity for three reasons: the ice bag is often not applied to the exact area of the wound; the heaviness of the ice tends to weigh down the hand and decrease elevation; and cooling often does not reach through the many layers of dressing or plaster to be of any benefit.

Slings

For ambulatory patients, we have generally abandoned the use of a sling because a sling encourages the dependency of the arm. We show the patients how to hold their hand high by resting their elbow on the arm of a chair when sitting with the forearm vertical or by resting their forearm on top of the head.

A sling also tends to make the patient feel complacent and lets him forget the importance of his own involvement in the rehabilitation process. Slings discourage the use of the upper extremity, thus encouraging muscle atrophy and edema. Patients should be encouraged to use the extremity even in the cast or dressing within limits that will not do further damage to the tissues or retard healing. A sling can also lead to joint stiffness from lack of use.

The doctor who applies the postoperative dressing or splint must apply it so that only the necessary joints are immobilized. It is disastrous for a patient to develop a frozen shoulder while immobilized for a median nerve laceration at the wrist because the extremity was placed in a sling and he was never told to move the shoulder until after the stiffness had developed.

Postoperative Splints

The nerve repair site must be protected for a minimum of three weeks postoperatively in a tension-free anastamosis. It must be protected up to six weeks if any tension has been used. However, extreme positioning of the joints, that is, greater than 30 to 40 degrees wrist flexion or greater than 90 degrees knee or elbow flexion, should be avoided to minimize the tendency to joint stiffness. If these extreme positions are necessary to close a nerve gap, interfascicular grafts should be used instead of direct repair.

Unnecessary joint immobilization will contribute to extra stiffness. For example, in a primary repair of an isolated, clean, median or ulnar nerve laceration at the wrist in an adult, we immobilize the wrist in nothing but a short arm cast at 30 degrees flexion because this relatively simple intervention will adequately relieve any nerve tension. The interphalangeal joints of the fingers have the greatest tendency to stiffness when immobilized in flexion, whereas the metacarpophalangeal joints tend to get stiffest in extension. Therefore after digital nerve repair, we flex the metacarpophalangeal joints to 60–80 degrees and then flex the interphalangeal joints in the least amount necessary to eliminate tension at the nerve anastamosis. Since 10–30 degrees proximal interphalangeal joint flexion is often all that is necessary, there will be less tendency to postoperative joint stiffness.

PATIENT EDUCATION

Early education of the patient about his role as an active participant in the rehabilitation process is essential to dispel the notion that somehow the physician and therapist will work magic to make his injured extremity as functional as before. It should be instilled in the patient from the onset to use the extremity whenever possible within the limits of disability. Before the patient is discharged, the physician should explain how to look for excessive edema and how to counteract it by constant elevation and active movement of the extremity as much as possible. The patient should know to seek attention and call if inordinate pain or a fever develops, or if the postoperative cast or dressing loosens or breaks.

The patient should be warned that since the protective mechanism of pain is lost, any anesthetic area is prone to injury and may actually be a liability to the patient until sensation is restored. He should be taught to recognize where the anesthetic area is located at all times. He should be particularly careful around any machinery, moving objects, or tools so as not to injure the hand. Because burns can easily occur, patients must be careful when cooking or checking water temperature and smokers should not use the anesthetic area to hold cigarettes. Patients with peroneal or sciatic nerve injury must always protect the anesthetic sole of their foot with a shoe. The anesthetic part is more prone to pressure sores from splints, so the patient should be taught to look for redness or blebs under splints or casts. Having the patient soak the dry and anesthetic part in water three times daily for 20 minutes and then oil with petrolatum will help eliminate dryness and cracking of the skin.

DESENSITIZATION

Hypersensitivity or hyperalgesia of the skin is a common corollary of nerve regeneration. It is possibly due to the increased sensitivities of immature nerve endings and sensory end organs to stimulation. The tendency of the patient is to avoid using the hypersensitive area because the stimuli are interpreted as being noxious. However, not using a part creates a habit of nonfunction as well as doing nothing to overcome the hypersensitivity. Contrary to what might seem rational, repeated stimulation is used to overcome the dysesthesia problem. Until the area is desensitized, it may be impossible to proceed with other modalities of therapy, such as splinting, sensory re-education, strengthening, and functional activities.

The desensitization program is really a two-part educational process. First the patient is told that the overreaction tendency is a natural phenomenon that occurs while the nerves are regrowing and that it will tend to lessen with time as the nerve endings mature. This knowledge will tend to calm the fears of the patient and thwart the development of a full-blown sympathetic dystrophy. Next, a gradually increasing gradient of stimulation is applied to the hypersensitive part. The patient should begin with non-irritating media and, as the area becomes desensitized, progress to different sorts of tactile stimulation. The desensitization program used at the Loma Linda University Hand Rehabilitation Center is outlined,[16] and the modalities listed can be used singularly or in combination.

> Whirlpool: 15 to 30 minutes. At low speed, this therapy can be used as the first stage of desensitization. It can be increased to high as the patient begins to tolerate the water turbulence.
> Massage: 10 minutes. Circular massage with lotion. With edema, elevate the extremity and "milk" in a downward direction. Concentrate the massage in the area of sensitivity.
> Textures: 10 to 30 minutes. Gradually the patient becomes able to tolerate the more irritating sources of tactile stimulation. Begin by rubbing the area on skin dowels covered with different media, such as fur, felt, and silk. Then have the patient roll, feel, and grasp such textures as pellets, bins of sand, Styrofoam, buckshot, rice, and macaroni (Fig. 19-4). Thera-plast is also a good medium for desensitization.

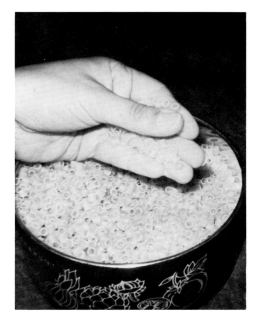

Fig. 19-4. This patient is manipulating dry macaroni shells as part of the desensitization program.

Vibration: Build up the patient's tolerance by increasing desensitization time. A hand vibrator is also available for a home program.
Percussion: Perform to tolerance, gradually increasing the time. Functional repetitive activity, such as hammering, is helpful, as is tapping over the area with a pencil or finger by the patient or therapist. Progress to heavier stimulation as tolerated.

SENSORY RE-EDUCATION

Few adults ever regain normal sensibility[5] or even close to normal sensibility following repair of peripheral nerves, especially the median or ulnar nerve. This failure may not only be due to incomplete and misdirected axon regrowth, but also to failure of the cerebral cortex to interpret correctly the altered profile of afferent impulses that come from the regenerated axons and sensory end organs. Accordingly, improved sensibility should result from a conscious effort of re-educating the brain to learn appropriate responses to the new stimulus patterns.[5] Wynn-Parry and Salter[19] advocate sensory education through sensory exercises using various objects that are placed in the injured hand of the patient who has been blindfolded. The program is begun by teaching the patient to identify various wooden blocks of different sizes and shapes. Teaching recognition of various textures is then begun, followed by familiar objects of daily life, such as safety pins, can openers, pencils, soap, and keys.

Dellon et al.[5] have developed a program of specific exercises to re-educate the perception of slowly and quickly adapting sensory fibers. (The slowly adapting fibers are those that respond to constant touch or pressure and are measured by 2PD. Fibers that adapt more quickly respond to moving touch.) It is important that the hand be desensitized before beginning sensory re-education.

Early Phase Exercises

Once the patient has developed some perception of constant touch or moving touch proximally in the hand, re-educating the slowly adapting fibers is done by touching the finger with a pencil eraser or other blunt object at varying pressures, first with and then without vision. The fast-adapting fibers are re-educated by repeatedly moving a blunt object across the sensorily deprived area, with or without vision.

Late Phase Exercises

Once the patient has the perception of constant and moving touch in the fingertips, exercises with variously shaped objects, especially coins, nuts, bolts, and familiar blunt objects, are used whether the patient is or is not blindfolded. The patient tries to discriminate among various objects by size, shape, weight, texture, and material. It is more meaningful for the patient to be subjected to objects in his sensory re-education program that he will use in his occupation or avocation.

Therapy should take place in a specific quiet place. The patient is introduced to the sensory re-education program by the therapist in 10–15 minute sessions. Once the patient understands the program, he will proceed on his own during several (three to five) sessions daily.

With this program, Dellon and associates[5] have found that measurably improved sensation occurs as early as four to five days after its initiation. They also found some long-standing nerve-injured cases who originally had no 2PD but who became functionally normal after two to six weeks of following a sensory re-education program.

MUSCLE TRAINING

Because muscle atrophy is a biological effect of denervation, it has seemed attractive to attempt to retard muscle atrophy by galvanic stimulation of the muscle. However, since there is little effect unless electrical stimulation remains almost constant, this modality has been abandoned as impractical.[18]

A muscle cannot be retrained until it shows some voluntary contraction. It is important to know the expected order of reinnervation following a nerve lesion. Standard methods of muscle strengthening are used once reinnervation has been detected. Progressive resistance exercises are given in the later stages. One versatile device for strengthening is the weight-well, shown in Figure 19-5A. Functional activities rather than routine boring exercises keep the patient's attention and interest (Fig. 19-5B).

Biofeedback has been successfully used as an adjunctive method for training reinnervated muscles. A hand-held box has been developed that will pick up an electromyographic signal from a muscle through a small surface electrode. Both

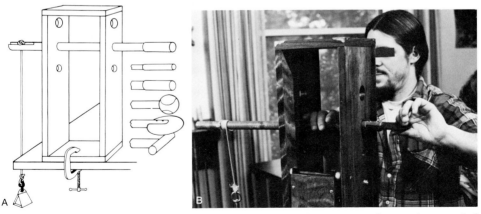

Fig. 19.5. (A) The weight-well is a wooden dowel placed through an open wooden stand. One end of the rod has a rope to which various weights can be attached. The handle on the other end of the rod is turned to wind up the rope and lift the weight and can be made to various sizes and shapes so that strengthening grasp, pinch, pronators, supinators, wrist flexors, or extensors can be emphasized. The weight-well was designed by Lois Barber of the Downey Community Hospital Hand Rehabilitation Center, Downey, Calif. (B) This patient is using the weight-well to strengthen the pinch of his left hand.

audio and visual signals are triggered when the threshold is exceeded. As more motor units become reinnervated, the threshold can be varied so that the device can train a patient to activate the muscle to a pre-set level. Conversely, the patient may need to inhibit an antagonist during certain actions. Biofeedback is not magic, nor is it a substitute for good physical and occupational therapy. It is, however, of practical assistance to patients who need an instant revelation of muscle action in learning to use muscles in the early stages of reinnervation.[1] It is simple and relatively easy to use and can speed voluntary control of reinnervated muscles.

SPLINTING PERIPHERAL NERVE INJURIES

Splints are very useful in peripheral nerve injuries but the purpose of each splint must be carefully thought out. Often nerve injuries occur in combination with tendon, vascular, and skeletal damage, so a splint may have to function in service of more than one isolated tissue injury.

There are three purposes for splinting peripheral nerve injuries:

> To prevent deformity. This may be done by providing an external power, such as a rubber band, to take the place of the paralyzed muscle until its function returns.
> To correct deformity. If joint or musculotendenous contractures have developed, dynamic splinting may be useful to stretch them out.
> To assist in function. By providing a force that is lost during muscle paralysis, dynamic splints may allow the patient to return to work before muscle reinnervation has begun.

Splints must be customized to fit each individual patient. A patient will not wear an uncomfortable splint. The patient must understand the purpose of the splint, how to apply it properly, and when and how long to wear it. He must be taught to look for pressure areas being made by the splint, particularly if it has been applied to an anesthetic area. All patients with identical nerve injury do not need the same splint. Indeed, some patients do not need a splint at all. It thus takes some cerebration on the part of the surgeon and therapist to identify clearly what purpose each splint will serve. Some patients with isolated, low ulnar nerve palsy will have little tendency to claw deformity and thus will not need a splint. It may only be necessary to teach the patient how to keep the joints passively supple. Some patients will need a splint to correct clawing in three fingers instead of just the usual ulnar two fingers. Many patients with low median nerve palsy do not need an opposition splint because the abductor pollicis brevis or opponens pollicis may receive enough innervation from the ulnar nerve to function satisfactorily.[13] Some patients have little opposition function, yet they are able to do everything they want to do with their hands. As long as they understand and practice keeping the first web space from developing an adduction contracture, a splint is unnecessary. Splint requirements change with time. It is poor patient care to make a splint, by definition, a temporary device, and not follow the patient to oversee its continued appropriateness, comfort, fit, and wear.

EARLY TENDON TRANSFERS

Early tendon transfer as an internal splint to allow earlier brace-free function should have a place in the care of the nerve-injured patient.[14] The following advantages are cited:

> It permits greater function of the nerve-injured extremity and perhaps more opportunity for spontaneous sensory re-education.
> It allows the patient to become brace-free sooner and is thus more convenient.
> It augments the eventual strength of the reinnervated muscles, which, following nerve repair in an adult, are not expected to regain their previous strength.
> It is particularly useful when eventual good recovery following neurorrhaphy is not expected, as for example, an opponensplasty performed early after a median nerve laceration repaired proximal to the elbow in which no thumb opposition recovery would be expected.
> It rebalances the hand earlier, thus lessening the potential for the development of contractures.

Early transfers are best performed within three months of nerve injury. We usually combine the tendon transfer with secondary neurorrhaphy to avoid an extra operation. The transferred muscle should be synergistic in order that little postoperative muscle training be necessary. The patient must be able to understand the nature of the transfer. The function of transferred muscle must be spared safely. Transfers for specific nerve loss are discussed as follows.

High Radial Nerve Palsy

The pronator teres transfer to the extensor carpi radialis brevis is an easily learned and useful transfer to correct the wrist drop deformity. Most patients can become brace-free through this transfer alone while they are awaiting return of finger and thumb extensor function. The pronation function of the muscle transfer is still maintained.

Median Nerve Palsy

In patients disabled by loss of the opposition function, early routine transfer of the flexor digitorum superficialis of the ring finger, palmaris longus, or extensor indicis proprius has been used.

Low Ulnar Nerve Palsy

The power grip can be restored early and the claw deformity eliminated by a transfer of the extensor carpi radialis extended by a graft through the dorsum of the hand's intermetacarpal space and lumbrical canal into the proximal phalanx. This operation creates a force that can flex the metacarpophalangeal joint. According to Burkhalter,[3] this transfer gives a greater increase in strength than transfer of the flexor digitorum superficialis of the ring finger.

RECONSTRUCTIVE SURGERY

Restoration of function following peripheral nerve injuries may be aided considerably by reconstructive surgery. An accurate and tension-free repair of the severed nerve is considered essential to aid the return of nerve function. Since many peripheral nerve injuries are not isolated injuries to the nerve, other tissue damage must be evaluated and considered in establishing the comprehensive rehabilitation program that may include reconstructive surgery.

Prior to nerve surgery, obtaining adequate skin coverage may be necessary to allow adequate joint motion and bring good nutrition to the injured area. Ensuring coverage may include grafting composite tissue flaps from the groin or elsewhere. It is necessary to have stable, united fractures and muscle and tendon damage may need to be corrected. Therapy to overcome joint stiffness may be required.

The goal of reconstructive surgery for nerve loss must be carefully thought out. Is it restoration of sensation or motor control or the elimination of neuroma hypersensitivity?

Neuromas

Painful and troublesome neuromas not responding to desensitization procedures cannot be desensitized. Removal of the neuroma and burying the end of the nerve deep in the tissues, where it is less likely to become irritated, will usually be successful.[13]

Sensory Loss

If adequate sensation has not returned to the denervated area, consideration of exploration and anastomosis of the nerve may be undertaken, depending on the nature, extent, and location of the nerve injury, the time elapsed since nerve injury or surgical repair, the age, profession, and desires of the patient, and the ability and experience of the surgeon.

If adequate sensibility in the median nerve distribution is not present, especially in the thumb and index finger, transfer of a neurovascular island's pedicle flap from an area with good sensation can be considered. Donor areas to cover a thumb without sensation include flaps from the ulnar side of the ring or middle finger. Taking a flap from the adjacent sides of the ring and little finger to cover the adjacent sides of the thumb and index finger also has merit.[13]

Muscle Paralysis

Irreversible motor paralysis may be overcome by redistributing the power from residual unparalyzed muscles. Tendon transfers have been worked out for all nerve injuries, and standard texts should be consulted for detailed information.[13] The prerequisites for tendon transfers are: the transferred muscle must be strong enough (grade fair [3] or greater strength),[4] it should have adequate excursion, a good gliding surface with minimal scar, and no sharp change in direction of pull. The muscle should be expendable and have adequate (or preferably normal) joint range. If these sound principles are adhered to closely, tendon transfers will give very satisfying results.

ACKNOWLEDGMENTS

The author thanks Ms. Janet Waylett, Supervising Therapist, Hand Rehabilitation Center, Loma Linda University, for her suggestions and assistance in preparing of the manuscript and Ms. Sharon Barnes for typing it.

REFERENCES

1. Basmajian, J. V.: Biofeedback. In Hunter, J. M., Schneider, L. M., Mackin, E. J., and Bell, J. A., Eds.: *Rehabilitation of the Hand,* pp. 523–525. C. V. Mosby, St. Louis, 1978.
2. Bell, J. A.: Sensibility evaluation. In Hunter, J. M., Schneider, L. M., Mackin, E. J., and Bell, J. A., Eds.: *Rehabilitation of the Hand,* pp. 273–291. C. V. Mosby, St. Louis, 1978.
3. Burkhalter, W. E.: Early tendon transfer in upper extremity peripheral nerve injury. Clin. Orthop. 104:68–79, 1974.
4. Daniels, L., Williams, M., and Worthingham, C.: *Muscle Testing,* pp. 3–4. W. B. Saunders, Philadelphia, 1956.
5. Dellon, A. L., Curtis, R. M., and Edgerton, M. T.: Reeducation of sensation in the hand after nerve injury and repair. Plast. Reconstr. Surg. 53:297–305, 1974.
6. Levin, S., Pearsall, G., and Ruderman, R. J.: Von Frey's method of measuring pressure sensibility in the hand: An engineering analysis of the Weinstein-Semmes pressure aesthesiometer. J. Hand. Surg. 3:211–216, 1978.
7. Moberg, E.: Criticism and study of methods for examining sensibility in the hand. Neurology 12:8–19, 1962.
8. Moberg, E.: Methods for examining sensibility in the hand. In Flynn, J. E., Ed.: *Hand Surgery,* pp. 295–304. Williams & Wilkins, Baltimore, 1975.
9. National Center of Health Statistics: Unpublished data.
10. Omer, G. E.: Assessment of peripheral nerve injuries. In *Symposium on the Hand,* vol. 3, pp. 1–11. C. V. Mosby, St. Louis, 1971.
11. Seddon, H.: *Surgical Disorders of the Peripheral Nerves,* pp. 36–54. Williams & Wilkins, Baltimore, 1972.
12. Semmes, J.: *Somatosensory Changes After Penetrating Brain Wounds in Man.* Harvard University Press, Cambridge, 1960.
13. Smith, J. R., and Graham, W. P.: Nerves. In Kilgore, E. S., and Graham, W. P., Eds.: *The Hand: Surgical and Non-surgical Management,* pp. 213–234. Lea & Febiger, Philadelphia, 1977.
14. Sunderland, S.: *Nerves and Nerve Injuries,* pp. 377–396. Churchill Livingstone, Edinburgh, 1968.
15. Von Prince, K., and Butler, B.: Measuring sensory function of the hand in peripheral nerve injuries. Am. J. Occup. Ther. 21:385–395, 1967.
16. Waylett, J. G.: *Hand Rehabilitation Center Procedure Manual and Teaching Syllabus,* 2nd ed., pp. 149–150. Fred Sammons, Brookfield, Il., 1979.
17. Werner, J. L., and Omer, G. E.: Evaluating cutaneous pressure sensation of the hand. Am. J. Occup. Ther. 23:345–355, 1970.
18. Wynn-Parry, C. B.: *Rehabilitation of the Hand,* 3rd ed., pp. 83–106. Butterworth, London, 1973.
19. Wynn-Parry, C. B., and Salter, M.: Sensory reeducation after median nerve lesions. Hand 8:250–257, 1976.

20

Brachial Plexus Injuries

Richard M. Braun, M.D.

Brachial plexus injuries involve the spinal roots, trunk, cords, and nerve elements, which all form a complex system of innervation of the upper limb. These brachial plexus elements emanate from the fifth cervical level and continue through the first thoracic root. They are responsible for all motor function and sensibility in the arm, forearm, and hand.

Brachial plexus palsy in adults originates from a full spectrum of injuries. The vast majority of the patients seen have a history of high-speed motorcycle or car accidents with occasional injuries caused by industrial trauma, direct penetrating injuries, and falls from substantial heights. Iatrogenic injuries from surgery or radiation therapy are rare. Special consideration is given to birth injuries in the department of pediatric orthopedics. Injuries associated with brachial plexus palsies may include head trauma with associated upper motor neuron disease, cervical spinal cord injuries, spinal and extremity fractures, burns or areas of skin loss, and frequent instances of combined neurological and vascular injury. The importance of these associated injuries cannot be overestimated in discussing rehabilitation planning. It is common for the entire effort of the acute-care facility and personnel to be oriented toward the patient's survival or restoration of limb viability, only to ignore areas of potential function that will be essential to the long-range rehabilitation of the patient. We have seen patients arrive after three months of excellent, intensive, acute care; nevertheless, they have joint contractures, limb edema, poorly united fractures, open wounds or pressure sores, and even unstable cervical spine injuries. The early evaluation of the entire problem is essential in the care of these complex injuries, but this is not always possible when a rehabilitation program begins only after an acute-care program is completed. Rehabilitation must begin *early* for optimal results to be attained in a seriously injured patient who will usually have significant residual physical impairment despite any treatment program now available. Two typical examples will illustrate this situation.

Case A, an adolescent boy, sustained a transection of his brachial plexus while skateboarding through a glass door. He was seen by an orthopedic surgeon in a nearby hospital emergency room. The patient was in deep shock because the axillary vessels were severed. Resuscitation with 4 liters of lactated Ringer's solution, emergency vessel ligation, packed cell transfusion, and antibiotic prophylaxis were started immediately. A vascular surgeon was called. The patient was ready for a general anesthetic within an hour and a repair of the artery and vein was performed successfully. Another surgeon was called to repair the brachial plexus. All the major nerve divisions were repaired in optimal fashion with the aid of optical magnification (Fig. 20-1) and modern suture technique. The wound was closed over suction drains and primary uncomplicated healing occurred. The patient's mother noted major swelling in the forearm three days after surgery; however, the patient had no pain and the vascular surgeon assured the mother that the radial pulse was of excellent quality. The surgeon who had repaired the nerves did not see the patient at that time, because the results of nerve repair would require months or even years of follow-up. The orthopedic

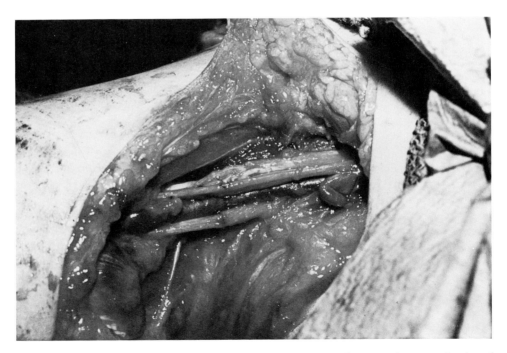

Fig. 20-1. A transection of the brachial plexus has been operatively repaired. Reconstitution of the brachial artery and vein as well as the major peripheral nerves is seen at the level of the axilla in a patient who sustained injury while skateboarding through a glass door.

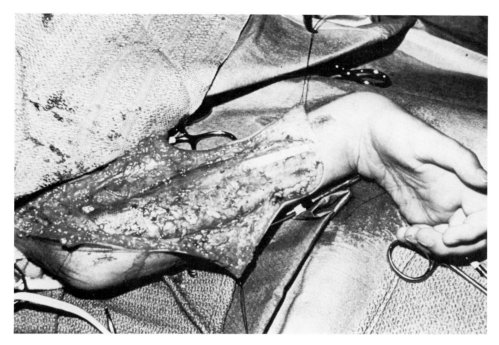

Fig. 20-2. A Volkmann's contracture with ischemic muscle in the volar compartment of the forearm is seen eight weeks after the initial injury noted in Figure 20-1. The patient had lost protective sensibility and was unable to complain of pain because of the nerve severance in his axilla. Necrotic muscle is noted in the forearm; it is associated with contracture in the wrist and fingers.

surgeon who saw the boy initially also reassured the parent that the patient would be started on a rehabilitation program as soon as possible.

The patient was seen "for splinting and rehabilitation" about eight weeks after the accident. He had been discharged by the vascular surgeon as a successful major vessel repair. A photograph of the forearm and hand is presented (Fig. 20-2) to illustrate the Volkmann's contracture the patient sustained. He had no complaint of pain because his nerve injury had destroyed his protective sensibility. His forearm and hand were completely anesthetic. Ischemic fibrosis and contracture of muscle had already resulted in a wrist flexion contracture and compensatory contractures in the fingers in the pernicious claw position. The limb was edematous and the joints were stiff. The rehabilitation program required total limb evaluation, surgery, dynamic and static splinting, elevation with intermittent compression splinting to reduce edema,[3] and an education program for appropriate instruction in this schedule for the patient and parent as well as instruction for one-handed activities. Tendon transfer surgery and therapy were later required to restore grasp function.

The patient's life had been saved but his rehabilitation was delayed for months by acute-phase factors that increased his final functional deficits.

Case B, a middle-aged, healthy, oil field worker, caught his hand in a drilling rig. His arm was pulled upward with great violence. Examination in the emergency room showed that the patient was in deep shock. A large hematoma was present in the periclavicular area, the hand was partially degloved, and the humerus had a displaced fracture of the midshaft. Resuscitation commenced with fluid replacement and a skilled vascular team performed an emergency subclavian-to-brachial artery graft.

The patient was seen two months later for rehabilitation. Initial examination at the Rancho Los Amigos Hospital was performed in conjunction with a distinguished visiting professor of orthopedic upper limb surgery who had more than four decades of experience with trauma of this type. His comment was appropriate: "It's too bad that so much has been done to save so little." The patient had a cool but viable limb with a barely palpable radial pulse. The limb was anesthetic, completely paralyzed, painful, swollen, with open hand wounds, and a displaced, angulated, ununited fracture of the humerus. Amputation through the humerus fracture site was advised with difficulty—the patient had already tolerated two months of pointless heroics. A postoperative program was designed to restore lost shoulder motion and begin prosthetic training.

In ideal cases, an appropriate diagnosis and a reasonable prognosis can be made at an early stage and the rehabilitation effort can begin as soon as possible. If the diagnosis is in doubt, or if the condition is changing, the program should be designed to anticipate these changes and assist recovery in every possible way.

An exact diagnosis of brachial plexus injury is often difficult to make when the patient is first seen. The usual mechanism of injury is a stretching type of trauma that injures the complex nerve cables in an irregular manner so that a distinct single level is often not seen. A complete transection may be present in some nerve fibers, whereas in another area of the same nerve or feeding tributary, there is only a neurapraxia due to a mild stretching force. The area of mild or moderate stretching will recover if further injury is prevented. The area of complete transection will not recover unless nerve ends are approximated by chance or by an operation. The reader is referred to descriptions of the technology of brachial plexus nerve repair and the relative indications for surgery.[4–6] The general areas of injury, however, do play an important role in the rehabilitation program and should be familiar to all physicians treating these patients. Injuries to the cephalad routes of C5 and C6 (+ C7), which spare the distal routes of C8 and T1, result in loss of shoulder and elbow control. Some of these cases may also lose portions of limb extension control in areas supplied by the radial nerve. Flexion and pronation of the forearm and hand as well as intrinsic hand muscles remain intact. Injuries to lower routes of (± C7) C8 and T1 result in preservation of shoulder and elbow flexion but loss of forearm and hand flexion, as well as loss of intrinsic muscle function. Loss of sensibility usually follows a familiar pattern, with C5 and C6 representing the thumb and index fingers, C7 the long finger, and C8 and T1 the ulnar fingers and forearm. An injury to the entire plexus results in an entirely anesthetic and paralyzed limb. However, an injury that appears complete at an early stage may show some spontaneous return of function at a later time. Factors with a poor prognosis for recovery include fractures of the cervical spine in the area of the cord, foramen, root egress area, or transverse processes. A Horner's sign (Fig. 20-3) or obvious atrophy in the thoracoscapular muscles or paralysis of the diaphragm also carry a poor prognosis, because they are the hallmarks of a proximal injury that cannot spontaneously improve. In our experience at Rancho

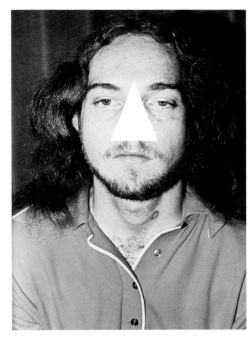

Fig. 20-3. A Horner's sign is demonstrated with ptosis of the eyelid, constriction of the pupil, and dryness of the face. A circle marked on the patient's neck indicates the approximate level of the stellate ganglion, which lies adjacent to the vertebral bodies. This sign carries a poor prognosis when associated with brachial plexus injury, because it defines a proximal nerve lesion in the region of the spinal cord and nerve root egress area.

Los Amigos Hospital, a functional diagnosis is quite adequate for rehabilitation purposes. Exact nerve testing may not be required for the patient's basic evaluation and treatment program.

The initial history of injury and primary treatment is obtained by the occupational therapist, who can easily learn the technical aspects of taking a basic and accurate medical history. The therapist then performs a sensory and muscle examination of the upper limb and records the findings on the chart along with the elapsed time since the initial injury. The therapist also palpates the area for the presence of point tenderness or a Tinel's sign and records other findings that may be significant, such as a Horner's sign indicating a stellate ganglion-level injury or the presence of severe pain in the limb, shoulder, or neck. The relationship between counterbalancing or elevating the arm and change in the pain pattern is noted, along with the presence of contracture in the joints, and skin condition. A well-motivated therapist can gain enough experience in this work to take a history, perform a regional physical examination, and make a major contribution to the rehabilitation plan for the patient.

The physician may augment this evaluation with his own. After discussion with the therapist, he may elect to request a myelogram or electromyogram. These tests do not replace the basic examination; rather, they may add an important depth of information. The presence of a meningocele seen on the cervical myelogram (Fig. 20-4) does not absolutely prove an irreparable nerve avulsion, because dural sleeve tears occasionally spare nerve elements, yet the presence of two or more meningoceles carries a very poor prognosis in combination with a history of major trauma and any findings of marked paralysis in the arm. Fasciculations on electromyograms may indicate areas of complete denerva-

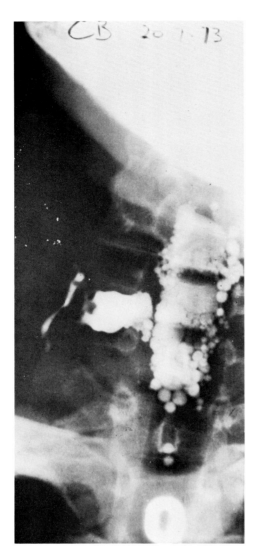

Fig. 20-4. A cervical myelogram demonstrates the presence of a large meningocele in the cervical area by the dye tracking into the region of a root avulsion. This usually carries a grim prognosis for irreparable nerve injury, but it does not always mean that the nerve root in this area has sustained avulsion.

tion. Sometimes electromyographic evidence may point out early electrical recovery that may even precede clinical evidence of returning muscle function. In these cases, continued splinting and exercises for preservation of joint range of motion plus the rest of the rehabilitation program must be continued under proper professional supervision.

REHABILITATION PLANNING

The basis of all rehabilitation is to allow the patient to attain maximal function with his residual permanent impairment. We attempt to minimize the effects of the injury and maximize the function remaining in the injured area and the untapped potential function in the remaining areas of normality. Neither of these objectives can be reached if the patient has a problem with residual pain in the area of injury. A painful limb will not be used or exercised. Contractures of joints and muscles compound the problem. Medications are frequently abused or overused. Vocational training and functional use of the injured limb are rarely accomplished. Psychological regression, dependence, and depression appear, and all chance for rehabilitation is dissolved in a sea of pills and pity.

We use four methods for dealing with the persistent pain problems seen in about 25 percent of our patients with brachial plexus injury. Three of these methods have given good results on occasion and may be used in conjunction with each other. The fourth, the use of analgesic medication, is considered a necessary evil to be avoided whenever possible. When drugs are given, it is only in moderation. Medication has never removed pain in a completely satisfactory manner in any patient we have treated. The long-term use of any narcotics or similar medication is obviously to be avoided.

Pain can occasionally be controlled by correct splinting. Splinting seems to work because it removes the traction effect of a paralyzed limb, which weighs about 9 kg and hangs without functional muscle counterbalance on the stretched nerves of the brachial plexus. This weight distracts those affected nerves that have already been stretched to the point of injury, which naturally results in pain. Several patients have gained early, satisfactory, and apparently permanent pain relief when the weight of the arm has been transferred directly onto the pelvis with our mobile forearm support splint with pelvic brim purchase (Figs. 20-5–20-8). This device may be rapidly fabricated to allow the weight of the arm to be transferred away from the shoulder-plexus-neck area and permit direct loading of the weight onto the pelvic brim.[8]

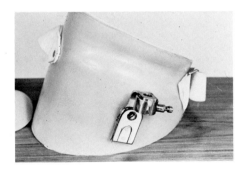

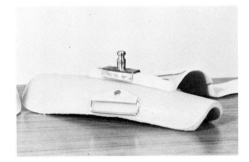

Fig. 20-5. A molded plastic pelvic support is used to transfer the weight of the arm directly onto the pelvis. Fabrication of this orthotic device is simple and relatively inexpensive. The contour of the pelvic portion allows for weight-bearing transfer onto the iliac crest.

Fig. 20-6. The forearm support of the orthotic device is seen in the inverted position. The metal peg fits into the socket on the pelvic portion. The forearm rests in the trough, as seen in Figure 20-7. The metal pin is adjusted along the length of the trough to provide for appropriate balance in the forearm. Most patients prefer this pin in the center of the forearm to allow for elevation of the hand and wrist by depression of the elbow and shoulder. This position is adjustable.

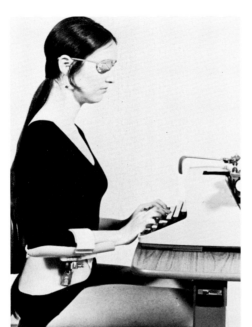

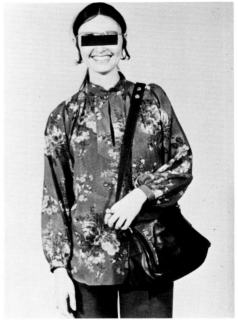

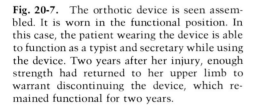

Fig. 20-7. The orthotic device is seen assembled. It is worn in the functional position. In this case, the patient wearing the device is able to function as a typist and secretary while using the device. Two years after her injury, enough strength had returned to her upper limb to warrant discontinuing the device, which remained functional for two years.

Fig. 20-8. The orthotic device is cosmetically concealed by the use of a slit in the patient's blouse. The metal prong protrudes through the slit. Another small slit in the undersurface of the sleeve allows for coupling to the forearm trough support. The fact that an orthotic device is used to support the injured limb is not readily revealed. This improves the probability that the device will be worn at work or in social situations. In the case shown, an ocular prosthesis was later applied to improve the appearance of this woman even further.

This principle is one traditionally used by hikers to carry heavy loads without transferring the weight of the pack to their shoulders, secured to the skeleton only by the thin strut of the clavicle and the thoracic muscles. If the shoulder straps sag, the hiker may experience brachial plexus injury as the clavicle is forced down onto the first rib by the weight of the pack. Relief of pain has been seen in several of these patients within days of splint fitting. The pelvic girdle of molded plastic has been used for back-pack type support if heavy loads are carried (Fig. 20-9). It can be modified easily to allow the patient both a back-pack and a forearm support splint. In most cases we attempt to fit the patient with this type of support shortly after injury; however, in one case a patient was fitted with the device two years after the date of injury. His pain subsided within a month and although his injured arm remained completely flail, his pain relief was extremely satisfying to both the patient and the members of the rehabilitation team, who are now able to teach him one-handed activities, retrain him for gainful employment, and gradu-

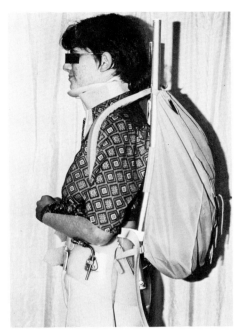

Fig. 20-9. This patient sustained a cervical and brachial plexus injury. Appropriate surgery stabilized the patient's neck. Spontaneous recovery was anticipated in the brachial plexus if further traction on the arm were avoided. She wished to attend college. An orthotic device was fabricated, allowing her to take all of the weight of her injured arm and transfer it to the pelvis through the mobile arm support. Her college books were placed in the backpack and were carried across campus without any transfer of weight onto the cervical spine, the clavicle, or the upper limb. The patient experienced no discomfort in her arm while carrying weights of up to 30 pounds and she was able to continue attending college while she recovered motor power in her arm spontaneously.

ally wean him from the pointless medications that impaired his level of awareness. This orthotic device is now routinely used on brachial plexus palsy patients who present with a painful upper limb following trauma or other injuries that have led to a neuritis in the brachial plexus.

Surgery may be effective in some problematic cases requiring pain control. Our operative procedures have included those for extraneural decompression, intraneural decompression, and sensory ablation. The decompression procedures may be quite effective in those cases with partial injury from such causes as impingement between the clavicle and the first rib[2] or compartment syndromes in the upper arm in the arterial sheath area of the brachial plexus.[1] Orthopedic surgical evaluation should be obtained in brachial plexus injuries to rule out possibilities that may yield to surgical intervention in the arm, the thoracic outlet, or even in the area of the cervical spine. It is common for cervical disc disease to commence with the same injury that directly injures the plexus. An acute, soft disc rupture proximal to the area of plexus injury may produce severe pain yet not result in diagnostic unilateral reflex loss or motor deprivation because the effect of more distal peripheral nerve injuries is masked. Special cervical x-rays may show reduced cervical motion, narrowed disc spaces, arthrosis, or fracture in the area of injury. Myelography or computerized axial tomography scanning may define a disc or cord lesion amenable to surgery. Intraneural neurolysis may be effective in pain management. Multiple branching within proximal nerve elements makes this procedure complex and not without risks. Nevertheless, a patient with a persistent, exquisitely tender mass in the neck who has not shown improvement over a period of several months may deserve exploration, internal neurolysis, and removal of scar and epineurium. The scarring will certainly recur, but it is rea-

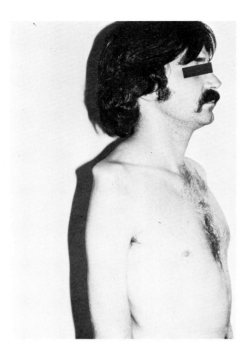

Fig. 20-10. This patient sustained a complete brachial plexus avulsion injury. Exploration of the plexus in the cervical area indicated an irreparable situation. The patient became addicted to narcotic medications because of his constant complaint of severe pain. His educational level and rehabilitation potential were good and it was elected to perform cervical laminectomy for coagulation of the dorsal root entry zone in the cervical area. The patient achieved virtually complete pain relief, discontinued medication, and has been restored to a useful life as a one-handed individual.

sonable to assume the scalpel is more gentle than the original stretching injury and diminished pain has been reported by several patients who have undergone this procedure. Good operative technique requires the knowledge of difficult anatomy, delicate microsurgical instruments, excellent illumination, and some type of suitable optical magnification.

Neurosurgical procedures designed to control pain, such as sensory rhizotomy and cordotomy, have usually been disappointing. However these procedures on the cord itself can be helpful in some carefully selected cases (Fig. 20-10). A neurosurgical consultant who is interested in this type of work is a valuable asset in such cases. Encouraging early postoperative results have been seen recently in patients with intractable pain from root avulsion injury. A surgical procedure using a controlled radio frequency to coagulate areas of the dorsal root entry zone has been described by Nashold and Ostdahl.[7] The procedure has been extremely helpful to several of our patients who received no significant benefit from stellate ganglion block, transcutaneous stimulation, narcotic medications, appropriate splinting, or a behavior modification program. Patient selection is not easy. The operations are difficult and carry substantial risk, which the patient must understand.

It is frequently necessary to have the patient with a painful brachial plexus injury seen in a "pain clinic." These clinics use behavior modification in assisting the affected patient to cope with pain. The risk in the use of these clinics is twofold. The referring physician may send a patient to the clinic simply because the patient has pain, takes excessive medication, and is difficult to deal with. The risk is that an area of potential intervention may have been missed because a thorough evaluation was not performed and an error of omission introduced. The risk is doubled in the pain clinic, where it may be assumed that the patient would not be there if any chance of an organic cause for the pain had been found. Therefore the patient is started on a psychologically oriented program without a basic medical evaluation and an error of omission is compounded by one of commission. The occupational therapist is ideally suited to keep communications open between the organically oriented physician directing the physical program and the representative of the pain program. The therapist may also act in a medically, psychologically, and socially supporting role to the patient, who has sustained major functional loss and has debilitating symptoms. The therapist is also the ideal person to work with the patient in the use of a cutaneous nerve stimulator for pain relief. The patient and the therapist form their own team to determine those anatomical areas, patterns of stimulation, and techniques that may prove helpful in assisting the patient to reduce medications, cope with painful stimuli, and continue to function in the re-education program.

THE ROLE OF ORTHOPEDIC SURGERY

Surgical treatment of the residual muscle weakness of brachial plexus palsy is oriented toward direct nerve repair or compensatory substitutions of unaffected muscle-tendon units for paralytic ones. The loss of deltoid and supraspinatus function is usually considered irreparable and glenohumeral arthrodesis may provide a shoulder that is stable and pain-free (Figs. 20-11, 20-12). Mobility due to pericapsular musculature will usually allow a patient to raise the arm to almost 90 degrees from the rest position at the side. Shoulder fusion should be the last step in upper limb reconstruction. It is extremely difficult to carry out effective forearm or chest-arm muscle transfers when the proximal shoulder joint is stiff and cannot be appropriately positioned to facilitate exposure of forearm muscle or the inner

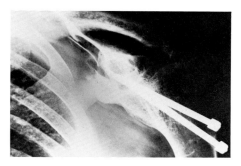

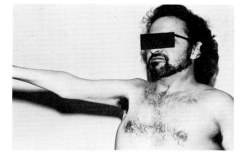

Fig. 20-11. Arthrodesis of the shoulder may prove helpful in cases with permanent paralysis of the deltoid and rotator cuff musculature. This stable platform allows periscapular musculature to elevate the upper limb. Intra-articular and extra-articular bony arthrodeses are seen on this radiograph.

Fig. 20-12. This patient has good scapular musculature with paralysis of the deltoid and rotator cuff. Shoulder arthrodesis enables him to elevate his arm to 90 degrees of abduction or forward flexion.

aspect of the upper arm in the area of the axilla. In addition, positioning the patient on the operating table when an arthrodesis is present in the shoulder may put excessive stress on the fused area. Fracture of the arthrodesis or the humerus may occur. Arthrodesis position is also dependent on the ability of the patient to flex his elbow and should therefore be determined after all attempts at elbow flexorplasty have been completed and the final range of elbow function is determined. In general, more shoulder abduction is required in cases of weak elbow flexion.

High lesions of C5–C6 routes frequently spare pectoral or forearm motor groups, yet they result in losses of elbow flexion. Transfer of the pectoral muscles and flexorplasty using forearm musculature are reliable procedures for restoring usable elbow flexion. Recent modifications of pectoral transfer for elbow flexion may obviate the need for shoulder arthrodesis if the tendon of the pectoral muscle is inserted on the scapular acromion. We prefer not to build motor power out beyond areas of good sensibility. In general, but not always, distal extremities with major sensory deprivation are not used for function even after motor power has been restored.

This chapter is not directed toward surgical technology and complete descriptions of the numerous practicable operations cannot be furnished. Nevertheless, the basic goal of surgery and its place in the rehabilitation program should be understood. An experienced therapist is frequently the best qualified team member to request a surgical evaluation. Competent therapists usually have a good relationship with the patient, know his goals and potential function, and are aware of the motor power available for transfer to an adjacent area of function with reasonable sensibility. The patient must understand what an operation has to offer and what he may risk in time, functional deficit, and emotional disappointment if the procedure fails to deliver the expected functional return. He must be willing to participate in a preoperative and a postoperative training program for muscle strengthening in functional use of the operated area. The new function must improve his activities of daily living and leave him with no additional functional loss.

As an example of a failure of preoperative evaluation, I will cite a personal experience. A girl who had lost her elbow flexion was operated on with transfer of the triceps anteriorly. She obtained an active range of elbow flexion from 30 to 95 degrees. I was pleased until the patient told me that she could no longer lift her arm out of the water during swimming, her favorite sport. The operation was a technical success and a functional failure. It is important not to simply perform "operative procedures" on patients who are already seriously disabled. A thorough understanding of the patient's activities and daily living patterns is the most important aspect of choosing the most appropriate surgical procedure. The patient with a low lesion may not be a candidate for any surgery due to impaired sensibility in the hand; nevertheless, if his job or an activity he enjoys calls for a helper hand function and he is intelligent and able to use some eye control, he may well derive real functional benefit from a procedure that restores function (Figs. 20-13–20-16). Our clinic's policy involves the patient, the family, and the therapist in this final aspect of surgical planning. All of these persons have spent many long hours wrestling with the patient's vocational and family situation, whereas the surgeon has usually not been so closely involved.

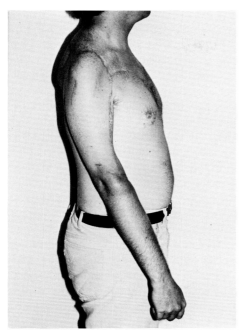

Fig. 20-13. This patient sustained a brachial plexus injury resulting in permanent loss of elbow flexion and shoulder abduction. Good sensibility and reasonably good motor power were present in the forearm and hand. He realized that a return to competitive motorcycle racing was unrealistic, but he had a great desire to return to riding a motorcycle and working in a motorcycle parts and repair facility. He is intelligent and well-motivated. Surgical reconstruction of the upper limb was undertaken and the patient was enrolled in a training program to become a motorcycle mechanic.

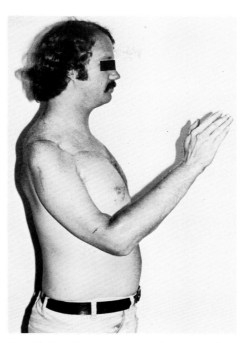

Fig. 20-14. Reconstruction of strong elbow flexion is accomplished by transfer of the pectoral muscle from the chest wall onto the arm and by proximal migration of the flexor carpi ulnaris to the distal aspect of the medial surface of the humerus. This patient required both pectoral and forearm flexorplasty. Good range of strong motion in flexion against gravity is demonstrated.

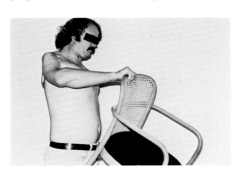

Fig. 20-15. Good strength in the remaining forearm muscles of the other limb, restoration of elbow flexion, and shoulder fusion stability resulted in the restoration of function with good strength.

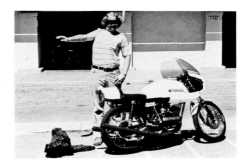

Fig. 20-16. The patient returned to his desired activity of riding motorcycles. His arm was functionally adequate to perform this activity. He completed a satisfactory training program in a junior college and now owns a shop for motorcycle repair.

VOCATIONAL REHABILITATION

The real measure of a rehabilitation program is the number of patients who return to society as integrated, related, and, ideally, as employed persons. It is obvious that all injured persons cannot return to a competitive labor market; nor can we expect a sociopath to return to productive society. Despite this fact, even a socially, psychologically, and intellectually deprived patient may become motivated after sustaining a serious, chronic, physical disability. This shift may occur because the individual is now totally separated from his former peer group environment or because he suddenly has a great deal of time to consider his values and his future in society. During these initial months, the patient relies heavily on the therapist as a friend, someone who cares and is interested in him when his peer group has disappeared. The physician is too far removed, too powerful an authority figure, and unfortunately "too busy" to form a basic supportive relationship with the patient, who definitely does need help from someone he can confide in. Vocational rehabilitation plays an important role in this phase of treatment, which requires restoration of self-esteem. Appropriate testing may uncover a previously unrecognized skill or talent. Educational training programs may not only allow the patient to become employable, but may also allow him to regain some faith in himself as a person. No rehabilitation program can succeed without restoration of patient motivation. Some patients can spur themselves on with minimal assistance and others require great strength, persistence, and reasonable prodding by all team members.

One anecdote may illustrate this situation. Gary, a 25-year-old patient, wandered phlegmatically around Rancho Los Amigos Hospital for two years. A vocational rehabilitation evaluation showed that he had a real talent for art and painting. His therapist felt that he would benefit from elbow surgery, and a flexorplasty was successful in restoring elbow flexion. Yet Gary did nothing. He had no motivation, but he continued attending the clinic every month without making up his mind about any future plans. All attempts at support and suggestion failed, so the rehabilitation team attempted a radical approach. At a formal conference in the clinic, he was told that the State of California had given him all that it could. He knew his exercise program and our recommendations and he also knew that he had done nothing about any of them. He was discharged from the clinic and given a dime for a telephone call. He was explicitly instructed that he could use that dime at any time to call vocational counseling at the hospital to request completion of his commercial art training and job placement. He was informed that the choice was his—he could either step forward and accept responsibility or remain "on the dole." He was told not to return unless he wished to help himself. A few days later the telephone rang. Gary is now gainfully employed as a commercial artist and paints for a hobby.

Vocational rehabilitation counselors have assisted in training one-handed typists who have passed civil service employment examinations, discovered talent in art and planning required for training in interior design, assisted in converting construction laborers into construction draftsmen, funded educational programs for a warehouseman to become a commercial property and real estate assessor, found baby tending and child care services to allow a disabled mother to return to finish her college education, and have even assisted an injured motorcycle racer to attain training to open his own motorcycle parts shop. The vocational counselor participates in the clinic and functions as a vital team member to prevent the patient from dropping out of a productive life during the initial period of disability.

SUMMARY

Rehabilitation of the brachial plexus palsy patient requires a combined effort of a team dedicated to assisting the patient to return to society with as much function as possible. An appropriate diagnosis of functional impairment is the initial requirement. Therapy to prevent contractures, assist in strengthening, and document returning functional areas continues throughout the program. Surgical intervention may assist the patient to recover some nerve function or to replace lost functional areas with transferred motor power. Pain control may be initiated through splinting or bracing methods, electrical cutaneous stimulation, or occasional surgical procedures. Prolonged narcotic medication should be avoided. Behavior modification programs have been beneficial to some patients but must be used judiciously.

The major factor in rehabilitating these patients is their own ability to become motivated to return to society as productive citizens.

REFERENCES

1. Braun, R. M.: Injury to the brachial plexus during brachial arteriography. J. Hand Surg. 3:90–94, 1978.
2. Braun, R. M.: Iatrogenic compression of the thoracic outlet. Johns Hopkins Med. J. 145:74–79, 1979.
3. Greenberg, S., and Braun, R. M.: Therapeutic use of the air bag splint for the injured hand. Am. J. Occup. Ther. 31:318–319, 1977.
4. Leffert, R. D.: Reconstruction of the shoulder and elbow following brachial plexus injury. In Omer, G., and Spinner, M., Eds.: *Management of Peripheral Nerve Problems,* pp. 805–816. W. B. Saunders, Philadelphia, 1980.
5. Millesi, H.: Surgical management of brachial plexus injuries. J. Hand Surg. 2:367–379, 1977.
6. Narakas, A.: Plexo braquial. Rev. Ortop. Traum. 16:855–920, 1972.
7. Nashold, B. S., and Ostdahl, R. H.: Dorsal root entry zone lesions for pain relief. J. Neurosurg. 51:59–69, 1979.
8. Perry, J.: Orthotic components and systems/prescription principles. In *Atlas of Orthotics, Biomechanical Principles, and Application,* pp. 81–129. American Academy of Orthopaedic Surgeons. C. V. Mosby, St. Louis, 1975.

21

The Painful Shoulder

Robert J. Neviaser, M.D.

The shoulder is a body area that has become a source of an increasing number of complaints. As more and more Americans have taken up regular physical exercise, the number of persons presenting with this type of musculoskeletal problem has multiplied, especially participants in racquet sports or other athletic activities requiring such overhead motions as throwing or swinging. Another reason patients are seen and treated is a greater awareness by physicians that disorders of the shoulder tendons cause real disability and can be helped by proper therapy.

ANATOMICAL CONSIDERATIONS

The shoulder is not a single joint. There are three distinct articulations involved in the shoulder girdle: the sternoclavicular joint, the acromioclavicular joint, and the glenohumeral joint.[2] The scapulothoracic relationship may also be considered as a joint. For the purposes of this discussion, only the glenohumeral and acromioclavicular joints will be considered.

The acromioclavicular joint is the lateral articulation of the clavicle with the acromion process of the scapula. It is supported by ligaments superiorly and inferiorly spanning the joint. It receives further support from two broad ligaments arising from the coracoid process inferior to the scapula and attaching to the clavicle. With maintenance of this normal joint alignment, the scapula and upper humerus are prevented from rotating anteriorly and inferiorly.

323

At first glance the glenohumeral joint appears to be a ball-and-socket arrangement; it does not, however, have the inherent stability of such a configuration. It resembles more closely a universal joint, allowing a great deal of motion in many directions. Its stability comes from supporting anterior and posterior ligaments. Of greater importance are the tendons and muscles comprising the rotator cuff—the supraspinatus, the infraspinatus, the teres minor, and the subscapularis. These tendons surround and blend with the articular capsule of the glenohumeral joint and attach to the tuberosities. The capsule has a redundant fold inferiorly when the arm is at the side; as the arm is abducted, this fold becomes taut. The joint lining, or synovium, covers the long head of the biceps brachii, which traverses the joint and passes through the tuberosities of the humerus.

The entire shoulder is covered by the deltoid muscle. As the rotator cuff muscles contract, they stabilize the humerus against the glenoid. With a fixed fulcrum thus provided, the deltoid can act to abduct the arm.

ETIOLOGY OF SHOULDER PAIN

In the younger patient, the most common cause of shoulder disorder is trauma, be it a single acute episode or a chronic repetitive process. A single, significant acute injury in a young person often produces an anterior glenohumeral dislocation or, in rare instances, a posterior dislocation. An acromioclavicular separation is another lesion commonly seen.

In an anterior dislocation of the shoulder, the most commonly seen process is a tearing of the capsular attachment from the anterior-inferior portion of the glenoid. If the first anterior dislocation occurs before the age of 20 years, the recurrence rate is more than 90 percent. If it occurs between the ages of 20 and 40, the rate of recurrence is nearly 75 percent. Later than age 40, the incidence of recurrence drops dramatically to 15 percent, but other associated problems will be seen more instead, including fractures of the greater tuberosity and tears of the rotator cuff.

Posterior traumatic dislocations are rare, comprising less than 5 percent of all shoulder dislocations. This type of lesion, however, is the most commonly missed. Any patient with a shoulder injury who has an internal rotation contracture and restricted abduction must be viewed as having a potential posterior dislocation. This is especially true in individuals with seizure disorders.[5]

Fractures of the shoulder are more frequent in the older patient. Fractures can involve the head, one or both tuberosities, or the surgical or anatomical necks. The clavicle, of course, is a common fracture in any age group.

Acromioclavicular separations are usually seen in younger, athletic persons who sustain a direct blow to the shoulder. The injury forces the acromion and humerus downward, rupturing the supporting ligaments of the clavicle and acromioclavicular joint. The lateral end of the clavicle then becomes prominent as the scapula falls inferiorly and rotates anteromedially. The long-term outcome is weakness in activities that involve reaching overhead.

Disorders of the tendons of the shoulder are seen in every age group. Before the age of 40, the history is usually one of progressively developing pain precipitated or aggravated by sports, especially tennis, swimming, or others requiring motions above shoulder level. Lifting or reaching is also painful. Active motion is often slightly limited, but passive motion can approach normal. This problem is due to inflammation of the rotator cuff and biceps tendons.[3] Patients in the fifth decade of life and beyond are also subject to tears of the rotator cuff due to degeneration, thinning, and eventual erosion of the tendon. This type of attritional tear is frequently found without any history of trauma.

Rotator cuff injuries do occur, of course, as a result of significant trauma. Acute ruptures cause weakness, especially in abduction, and pain, often at night. It is important to recognize, however, that the patient need *not* have complete loss of abduction for a rotator cuff tear to exist. It is this myth that accounts for these lesions being missed.

An overused diagnosis for a condition presently seen infrequently is adhesive capsulitis. This is an inflammatory contracture involving the capsule, especially the dependent fold. It is painful and restricts abduction and internal rotation. Often it is seen in women, in the nondominant arm.

Arthritis, either rheumatoid or degenerative, does not often involve the shoulder. It is surprising how much change in the joint brought about by arthritic processes can be tolerated by patients and how well they adjust to this functionally. In a small number of cases, pain and loss of motion will be severe enough to warrant a surgical approach.

DIAGNOSIS

The diagnosis of shoulder disorders can usually be made by history, physical examination, and roentgenographic evaluation. The history should reveal the presence of major trauma and the nature of the functional disability, for instance, what motions are lost or painful, the nature of the pain, and if there is night pain.

The physical examination can serve to narrow the differential diagnoses. Localized tenderness over the cuff or biceps tendons (Fig. 21-1) should be sought.

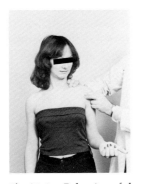

Fig. 21-1. Palpation of the biceps tendon performed with the hand supinated and the shoulder in some external rotation.

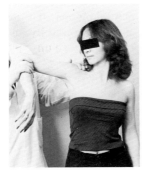

Fig. 21-2. Compressing the rotator cuff against the acromion and coracoacromial ligament.

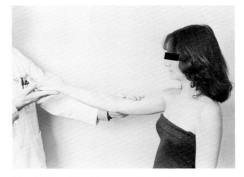

Fig. 21-3. The biceps resistance test.

Pain with palm-down abduction (Fig. 21-2) directs attention to the rotator cuff, whereas pain on resisted forward flexion (Fig. 21-3) suggests involvement of the biceps. Restriction of passive abduction and internal rotation should alert the physician to the presence of adhesive capsulitis.

Roentgenographic evaluation should take two forms. Routine films must be done with any shoulder problem and should include an axillary view, which is essential to rule out any dislocation.

For lesions of the tendons, arthrography is of great value. It will establish a definitive diagnosis in ruptures of the rotator cuff and in tendinitis, subluxation, or dislocation of the biceps tendon. Arthrography is also necessary to establish a diagnosis of adhesive capsulitis.

TREATMENT

For acute anterior dislocations, the need for prompt closed reduction is obvious. After the first episode, immobilization of the arm at the side and in internal rotation for three weeks is advisable. For recurrent anterior dislocations, prolonged immobilization or exercises have *no* effect on the prevention of future recurrences. The single most important determining factor is the age of initial dislocation. Surgical repair of the capsular defect is the treatment of choice, as it is for recurrent posterior dislocations.

The treatment of shoulder fractures depends on the type of fracture and the patient's age. For impacted or undisplaced fractures, immobilization is all that is needed. For displaced fractures, surgical reduction may be required. For acromioclavicular injuries, surgical repair may be useful in young, active patients with complete or nearly complete separations. In more sedentary individuals, symptomatic treatment may be acceptable, that is, rest in a sling until the pain subsides (about 10–14 days), followed by a progressive increase in active and passive motion.

Tears of the rotator cuff, especially the acute, massive, complete ruptures or the painful, chronic ones, need surgical reconstruction.[1] It is fallacious to believe that these lesions will respond to physical therapy alone.[4] Disorders of the biceps, particularly the subluxing or dislocated biceps, should also be managed surgically. Tendinitis of the cuff and biceps can be treated by anti-inflammatory medications and gentle stretching exercises, but if they are unresponsive, surgical intervention may be required.

For the true adhesive capsulitis with restriction of active and passive abduction as well as internal rotation, treatment is dependent on the severity of the loss of abduction. For patients who can abduct to 90 degrees or more, therapy is instituted directly. For those with less than 90 degrees of abduction, manipulation under anesthesia is required before therapy is begun.

Physical Therapy

The role of physical therapy in the rehabilitation of the shoulder is extremely important. It is valuable in treating lesions that do not require an operation as well as rehabilitating those that do.

The important aspect of shoulder physical therapy is the gaining of motion. Strength is of very secondary importance.

The formalized rehabilitation program is supervised by the therapist, but it is only a basis on which the entire treatment is built. A home program is very important as well. For patients who have been immobilized, to allow a fracture to heal or to recuperate from an operation, the first week is spent doing pendulum exercises in a sling. The patient faces a table or counter, bends at the waist and swings the extremity to and fro as well as in circles. The circles are made in both clockwise and counterclockwise fashion with progressively larger diameters.

Following this introductory program, a more formal regimen is begun. Often the application of moist heat is effective in giving a sense of freedom to the joint. To improve mobility, certain techniques are used. The wheel on the wall is valuable in increasing abduction as well as flexion, extension, and external rotation. It can be started with a small-diameter circle, which is then increased. It is important that the patient's hand be placed on the handle so that the arm is in external rotation (Fig. 21-4). This allows the motion to occur at the glenohumeral joint primarily, without compressing the rotator cuff and biceps tendons under the acromial arch.

Flexion can be gained by assisting with the opposite arm. It is also aided by having the patient face a wall and "walk up" it with the fingers of the affected arm (Fig. 21-5). If the patient stands sideways or perpendicular to the wall, abduction is achieved.

Extension and external rotation of the shoulder are produced by passing the hand across the occiput and upper neck to touch the ear on the opposite side. This is a more effective movement than going across the top of the head. These same

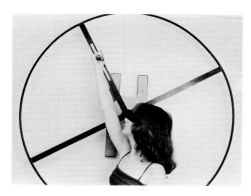

Fig. 21-4. Proper use of the wheel. Note the position of the hand—in supination with the shoulder in external rotation. This position should be used whenever possible.

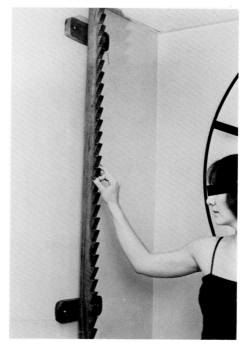

Fig. 21-5. Wall walking, here illustrated with a finger board.

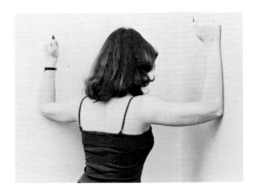

Fig. 21-6. Passive exercise to increase extension and external rotation in abduction. It can be performed in a doorway as well.

motions can be achieved by having the patient stand in a doorway, place both hands on the door frame overhead, and lean forward through the doorway (Fig. 21-6).

Internal rotation can be improved by assisting the affected arm in reaching the intrascapular region with the opposite hand. A good exercise for both internal and external rotation is pulling a towel back and forth in a back-drying motion. If internal rotation needs work, then the involved extremity is the lower arm. If external rotation is restricted, the affected part is the upper arm (Figs. 21-7A, B).

The postoperative rehabilitation on the tendons of the shoulder, especially those of the rotator cuff, differs somewhat from what has just been described. Of course, regaining motion is important, but muscle retraining is also needed. The

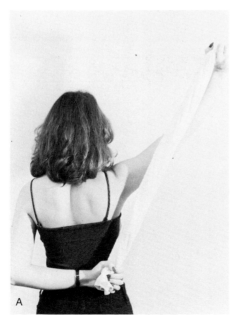
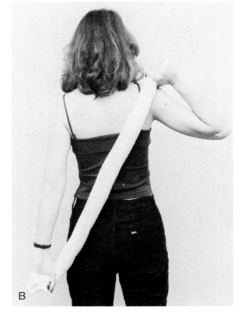

Fig. 21-7. (A) Back-drying maneuver to assist internal rotation. (B) The same exercise also can improve external rotation.

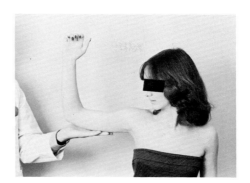

Fig. 21-8. The key exercise to establish function early in rehabilitating the rotator cuff.

following program is used. The affected arm is held by the therapist at 90 degrees of abduction; the patient then tries to raise the arm higher, away from the supporting hands (Fig. 21-8). This is done with the elbow flexed to a right angle and the hand pointed forward and then toward the ceiling. This exercise is the keystone to restoring rotator cuff function. It is also practiced at home by the patient, who can be assisted by someone or, if by himself, can rest his arm on top of a bureau or a shelf and raise it from there. Once the patient can accomplish active abduction from 90 degrees upward, then abduction from the side is emphasized.

Resistive exercises are designed to increase strength. They should be used only after active motion has been accomplished satisfactorily, which comes at least 12 weeks after tendon surgery or after a fracture of the shoulder.

In summary, the role of physical therapy in the rehabilitation of the shoulder is important. It should primarily emphasize motion and strength secondarily. It should not be considered an alternative to surgery but an adjunct to proper treatment, which often includes an operation.

REFERENCES

1. Neviaser, J. S., Neviaser, R. J., and Neviaser, T. J.: The repair of chronic massive ruptures of the rotator cuff of the shoulder by use of a freeze-dried rotator cuff. J. Bone Joint Surg. 60A:681–684, 1978.
2. Neviaser, R. J.: Anatomic considerations and examination of the shoulder. Orthop. Clin. North Am. 11:187–195, 1980.
3. Neviaser, R. J.: Lesions of the biceps and tendinitis of the shoulder. Orthop. Clin. North Am. 11:343–348, 1980.
4. Neviaser, R. J.: Tears of the rotator cuff. Orthop. Clin. North Am. 11:295–306, 1980.
5. Neviaser, R. J., Neviaser, J. S., Neviaser, T. J., and Neviaser, J. S.: A simple technique for internal fixation of the clavicle. Clin. Orthop. 109:103–107, 1975.

22

Major Fractures

Vert Mooney, M.D.

The specifics of fracture care can fill many textbooks. There is still considerable controversy over ideal techniques, materials, and even the most significant determinants of healing. Thus the purpose of this discussion is not to recommend any particular method of care over another, but rather to advocate the philosophy of mobilization. The goal of fracture rehabilitation is to mobilize the injured tissues, skeletal and soft, as rapidly as is consistent with the healing process. To do this, union of the fracture must be achieved as rapidly as possible. Muscle strength must be returned to even greater than normal levels during the rehabilitation phase. Finally, the range of motion in the joints must be preserved or enhanced by whatever methods possible.

In that mobilization is the theme of rehabilitation, most of the discussion centers on significant lower extremity fractures and their post-acute care. Hospital inpatient stays that are as short as possible should be a primary goal, as is avoiding the habituation to disability by prolonged off-work time. Returning the individual to the highest level of function consistent with his injuries—returning to the pleasure of a contributing role in society—is the ultimate goal.

HISTORICAL CONSIDERATIONS

Rest and movement, those two diverse concepts, are the key factors that accelerate or confound fracture rehabilitation. For at least a century, the relative roles of each has been debated. Of considerable significance to our current attitude of fracture care is that the advocacy of rest grew primarily out of the English school. The advocates of motion usually derived from the Continental school of care. And because the intellectual base of orthopedic care is largely an outgrowth of the English philosophy, for many years rest has been the primary method of fracture care. The positive claims of rest as a method of care date back over 100 years to John Hilton and Hugh Owens Thomas.[8] Certainly the major textbook of fracture care until recently was that by Sir Reginald Watson-Jones[9] who, as a disciple of the school of rest, continued to base his treatment on that classical method of rehabilitation. Once the care of skeletal trauma in America gradually fell into the hands of disciples of the English school, prolonged rest certainly had its day as a mechanism of care.

Yet it was the method of mobilization and rehabilitation that brought orthopedists into the field of skeletal-trauma care. The father of orthopedics, Robert Jones, achieved his reputation in the early care of lower extremity fractures by the use of his uncle's famous device, the Thomas splint. This device was used to transport and eventually suspend in traction femoral fractures sustained by soldiers during World War I and it was later adopted for industrial injuries. The splint had originally been used to mobilize the resting tubercular knee. Thus, again it is not surprising that the philosophical stance of tuberculosis treatment, rest, became engrained in the therapy of skeletal trauma.

The opposing point of view was best expressed early by Lucas-Championiere.[3] In 1910, he advocated supervised active motion soon after injury, with the addition of friction massage to control discomfort. "Action is life," was the motto of this school, contrasted to continued and enforced rest advocated by the English. This controversy was summed up best in the Robert Jones lecture of 1952, given by George Perkins.[6]

At a surprisingly early date, an American advocate of mobilization emerged. In 1855, Dr. H. H. Smith of Philadelphia applied braces, which he called "artificial limbs," to ununited fractures. In a tentative rebuttal to then prevailing practice, he stated, "It is an inquiry worthy of note in passing whether in the treatment of fractures very perfect rest may not be one cause of the deficiency of the new bone union."[7] It took more than 100 years before his concept of ambulatory care for fractures to be rediscovered by Ernst Dehne,[1] who reported a perfect record of union in the case of cast treatment for fractures with immediate weight-bearing. His father, an Austrian physician, had used Smith's braces, so the positive results of mobilization had been demonstrated to Dehne as a youth.

In America, the surgical care of fractures with internal fixation had been adopted by general surgeons once improved metallurgy made stainless steel available. Such celebrated surgeons as William O'Neal Sherman of Pittsburgh, Preston Wade at New York Hospital, and Harrison McLaughlin at Columbia-Presbyterian were strong advocates of the surgical fixation of fractures during the 1940s and 1950s. However, high incidences of failure and disastrous infection due to poor understanding of mechanical principles allowed the more "conservative" approach of the orthopedists eventually to succeed the general surgeons' view in responsibility for fracture care. The surgical approach for skeletal reconstruction was considered proper, but the same surgery to enhance mobilization of fractures was considered destructive to the principles of continued and prolonged rest so strongly developed by the English school.

Since the 1970s, the pendulum in fracture care has swung toward the surgical fixation of skeletal trauma according to the Swiss AO technique. In response to the "cast disease" caused by prolonged rest, Maurice Müller and his colleagues[4] developed a whole new technique of fracture fixation based on sounder scientific principles than had ever been practiced before. In Europe, fracture care had developed somewhat differently from an administrative standpoint. The concept of traumatology, as opposed to orthopedics, was more highly developed. In many areas orthopedics stayed strictly in the area of reconstruction, whereas traumatology, which included all aspects of surgical care for trauma, was the standard of care. Out of this concept grew the now very acceptable methods of rigid internal fixation, the entire basis of the AO system of fracture care.

Thus, the two principles of care, rest and motion, have now been joined in the Swiss method of fracture care. Profound rest to the skeletal system of rigid internal fixation allows primary union of the bone. By replacing the structural integrity of the skeletal system with plates and screws, rapid mobilization of the limb is possible. Motion of the soft tissues is allowed, yet rest of the skeletal tissues is enforced. The goal of excellent surgical care of fractures in this system is sufficient stabilization of the skeletal system to allow rapid mobilization of the joints and muscles and the return of normal function as soon as possible. The two basic conceptual flaws of that approach are the "overkill" of stabilization, which may be so efficient as to diminish stresses to the skeletal system that it is no longer strong enough to carry out its appropriate function, and the other side of that problem, the need to remove internal fixations surgically at some time after injury. Another flaw in the AO concept is the higher level of surgical skill and mechanical understanding necessary in the care of fractures. The risks of failure are greater when the treatment program is poorly administered on a technical basis than in the nonoperative care. To a large extent this final flaw should be resolvable by increasing the surgical technician's skill and understanding of the mechanical principles involved. Certainly everything favors effective fracture rehabilitation by the appropriate application of AO internal fixation methods, but the risks taken and the skills necessary to achieve them are higher.

Probably the clinician who best stated the appropriate orthopedic philosophy for fracture care was Joel Goldthwaite,[2] who in the Robert Jones lecture of 1932 suggested the principle upon which fracture rehabilitation must be based: "the orthopedic surgeon is most qualified to provide fracture care from acute onset through rehabilitation because it is a basic principle of his training that from the very beginning, he has the end result in mind." This view of the end result is the principle that forces us to mobilize all resources in the rehabilitation program. Ironically, Goldthwaite's words were spoken against operative care for fractures, or even for reconstructive chronic orthopedic problems. Thus, by taking his words out of context, we will look to the principles in achieving the ideal end result.

REHABILITATION OF FRACTURES

Relationship to Acute Care

The urgencies of acute care for fractures regulate the ultimate result and the in-hospital time expected. There is a constant trade-off between immediate or early surgical care versus delayed or closed methods of care. To a certain extent, the technical and institutional skills available in a community control the role of surgical care for fractures. An excellent example of this phenomenon at work is the experience of femoral fractures cared for in the Seattle area. With the development of a highly skilled team of surgeons at Harbor View Hospital (and the investment in an extensive inventory of instruments, femoral rods, and ancillary equipment), the standard of care in that community is now closed rodding of femoral shaft fractures. Alleged negligence suits have even been considered when femoral shaft fractures were treated by the traditional skeletal traction and cast brace methods. The in-hospital stay for patients referred to Harbor View Hospital from other locations is only a few days and then they are referred back to their primary hospital for continued care, thus decreasing hospital stays. In other communities without this high level of teamwork and institutional cooperation, it would be foolhardy to attempt all femoral-shaft fracture care by closed rodding methods.

The patient's safety at the specific time and place where he finds his care is, of course, the ultimate priority. If a less demanding and specialized method of care can offer a similar level of favorable result with the same effective rate of return to work as that of a highly demanding surgical method, in certain circumstances the simpler approach may well be quite suitable.

An example of another mode for the care of fractured femoral shafts that can offer a fairly similar rate of healing and return to work with about the same in-hospital time is that of fracture bracing combined with Neufeld roller traction.[5] Figures 22-1–22-3 present this method of immediate care as it blends into a rehabilitation program for fracture care. The important element of this method is the utilization of traditional skeletal traction to achieve alignment, elevation, and relative immobilization of the injured limb. This method offers relatively low risks to the injured part and allows gradual motion as the healing process develops. If other factors are operating, the patient can be mobilized out of bed quite rapidly and become ambulatory as feasible. Because he may go in and out of traction, to a

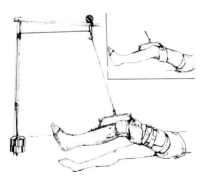

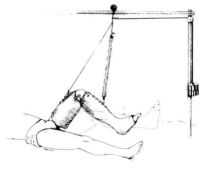

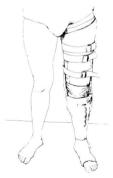

Fig. 22-1. Neufeld roller traction demonstrating a traction suspension system that can use a fracture brace. The inset drawing shows how the system may be used for a long leg cast. An adjustable thigh corset with plastic hinges provides fracture brace mobility and can be applied later.

Fig. 22-2. The roller traction system with the addition of a counterbalanced spring can furnish an exercise program that begins while the patient remains in traction.

Fig. 22-3. The fracture brace in the ambulatory phase, using an adjustable plastic thigh corset.

certain extent according to his own needs, many other aspects of rehabilitation can be achieved, such as progressive independence and the strengthening of other limbs. By avoiding prolonged recumbancy, appropriate drainage of the urinary system is achievable, pulmonary and visceral functions are considerably assisted, and finally, chronic tissue trauma and pressure areas caused by prolonged recumbancy are circumvented. This method of care certainly obeys the basic principle of intelligent rehabilitation—controlling early factors in a disease process to prevent complications and reduce the need for correcting them in the post-acute phase. Figure 22-2 represents an exercise program that can be instituted while the patient is in bed and that, of course, also responds to the principles of effective rehabilitation. Active motor function and joint range of motion as soon as it is possible, considering the degree of trauma suffered, are important aspects in early return of normal activity to a limb.

Figure 22-3 demonstrates the use of a fracture brace in the post-acute phase. The brace allows the muscle activity to continue to stabilize the "plastic" skeletal system in this maturation phase of bone union. The adjustable thigh corset is a considerable improvement over the static cast brace. A fracture brace is a significant improvement over the now passé use of a spica cast for a fractured femur. The spica cast exemplifies all the negative characteristics of effective fracture rehabilitation. It forces the knee to be immobilized for a prolonged period. It requires prolonged recumbancy, with all of the complications suggested by that condition, yet still does not adequately immobilize the fracture site. Most significantly, it enforces on the patient a condition of dependence and frustration with his own state, which militate against healthy behavior and early return to functional activity. Yet the fracture brace and roller traction system also has considerable limitations. This system cannot restore full length to the limb. Some shortening would have to be accepted in treating the type of fracture for which this is most appropriate—the severely comminuted femoral shaft fracture. The more aged and infirm the patient and the greater number of other fractures involved, the less applicable in this system. Even in the very simple fracture with only a small opportunity for callus formation, closed systems probably take four to five months to achieve complete union (in severely comminuted fractures complete union might be expected in three to four months). Femoral shaft rodding, either closed or by retrograde method, probably is a better method of treating the very simple shaft fractures from the standpoint of offering more of an opportunity than does the cast brace alone for rapid mobilization of the patient.

Here is therefore an example of two different systems of care for the femoral shaft fracture, each with the same goal. Both the roller traction and the closed rodding systems point to the need for rapid mobilization of the patient. Both allow early active motion to the joints above and below the fracture. With minimal additional mobility to the injured party, rapid progress out of the hospital and return to home and work can be expected. One might expect the same moderately comminuted shaft fracture treated by roller traction to take four months before the patient was free of all appliances, whereas with the closed rodding method the event transpires within a month, although some of this advantage is lost to rod removal. Nonetheless, in both settings the view of early mobilization is the urgency driving the clinician toward effective fracture rehabilitation.

One of the most complex problems to treat is the pelvic fracture. Not only is surgical care for these fractures difficult, but even under the best of circumstances mobilization of the individual is delayed. It seems clear, however, that with a greater understanding of biomechanics and our improved methods of fixation, the prolonged recumbancy once believed to be necessary for the treatment of these fractures is no longer necessary.

Figures 22-4A and B illustrate a complex pelvic fracture with an extremely unstable hip. Maintaining this individual in traction for a prolonged period of time certainly delays the opportunity for rehabilitation. More than that, for this particular type of fracture, even lateral traction and distal traction do not have the opportunity of restoring near normal architecture. No traction method can bring the inner wall of the pelvis into a normal articular relationship with the femoral head. Thus, any period of time spent lying in the more traditional traction systems would be wasted. Even a later reconstruction with a total hip would be made extremely difficult with the inner acetabular wall so medially displaced.

Thus, surgical care as shown in Figure 22-5 is a reasonable method of rehabilitation for pelvic fracture. Even if the reconstruction of the acetabulum is incomplete and inadequate, the individuals are still better off by being allowed to mobilize slowly with increasing stress gradually applied to the acetabulum. Figure 22-6 demonstrates this patient convalescing in a roller traction-distraction suspension system. The advantage of the system to the patient is that it allows far more comfortable traction. The roller traction system avoids the peak loading typical of other traction systems. The traction system now flows with the system and thus allows the patient to move comfortably in bed. With the reduction of peak loading, the acute response of reactive muscle spasm is also avoided. The patients are far more comfortable in this system of traction. Eventually, gradual mobilization with progressive weight-bearing can be instituted.

Mobilization and ambulatory activity, of course, are the goals for lower extremity fracture care. In the delayed union of shaft fracture, there is a frequent

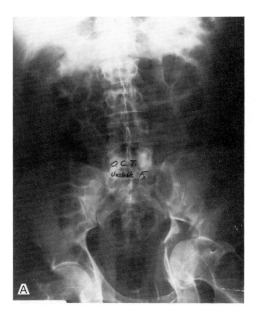
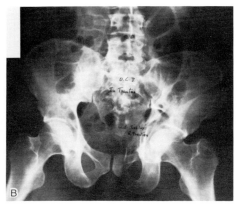

Fig. 22-4. (A) This x-ray reveals an extremely unstable acetabular fracture. (B) At this stage reduction is available, but instability will occur when the patient is out of traction.

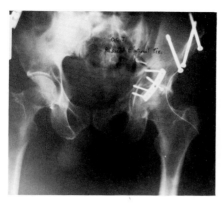
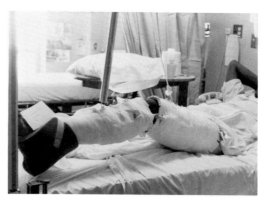

Fig. 22-5. Surgical status after open reduction and internal fixation. The hip is
now stable.

Fig. 22-6. Having the patient lie in roller traction
allows early mobilization following an acetabular
fracture.

dilemma. Should more surgical care be given or additional delay be offered the
patient as clinicians await a union that experience has predicted will eventually
occur? We must remember that for an individual who must return to some work
activity, the delay is a severe financial burden. The car payments, the children's
medical bills, must await eventual resolution of the fracture. Figure 22-7 presents a
typical fracture that is lethargic in union but that has an excellent potential of
eventually uniting without additional surgical care. The patient is anxious to
return to his job requiring hard physical activity, but his physicians fear that at
work he will refracture the limb. An alternative to additional surgery or prolonged
off-work time is the construction of a total-contact plastic orthosis. This type of
custom-fitted protection device will allow rapid return to activity. It fits inside a
work shoe and allows sufficient mobility for the patient to return to construction
work. The question of additional surgery is avoided, yet the patient is productive

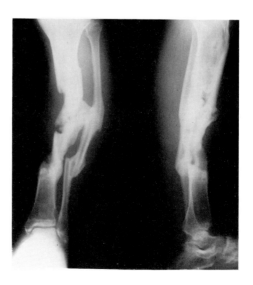

Fig. 22-7. This x-ray demonstrates a complex
open comminuted fracture. Its delayed union
requires prolonged protection.

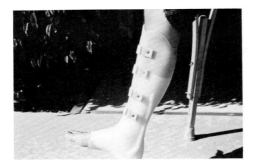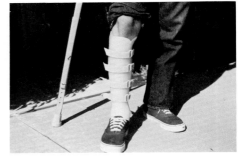

Fig. 22-8A, B. A custom-fit, molded plastic ankle-foot orthosis. No special footwear need be worn with it.

and truly rehabilitated. To achieve this sort of rehabilitation, however, the orthotist must have sufficient experience in constructing vacuum-formed plastics in order to provide superior custom-fitted devices (Figs. 22-8A and B).

The ultimate goal in fracture rehabilitation is to avoid having the patient lose any time from work. Many minor fractures can be treated in this manner, but certain accommodations to vocational demands must be made. A carponavicular fracture of an operating room nurse may be a minimal fracture, but the traditional method of care, using a plaster cast, is entirely incompatible with the work environment of an operating room. Figure 22-9 shows the plastic orthosis that was constructed for her to immobilize the wrist joint and avoid the torque forces of the thumb. The material used to construct it was Surlyn. Because it is a clear plastic, it offers some cosmetic and hygienic advantages. The nurse lost no time from work (although she had to function as a circulating nurse only and not as a scrub nurse), and once union was achieved we could identify no disability.

Sometimes the rehabilitation effort must accept compromises. Figure 22-10 presents the femoral shaft fracture of a young woman who also sustained severe back and buttock burns. Treating the fracture would be relatively simple on its own, but because the surgical site has second- and third-degree burns, an operation would be threatened by the potential for infection. Yet traction care would be impossible for this patient in that a supine position would be unacceptable from the standpoint of burn care to the back and buttock, so she had to be mobilized in some device.

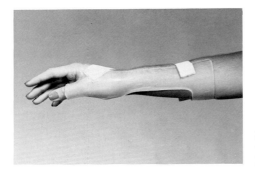

Fig. 22-9. This molded plastic orthosis provides long-term mobilization for a carponavicular fracture.

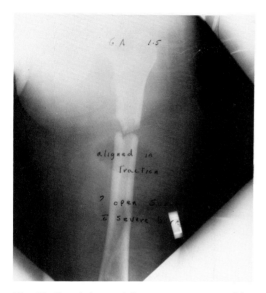

Fig. 22-10. A femoral fracture accompanied by severe burns that prevent surgery.

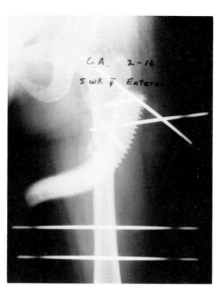

Fig. 22-11. External fixation has been used to immobilize the fracture, allow mobilization of the patient, and permit the burns to heal. In this case, the fixation was provided by epoxy-filled plastic tubes fixed to pins above and below the fracture site.

An external fixation device with pins passing through the area of skin involvement was used. It was recognized that these pins probably would become loose and infected with the passage of time, but the mobilization of the patient was paramount in her ultimate rehabilitation. Figure 22-11 reveals the alignment of the fracture, which did unite.

Continuing Care

In the post-acute and chronic phases of fracture care, rehabilitation often falls to the therapist or other allied health personnel to educate, motivate, and guide the patient via an exercise program. All allied health personnel who participate in fracture rehabilitation need to understand the fracture itself, the limitations of physical treatment programs, and the prognosis of the fracture as perceived by the surgeon. Thus the therapist should see the x-rays and be in on any discussions of the patient's treatment before progressing into extensive therapy.

Under ideal circumstances wherein a team approach is used for the rehabilitation of fractures, the therapist is also aware of the social context of treatment and any disease factors that may limit progress. In the case of complex problems, a conference should be held for all interested and participating staff. Accounts of continency of bowel and bladder, medications, assistance and support expected from family members, and motivation for self-care would all be reported by the nurse caring for a person with complex fractures. In some circumstances the report of a social worker would be valuable to identify financial resources, vocational problems, the status of continuing care in the home environment, and community resources available to the patient. A therapist would report the patient's muscle strength and range of motion and mobility status. In each report, status should be defined by specific phrases, each with a constant meaning. Assisted ambulation is different from supervised ambulation. Assisted with crutch is different from assisted with cane. The therapist should be prepared to identify some aspect of the functional capacity of the patient, that is, ability to walk 6 m. In cases of upper extremity trauma, occupational therapists are frequently helpful in identifying hand function and expectation for its continued use.

Upper Extremity Trauma.   Patients with significant upper extremity trauma frequently have associated neurological impairment. Thus rehabilitation should not only focus on increasing range of motion and strength to the hand and elbow, but perhaps must include some sensory retraining. Accordingly, any reports made should identify sensory deficits on both neurological and functional levels. This means the rehabilitation team must be aware of fairly well understood and effective systems for retraining sensory deficits. These methods are based on exposing the patient to various textures for training hand function or using various weights and functional implements in a prescribed method. By using retraining methods, marked expansion in function is possible, even in people sustaining significant neurological deficits.

There is no question that the leader of the fracture rehabilitation team must be the surgeon who was responsible for the acute care. It is extremely difficult for any other physician to have sufficient background and knowledge to guide the rehabilitation effort if he did not participate in the earlier care of the fracture and have understanding of the choice of initial treatment program. It is inappropriate for the surgeon to tell the therapist specifically, in terms of numbers of exercises and weights, what should be done. For medical and legal protection, the order should include expected limitations and it should certainly identify the fracture problem for which training is necessary. But since the physical rehabilitation of fractures is essentially a problem in coaching the individual to match his achievement with his potential, the treatment program must be quite dynamic. It is difficult, for instance, to prescribe the precise number of quadriceps exercises that would be ideal on any given day for a fractured distal femur. The therapist, as coach, can identify the point at which fatigue is confounding motivation and when muscle activity is being inhibited by pain or increasing fatigue. The therapist does document the patient's achievement, so the rate and amount of progress can be observed in a retrospective analysis. Out of this retrospective analysis projections of continuing progress become more and more valid. Empirical investigations of hospital benefit and physical therapy coaching also become possible, based on analysis of progress. The therapist will be able to see when therapy has reached the point of diminishing returns.

There are useful adjuncts to physical exercise programs for the post-fractured individual. Transcutaneous electrical nerve stimulation (TENS) has a useful role to play. By various forms of electrical stimulation to the limb being treated for fracture, the nervous system can to a certain extent be distracted and take less note from the noxious stimuli arising from the injured site. Massage, vibration, heat, and cold—other mechanisms that enhance sensory input—may also be beneficial in these situations.

Re-education

In motor training after fracture and/or joint injury, the balance of facilitation and inhibition at the anterior horn cells is a useful concept. At the appropriate segmental level in the cord, the anterior horn cell functions as a response between facilitative and inhibitor influences impinging upon the cell wall. The summation of facilitation versus inhibition finally achieves a critical level and the cell wall and axon are depolarized. Depolarization triggers the transmittal of a signal to the motor end-plates. Pain may inhibit the anterior horn cells, when the source of the pain is the injured site motored by the anterior horn cell in question. In spite of vigorous facilitative messages from the cerebrum, the anterior horn cell cannot be fired. If the inhibitive signals from the noxious stimuli at the site of pain can be diminished, then motor functioning can occur. For example, after an arthrotomy, the painful knee is distended with blood and it cannot be made to function despite the strong input from the brain. If this bloody effusion is drained and the joint is filled to the same degree of distension with a local anesthetic, motor function returns readily. Primitive reflexes force pain to facilitate flexor activity as a protective reflex. Extensor function must actively fight against these reflexes.

Many other influences aid or thwart the anterior horn cells. Posture, for instance, has an appreciable effect. The reflex activity of posture can easily be demonstrated in the stroke patient, who, when sitting, may have a flexor pattern that makes extension activity of the lower limb muscles impossible. However, when the stroke victim is stood up, the flexor pattern may suddenly reverse to one of extension, wherein the quadriceps fires vigorously, as does the gastrocsoleus, which extends the knee and places the foot in a plantar fixed position. The therapist can take advantage of these reflexes while retraining muscles. It is evidently more difficult to retrain a quadriceps mechanism when the patient is sitting because the reflexes that reinforce stance phase stability are not operating. If the individual is stood up, quadriceps function may become more readily available. Thus, retraining lower extremity in an erect, direct posture has the potential to be more efficient.

Ambulatory gaits that develop after fractures are frequently a source of some concern. Therapists are often instructed to train patients in activities that do not put weight on the injured limb. However, to me, such instruction seems unrealistic in that crutch walking without weight bearing is difficult to achieve. Even if pain is not a constant reminder, I think the gait may become an unsafe and even a potentially destructive pattern. Especially in older persons with less precise balance and motor control, instructions to favor the injury after an internal fixation of a fractured hip forces the individual to carry on walking activity while constantly thinking of what he is doing. Such concentration is not realistic, as when the person comes upon a door or an elevator or crosses a street. He is more concerned about the objects before him than about his gait pattern. He suddenly will recall that he is supposed to be non-weight-bearing and make a misstep that may, in turn, lead to loss of control and far more significant loading of the fracture site than is desired. A wiser alternative would seem to be partial weight-bearing determined by the patient's tolerance. This would allow him to achieve some stance phase stability on the injured limb while avoiding peak loading of the fracture by correct use of the crutch. Three-point gaits seem more realistic for patients with lower extremity fractures than non-weight-bearing gaits in order to avoid potentially destructive pressure on the fracture site.

Finally, the value of the external support device around the limb needs to be considered in terms of effective muscle control. Clinical experience suggests that people can use their muscles more effectively if they are firmly supported. The ultimate example is the weight lifter, who is far more effective in performing his Valsalva's maneuver if he is wearing a belt against which the abdominal muscles can work. A more apt demonstration of this phenomenon, however, is found in the individual who has been freely walking in a short leg cast without distress or limitation. Yet, immediately after removing the cast his leg and ankle will feel weak and unstable; because his muscles were able to work against a firm support of a cast, they had gotten used to "loafing." Once the full stresses of function were displayed to them again, they were no longer able to respond fully and immediately to functional demands. This as yet unproved hypothesis does, however, offer some justification for using firm limb supports in the rehabilitation of fractures. It does explain why various types of adjustable fracture braces allow the muscles to achieve a stability to the fractured limb that was not accomplished when unsupported. This concept does provide a rationale for the continuing use of adjustable limb supports made of firm plastic material against which muscles can work and gain effective function despite the injury and reduced functional capacity.

As indicated earlier, the effectiveness of fracture rehabilitation is greatly dependent upon the early reconstruction of initial damage. Significant joint irregularities cannot be tolerated if a joint is to return to normal function. There is some potential for joint remodeling in early phases of the healing process. As repair tissue becomes aligned under the stresses of function, the collagen of the repaired joint may respond to the forces of function through a fiber cartilagenous surfacing with some characteristics of true articular cartilage. The timing for this phenomenon, however, occurs within narrow limits. If the stresses of function are displayed to the healing joint too early, the opportunity for collecting connected tissue-building cells is limited. If the function of the joint is delayed for a prolonged period of time, scar will fill the vacuum of activity, but it will be aligned along random or improper lines of stress. The stimulus for fiber cartilagenous development will have been lost and the glue of fibro-orthosis arthrosis will have set it. Every opportunity consistent with nondestructive motion should be taken to provide injured joints an early opportunity to function.

SUMMARY

Certain historical aspects of fracture rehabilitation have been reviewed and a few examples of methods of care that affect rehabilitation have been provided. One cannot emphasize enough the importance of Goldthwaite's words concerning long-term results. The surgeon must keep in mind the end result as he approaches the initial fracture care. Rehabilitation implies knowledge of disability to the whole system, not just the fracture involved. It also implies understanding the humanistic aspects of return to work, return to home, and reasons to return to healthy behavior. The complete fracture surgeon cannot delegate responsibility for this general knowledge to other individuals. But he must be prepared to seek more than the advice of other specialists and clinicians; he must also turn to allied health professionals who have more technical knowledge than he has. Psychologists, social workers, and therapists all contribute significantly to the rehabilitation of complex fractures. To not benefit from their experience and assistance is to make greater demands in time and knowledge upon the surgeon himself, while leaving open the potential for the development of complications that need not have occurred.

REFERENCES

1. Dehne, E.: The ambulatory treatment of the fractured tibia. Clin. Orthop. 105:159–173, 1975.
2. Goldthwaite, J. E.: The background and foregrounds of orthopedics. J. Bone Joint Surg. 15A:279–301, 1933.
3. Lucas-Championiere, J. M. M.: *Precis du Traitement des Fractures Par le Massage et la Mobilisation.* G. Steinheil, Paris, 1910.
4. Müller, M. E., Allgower, M., and Willenegger, H.: *Manual of Internal Fixation.* Springer-Verlag, Berlin, 1970.
5. Neufeld, A. J., and Mays, J.: Skeletal traction methods. Clin. Orthop. 102:144–149, 1974.
6. Perkins, G.: Rest and movement. J. Bone Joint Surg. 35B:521–539, 1953.
7. Smith, H. H.: On the treatment of ununited fracture by means of artificial limbs. Am. J. Med. Sci.: January, 1855.
8. Thomas, H. O.: Diseases of the hip, knee and ankle joints and their deformities treated by a new and efficient method. Clin. Orthop. 102:4–9, 1974. (Reprint of the 1876 original.)
9. Watson-Jones, R.: *Fractures and Joint Injuries,* 4th ed. Williams & Wilkins, Baltimore, 1960.

23

Burns

E. Burke Evans, M.D.
Donald H. Parks, M.D., F.R.C.S.(C), F.A.C.S.

Thermal burns mainly affect the skin, and most severely burned persons develop scars and soft tissue contractures that cause transient or permanent limitation of joint motion. A few are affected by direct exposure of bones, joints, and muscles or by later changes in these structures. However, among post-burn changes, it is scar contractures that are the most deforming and have the greatest adverse functional effect. Thus, in all phases of burn care, rehabilitation measures are directed for the greater part toward prevention or correction of contracture and maintenance or restoration of joint motion. We believe that functional care of burns, exclusive of specific life-saving measures and surgical reconstruction, must involve aggressive wound management, efficient positioning and splinting, skeletal suspension and traction, pressure wrapping, early mobilization and exercise, and extended observation.

A burn rehabilitation program, such as that just outlined, requires no special facility. It does require, however, an experienced and dedicated team of physicians, nurses, physical and occupational therapists, aides, and technicians. The program begins when the patient enters the hospital and ends when maximum function is recovered.

WOUND MANAGEMENT

There has been a recent trend in burn care toward early surgical excision of the burn wound.[2,10,13] The advent of newer anesthetic techniques, the availability of blood for transfusion, and increasing support from the multidisciplinary burn team have contributed to the success of excisional therapy. This treatment has led to decreased morbidity in burn patients and allowed earlier wound closure, facilitating and accelerating rehabilitation.

First- and superficial second-degree burn wounds are treated with topical agents and allowed to heal spontaneously. Deep second- and third-degree burns are treated surgically in most circumstances. Three basic techniques are used: tangential excision, tangential debridement, and excision to fascia.

Tangential Excision

Tangential excision applies to deep second-degree burn wounds and is usually performed two to five days following the burn. It involves sequential shaving of layers of burned tissue until uniform pinpoint bleeding is recognized and immediate grafting with split-thickness autografts follows. This technique of early definitive wound closure allows early joint motion, shortens the hospital stay, and probably decreases hypertrophic scar formation.

Tangential Debridement

Tangential debridement involves the sequential shaving of wound eschar in third-degree burns (Fig. 23-7). The procedure is carried out early in the post-burn period when resuscitation has been achieved and the patient shows cardiovascular stability. Following debridement, wounds are dressed with topical antimicrobial-impregnated dressings and biological dressings, such as pigskin or amnion, or autografts. We prefer to apply dressings and follow with daily hydrotherapy or to cover the wounds with biological dressings. The procedure facilitates sloughing, promotes healthy granulations, and permits early autografting.

Excision to Fascia

Excision of the burn wound may be indicated for localized, deep third-degree wounds, such as hot press injuries of the hand, or in full-thickness burns involving 50 percent or more of the body surface, wherein early autografting on an acceptable recipient site is required to reduce the size of the burn.

As soon as the general state permits, patients with open wounds are tubbed daily in hypochlorite or another suitable solution for wound cleansing and dressing change. Tubbing allows early water-supported motion of involved extremities.

With these three techniques, early wound closure is achieved and the period of confinement previously required for spontaneous separation of burned tissue is avoided. From a rehabilitative standpoint, patients can be mobilized and ambulated quickly.

POSITIONING AND SPLINTING

It is the nature of the burn wound to contract and the burned patient to position himself so as to relieve tension on the wound. Therefore, accurate positioning is essential throughout the acute phase of burn treatment, that is, until the wounds

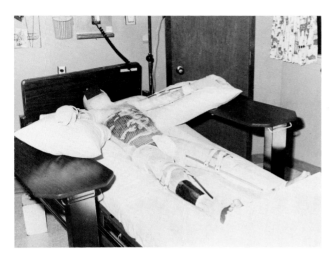

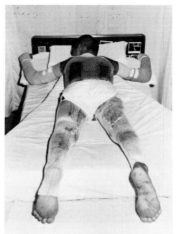

Fig. 23-1. Proper supine positioning of a 16-year-old boy with 60 percent third-degree burns involving neck, trunk, and all extremities. Neck: midline in slight extension. Shoulders: slight scapulothoracic retraction, 80 degrees glenohumeral abduction, and 20 degrees glenohumeral flexion. Elbows: extension. Wrists: neutral or slight extension. Metacarpophalangeal joints (2 through 5): 80 degrees flexion. Proximal and distal interphalangeal joints: full extension. Thumbs: carpometacarpal flexion and abduction, slight metacarpophalangeal flexion, and interphalangeal extension. Spine: straight. Hips: extension, 15 degrees symmetrical abduction, slight external rotation. Knees: extension. Ankles: neutral. Feet: neutral. The patient is wearing an orthoplast neck conformer splint, three-point aluminum and orthoplast splints for elbows and knees, and orthoplast splints for wrists and hands. Ankles and feet are held at neutral against a padded foot box. There is a towel roll between his shoulders. Silver sulfadiazine dressings are held in place by Surgifix tubular net.

Fig. 23-2. Four weeks later the same patient was nursed prone on a 20 cm foam mattress cut to allow arms to drop forward and feet to hang clear of the end. Upper extremities were being actively exercised and wrapped free of splints. Lower extremities required no splints with prone nursing because of gravitational extension of the knees.

have healed and the patient is mobile (Figs. 23-1 and 23-2). Splinting of involved parts may be required for an extended period of time. The matter of positioning and splinting will be considered in relation to specific joints or regions.

Neck, Shoulder, and Upper Chest Burns

Anterior neck, shoulder, and upper chest burns lead to flexion of the neck, elevation and protraction of the scapulae, adduction of the arms, and accentuation of thoracic kyphosis (Fig. 23-3A). The neck should be positioned at neutral or in just a few degrees of extension (Fig. 23-1). With hyperextension, the lips will not easily occlude and the chin will drop, thus defeating the purpose of positioning.

A thermoplastic splint made expressly for the patient may be applied over burn dressings or on stable grafts. The pressure of the conforming splint prevents hypertrophic scar and contracture and will reduce established scar and correct deformity (Figs. 23-4A–C).[11,12,19]

Forward drift of scapulae can be impeded with a firm mattress and a tight

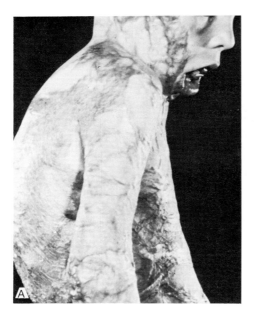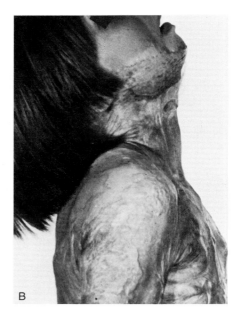

Fig. 23-3. (A) A 10-year-old boy with flexion of the neck, protraction of the scapulae, and accentuation of the thoracic kyphosis due to scar contracture from third-degree burns of the chest, neck, and axillae. (B) Twenty months later there had been surgical release of neck and axillary contractures, after which a conformer orthoplast splint was used to prevent further contracture. The shoulders remain slightly protracted.

towel or felt roll placed vertically between the scapulae. A degree of persisting forward drift is inevitable with severe anterior chest burns (Fig. 23-3B), but the deformity eventually disappears.

Arms are abducted no more than 75–80 degrees in the plane of the scapulae or in 20–30 degrees of flexion (Fig. 23-1). Abduction in the coronal plane places the arm in glenohumeral extension and predisposes the head of the humerus to subluxation. Glenohumeral abduction beyond 80 degrees causes upward rotation and elevation of the scapulae from passive displacement of the scapulae and from the patient's voluntary shrugging to relieve axillary tension. Elevation of the scapulae narrows the shoulders and shortens the neck, accentuating neck contracture.

Axillary contracture can be controlled by firm elastic figure-eight wrapping over 7.5 cm foam padding cut to conform to the axilla (Figs. 23-5A, B).

Torso Burns

When the trunk is burned, the spine must be kept straight (Figs. 23-1 and 23-2). Contracture resulting from asymmetrical burns of the trunk causes a temporary scoliosis. But it is ordinarily corrected when the burn scar has softened or has been surgically relieved. Structural scoliosis will result if contracture is not corrected.

Girdle or groin burns cause flexion and adduction of the thighs. If the patient experiences prolonged flexion and adduction posture, the femoral head may tend

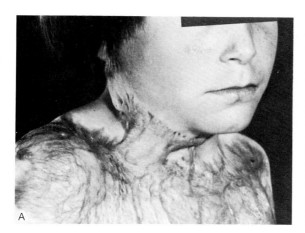
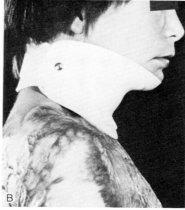
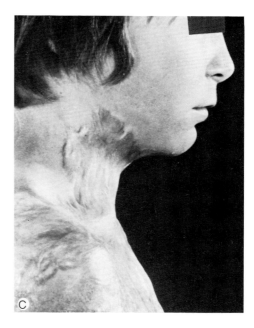

Fig. 23-4. (A) A 7-year-old girl with thick, constrictive, hypertrophic scar of the neck. (B) The scar was treated with orthoplast conformer splint pressure only. (C) After 12 weeks of pressure, the scar is flat, the contour of the neck has been restored, and there is no flexion contracture.

to drift away from the acetabulum. Hips should thus be positioned in extension and in symmetrical abduction of 15–20 degrees.

Burns of the Upper and Lower Extremities

Burns of the extremities, regardless of distribution, tend to cause flexion contractures of elbows and knees. These joints are therefore positioned in full extension. Unarticulated three-point aluminum and thermoplastic splints can be used to maintain extension (Fig. 23-1).[11,12,19] Open splints are preferred to occlusive ones because they are more favorable to wound care. Patients who are voluntarily able to keep their limbs straight can often be managed without splints.

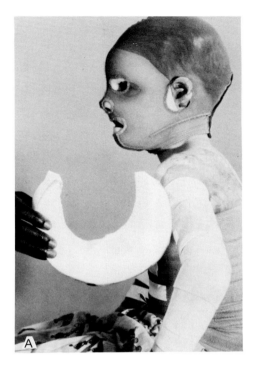
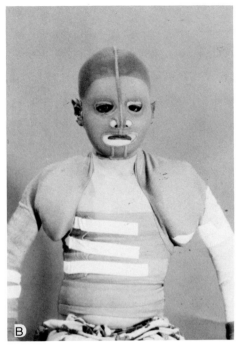

Figs. 23-5A, B. Axillary scar contractures controlled by elastic figure-eight bandages over 7.5 cm foam padding cut to conform to the axillae. The silicone rubber face mask and Jobst elastic head stocking are custom-made.

Ankles of burned patients become plantar-flexed and their feet become inverted. Firm foot boards are needed to hold ankles and feet in neutral position (Fig. 23-1). Established equinus deformity is difficult to correct. Modified surgical boots or fleece-lined shoes permit patients with even severe equinus deformity to ambulate soon. Lengthening of the Achilles tendon is rarely indicated because the muscle is normal although shortened. The deformity corrects with weight-bearing as the scar softens or after scar release. Skeletal traction through a pin placed posteriorly in the calcaneus will often correct an equinus deformity.

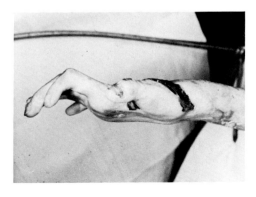

Fig. 23-6. Typical hand deformity in a 10-year-old girl with extensive upper extremity burns. No splint was used in early treatment.

Contractures after dorsal burns of the feet may cause extreme digital extension that will require surgical correction.[9] The deformity can be prevented with toe traction at time of grafting and with shoes with metatarsal bars.

In the usual deformity that occurs from burns of the unsupported forearm, wrist, and hand, the wrist is flexed, the metacarpophalangeal joints of the medial four digits are extended, the proximal interphalangeal joints are flexed, and the distal interphalangeal joints may be flexed or extended. The thumb is in metacarpal adduction and extension, metacarpophalangeal extension or flexion, and interphalangeal flexion. The hands, thus, are much like those of patients with intrinsic muscle loss (Fig. 23-6).

An orthoplast splint applied shortly after the burn will maintain proper position with the wrist neutral or slightly extended, the metacarpophalangeal joints moderately flexed, and the proximal and distal interphalangeal joints extended. The thumb is held in metacarpal abduction and flexion, slight metacarpophalangeal flexion, and interphalangeal extension (Fig. 23-1). The splints are fabricated for each patient.[19] They may be applied over burn dressings or stable grafts (Figs. 23-1 and 23-7A–H).

SKELETAL SUSPENSION AND TRACTION

When extremities are burned extensively, skeletal suspension permits circumferential grafting and dressing of all surfaces, maintains position, and leaves the extremity free for motion, exercise, and tubbing.[4] In the lower extremity, suspension pins may be placed in distal femur, proximal and distal tibia, calcaneus, metatarsals, and digits. In the upper extremity pins may be placed in the olecranon, distal radius, metacarpals, and digits (Figs. 23-7A–H). Pins may be inserted directly through cleaned burned skin, eschar, or granulation tissue. Threaded pins are preferred because they do not slip. Two weeks is the average maximum period of skeletal suspension or traction. In cases of prolonged suspension, cylindrical sequestra may develop and there may be occasional local osteomyelitis that will clear promptly with local debridement and proper antibiotic therapy.

Skeletal traction may be used in the acute phase of burn care to straighten extremities that have developed early positional contractures and cannot be properly positioned by other means. It is used in the later phase of burn care to correct established contractures (Figs. 23-8A–C).[6]

Special skeletal suspension splints have been designed for hands. The splints are anchored proximally with a threaded Steinmann pin in the distal radius. The radial pin is introduced dorsally and removed from the volar surface to avoid entrapment of the radial artery. Digits are controlled with Kirschner wires attached to finger bows and thence by rubber bands to the splint frame. The wires are inserted through the nail and distal phalanx. These splints are used for positioning digits for grafting and for correcting digital contractures (Figs. 23-7C–E).

A more elaborate hay-rake splint, so named because of its design, corrects severe, established contractures alone or in conjunction with surgical release

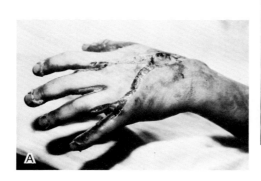
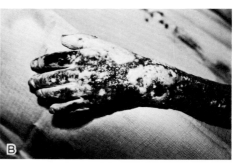
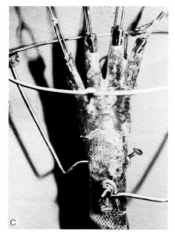
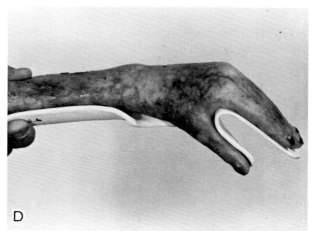

Fig. 23-7. (A) Third-degree burn of the dorsum of the left hand of a 7-year-old boy with third-degree burns on both upper extremities. The escharotomy was performed for relief of tension on the second post-burn day. (B) On the 22nd post-burn day, after a series of tangential debridements, there were healthy bleeding surfaces. (C) The hand was positioned in a halo splint at the time of application of thin split-thickness and mesh autogenous grafts on the 22nd post-burn day. The thumb is in full metacarpal abduction and flexion and is thus not seen. (D) After grafts were stable,

(Figs. 23-9A–C). The hay-rake splint has been modified for use in the foot. The anchor pin is placed in the calcaneus.

Established contractures can be corrected by static splinting. The occupational or physical therapist who makes the orthoplast splints must see the patient often for splint modification and for supervision of active and passive exercise of the extremity.

PRESSURE DRESSINGS

Consistent local pressure of 25 mm mercury or more is effective in preventing hypertrophic scars and contracture and in reducing them once established.[11]

Pressure may be applied with elastic bandages (Figs. 23-5A, B and 23-7E), with special Jobst garments for trunk, extremities, and face, and with orthoplast conforming splints (Figs. 23-3B and 24A–C). Pressure is applied early in the

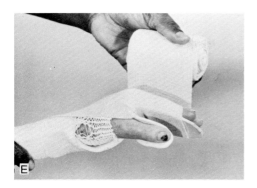

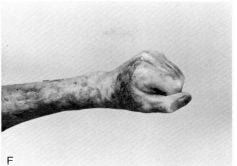

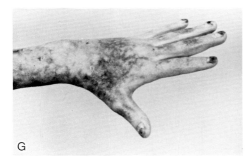

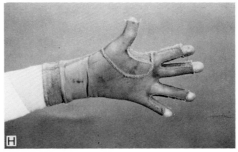

the hand was returned to an orthoplast splint. The wrist is held in neutral, the metacarpophalan-geal joints in flexion, and the interphalangeal joints in extension. The thumb is in metacarpal abduction and flexion and metacarpophalangeal and interphalangeal extension. (E) The splint is wrapped with elastic bandage to hold it snugly in place and distribute pressure evenly. (F,G) Digital range of motion on 46th post-burn day. (H) Jobst glove applied two months after burn.

postgraft period with elastic bandages and splints. Elastic bandages are replaced with Jobst garments when the weight of the patient and the dimension of the affected extremity are stable. Hand splints are applied with a special technique so as to seat the splint well and distribute pressure evenly (Figs. 23-7C–H). For control of scar hypertrophy, pressure must be applied as long as the scar is raised and hyperemic or until the area being treated is soft and flat and approaches normal skin in color.

MOBILIZATION AND EXERCISE

Programmed active, passive, and assistive exercising of both burned and un-burned extremities begins as soon as the general state of the patient permits. If the patient is on a tubbing routine, involved extremities and digits can be moved with

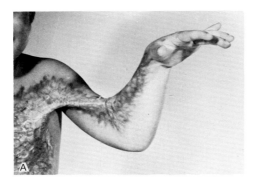
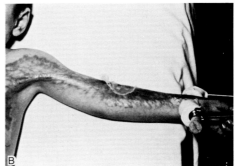
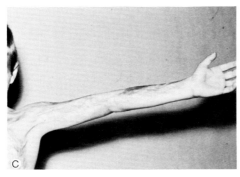

Fig. 23-8. (A) One of two upper extremities with severe axillary and cubital contractures in a 4-year-old boy three months after burn. The scar is still red and hypertrophic. (B) Five days after constant 2.25 kg skeletal traction, the elbow is straight and the axillary contracture is reduced. (C) The appearance three years later. A small local flap was required in the cubital fossa.

water support. Splints should be removed regularly for exercise; digits and extremities in traction should be freed for the same purpose.

Patients may stand and walk prior to grafting, provided burned lower extremities are properly wrapped with elastic bandages. Fresh grafts on the lower extremities will confine a patient to bed, but walking may be resumed as soon as these grafts are stable, which usually occurs on about the tenth post-graft day. Elastic wrapping of the lower extremities is essential (Figs. 23-5A, B).

Because of early mobilization and exercise, the complications of osteoporosis and heterotopic bone formation are now rarely observed.

SPECIAL PROBLEMS

Formation of Heterotopic Bone

Heterotopic bone occurs infrequently but it seriously affects the function of those few patients who develop it. Joint motion may be limited or completely blocked by heterotopic bone formation. This phenomenon has been observed most often in patients with third-degree burns involving 30 percent or more of body surface.[5-7] When it occurs, it will tend to increase in dimension until the burn wound has healed, following which, if it has not bridged the joint, it will decrease in dimension. In children it may completely disappear. If heterotopic bone remains to ankylose a joint or to interfere with its motion, it can usually be successfully excised.[4,5] If it involves the pericapsular structures in more than one

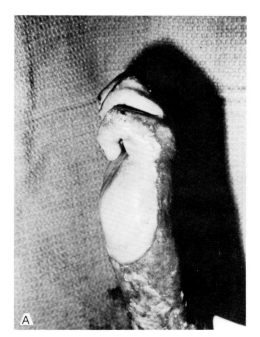
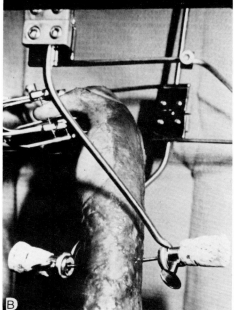
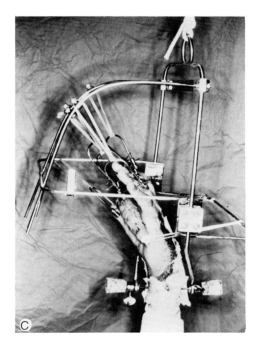

Figs. 23-9 A, B, and C. Severe metacarpophalangeal and digital contractures in an 11-year-
old boy were corrected in 11 days in a hay-rake
splint. As correction proceeded, the traction
collars were advanced up the curved rods to
bring the digits into the fully extended position.
Palmar resistance was accomplished through a
tapered cork anchored on the posterior bar.

plane, the chances for mobilization of the joint by surgical means are proportionately diminished.

Heterotopic bone is important to monitor in rehabilitating burns for more
than its compromise of function. There is good, although anecdotal, evidence in

our experience and that of others[15] that superimposed trauma or early, over-aggressive, passive mobilization of joints in burned persons predisposed to heterotopic bone formation will lead to its rapid proliferation in the pericapsular structures damaged by the forced motion. Thus passive mobilization of burned extremities should not be forceful, particularly when there are open wounds.

Exposed Joints

The knee and the elbow and the proximal interphalangeal joints of the medial four fingers are likely to be exposed on their extensor surfaces to full-thickness burns. The measures taken to preserve these joints are simple. The joint is held in extension by skeletal traction or by external splint (Figs. 23-10A–C). The joint is irrigated daily in the tub with hypochlorite solution and is progressively debrided. Dead bone at the knees and elbows is removed and exposed bone is drilled as indicated. Granulation tissue eventually bridges the joint, so it is possible to apply a split-thickness autogenous graft.

The joints of adolescents and children managed this way will remain functional. Exposed joints in adults are not always so forgiving. In children and adults, ankylosis may occur or operative fusion may be necessary.

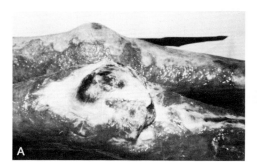
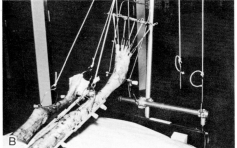

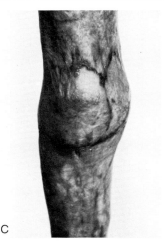

Fig. 23-10. (A) The right knee joint and proximal tibia were exposed by a full-thickness burn in a 12-year-old girl. The knee joint and surrounding granulation tissue were suppurant at the time of admission. (B) After six weeks of daily tubbing in hypochlorite solution and regular lavage and debridement, autogenous grafts were placed on healthy granulation tissue, bridging the joint. Throughout this time, the extremity was skeletally suspended, the knee was held in extension with an adjustable external metal splint transfixed to bone with Steinmann pins, and the foot positioned for grafting with a modified hay-rake splint. The exposed bone required tangential partial decortication to punctate bleeding and encourage granulation tissue, which was then covered with skin grafts. (C) Two years later, knee function is satisfactory with weak quadriceps. It was protected by a brace for six months.

Septic arthritis of hematogenous origin in burn cases may be difficult to detect because of the overlying burn and already existing septicemia. Once the condition is recognized, the joint should be opened widely and regularly irrigated. The management from then on is the same as for joints exposed at the time of the burn.

Fractures

Fractures of extremities occurring at the time of a severe burn are managed with skeletal traction if the affected extremity has a third- or deep second-degree burn. Although skeletal traction interferes with mobilization, treatment can otherwise be carried out as usual.

Amputations

The level of amputation in thermal burns is determined by the lack of viability of the part, not by the level of full-thickness burn. Split-thickness grafts mature well under prostheses. Thus, the stump should be left as long as the muscles will allow. A grafted stump may break down along the edges of grafts where scars remain friable, but these scars will respond favorably to the pressure of a well-fitted socket.

The problem is quite different in electrical burns. The skin may survive, whereas the muscle will die from proximal disintegration of damaged blood vessels. The amputation level is determined nonetheless by the viability of muscle. Extremity loss is the most serious functional consequence of electrical burns. Once the amputations have been performed, rehabilitation measures are the same as for any amputee.

Other Musculoskeletal Changes

Other musculoskeletal changes affect function adversely, but they occur infrequently. The following list, categories of skeletal changes that can accompany burns, is drawn from the literature.[4,5]

Alterations limited to bone:

> Osteoporosis[2,3,7,14]
> Periosteal new-bone formation
> Irregular ossification
> Diaphyseal exostoses
> Acromutilation of fingers[16]
> Pathological fractures[5]
> Osteomyelitis[5]
> Necrosis and tangential sequestration

Alterations involving pericapsular structures:

> Pericapsular calcification
> Heterotopic para-articular ossification
> Osteophytes

Alterations involving the joint proper:

>   Dislocation
>   Septic arthritis[5]
>   Spontaneous dissolution
>   Ankylosis

Alterations involving muscles and tendons:

>   Desiccation of tendons
>   Fibrosis of muscles[18]

Alterations secondary to soft tissue contractures:

>   Muscle contractures
>   Malposition of joints
>   Scoliosis

Abnormalities of growth:[1,8,17]

>   Acceleration
>   Destruction of growth plate

Nonviability of extremity leading to amputation

RECURRENCE OF DEFORMITY

We cannot state too strongly that closely supervised rehabilitation programming for severely burned persons, and even for those with limited but critically located burns, must begin as soon as possible after the burn. It must continue until all scars are soft and pliant and the patient can easily manage his own program. Family members must be coached by therapists in exercise routines and in the proper use and application of splints and pressure wraps or garments. Any interruption of a program while scar is still active, thick, or red will lead to recurrence of deformity or even to its development where none previously existed.

REFERENCES

1. Artz, C. P., and Moncrief, J. A.: *The Treatment of Burns,* 2nd ed. W. B. Saunders, Philadelphia, 1969.
2. Burke, J. F., Bondoc, C. C., and Quinby, W. C.: Primary burn excision and immediate grafting: A method of shortening illness. J. Trauma 14:389–395, 1974.
3. Colson, P., Stagnara, P., and Houot H.: L'ostéoporose chez les brûlés des membres. Lyon Chir. 48:950–956, 1953.
4. Evans, E. B.: Orthopaedic measures in the treatment of severe burns. J. Bone Joint Surg. 48A:643–669, 1966.
5. Evans, E. B.: Musculoskeletal changes complicating burns. In Epps, C. H., Jr., Ed.: *Complications in Orthopcedic Surgery,* vol. 2, pp. 1133–1158. J. B. Lippincott, Philadelphia, 1978.

6. Evans, E. B., Larson, D. L., Abston, S., and Willis, B.: Prevention and correction of deformity after severe burns. Surg. Clin. North Am. 50:1361–1375, 1970.

7. Evans, E. B., and Smith, J. R.: Bone and joint changes following burns. J. Bone Joint Surg. 41A:785–799, 1959.

8. Frantz, C. H., and Delgado, S.: Limb-length discrepancy after third-degree burns about the foot and ankle. J. Bone Joint Surg. 48A:443–450, 1966.

9. Heimberger, R. A., Marten, E., Larson, D. L., et al.: Burned feet in children—acute and reconstructive care. Am. J. Surg. 125:575–579, 1973.

10. Janzekovic, Z.: A new concept in the early excision and immediate grafting of burns. J. Trauma 10:1103–1108, 1970.

11. Larson, D. L., Abston, S., Evans, E. B., et al.: Techniques for decreasing scar formation and contractures in the burned patient. J. Trauma 11:807–823, 1971.

12. Larson, D. L., Abston, S., Willis, B., et al.: Contracture and scar formation in the burn patient. Clin. Plast. Surg. 1:653–666, 1974.

13. Mahler, D., and Watson, J.: The early excision of burns. Burns 1:65–69, 1974–1975.

14. Owens, N.: Osteoporosis following burns. Br. J. Plast. Surg. 1:245–256, 1949.

15. Pruitt, B. A.: Personal communication.

16. Rabinov, D.: Acromutilation of the fingers following severe burns. Radiology 77:968–973, 1961.

17. Ritsila, V., Sundell, B., and Alhopuro, S.: Severe growth retardation of the upper extremity resulting from burn contracture and its full recovery after release of the contracture. Br. J. Plast. Surg. 29:53–58, 1976.

18. Salisbury, R. E., McKeel, D. W., and Mason, A. D.: Ischemic necrosis of the intrinsic muscles of the hand after thermal injuries. J. Bone Joint Surg. 56A:1701–1707, 1974.

19. Willis, B. A., Larson, D. L., and Abston, S.: Positioning and splinting the burned patient. Heart Lung 2:696–700, 1973.

24

Amputations of the Upper Extremities

Robert D. Keagy, M.D.

The ideal goal of rehabilitation of the patient with upper extremity disease or injury is the restoration of full, normal, bimanual capabilities.

The upper extremities have value to the human in three spheres: the prehension and positioning of objects; the perception of touching and being touched; and the cosmetic values of symmetry of form and softness of contact. The ability to grip and feel is commonly understood and accepted. The need for symmetry of form and softness for human contact is less commonly appreciated. The combined assets of the extremity are needed to achieve activities of self-care, household tasks, and occupational duties. When disease or injury damages any or all of these capabilities, rehabilitation is needed. Amputation represents a combined loss of form, function, and feeling.

Amputation can occur traumatically and be an accomplished fact before the patient presents himself to the physician. Frequently, however, the patient presents with his extremity present but so diseased or damaged that restoration of function, feeling, and form will not be possible. The natural, initial tendency is to be concerned with restoration of form as the basic requirement to the restoration of function and feeling. However, scarring and denervation can produce an extremity that is functionless, insensitive, and stiff. These problems can completely subvert any cosmetic or emotional value of the retained extremity. At this point, elective amputation may disencumber the patient of a burdensome appendage.

Decisions concerning elective amputation can be greatly facilitated if the attending physician is familiar with the capabilities and problems of amputees and the use of prostheses. Generally, this is best achieved by personal observation of amputees. It cannot be attained by simply studying the components of artificial limbs or the techniques of amputation surgery.

There are limits to the use of prostheses. First, it is important to consider whether the amputation is unilateral or bilateral, and, if unilateral, whether the remaining extremity is the dominant or nondominant one. The activities of daily living concerning self-care, as well as many household and occupational tasks, can be well performed with one hand if it is the dominant hand. Many assistive devices are available to abet the one-handed person. Some patients are sufficiently ambidextrous to be able to convert their dominance, and others can appreciably upgrade the performance of the originally nondominant hand with the skilled assistance of an occupational therapist.

Despite one-handed skills and the availability of assistive devices for the one-handed, there are many tasks that require two hands, for example, the use of a zipper or paper clip. The exigencies of daily living are such that the need for bimanual activity is recurrent through the day. At these times, the unilateral amputee may find the grasp capabilities of a prosthesis to be a useful "helping hand." The prosthetic split hook can be so useful that patients accept and use it regularly despite its definite lack of cosmetic form.

These considerations help to explain why almost all bilateral amputees use their prostheses and why some unilateral amputees do not use any prosthesis.

Additional considerations concerning the use of prostheses involve "fit" and cosmesis. Before an amputee will use a prosthesis, there must be a comfortable fit of the stump in the socket. Therefore, the surgical considerations that lead to nontender, easily fitted stumps, as well as the prosthetic techniques to achieve socket congruence and tolerance have a significance in terms of ultimate rehabilitation.

All patients initially picture a completely cosmetic limb. They cannot appreciate that form without function is rarely adequately cosmetic. Yet only an occasional patient will continue to wear a purely cosmetic arm or hand for very long or in private. However, if even the simplest cosmetic arm has a passively positionable elbow and a stable socket, the prosthetic hand can be usefully employed as a "paperweight" to stabilize writing materials, to carry a purse, coat, or umbrella, or to act as a backstop to stabilize objects for the remaining hand.

To rehabilitate the amputee prosthetically, the residual limb must have maximal joint excursion and strength. Optimal selection of the level of the amputation and appropriately prompt initiation of exercise will maximize the rehabilitation potential of the patient.

Optimum rehabilitation starts immediately after the patient is injured or the disease is recognized. Rehabilitation is a sequence of processes simultaneously pertinent to the injured or diseased part and to the patient as a whole entity. All elements of treatment are a part of the process and must be chosen and applied in terms compatible with the whole patient as well as the residual limb. Rehabilitation may require surgery, even amputation, as a prime step in reducing residual dysfunction and restoring ability. Because no normally useful part is ever amputated, it is illogical to refer to the rehabilitation of an amputee as if the amputation were the primary problem rather than a part of the rehabilitation process. To approach amputation as a salvage procedure is pejorative.[1] The onerous concept of salvage too frequently causes the entire medical team to behave as if the amputation were a disaster, and this, in turn, colors the whole course of the rehabilitation process. When appropriately applied, amputation is a rescue procedure that starts the rehabilitation process. Both the patient and the team can improve their outlook if they realize that the major initial step to rehabilitation of the patient may have been the definitive amputation operation.

Rehabilitation is a time-related problem. Each step in the sequential process succeeds best if it is timely. Delays lead to stiffness, atrophy, loss of skills, discouragement, and loss of morale. A delay at one point in the process usually means that each subsequent step in treatment will be more lengthy and possibly less successful.

Initial approaches to the traumatically damaged limb should be conservative in terms of saving functional units rather than just saving viable tissue. Amputation decisions and procedures should leave a residual limb that retains maximum function and not just maximum tissue. A conservative approach to the damaged upper extremity, which zealously applies surgical technology, can salvage unusable tissue and parts. If the residual limb is stiff, tender, or insensate in any part, the use of the entire limb will be compromised. If initial attempts to save functioning tissue fail, amputation may be the optimum way to re-initiate the rehabilitation process.

Conservatism in terms of tissue salvage is not wise in itself. Wise conservatism is a more sophisticated goal. The wisdom is to provide the most useful residual limb, rather than simply saving everything that can be saved without concern for further use capability. Salvage without function is a technical fraud. The operation may succeed, but the patient will fail.

Kindly considerations of future cosmesis, body image, and performance capabilities are difficult to balance. Figure 24-1 illustrates a patient who suffered electrical burns to both upper extremities. The left, nondominant arm was amputated initially. Extensive efforts were expended to salvage the right arm, which was, in the end, simply stiff, anesthetic, and useless below the shoulder. This patient could be much more competent if he were converted to the status of a bilateral, above-elbow amputee.

The patient who has had an amputation has innumerable reasons to be discouraged. He has probably not previously had any real familiarity with another amputee. Lacking the opportunity to observe other amputees, there is heightened receptivity to the lore of the streets, which tends to propagate depression or induce bionic fantasies.

Attendance at an amputee clinic offers the patient several real benefits, not the least of which is the opportunity to observe many other amputees, newcomers as well as more accomplished individuals. The feeling of being alone is dissipated. The patient acquires precedents for achievement techniques and levels of accomplishment. The word of the surgeon is now reinforced by visible, tangible examples.

Simultaneously, the fact of a clinic allows the clinic team to develop an expertise based on experience. The several disciplines not only serve the patient in an organized fashion, but also serve each other by an interaction of the disciplines in broadening knowledge and developing new techniques.

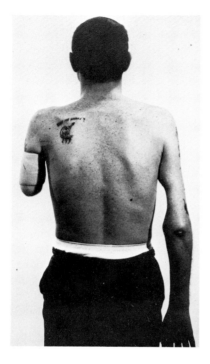

Fig. 24-1. Retained right upper extremity has lost all innervation below the shoulder. It is stiff, insensate, and encumbering.

The optimal clinic team consists of an orthopedic surgeon, a physiatrist, an occupational therapist, a physical therapist, a prosthetist, and a social worker.

The orthopedist provides information and evaluation of the patient from the standpoint of the surgical past and possibilities for the future. The physiatrist and therapist lend their skills to training and use problems. The prosthetist contributes knowledge of materials, components, and fitting techniques.

The social worker is usually the team member who resolves the emotional problems of the patient and the family, and solves the socioeconomic problems of procuring funding for the rehabilitation process. Psychological counseling and vocational counseling are additional services that are frequently needed. No individual physician or therapist can know or achieve enough to meet the highly individualized needs of every amputee.

The initial prescription is usually formulated by combining the surgeon's knowledge of the residual limb with the prosthetist's knowledge of fitting techniques, the characteristics of various prosthetic components, and available materials. The therapist's awareness of the patient's pre-prosthetic performance capabilities can help to establish attainable goals for the amputee through the use of his prosthesis.

If the amputating surgeon chooses not to formulate and coordinate a prescription and the necessary training, it would be well to refer the patient to an amputee clinic. The clinic should be considered a resource to which responsibility is delegated, rather than a place to which a patient is relegated. The greatest disservice that can be done to a patient is simply to remove the final dressing and send him off to look for an artificial limb without provision for prescription, training, or follow-up.

GENERAL PRINCIPLES PERTINENT TO AMPUTATION SURGERY

Certain principles of surgery apply to amputations at any level.

Skin Flaps

Skin flaps are planned so that the net length, after skin retraction has occurred, will equal the diameter of the limb at the site of the proposed transection. This requires some surgical judgment to estimate skin turgor and elasticity, but that is part of surgery. One should allow for additional length to accommodate the thickness of the subcutaneous fat. Actual scar placement is not often a problem if there is any subcutaneous tissue between the bone and the skin. Exceptions to this rule will be given as each level is discussed.

When the outlined skin flaps are incised, the skin and subcutaneous tissues retract. The deep fascia is incised in line with and at the level to which the skin has retracted. Muscles and tendons are transected transversely so they will retract to a point just about 0.5 cm distal to the planned site of bone transection.

Periosteum and Bone Section

The periosteum of the bone is incised with a sharp knife. Periosteum should be stripped only distally in order that spurs of periosteal new bone will not form in the stump. The bone is easily transected with a sharp handsaw. If a power saw is used, the blade and bone should be copiously cooled with irrigating fluid to prevent burning the bone and causing a "ring" sequestrum to form on the retained bone end. If the bone ends will not have reasonably thick coverage by soft tissue, the margins may be rasped to avoid sharp edges. Before doing this, however, the periosteum should be resected 0.5 cm more proximally to avoid mechanical induction of a periosteal response with the rasp.

Nerve and Neuroma

A neuroma always forms at the end of a cut nerve. There is no way to prevent this, although there have been innumerable efforts to do so. All amputees have a neuroma on each cut nerve. However, a neuroma, although usually detectable on examination, is uncommon as a cause of trouble for the amputee. Pressure on a neuroma causes discomfort and dysesthesias radiating into the originally inner-vated area of the phantom. The fibers in the neuroma are predominantly fibers that transmit pain. However, even a painful or touchy neuroma never causes a stocking or glove pattern of pain referral or diffuse stump tenderness. Neuroma problems are just as definitely identifiable in a residual limb as they are in an intact limb because the dysesthesia resulting from pressure is referred into the original nerve pattern in the phantom limb.

Neuromas should not be spoken of as of some abstract, unmanageable evil. They usually give trouble only if adherent to the end of a bone, or if they are placed at a socket brim level or at a site of major force transmission in the stump.

Most neuromas can be accommodated in the prosthesis by providing a slightly hollowed area of relief in the socket.

It is easier to handle the stump if the nerves are cut to make neuromas form away from the bone end and deep within muscle. Troublesome neuromas most commonly occur in partial hand amputations. The troublesome neuroma can be treated by resection and repositioning into deeper tissue. Neuromas of the ulnar nerve below the elbow can be treated by resection of the nerve at any site above the elbow, allowing the stump to remain undisturbed.

Wound Closure

Blood vessels require only ordinary ligation adequate for the size of the vessel. The wound can be closed in layers, approximating the deep fascia, the subcutaneous tissue, and skin. A drain should be left beneath the deep fascia. A compression dressing should be applied in surgery. More will be said of this in the section on stump care.

Split skin grafts are quite durable within a prosthesis, providing they are not adherent to bone or tendons. Well placed, that is, over fatty tissue or muscle bellies, they give little trouble, even inside sockets. Bone ends or other exposed bone should not be covered with split grafts. Local skin flaps should be used to cover the bone ends, leaving split graft coverage for muscular areas. The amputated part is sometimes a good source of split or free full-thickness grafts. Pedicle skin flaps can be used to produce wound closure, but the fat of the trunk is relatively unstable on the stump, and changes in body weight will cause unequal weight gain in the flap on the stump. The time required for the stump to be attached to the torso can lead to stiffness of all of the joints of the extremity.

Transverse circular (Guillotine) amputations frequently result from trauma. Additional resection of enough bone to permit primary closure with local skin can result in major shortening. Whenever the stump cannot be closed primarily, skin traction can be used, sometimes with local undermining of the skin edges to stretch the surrounding skin and thus produce gradual closure. Wound contraction does not occur in the extremities in the first few weeks after injury. The initial reaction of all of the tissues is progressive retraction unless the wound is closed. However, if skin traction is applied and maintained more or less continuously, a marvelous closure can result without additional surgery.

Skin traction is accomplished by applying any medical adhesive to the skin for several centimeters proximal to the wound edges. A stockinette is rolled up onto the cemented area. Dressings must be applied to the open wound through a slit in the stockinette. The whole stump is then wrapped with an elastic bandage and 1.35–2.25 kg of traction weight is then applied to the end of the stockinette. Gradual stretching of the skin will occur and the wound will close in approximately six weeks. The skin of the resulting closure will have good sensation. This traction need not be bed-confining or continuous. The patient may unhook the traction to go to the bathroom or to physical therapy for range of motion or strengthening exercises. Skin traction should also be used when there is tension on a sutured wound.

COMPLICATIONS

Choking of the stump is the most common and pernicious preventable complication in the postoperative period. It occurs when the stump is more compressed proximally than distally. This unfavorable pressure differential, aggravated by dependency, results in terminal swelling, induration, erythema, and even vesication of the stump. Edema fluid will ooze through the wound. On palpation, the stump feels like an orange on the end of a broomstick. The erythema, induration, oozing, and tenderness suggest infection.

Treatment consists of providing compression to the end of the stump with lesser degrees of compression more proximally. Elevation of the limb helps but cannot be used much in an ambulatory patient.

The time-honored technique of applying graduated pressure to the stump is done with an elastic bandage wrap. The turns of the bandage are applied obliquely, never circumferentially. A properly applied dressing always extends well above the joint proximal to the surgical site. Since the greatest compression (tolerable pressure) is applied to the terminal end of the residual limb, the dressing will tend to slip off after a few hours. It must, then, be reapplied to re-establish the compression gradient.

The compression dressing has an additional function besides that of controlling edema: it facilitates the shrinkage of the subcutaneous and intramuscular fatty tissue. Such tissues always shrink under compression, and since the socket of a prosthesis will apply pressure, the stump must be preshrunk before the definitive socket is fitted. Failure to preshrink the stump will result in a misfitting, loose socket shortly after fitting and training begin. This is expensive and new sockets or socket adjustments cause delays in what should be a natural sequence of events. Optimum wrapping techniques produce a stump that is ready for definitive fitting at three to six weeks. Even after the definitive socket is fitted, the stump should be wrapped at night or whenever the socket is not worn for at least three more weeks.

Rigid dressings in the form of socket-like plaster casts can be superior to an elastic wrap. The rigid dressing can simultaneously control edema, splint and protect the wound, and induce shrinkage.

A rigid dressing is usually applied over a light wound dressing by using a five-ply, wool stump sock and one or two rolls of elastic plaster. The anterior trim line at the elbow should be cut low enough to permit elbow flexion. If the end of the stump is larger in circumference than the mid portion, as in wrist and elbow disarticulations, the socket may be self-suspending. At any rate, it cannot then be simply slipped off over the end. However, being light and easily fashioned, a new cast can be made in just a few minutes whenever one becomes loose.

The problem of suspending the socket is very important because if the rigid dressing slips distally, there will not be compression on the end of the stump, and terminal swelling will occur just as with any other dressing. A prosthetic harness can be used for suspension of the plaster cast. The harness still permits removal for wound inspection or, as the stump shrinks, the addition of extra stump socks to restore snugness.

Immediate post-surgical fitting pertains to the provision of a prosthesis in the operation room. Childress et al.[3] fitted patients at surgery with temporary myoelectric prostheses for below-elbow amputations. The patients were able to use the electric hand remarkably well as soon as they recovered from anesthesia. Nevertheless, immediate postoperative fitting has not been widely practiced on the upper extremity, since use of the prosthesis (particularly body-powered, cable-controlled devices) requires forces between the socket and the end of the stump that may be too painful to be practical in the immediate postoperative period. The biggest problem with immediate fitting, besides the added weight of the device on a new wound and stump, is that, at three months, no significant difference exists between patients with an immediate postoperative fit and those who merely have had good care in a rigid dressing. Rigid dressings are the most regularly useful part of the immediate fitting technique.[10]

SURGICAL DECISIONS AND LEVELS

The performance capabilities of a hand are so valuable that the surgeon tries to avoid losing any functional part. However, it is function, not form, that is ultimately useful and finally cosmetic. Considerations of salvage must be primarily related to future function, rather than the preservation of form.

The Partial Hand

If part of a hand is mobile and sensate, while another part of the same hand is insensate, tender, or not mobile, only the mobile, sensate part of the hand will be used. Such hands are rarely cosmetic or functionally acceptable even if all of the components are present. The use of the hand is often compromised and the patient encumbered by the need to avoid or protect the rest of the hand. At times, the removal of such stiff, insensate, or tender parts will disencumber the patient and appreciably enhance the patient's performance capabilities.

The Carpometacarpal Level

Carpometacarpal amputation leaves a long stump and is not better than a wrist disarticulation in a laborer. It is very useful, especially on the dominant side, for bilateral amputees or patients accustomed to precision hand work.

If possible, the bases of the second and third metacarpals should be saved because they bear the insertions of the wrist's major control tendons. If these metacarpals are completely gone, an effort should be made to reattach the wrist extensors and flexors to the distal row of carpal bones.

If the carpal bones are covered with good skin and the carpal area is free of neuromas, the carpal stump may be fitted with a small prosthetic cap suspended from a forearm cuff by flexible Dacron hinges. The terminal device can be a hand or a hook permanently mounted on the small cap and controlled by the usual prosthetic harness. The preservation of wrist flexion and extension, along with full pronation and supination, gives great freedom and permits very precise positioning of the terminal device of the prosthesis, which is of use not only for fine work, but also for self-care.

Amputation at the midcarpal level is not useful. It produces a wrist disarticulation that is too long. Such stumps can be fitted, but the patients would be better served if the proximal row of carpal bones were excised.

Wrist Disarticulation

Wrist disarticulation is a very useful level. The amputee can usually achieve about 50 degrees of active pronation and supination in a well-fitted prosthesis. This is a very real contribution to the patient's performance possibilities.

During most usage situations, the elbow is flexed to some extent to place the hand forward. The weight of the hand and forearm is supported by the elbow flexors acting about the rotation center of the elbow joint. The weight of the prosthetic socket is carried on the volar and radial surface of the stump. It is important to have good skin on this surface.

Wrist disarticulation is accomplished by forming adequate flaps for closure and transecting the tendons to allow them to retract to the level of the bone ends. Because there are no muscle bellies to cushion the bone ends, neuromas can be troublesome. The median and ulnar nerves should be gently pulled distally and transected so that the cut nerve ends will retract proximally to a site about 5 cm above the bone ends. The small sensory branches of the radial nerve and the palmar cutaneous branch of the median nerve should be identified and similarly transected.

Articular cartilage should not be disturbed. The ulnar styloid can be resected and smoothed usefully, and the tip of the radial styloid can be rounded off and the cut bone edges smoothed. The radioulnar joint should not be disturbed because pronation-supination motions may become painful.

Forearm Amputations

Amputation through the forearm can be accomplished at any level. The major force reactions between the stump and a socket will occur on the volar-radial area, and reasonable attention should be given to cover this surface with good skin, placing grafts elsewhere, if possible. "Useful" length is that portion of the forearm that is distal to the biceps tendon when the elbow is flexed 90 degrees. A minimum of 2.5 cm of bone covered by healthy skin is necessary at this area to achieve reasonable prosthetic function. If the residual will provide less than this length, the biceps tendon should be released from the radius and allowed to retract. The brachialis can adequately flex the stump, and performance will be better than an elbow disarticulation or an above-elbow level. This pertains to arms that are not massively obese. If, despite the biceps release, there will not be 2.5 or more cm of forearm surface distal to the antecubital crease, then the radius and ulna should be completely resected to the elbow disarticulation level, which will be much less trouble to the amputee than the "too short," below-elbow level.

At the below-elbow levels, skin flaps can be fashioned in any convenient way, but, if possible, placing the scar on the volar or lateral aspects of the distal radius should be avoided. As is customary, the skin flaps are outlined and allowed to retract, while the fascia is cut on the line to which the skin flaps retract. Muscle resection proceeds as usual, except that enough of the flexor sublimis can sometimes be saved to pull it (and only it) over the bone ends to attach it to the dorsal fascia. Suturing more muscle over the bone ends is unnecessary and sometimes troublesome.

MYOELECTRIC DEVICES

Myoelectric devices are most useful for the below-elbow amputee. Good and regularly useful systems are available through certified prosthetic facilities. There are electric hands in male, female, and child sizes. The motor and batteries are usually in the wrist area. This makes the device heavy, and a good lifting surface of sound skin with adequate stump length is essential for satisfactory use. The optimum length is at the distal third of the forearm. Electrodes are placed in the wall of the socket so that they contact the skin over the flexor and extensor muscles of the forearm. The circuitry provides that impulses received from the flexor mass will cause the prosthetic hand to close, while impulses from the extensor muscles will cause the hand to open.

Since contact with the skin must be good, the socket must fit well, and the fit cannot vary. A stump sock cannot be used. Therefore the amputee should initially be fitted with a conventional body-powered, cable-controlled prosthesis. After it has been worn for six months, definitive shrinkage will have occurred and tenderness largely abated. The stump will be mature. Then a definitive myoelectric device can be fitted. Myoelectric devices work only if the patient produces a good signal for the electrodes to detect. The patient should be "myotested" before hopes are raised or a prosthesis ordered.

Distant myoelectric sites are not generally used now because the net result is not superior to a switch-controlled device or to body-powered cable systems.

After the prehension release mechanism of the electric hand, the next most useful electric device is a wrist rotator. The usual control mechanism is pronation and supination of the stump against mechanical switches within the below-elbow socket. A wrist rotator working on mechanical switches can be used in the same socket with a myoelectric terminal device. The stump must be long enough (mid- or distal forearm) to support the extra weight of these devices.

Myoelectric hands are very useful for light activity. However, the cosmetic cover is not durable and the machinery will not permit heavy use. Most male below-elbow amputees should have two prostheses; one cable-driven with a hook for heavy duty use and the other a myoelectric prosthesis with a hand for lighter uses.

The below-elbow amputee is the only person for whom a good myoelectric system is regularly used. Experimentation is under way at several centers on electric elbows, but the present units are slow, noisy, and drain the batteries rapidly. Other experiments pertain to myoelectric control sites. Proportional control of the electric motor is now a reality.[2] New studies report the use of patterns of electromyographic activity to produce more control modes than there are pick-up sites.[5] This technique requires a small computer to be worn at the waist but will permit control of multifunctional prostheses from relatively limited pick-up points.

Elbow Disarticulation

Disarticulation at the elbow differs little from other amputation techniques. Because major interactions between the stump and the socket will occur at the anterior distal end of the stump, the flaps should be fashioned to position the scar on the posterior aspect of the stump, if possible. The biceps and triceps tendons can be sutured together and both covered and anchored by turning a flap of the brachioradialis from lateral to medial and attaching it to the medial epicondylar ridge in order to pad the end of the humerus. The median and ulnar nerves should be sectioned 5 cm above the bone end.

Above-Elbow Amputation

If an above-elbow stump is not longer than 5 cm below the anterior axillary fold, it cannot be fitted with an above-elbow prosthesis and will require a shoulder disarticulation type of prosthesis. This length is necessary because the mass of the hand and forearm is such that forward placement of the hand in relation to the shoulder axis, for example, elbow flexion, will exert, gravitationally, an extension movement at the shoulder. This is ordinarily resisted by the shoulder flexors acting through the humerus. For the above-elbow amputee, forward hand placement requires not only scapulohumeral flexors, but an adequate area for force transmission between the anterior aspect of the residual limb and the socket. Although the required reaction force can be reduced prosthetically by using lightweight forearm, wrist, and terminal device components, minimally efficient force transmission by the stump within the socket requires that at least 5 cm of humerus be present distal to the anterior axillary fold. This level is just distal to the insertion of the deltoid. This minimum level is as high as one can resect the humerus and yet restore the patient to useful function with an above-elbow prosthesis.

The need for adequate, pain-free, force transmission requires that the surgeon provide good muscle padding and skin coverage on the anterior aspect of the humerus. Flaps may be rotated, if necessary, so that scars and split grafts occur elsewhere. Nerve resection in the arm should place the neuromas medially or posteriorly, never anteriorly. The median and ulnar nerve sections should be staggered to avoid a large confluent neuroma. The neuromas should be placed well away from the scar and the bone end.

The standard anterior and posterior fish-mouth flaps are quite satisfactory. However, the scar may be anywhere if it is separated from the anterior surface of the humerus by muscle and if no nerve is adherent to it.

Shoulder Level Amputations

If amputation requires resection of the humerus above the anterior axillary fold, the patient will have a functional disability equivalent to a shoulder disarticulation. However, retention of the proximal humerus will retain the symmetry of the shoulder girdle and is quite desirable from a cosmetic standpoint. The deltoid should be attached over the end of the humerus to the serratus. This placement gives a nicely acceptable configuration to the stump, because the presence of the humeral head beneath the acromion gives the shoulder fullness, and a cosmetic shoulder cap is rarely necessary (Fig. 24-2). Such patients can wear clothes well without any prosthesis. However, if the insertions of the pectoralis major and the latissimus dorsi are not preserved, the residual humerus will abduct and distort the stump. This situation should be prevented by rearrangement of residual musculature to avoid unwarranted abduction or flexion.

The need for an anatomical shoulder disarticulation poses several difficult problems for the surgeon. Vasconcelos[11] describes shoulder disarticulation as an "orthopedic failure" and considers it a "bad operation." The unmodified residual of the operation is generally quite unsightly. The shoulder and scapulothoracic muscles atrophy, leaving the bony acromion and coracoid protruding beneath the skin. The residual is unlovely in the bedroom and is not sufficiently full to cause clothing to hang symmetrically. At the least, a cosmetic shoulder cap will be required. Any scar or skin graft over the acromion can cause trouble due to tenderness or a tendency to break down if a functional prosthesis is worn. The coracoid process can also become quite tender if it is allowed to become prominent or if the cutaneous scar adheres to it.

Nevertheless, the scapula is highly mobile if the serratus anterior, pectoralis minor, and trapezius muscles are intact and scapulothoracic motion is unrestricted by adherent scars. This mobility permits movement of the acromion within a prosthetic shoulder cap to be used to activate switches of an electrically powered arm. Such devices are currently experimental but may well become practical within the lifetime of a young amputee. Switch-controlled electric hands and wrist rotators are available, but a dependable electric elbow is not. Generally, a passive cosmetic arm with passively positioned joints is indicated in an appropriately motivated young patient and may permit him to pursue light activities.

If the use of an electric arm is not reasonably probable, as in patients older than 30 years of age or with resections of the nondominant arm, then the residual shoulder should be made as cosmetically smooth as possible. The acromion can be osteotomized and bent down. The tendons of the rotator cuff and teres major should be sutured together over the glenoid to help fill the subacromial gap. The scapula will ride upward and backward if all of the shoulder depressors are

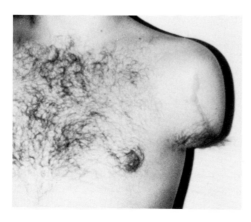

Fig. 24-2. Neat configuration of functional shoulder disarticulation stump, with the head of the humerus retained (post-traumatic).

resected or denervated, which in turn will lead to additional asymmetry of appearance not remediable by a shoulder prosthesis. Therefore the latissimus and pectoralis major should be reattached to the mass of tendons over the glenoid, particularly if the pectoralis minor is compromised. If the deltoid muscle, and axillary nerve, can be saved, it should be sutured to the serratus to attenuate further the otherwise bony contour of the shoulder.

Forequarter Amputation

Forequarter amputation is not a difficult procedure. There are well-described surgical techniques to accomplish the amputation by an anterior (Berger) or posterior (Littlewood)[8] approach. The posterior approach is much easier. Pertinent details include careful section of the nerves to make certain that the neuromas lie within the scalenes rather than upon the muscles or first rib.

If at all possible, the medial 2.5 cm of the clavicle should be conserved. The subclavian vein is adherent to the bone at this site and is easily torn. Furthermore, the sternocleidomastoid muscle attaches at this site, and removal of this part of the clavicle results in significant and unsightly distortion of the neck, a disfigurement difficult to camouflage.

Skin grafts are applied as needed. The amputated limb is a good source of split and free full-thickness grafts.

Postoperatively, the patient may be mobilized as rapidly as possible. All of the know-how of the occupational therapist should be utilized to develop the patient's skills in one-handed activities of daily living. Work simplification techniques should be explored.

A cosmetic shoulder cap made of light, washable plastic is fitted as soon as the wound permits so that the patient's clothes hang symmetrically. The patient should be informed and reassured about the inevitable but asymptomatic and nonprogressive scoliosis that occurs immediately after this and other major upper extremity amputations.

At present we have no functional prosthetic limb restoration at this level. The rehabilitation team must be firm about this. "Cosmetic" limbs are only marginally cosmetic. The absolute absence of spontaneous activity introduces an artificial mannequin-like quality that is actually anti-cosmetic. The presence of such cosmetic limbs further encumbers and constrains all of the activities of the patient. Occasionally, however, an amputee will be totally unreceptive to this advice, and for these patients, well-designed cosmetic prostheses are available. These devices generally have "passive" elbows that may be positioned by using the remaining hand. Positioning of the elbow is retained by friction or by a lock in the prosthetic elbow joint. With the forearm flexed, the prosthetic hand may be used for pushing or holding light objects, or a purse or coat may be suspended from the forearm. A joint allowing passive abduction of the shoulder will facilitate dressing.

Electric or cable-driven devices can be fabricated for the forequarter amputee, but these are seldom of real use. Prescriptions can be formulated for the adamant patient, allowing the patient to discover for himself the usefulness or encumbrance of the device.

Intercalary Resections

Scapulectomy is rarely the amputation of choice when "cure" is the goal of cancer surgery.[6] The scapula is accessible to radiation. Scapulectomy may be indicated for osteomyelitis, the residuals of radiation therapy, or lesions of limited malignancy.

The incision can sweep from the inferior angle of the scapula upward, toward, and then along the spine of the scapula. The skin of the region tolerates the raising of large flaps. By detaching the latissimus, the scapula can be tilted upward, so that the plane of the scapulocostal space is easily accessible. The trapezius, rhomboids, and levator scapulae are easily detached and the acromion and coracoid are disarticulated. De Palma[4] describes a technique for sectioning the rotator cuff at the neck of the scapula. His method permits the remnants of the cuff to be used to suspend the humerus from the clavicle. Some form of suspension is highly desirable to avoid later traction lesions of the brachial plexus.

The Tikhor-Linberg[7] procedure (Figs. 24-3 and 24-4) is an even more massive resection of the bone and muscles of the shoulder girdle, which preserves the more distal elements of the extremity, leaving them suspended solely by the neurovascular bundle. The configuration of the shoulder girdle is lost, and the extremity usually shortens and tends to flap if the patient is active. There is no proximal stability and the hand cannot be "placed" for effective use except near the waist. The patient cannot get his hand to his mouth or hold more than a few ounces. A suspension harness may be necessary to relieve the weight of the arm from the brachial plexus.

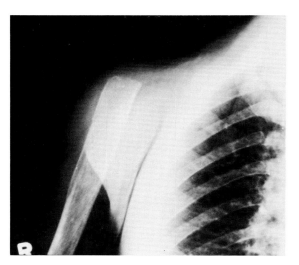

Fig. 24-3. Postoperative roentgenogram following Tikhor-Linberg resection of the shoulder girdle.

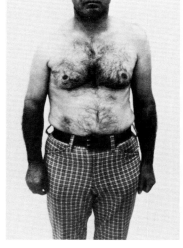

Fig. 24-4. This patient has had a Tikhor-Linberg resection of his shoulder girdle. Hand function is normal, but the hand can only be placed to the upper abdominal area.

FUTURE DIRECTIONS

The obvious goal for the future is further development of techniques of tissue retention that will preserve function with form yet without unsightly scarring or deformity. The era of surgery at the microscopic level has just begun and seems to be expanding. The restoration of function is not solely a structural problem, however. There is a chemistry of wound repair to address. The use of enzymes to facilitate tissue gliding, as investigated by Peacock and Van Winkle,[9] is an example.

Despite expected advances along these lines, amputations and amputees will be with us for the foreseeable future. New prosthetic fitting techniques to achieve more comfortable and more stable sockets are in constant development. Research is finding lighter and more durable materials. External power sources, such as miniaturized electric motors, myoelectrical pick-up and amplification techniques, and microswitches are all in various experimental stages. The future upper extremity prosthesis will probably be largely powered by self-contained electrical units. Perception and feedback possibilities are under exploration. Cosmetic covers and soft padding are available but not yet satisfactory. There is an almost unlimited opportunity for research along any of these lines.

REFERENCES

1. Burgess, E. M.: Sites of amputation election according to modern practice. In De Palma, A. F., Ed.: *Clinical Orthopaedics and Related Research,* vol. 37, p. 17. J. B. Lippincott, Philadelphia, 1964.

2. Childress, D. S.: An approach to powered grasp. In *Advances in External Control of Human Extremities,* pp. 159–167. Proceedings of the Fouth International Symposium on External Control of Human Extremities, Dubrovnik, Yugoslavia, August 28–September 2, 1972. Yugoslav Committee for Electronics and Automation, Belgrade, 1973.

3. Childress, D. S.: Hampton, F. L., Lambert, C. N., et al.: Myoelectric immediate postsurgical procedure: A concept for fitting the upper extremity amputee. Artif. Limbs 13(2):55–60, 1969.

4. De Palma, A.F.: Scapulectomy and a method of preserving the normal configuration of the shoulder. Clin. Orthop. 4:217–224, 1954.

5. Herberts, P., Almstrom, C., and Caine, K.: Clinical application study of multifunctional prosthetic hands. J. Bone Joint Surg. 60B:552–560, 1978.

6. Keagy, R. D.: Amputation about the shoulder girdle. In Post, M., Ed.: *The Shoulder–Surgical and Nonsurgical Management,* pp. 547–554. Lea & Febiger, Philadelphia, 1978.

7. Linberg, B. E.: Interscapulothoracic resection for malignant tumors of the shoulder joint region. J. Bone Joint Surg. 10:344–349, 1928.

8. Littlewood, H.: Amputations of the shoulder and at the hip. Br. Med. J. 1:381, 1922.

9. Peacock, E. E., Jr., and Van Winkle, W., Jr.: *Wound Repair,* 2nd ed., pp. 462–463. W. B. Saunders, Philadelphia, 1976.

10. Tooms, R. E.: Amputations. In Crenshaw, A. H., Ed.: *Campbell's Operative Orthopedics,* vol 1, pp. 881–883. C. V. Mosby, St. Louis, 1971.

11. Vasconcelos, E.: *Modern Methods of Amputation,* p. 23. Philosophical Library of New York, New York, 1945.

25

Amputations of the Lower Extremities

Ernest M. Burgess, M.D.

Amputation surgery is an area of major responsibility for orthopedic surgeons. Because loss of function in the ablated portion of the limb is complete, the surgery is unique. Function must be replaced by a mechanical substitute, the prosthesis. Since in a sense the surgery is completely destructive, it is often looked upon as dull and unrewarding. This attitude has, to some degree, limited interest in surgical research and progress.

Most amputation surgery is actually reconstructive. Conservation and appropriate surgical management of residual limb tissues permit the surgeon to construct out of the amputation, a terminal end-organ for obtaining the most effective control of the prosthesis and the most satisfactory man-machine interface (Figs. 25-1 and 25-2). Viewed in this light, the amputation is a more challenging surgery. Proper management of stump tissues such as muscle and nerve through biofeedback and available myoelectric energy in the residual limb can even harness and retain by neurophysiological transfer mechanisms, certain functional capabilities of that portion of the limb which has been removed. These reconstructive aspects of amputation surgery are particularly important for function, comfort, and appearance when they can be incorporated with the high technology engineering possible in modern prostheses.

The surgical and engineering challenge of total functional loss is indeed great. No other surgery of the extremities even approaches this rehabilitation engineering demand. The surgeon and other members of the amputee team are further confronted by vocational and psychological potentials, even the ability to assist

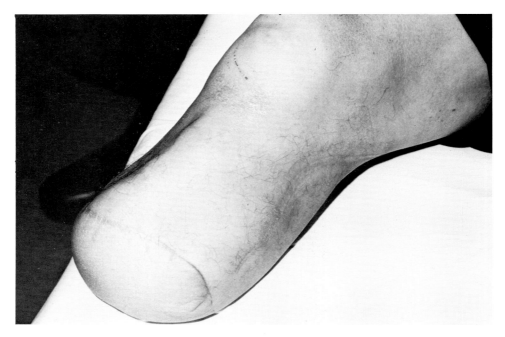

Fig. 25-1. Physiological below-knee amputation. The muscles have been stabilized. Residual limb contours permit excellent interface and total contact with the prosthesis.

the amputee to high and rewarding levels of physical accomplishment in recreation and sports. Amputation surgery is neither intellectually nor technically unrewarding.

Existing attitudes about amputation surgery and the fact that it is necessitated by a wide variety of pathological states—peripheral vascular disease, trauma, congenital limb deficits, infection, and malignancies—result in its being performed by surgeons with a variety of training backgrounds. The surgery is only the initial step in restoration of function. Without a working knowledge of prosthetics—which includes the rapid technical advances in the field of limb substitutes—and without understanding rehabilitation and training techniques, the surgeon is not fully qualified to amputate. This lack of knowledge and interest in rehabilitation cannot justify the common practice of referral and transfer of all postoperative care to others. This practice deprives the surgeon not only of the satisfaction of observing functional progress and rehabilitation of the patient, but also an awareness of what exactly is required by the surgical reconstruction itself.

The requirements for successfully performing amputation surgery need not fall within specific territorial guidelines. Orthopedic surgeons, vascular surgeons, general surgeons, and plastic surgeons can all work successfully in this field if they are willing to equip themselves with the necessary information and abide by the temporal requirements for amputee rehabilitation. In general, orthopedic surgeons have best qualified themselves by interest and training to perform modern amputation surgery. Their basic interest in extremity function and their knowledge of biomechanics provide a natural background. Attendance lists for post-graduate workshops and courses on amputations and prosthetics show that orthopedic

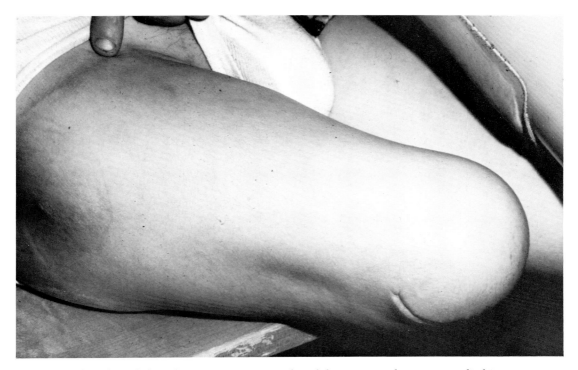

Fig. 25-2. Physiological above-knee amputation. Muscle stabilization provides a strong, cylindrical residual limb for prosthetic control.

surgeons are almost exclusively the surgical attendees. However, there has been a definite recent increase in interest in amputation on the part of vascular surgeons. The high level of surgical skill they possess, along with their knowledge of ischemic limbs, qualifies them to incorporate amputation surgery and rehabilitation into their area of expertise. It is hoped that this trend will continue.

Many times throughout this text orthopedic rehabilitation will accent the need for team service. The team approach is not only desirable, it is essential for amputee rehabilitation. The surgeon is not qualified to design and fabricate a prosthesis: the prosthetist has no surgical training. With few exceptions, adequate amputee management can be successful only when it is carried out in a team setting. Each participant and member of the team is of equal importance. This includes the surgeon, prosthetist, rehabilitation personnel, social workers, psychologists, and others as their services are required. However, because of the responsibilities involved, the surgeon is the team leader.

DEMOGRAPHY OF LOWER EXTREMITY AMPUTATIONS

For centuries, amputations have been associated with trauma, especially war. Napoleon's personal surgeon, Baron Varrey, described his performance of 200 amputations in a 24-hour period during the Smolensk campaign. Medical writings from the American Civil War record the treatment of thousands of amputations occurring over a period of a few days in the course of this particularly violent conflict. Weiss of Warsaw, in a personal communication, describes the unnumbered amputees, many unhealed, struggling about with makeshift crutches and sticks in the Warsaw area following World War II. The recent military actions in Korea and Vietnam left substantial numbers of combatants with complicated and multi-membral amputations. Field medical service was of such an expert and life-saving quality that severely traumatized individuals survived who would have otherwise died.

Civilian amputations throughout the Western world at the present time are necessitated in the most part by limb ischemia. Recent statistics from a number of European countries and from the United States indicate that approximately 75–85 percent of all major amputations of the lower extremities result from peripheral vascular disease (Fig. 25-3). One third of these individuals have diabetes (Fig. 25-4). A large majority are 50 years of age or older. Lower extremity amputations for trauma, infection, neoplasm, congential limb deficiencies, and other causes make up the remaining percentage of the amputation load.

Amputations for peripheral vascular disease are not only the most frequent, they are increasing in number. The aging population and the increase in diabetes and degenerative arterial disease of all types account for this greater number of amputations each year. Vascular reconstructive surgical techniques have salvaged many ischemic limbs that would otherwise have come to amputation. These procedures operate by mechanically increasing blood flow to the threatened extremity. They do not alter the basic pathological nature of the underlying disease, and they are palliative rather than prophylactic or curative. Therefore

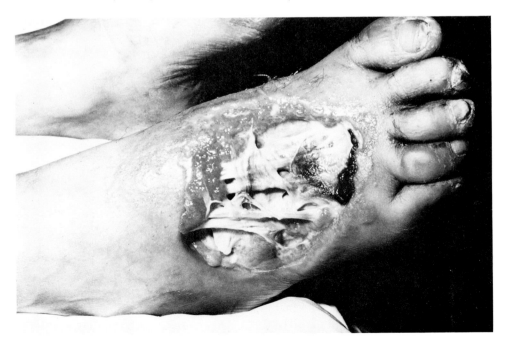

Fig. 25-3. Diabetic gangrene with infection and neuropathy. A below-knee amputation is necessary.

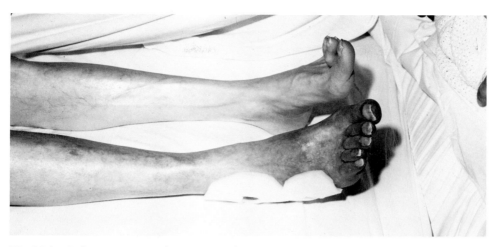

Fig. 25-4. Ischemic gangrene from arteriosclerosis. Vascular reconstructive surgery is not indicated. Below-knee amputation is required.

vascular reconstruction is by itself limited in effectiveness when plotted against time. Old and failed reconstructions are increasingly coming to amputation, adding to the load of unreconstructable ischemic limbs (Fig. 25-5). The economic cost of these disease states is large. The American Diabetes Association estimates that the cost in time loss and treatment for this one condition exceeded $16 billion in the year 1979. During that year, 1.2 million new diabetics were diagnosed in the United States. Appreciable numbers of these patients are at risk for lower limb amputation.

While many of these older people who require amputation for vascular disease present a low rehabilitation potential, the majority who are able to walk with a prosthesis can be returned to a home setting. They can continue to enjoy a satisfactory quality of life. These individuals constitute the primary peacetime amputation challenge.

Rehabilitation potential is in most cases related directly to the level of amputation. The single most important accomplishment in amputation surgery during the last decade has been the achieving of lower levels of amputation in patients with ischemic limbs. It is possible to achieve below-knee primary healing and successful prosthetic rehabilitation in three-fourths of all individuals who lose legs and feet from peripheral vascular disease. This is not an isolated or limited accomplishment. Results of this quality are reported throughout the world.

The factors responsible for lower-level healed amputations are primarily technical. These will be discussed in terms of current knowledge of limb viability and the technical aspects of preoperative, surgical, and postoperative management.

LOWER EXTREMITY AMPUTATIONS FOR ISCHEMIA

Most patients requiring amputation for peripheral vascular disease are elderly. They present the many pathological states generally associated with aging.

A careful general history and physical examination are essential. They pro-

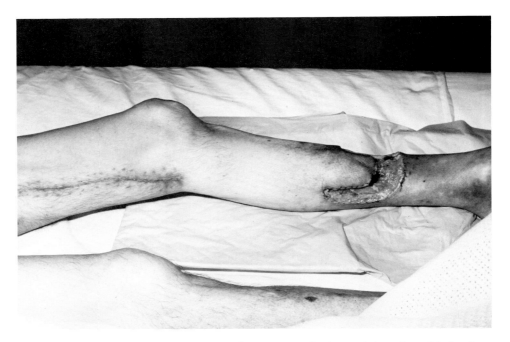

Fig. 25-5. Failed vascular reconstruction with gangrene, infection, and tissue loss. A below-knee amputation with prosthetic rehabilitation was successful.

vide by far the most important facts needed for preoperative evaluation. The need for amputation and the appropriate level and type of surgery may be obvious. Many patients, however, will fall into a gray zone requiring additional information to establish appropriate treatment. A complete, standard vascular diagnostic work-up should be a part of every preoperative survey except in severe emergency. This work-up will extend to include specific laboratory information in addition to the history, careful physical examination, and routine laboratory data.

LABORATORY TESTS FOR LIMB VIABILITY (Fig. 25-6)

Arteriography

Injection of radio-opaque material into the arterial circulation is the basic diagnostic means of outlining the mechanical state of arteries. The technique is well established.[12,15,22,23] It can be performed in any well equipped x-ray department. Its primary value is not only to diagnose and visualize the position and patency of limb arteries; it also provides the vascular geography through and around which all arterial reconstructive surgery is conducted.

This visual description of limb arteries is absolutely essential to the vascular surgeon. It is of considerably less value and can be misleading when amputation is

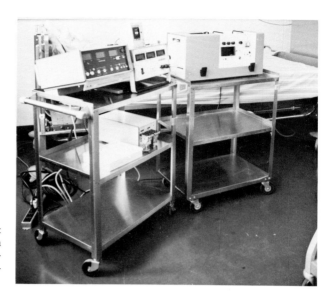

Fig. 25-6. Non-invasive diagnostic equipment in a clinical limb viability laboratory. Shown are the transcutaneous PO_2 monitor, laser Doppler instrument, and the multispectral analysis device.

being considered. There is no direct, constant, or predictable relationship between tissue viability and vessel patency as seen by x-ray. The arteriogram then will reveal a wealth of important information about the arteries, but it cannot be used as a guide to determine the level of amputation. When viewed in this context, it is useful although not critical information for the amputating surgeon.

One interesting area of specific value is the opportunity under some circumstances to re-vascularize by surgery an ischemic limb at risk for high-level amputation. Functional salvage of the entire limb is not the surgical goal under these circumstances. The re-vascularization is performed to permit lower levels of amputation, primarily from above the knee to below the knee. Occasionally, well planned vascular surgery will allow knee salvage although the amputation cannot be avoided.

Current technology has made the arteriogram a practicable test, but a small hazard still exists with its use. Vascular surgeons and others have seen acute arterial occlusions immediately following the dye injection. These circumstances are fortunately rare.

Limb Blood Pressure

Segmental blood pressure measurements along the limb are valuable as a measure of viability. The test is non-invasive and can be performed by a well trained technician. Blood pressure readings are obtained segmentally using a proximally placed pneumatic cuff with ultrasound Doppler recordings to hear and record blood flow. Segmental blood pressures can be obtained with this method down to and including toe levels. Wagner has established an ischemic index taken from blood pressure readings at segments along the leg by comparing these readings to the brachial (central) blood pressure obtained in the arm.[27] The mathematical relationship between the two readings is called the ischemic index.

The critical level is .35 to .45. An index below this level indicates that the segment tested has a poor chance of healing primarily following amputation.

Doppler ultrasound recording of segmental blood pressures is a simple, non-invasive, and inexpensive test. Its use is recommended, but as with most laboratory tests, it is not infallible. Hard, sclerotic arteries that are difficult to compress will give false readings. Patients with arterial pathology of this type can generally be identified and then the results of segmental blood pressure, Doppler ultrasound, or ischemic index data might be considered unreliable.

Some emphasis has been placed on wave form changes using the Doppler ultrasound equipment.[3] At this time, variations in wave form are of more theoretical than practical value. The vascular work-up should include, however, the segmental blood pressure and the standard Doppler reading of wave form characteristics.

Skin Temperature

Skin temperature is related directly to local blood flow and perfusion. It is an important measure of skin viability and healing potential. The skin circulation is also sensitive to challenge by local application of heat and cold, by positioning relative to heart level, and by pressure. Routine physical examination of the ischemic limb includes an estimate of the skin temperature. More accurate measurements can be obtained by a variety of types of equipment, including the thermograph, skin thermistors, radiometry, and crystallography. Every ischemic limb considered for amputation should have the skin temperature evaluated. Areas of temperature change should be noted and compared to the opposite extremity and to other parts of the body. While it is not possible to rely on skin temperature alone as a direct indicator of local tissue viability, it is a very useful prognosticator of wound healing.

Practically all of the temperature measurements on the limbs are surface readings. It is possible by minimally invasive techniques to measure temperature in the deeper structures, particularly muscles. Such studies are not generally used. Rather, they are reserved for special circumstances such as localized compartmental ischemia with possible necrosis. Refined skin temperature measurements, such as by thermography, will be increasingly important for determining appropriate amputation levels in ischemic limbs. At present, this information is supportive, not absolute.

Skin Color

Color changes in the skin can reflect its vascular state. Normal variations in skin pigmentation complicate the use of color changes as an important diagnostic tool. For many years, blanching on elevation and rubor with dependency plotted against time have been looked on as useful tests for the degree of limb ischemia present. Of more specific value is the reflection by the skin of color wavelengths. This determination is known as monospectral and multispectral analysis. There is now available a multispectral technique that can be successfully used to identify areas of viability and of tissue death in surface burns.[2] This multispectral technique can accurately define burned areas that will heal spontaneously as compared with those that will require skin grafting. It is possible to adopt similar methods for the study of reflected light from the skin itself. Present experimental equipment uses three wave lengths: green, red, and infrared. Coordinated study of the reflected light wave is thought to be a measure of oxygenated hemoglobin in the skin. The multiple wavelength spectral scope is placed directly on the skin and, under constant temperature, the reflected light waves are analyzed and digitalized immediately. At this time, multispectral analysis is still in the investigative stage.

Skin Diffusion of Metabolized and Unmetabolized Gases

Oxygen (diffusion) through the skin is a direct measure of skin viability. Its determination by an electrical surface probe is simple, non-invasive, and easily obtained by a skilled technician. The skin is carefully heated to a constant temperature of 44–45°C and then the oxygen level is determined. Transcutaneous oxygen tension ($TcPO_2$) is now being used to establish amputation level. It may become one of the most practical and useful of laboratory tests. One drawback is the amount of time required to conduct the test at each single area on the skin. At present about 20 minutes is required to establish temperature level and record the oxygen diffusion. When a number of sites are being measured, the time involved becomes a factor. Progress is being made in conducting multiple site readings simultaneously.

A local measurement of such inhaled and unmetabolized gases as helium, hydrogen, and argon also indicates the local state of circulation, as can 100% oxygen inhalation with measured $TcPO_2$ skin excess. The entire area of transcutaneous gas measurement for this purpose is under thorough investigation both in the animal laboratory and in human limbs.[1,21] By the time this text is in print, $TcPO_2$ should be clinically calibrated and practical.

Radioactive Isotopes

The local uptake and diffusion of radioactive isotopes are measures of local microcirculation. Standards have been established by Moore and others[12,19,20] who used xenon-133 to determine amputation level preoperatively (Fig. 25-7). A high degree of predictable accuracy is reported by these investigators. The technique requires availability of the isotopes and counter capacity. Use of these techniques will be limited to available facilities. They do provide an excellent research tool and can be cross-referenced with simpler methods.

Pulsatile Blood Flow

Equipment is available to measure pulsatile blood flow in the larger arteries and in the skin microcirculation. Sound and light waves are backscattered from moving blood cells within the arteries and arterioles. The dynamics of limb blood flow are thus demonstrated. Of particular interest is the laser Doppler instrument, which backscatters a single beam of laser light from moving blood cells in the microcirculation to a depth of approximately 1.5 mm through the skin surface.

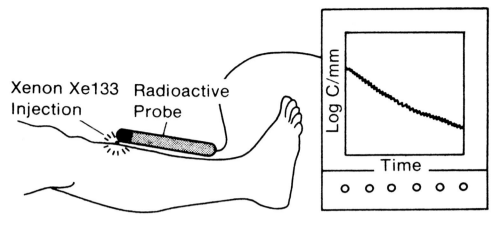

Fig. 25-7. Diagram of the radioactive isotope system for measuring microcirculation in the skin.

This sensitive, portable, and non-invasive equipment has just recently been standardized for commercial manufacture and use.[14,16]

Electromagnetic flowmetry is a somewhat more complicated technique used to determine pulsatile blood flow through the larger vessels. It has not yet gained wide acceptance for determining levels of amputation.

PREPARATION OF THE PATIENT FOR SURGERY

Most patients coming to amputation for limb ischemia are in poor health. Age and associated illness require a thorough preoperative medical evaluation and close supervision. The timing of the amputation will to a degree be determined by the surgical risk. An individual with poorly controlled diabetes and a severely infected, ischemic foot may require emergency open-ankle disarticulation for infection control and for stabilizing the patient's general condition. A few days later, a definitive, higher-level amputation can be performed. Once the decision to amputate has been made, the surgeon and the internist cooperate to minimize operative risk.

The physical therapist can be especially helpful by teaching preoperative exercise, crutch use, transfer techniques, and other physical activities.

Psychological support is, of course, helpful. The patient and family need to understand what is going to take place and how it will affect physical activities and social relationships. A useful practice is the preoperative visit from amputees with a similar type of disability who are doing well. Knowledge of the positive aspects of the surgery—relief of pain, increased mobility, improved general health—are all supportive.

Local Management

Ischemic tissues heal poorly. The skin of the limb should be carefully prepared for surgery by gentle mechanical washing with a non-irritating soap. Harsh chemicals are not used in the preoperative preparation of the skin or at the time of surgery. Elderly people are at greater risk for anesthesia and surgery. Operative and immediate postoperative mortality and morbidity will be very low when the patient comes to surgery properly prepared, with the physiological state well understood.

THE SURGERY

The amputation is conducted without a tourniquet unless some unusual circumstance should warrant its use for a short period of time during the operation. A pneumatic tourniquet can be applied loosely. It is to be inflated only if circumstances absolutely require its use. Blood loss at surgery is seldom a troublesome problem.

The principles of good surgery—gentleness, careful handling of tissues, and adequate hemostasis—apply to an even greater degree when operating on ischemic tissues, which are low in vitality compared to more normal structures. Harsh retraction is avoided. Local circulation should not be further compromised by wide dissection of tissue planes. Skin flaps should not be dissected up from deeper tissues, nor their blood supply disturbed more than absolutely necessary. Large nerves are carefully ligated, as are all major vessels. Cautery can be judiciously used on tiny bleeding points. Bone surfaces are appropriately bevelled and carefully rounded. Closure is carried out in layers so as to avoid undue tension. Most wounds should be drained for 24–48 hours. Sharp dissection is used throughout.

The quality of the surgery is a major determining factor in wound healing. When operating on ischemic tissues, the surgeon enjoys no latitude or margin of technical error. Skill and surgical excellence are directly related to the degree and the type of healing response. A poor wound closure carried out in the presence of healthy, well-vascularized tissues will be compensated by the vital genetic healing capacity present. A poor wound closure through devitalized and poorly nourished tissues encourages wound breakdown and infection before the slow healing process can effectively seal wound surfaces together. Application of these general surgical principles will be further considered at each of the amputation levels.

POSTOPERATIVE CARE

Immediately following surgery, the surgeon focuses on establishing optimal physical and metabolic circumstances for wound healing. Since the amputation is terminal, control of the external environment is not limited to concern for limb tissue beyond the site of the operation. This unique circumstance is particularly helpful. Temperature, humidity, pressure, splinting, and sterility are all controllable. The value of immobilization and tissue rest has long been recognized as beneficial during the early stages of wound healing. Proper attention to these external environmental forces assists healing.

The internal wound environment is less easily controlled and more dependent upon the physiological state of the patient. Fluid balance, edema control, prevention of stasis, appropriate nutrition, and mobilizing of the patient with exercise all relate to postoperative well being. These elderly and often debilitated patients require great attention to detail if morbidity and mortality rates are to be kept low.

Postoperative Soft-Wound Dressings

Soft dressings provide the least effective postoperative wound management. They provide some protection and cleanliness, yet they do not immobilize, control pressure, or permit an appreciable degree of patient mobility without pain.

Additional stump wrapping with supportive elastic or cotton dressings or with a tapered stump stocking improves the support and partially controls edema. Care must be taken in the application of the soft-pressure dressing in order to avoid proximal constriction. The techniques for wrapping stumps after surgery are well demonstrated in nursing and physical therapy texts and manuals.

Postoperative Rigid Wound Dressings

Splinting of tissue wounds by rigid dressings is a practice that has been accepted for centuries. Availability of blood, antibiotics, improved anesthesia, and the physiological response of the body to trauma have not decreased the need for immobilization as a basic principle of wound healing. The amputation is particularly suitable for management by rigid dressings. Because the surgery is terminal, it is possible to incorporate a distal pressure interface in the dressing that will limit edema, yet not constrict blood flow and fluid exchange. Plaster of Paris of either the elastic or standard type is available everywhere and is generally used. A wide variety of other cast materials can also be used as long as they do not retain heat or moisture. A semi-rigid material like unna paste is also used successfully.

Application of a rigid dressing immediately following surgery is a precise technique (Figs. 25-8–25-12). Careless application defeats its advantages. Pressure-

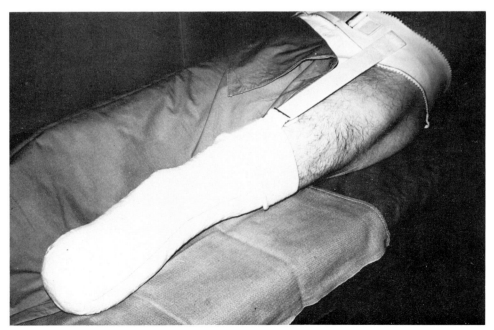

Fig. 25-8. The below-knee plaster of Paris rigid-wound dressing.

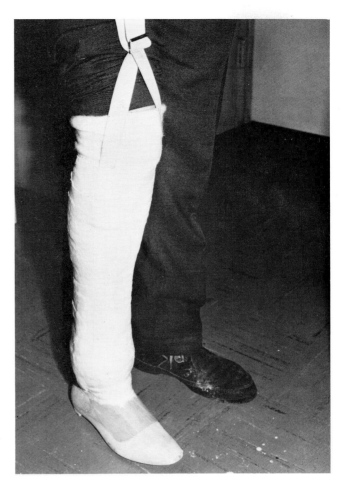

Fig. 25-9. The plaster of Paris immediate post-surgical prosthetic fitting for the Syme amputation.

sensitive areas will break down within hours under a cast improperly padded and contoured. Surgeons, prosthetists, cast technicians, physical therapists, and nurses are, when properly trained, all qualified to apply immediate post-surgical rigid dressings. The trained person can apply hundreds of post-amputation rigid dressings without complication when established techniques are understood and used. The technique of rigid dressing application following amputation of lower extremities is well documented by manuals, visual aids, and courses taught throughout the United States, Canada, and elsewhere. The skills in application can be promptly acquired. Actually, it is technically easier to apply a proper rigid dressing than to teach soft-pressure dressing and bandaging. Skill in applying post-surgical rigid dressings should be generally acquirable by any individual involved in amputations.

Critics point out that the closed rigid dressing prevents frequent inspection of the wound. This feature is an advantage rather than a disadvantage. Frequent dressings of the wound, particularly among the older age groups, are best avoided. The advantages of an improved wound healing environment, comfort, prevention of joint contractures, control of edema, and easy mobility of the patients far

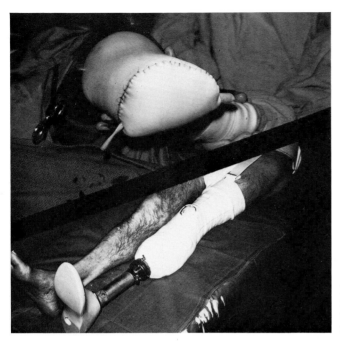

Fig. 25-10. The immediate post-surgical rigid dressing and attached adjustable prosthetic unit for early, limited weight-bearing in the below-knee amputation.

outweigh any disadvantages—which are primarily iatrogenic. Modern amputation management dictates a knowledge of and proper use of rigid dressing techniques.

Controlled Environment Treatment and Air Splints

Airbag dressings have been used for years to splint injured limbs temporarily. Long-term use has been avoided because the bags retain heat and moisture. Sealing of the bags, even those with double wall construction, may be constricting to fluid exchange. Newer designs minimize some of these faults.

The British Biomechanical Research and Development Unit at Roehampton has devised a treatment system (Fig. 25-13) with a flow-through polyvinyl bag that permits proximal venting of air or other selected gas.[6,17] This system allows sterile, filtered air to pass through the bag at a controlled temperature and humidity. Pressure on the remaining part of the leg or arm can be either constant or intermittent and controlled mechanically by the console. Gas composition can be altered to include high concentrations of oxygen. The bag can be applied to the amputation immediately following surgery and without dressings so that the operative site can be visualized during the early healing period. The bags are disposable and relatively inexpensive. Earlier models of the equipment for controlled environment were large, relatively cumbersome, and noisy. Today the units are small and portable, and most of the other disadvantages have been eliminated. It is necessary to maintain the bag in position by comfortable suspension straps. Otherwise it is blown off by the force of the air passing proximally to the vent on the leg near the pelvis, or the shoulder in the upper limb.

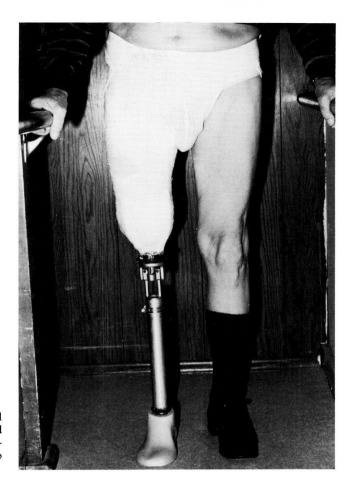

Fig. 25-11. The immediate post-surgical rigid dressing for knee disarticulation and above-knee amputations. The cast is suspended by a soft spica, which permits hip movement. A prosthetic unit is attached.

The controlled environment treatment system does not permit weight bearing, nor is the immobilization as adequate as in a rigid dressing. Both of these objections can be overcome by placing the postoperative limb in a light rigid dressing and then enclosing the entire limb with cast in the airbag. Patients can be up and about in a chair and with crutches. It is also possible to attach a yoke device to the bag to permit limited weight bearing.

A number of modifications of the airbag principle have been developed in Australia, the United States, and elsewhere.[18,26] It is a particularly useful device for preventing and controlling edema. Excess tissue fluid can be forced out of the limb rapidly as air under pressure flows through system. Pain specifically related to edema and tissue tension responds remarkably.

Contrary indications to postoperative airbag management are infection, thrombosis, thrombophlebitis, and related pathology that could be aggravated by the application of external pressure.

The pressurized airbag can be used to contour casts, including post-amputation rigid dressings. The plaster or other material is applied in a nearly liquid state.

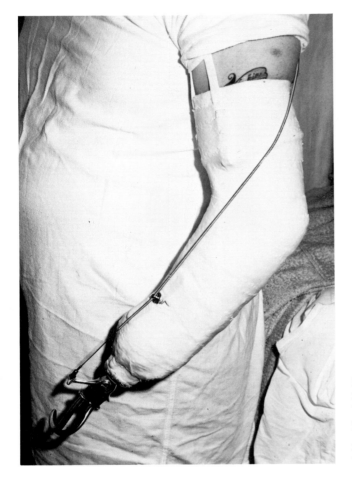

Fig. 25-12. The rigid plaster of Paris dressing with attached functional terminal device for below-elbow amputation. Immediate post-surgical terminal device control can be obtained by conventional harnessing (as in this illustration) or by a myoelectric system.

Then the entire limb and soft cast are inserted into the bag as pressure is applied to contour the cast. A remarkably smooth and fitted cast is obtained. Pressure-sensitive areas are protected by padding. Casts applied by the onset of pressure fit intimately and are comfortable. Cast technicians, surgeons, and others can easily learn the technique of cast application through pressure.

The use of air splints and pressure casting will increase as the technique becomes better understood and equipment more generally available.

TISSUE MATURATION AND PROSTHETIC FITTING

A major weakness of amputee management is the length of time between surgery and the fitting of the definitive prosthesis. Every day of unjustified delay diminishes effective rehabilitation. Most lower extremity amputees who heal without complications will be ready for a prosthesis within 4–8 weeks after the operation.

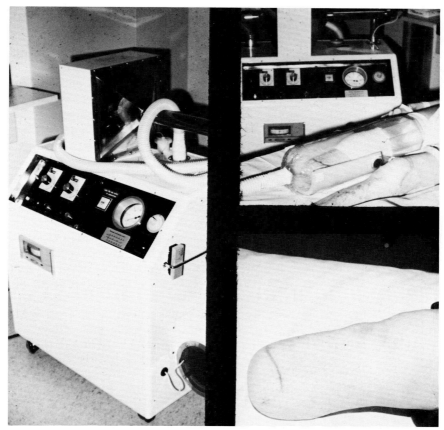

Fig. 25-13. The controlled environment treatment (CET) console and dressing bag. This unit is applied in the operating room immediately following surgery.

A provisional or temporary inexpensive, light prosthesis should be applied as early as the physical circumstances permit. Delay in obtaining the prosthesis is unjustified and uneconomical. The amputee team is specifically charged with prompt, progressive rehabilitation. The practice of waiting weeks or months for an artificial limb can and should be changed.

Methods used to stabilize stump size include rigid dressings, pressure bandaging, and exercise. Early and limited weight-bearing in a rigid dressing, be it with temporary pylon or a provisional prosthesis, will condition and stabilize the stump faster than any of the other standard techniques.

Rigid Dressing For Stump Maturation

Rigid and semi-rigid dressings using plaster of Paris, synthetic cast materials, unna paste, or splints all provide immobilization. The ideal rigid dressing immobilizes the amputation site and the closest proximal tissues, maintains distal contact and pressure without being tight or proximally constricting, and protects the operative site from injury. The dressing immediately over the closure wound should not seal the wound nor retain heat and moisture. Maceration and local bacterial growth are encouraged by warm, moist, occlusive dressings.

A wide variety of rigid and semi-rigid dressings are used throughout the world. The author popularized the closed, elastic plaster cast placed over a sterile Orlon-type stump stocking with a sterile polyurethane foam endpadding.[5,8-11] Polyurethane padding is also used to bridge and protect pressure-sensitive areas such as the patella and the anterior tibia. Cast suspension is important to maintain distal contact and end pressure. This suspension is obtained by auxillary strapping, proximal adhering of the Orlon stocking to the skin with a biologically compatible adhesive, and contouring the cast. Many thousands of rigid dressings of this type have been successfully used at all levels of amputations. When the wound has been drained, the drains are removed 2–3 days after the operation without removing the cast or disturbing its support. Limb and body activity is encouraged immediately after surgery and progressively increased throughout the early postoperative period. Most patients can be up in a wheelchair the day after amputation. The rehabilitation process that begins before surgery is carried out immediately following surgery from the time of the wound closure.

Unless they loosen or there is indication of some complication developing, rigid dressings are generally removed 10–14 days following the operation. During these first 2 or 3 weeks after surgery, no weight bearing is allowed through the rigid dressing in ischemic limbs, but the cast can be intermittently pulled tight against the amputation site and then relaxed on a regular schedule to simulate the action of a pump. A folded towel or strap around the end of the cast allows the patient to apply the intermittent pressure.

A second rigid dressing is applied immediately after removal of the initial postoperative cast and wound inspection. Sutures are left in place until the wound is well healed. Immediate and early partial weight-bearing through a terminal device applied to the cast is withheld in the ischemic amputation until wound healing is secure. The wait may involve several weeks or it may be possible to ambulate the patient with very light weight-bearing and simulated walking after the first cast change. Under no circumstances should healing be compromised by attempted partial or complete weight-bearing through the rigid dressing until wound healing is secure. The whole rehabilitation process is directed toward prompt wound healing.

The normal course of rehabilitation using the rigid dressing technique brings the patient through the immediate postoperative period to a partial weight-bearing cast or temporary prosthesis. Stump maturation is rapid within the rigid dressing and with early partial weight-bearing.

As soon as wound healing is secure and the shape of the stump reasonably well stabilized, a semi-permanent or permanent limb can be fit. Further rehabilitation will be individualized according to the established goal for each patient. If the patient is going to be confined to a wheelchair and not wear a prosthesis, the effort will then be directed toward teaching transfer techniques, good general health, and maintaining joint mobility and muscle strength. A tapered stump stocking may be permanently required except at night.

As rehabilitation progresses, decisions are required of the entire amputee team. It is necessary to establish carefully planned individual levels of accomplishment early in the postoperative period. Therapy is directed toward obtaining this goal.

Application of a prosthesis to the rigid dressing is delayed in the presence of peripheral vascular disease. These indolent, slow-healing incisions cannot undergo excessive mechanical stress. Early ambulation with partial weight bearing is encouraged, but only after wound healing is secure. Careful supervision is necessary to control the degree of weight borne and the amount of walking. Weak, elderly individuals cannot dependably use walkers when they are unsupervised. A tilt table is an effective device to promote some longitudinal weight-bearing force for both bilateral and unilateral leg amputees early in the postoperative period.

LEVELS OF AMPUTATION FOR PERIPHERAL VASCULAR DISEASE

The level of amputation is the single most critical factor in patients undergoing surgery for peripheral vascular disease. When the knee is functional and the patient can be expected to walk, the amputation should be performed below the knee level whenever possible. Limb viability studies, improved surgical techniques, and watching the patient's physiological state after surgery have in the last decade salvaged large number of knees that would have otherwise been lost with a more cautious approach to wound healing. Communications from widely separated areas throughout the world indicate that 60–80 percent of all lower extremity amputations can be performed below the knee; they will heal, and in most instances, permit the use of a prosthesis. The trend to low levels of amputation is continuing. The long-established practice of routine through-knee and above-knee amputations is being replaced by more careful preoperative study of the patient and, occasionally, by the use of vascular reconstructive surgery to lower the amputation level to below the knee. The techniques for low levels of amputation are available and the indications are well defined. Education is now needed for the more general acceptance of knee salvage as a fundamental principle.

Rigid established rules for specific amputation levels have largely disappeared. Modern prosthetic substitution at the below-knee, Syme, and partial foot levels is routinely successful. Except for certain hindfoot amputations, the lower fourth of the leg, and at the very short below-knee level, the surgeon selects the lowest level at which successful healing can be expected with a physiological residual limb.

Forefoot and Midfoot Amputations (Fig. 25-14)

Toe, ray, transmetatarsal, and midfoot amputations are indicated when healing can be expected. It is a mistake, however, to conduct repetitive surgery through tissue with a low healing potential. Dry gangrene of the toes invites local removal, but the operation will be unsuccessful unless blood supply is adequate. This is particularly true of patients with classical types of arteriosclerosis. Patients with diabetic ischemia are more likely to heal at these distal levels, providing the gangrene is not complicated by deep infection. Healing is slow; patience is required. Excellent protective footwear, modern partial foot substitutes, and

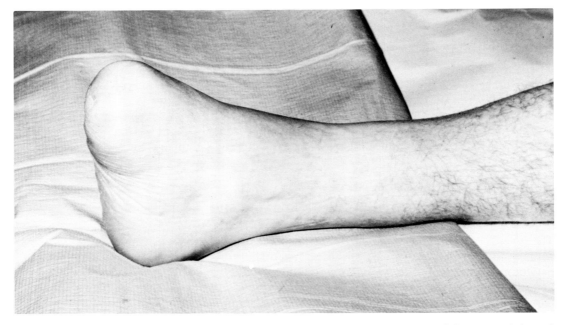

Fig. 25-14. Midfoot amputation performed for ischemia. Amputations of the toes and through the foot are increasingly effective for peripheral vascular disease. Improvements in prosthetic substitution as well as surgical techniques are responsible for the success at these levels.

careful foot hygiene will allow prolonged weight bearing and function in these minor level amputations.

Amputations through the hindfoot are generally avoided in the presence of impaired circulation. Delayed healing, residual ankle equinus, and related problems occur frequently and, for all practical purposes, eliminate these levels.

Syme Amputation (Fig. 25-15)

Until recently the Syme amputation has been considered an unsatisfactory level for peripheral vascular disease. A high failure rate could be expected using the standard one-stage technique. This amputation level nonetheless has certain advantages over higher amputations, including the below-knee level. Less energy consumption is required with the Syme amputation, a large degree of end-bearing is characteristic, the amputation is generally durable, and patients show few problems with pain. Earlier Syme prostheses were cumbersome and unsightly. Several recent prosthetic designs are not only cosmetic but light, functional, and comfortable.

The two-stage technique as used by Wagner[28] has re-established the Syme amputation as a valuable level for ischemia. The initial stage is essentially a closed ankle disarticulation over an irrigation drainage system using the classical heel skin end-pad. The skin flaps are made slightly longer to accommodate the malleoli. Several weeks after healing of the initial amputation, the malleoli are removed through two small incisions, one lateral and one medial. The next stage depends on

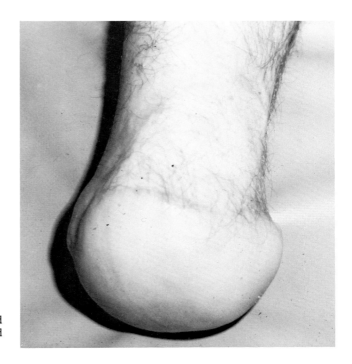

Fig. 25-15. Syme amputation. The heel pad is well centered over the distal tibia and firmly in place.

the score of the ischemic index described earlier in the chapter. When local skin and other tissues are satisfactory and the ischemic index level is 35 percent or above, Wagner and his associates have achieved more than a 90 percent primary healing rate in this two-stage Syme technique.

The Syme amputation does not replace the below-knee level as the major level of choice for peripheral vascular disease. Yet it has become a useful primary site for a significant number of patients, especially those with diabetes. Early rehabilitation is somewhat delayed by the two stages of surgery. Comparatively early postoperative partial weight-bearing can be accomplished in a temporary device, however, and early fitting with provisional prostheses is also successful. The Syme amputation is particularly valuable when the limb loss is bilateral.

Below-Knee Amputation (Fig. 25-16)

Below-knee amputation is the most important level for ischemia. The success in establishing operative and postoperative techniques that salvage the knee represents the single most important recent advance in amputation surgery for ischemia. The surgery is not difficult, but it does demand judgment, experience, careful tissue management, and meticulous attention to early postoperative care. The thousands of patients whose knees have been saved by successful below-knee surgery, along with the quality of life many of them enjoy, mandate a critical evaluation of each patient before routinely proceeding to amputation at a higher level.

Skin and subcutaneous tissue over the anterior lower leg are generally of poorer quality than the skin covering the calf. Cutaneous blood flow, even in the

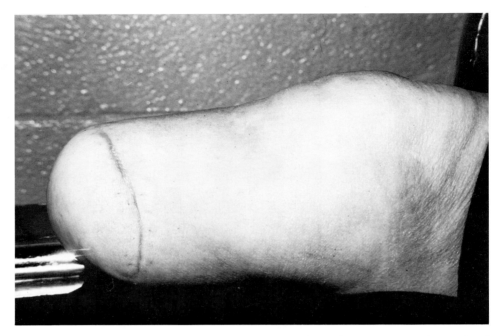

Fig. 25-16. Classical long posterior flap (Burgess technique) below-knee amputation for peripheral vascular disease. This amputation is effective up to the insertion of the patellar tendon when the knee joint is normal.

presence of impaired circulation, is also generally better over the posterior leg area. Classical earlier below-knee amputation techniques utilized a long anterior flap with the closure wound posterior. Reversal of the skin flap to eliminate the anterior flap and create a more desirable posterior skin and myofascial flap with the incision placed anteriorly has overcome most of the healing problems. Improved below-knee socket design and suspension allowed successful prosthesis use with shorter below-knee stumps. These two changes in surgical technique are complemented by the posterior flap support and immobilization of the immediate post-surgical rigid dressing. This combination of the long posterior myofascial-skin flap and the postoperative rigid-pressure dressing have established the below-knee level as appropriate for at least two-thirds of all major amputations for peripheral vascular disease. The surgical and post-surgical details of management are well documented.[7,8,11]

The rigid-dressing technique is especially suitable at the below-knee level. Pressure-sensitive areas on the residual limb at and about the knee must be properly padded and relieved. Suspension of the dressing is secured by using a strap and waist belt with contouring of the cast at the time of its application. Early, not immediate, weight bearing is practical with temporary prosthetic attachments. Since the rigid dressing immobilizes the knee in extension during the early weeks following surgery, flexion contractures and stiffness of the knees are avoided. The entire rehabilitation process, including stump maturation and early limb fit, makes the below-knee level a successful and gratifying rehabilitation experience for both the amputee team and the patient.

Unhealed or partially healed amputations can still be managed in rigid dressings with closed-cast treatment and partial weight-bearing. Experience in treating
open, unhealed, and infected amputations by this method dates back to World
War I. Berlemont revived this treatment after World War II and from his experience, Weiss, Burgess, Gulbranson, and others developed the rigid dressing, immediate post-surgical fitting systems that are now used around the world.[4,9,13,25,29]

Knee Disarticulation (Fig. 25-17)

Knee disarticulation is a perferred level to above-knee amputation when the
choice lies between the two. Some surgeons, particularly in England and Europe,
amputate through the knee as the level of choice. The operation is well tolerated by

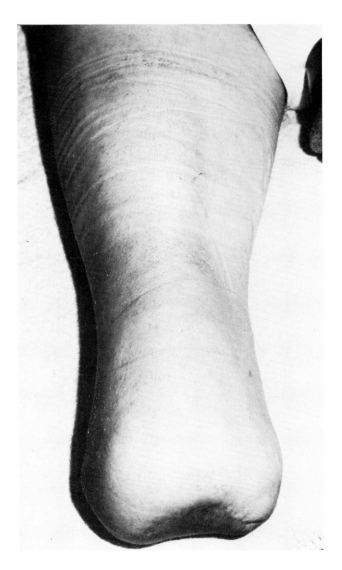

Fig. 25-17. Knee disarticulation with removal of the patella and stabilization of the
flexor and extensor muscles.

older people, bleeding is easily controlled, and surgical complications are few when the skin is sufficiently healthy to heal. The long anterior flap technique, standard for many years, has been replaced by more nearly equal anterior-posterior skin flaps, or by sagittal flaps. The quadriceps mechanism is stabilized by suture of the patellar tendon to the remaining portion of the cruciate ligaments in the intercondylar notch. The hamstring tendons can also be pulled into the notch and stabilized. The patella is generally not disturbed during the performance of knee disarticulation for ischemia.

Rehabilitation of the patient with a knee disarticulation is associated with the same disadvantages that occur at the above-knee level. An artificial knee joint is required: either the simple side joints or the more physiological prostheses such as the polycentric, four-bar, and six-bar linkage mechanisms and the intrinsic knees, which include hydraulic units. None of these prosthetic knees, however, even remotely approaches the control and stability provided by the patient's own knee.

As below-knee amputation has increased in popularity, fewer knee disarticulations are being performed. It nevertheless is a good amputation level when the patient is wheelchair- or bed-confined and not expected to wear a prosthesis or walk. Prosthetic rehabilitation can occur with many knee disarticulation patients, but energy requirements are high and present prostheses are still perceived to be cumbersome and heavy. When the patient's mobility is by wheelchair and no prosthesis is worn, the long-lever arm and increased thigh surface will improve wheelchair sitting, and there will be less of a tendency for fixed hip flexion contractures. It can be expected that through-knee amputations will be performed less frequently as a primary site of election.

Above-Knee Amputation

Formerly the level of choice, the through-thigh amputation is now reserved for patients whose vascular disease is so severe that lower levels cannot be expected to heal and also, of course, for patients whose amputations have failed at the through-knee and below-knee levels. Amputation at this level is also advisable when patients are not ambulatory or have severe knee flexion contractures. Elderly, debilitated patients who are bed-confined and who require major limb ablation will be more easily cared for and have fewer complications at the above-knee level when both unilateral or bilateral amputation is necessary.

The site of above-knee surgery is generally through the mid-thigh. Anterior, posterior, or saggital skin flaps are formed, all equal in length. Extensive muscle stabilizing procedures are avoided; the periosteum and fascia are closed in layers with care to cover the well-rounded bone end adequately and the amputation is made as cylindrical as possible. The overriding consideration is primary healing. Rigid dressings provide an excellent wound environment, although they may become soiled by feces and urine and cause pressure areas around the brim of the cast. Supportive soft-tissue dressings may be more applicable, particularly if the patient is not a potential walker.

Rehabilitation of the potentially ambulatory, elderly patient with above-knee amputation challenges the amputee team. Modern lightweight limbs with safety knees have increased the number of this population who can walk, usually with external aids, but most institutions report one-third or less of these patients becoming functional walkers. Some amputees can wear a provisional limb a few

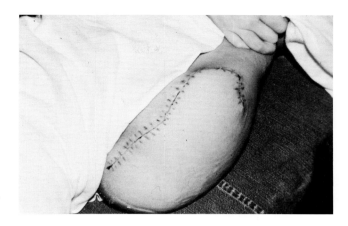

Fig. 25-18. Hip disarticulation with anterior closure.

hours each day for appearance and for stability when sitting. More than any other single group of lower limb amputees, the older above-knee patient needs in-depth evaluation as to rehabilitation potential. Relatives and friends often request a limb when it will not be used. On the other hand, the level of amputation itself should not discourage rehabilitation efforts. It is a gratifying experience to accomplish walking independence with this degree of major limb loss.

Hip Disarticulation (Fig. 25-18)

Severe and total occlusive arterial disease below the level of the renal arteries may occasionally necessitate unilateral or bilateral hip disarticulation. Healing problems are severe, these patients are routinely bed- and wheelchair-confined, and the majority do not survive the disease and the subsequent surgery. Rehabilitation potential is limited to bed care and to occasional sitting. Anticipated longevity is short.

AMPUTATIONS FOR CONDITIONS OTHER THAN PERIPHERAL VASCULAR DISEASE (Figs. 25-19A and 25-19B)

Approximately 20 percent of amputations result from trauma, tumors, and infections. A small number of limb-deficient children also require amputation or revision surgery. Most of these individuals are young or of working age. Rehabilitation offers an unusual opportunity for functional restoration. Physically active lower-extremity amputees can ski, climb mountains, play baseball, basketball, and all racquet sports, swim, ride horses, race motorcycles, run marathons, sky dive, and golf, to name but a few of their recreational activities. They operate heavy construction and farm equipment, drive trucks, build houses, sit in Congress, and are presidents of corporations. Much of this broad scope of physical activity has come about in the last two decades as a result of better amputation surgery and especially because of the great improvement in artificial limbs.

Rehabilitation of these amputees begins with preoperative evaluation and especially with surgery. The so-called conventional or traditional surgical tech-

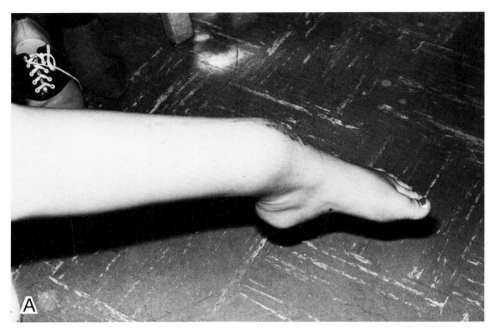

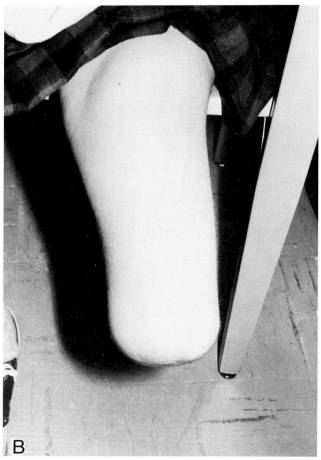

Fig. 25-19. (A) Congenital pseudoarthrosis of the tibia and fibula, multiply operated upon and now requiring below-knee amputation. (B) Healed, muscle-stabilized amputation.

niques are inadequate to prepare the residual limb as a functional organ capable of using a modern prosthesis and thus fully exploiting available functional restoration. Amputation surgery under these circumstances must be considered plastic and especially reconstructive, with emphasis on conservation of length and all useful remaining tissues, especially muscle.

Skin management is planned to provide a healthy, non-adherent, non-tender covering with good sensibility. Placement of the scar is generally irrelevant because the residual limbs will be in total contact with the inside of the socket. Muscles are routinely stabilized near or at the distal end of the stump. In this way the muscles can provide strength, contour, mass, and control. Functioning stump muscles also greatly enhance prosthetic use by normal afferentation, which means proprioception and biofeedback. When properly conditioned, these active residual stump muscles can improve prosthetic suspension and even signal to the amputee both consciously and subconsciously on how to position the leg and the prosthesis more naturally. Many well-muscled amputees relate that use of residual limb muscles within the prosthesis gives them a sense of position and movement of the absent portion of the leg and foot.

Blood vessels are ligated so as to retain maximum blood supply to the limb. Nerves are carefully ligated under gentle traction and allowed to retract into areas surrounded by soft tissue, where they will not be a source of pressure, friction, or irritation. Exteriorizing of certain sensory nerves is being considered as a way of improving pressure information in limb control,[24] although the idea is not practical at this time. The bone is carefully rounded to avoid areas of high pressure and the periosteum is generally closed over the open end of the divided bones.

Amputations performed in this manner require careful, intelligent surgery. Such surgery is as great a challenge as other extremity reconstruction procedures, including joint reconstructions and vascular surgery. It is not casual and should not be performed as a surgical teaching exercise by the least experienced members of the staff.

Amputations and Conversion of Congenital Limb Deficiencies in Children

Amputation surgery for acquired conditions (including trauma and tumors) in the immature skeleton require especially careful planning. The surgeon must project the residual limb to skeletal maturity. These amputations are generally carried out through joints to preserve epiphyses. When diaphyseal surgery is necessary, care must be taken to avoid complications of bone overgrowth. Staged operations in children may be required during the growth period to secure the best possible result at maturity. There is no extremity surgery that requires greater ingenuity, knowledge of the circumstances, and skill than conversion amputations in such complicated limb deficit problems such as proximal focal femoral dysplasia or partial longitudinal absence of the tibia.

Open and Special Amputations

Infected, contaminated, and open amputations are treated as is consistent with the individual pathology. Delayed closures, skin grafts, and revision when necessary employ the same principles of surgery and rehabilitation that have already been outlined. There is still a useful place for skin traction under specific circumstances. The amputee team is constantly aware of the value of early rehabilitation so that the time between amputation and prosthetic fitting is of critical concern for appropriate, long-range rehabilitation.

Atypical residual limbs are occasionally encountered, especially in congenital limb deficits, complicated trauma, and paralytic disorders. Specialized management is required. Close cooperation between the members of the amputee team and the patient and family will achieve planned functional goals.

Postoperative Care

Amputations through relatively healthy and well-vascularized tissue present no healing problem. Immediate rigid dressing and post-surgical prosthetic fitting are by far the best system for routine management. With the exception of complicated cases, such as patients suffering multiple trauma and extensive burns, the immediate post-surgical prosthetic rigid dressing technique permits the amputee

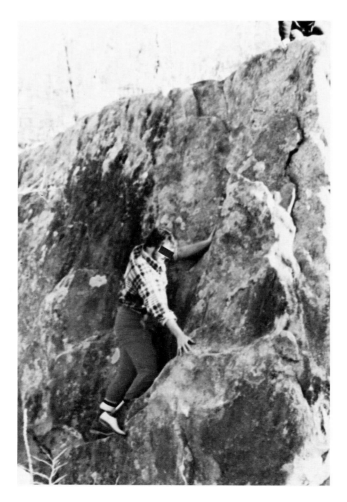

Fig. 25-20. Below-knee amputee is able to enjoy mountain climbing by using a specially designed prosthesis. High levels of physical accomplishment are possible after many types of amputations.

to be up shortly after surgery, assume bipedal activities, and progress rapidly to definitive limb fit. The surgeon cannot justify less effective postoperative management by considering immediate postsurgical prosthetic dressing too technical and complicated to use as compared to simple soft dressings. Alternatives such as the controlled environment chamber, airbags of various types, and semi-rigid dressings are acceptable. The surgeon needs all of the effective modern postoperative management systems and should use them as indicated.

Members of the amputee team are best qualified when they understand and participate in all stages of the rehabilitation process. There is no reason why physical therapists, prosthetists, and engineers should not see the patient prior to surgery and have the opportunity to view the operation itself. The surgeon, likewise, must not relinquish responsibility, care, or interest in the patient following closure of the wound. This total involvement in functional restoration should carry through at least to definitive limb fit. Only when these circumstances exist can the patient, the focal point of the entire amputation team effort, be best served (Fig. 25-20).

Lower extremity amputation, with its accompanying loss and impairment of mobility, severely changes the quality of life. Cosmetic disfigurement is a constant reminder of social and functional disability. Yet high standards of orthopedic rehabilitation are possible even in elderly individuals with limb loss. The amputee rehabilitation team has the great opportunity to perform a rich and rewarding human service to others.

REFERENCES

1. Achauer, B. M., Black, K. S., and Litke, D. K.: Transcutaneous PO_2 in flaps: A new method of survival prediction. Plast. Reconstruct. Surg. 65:738–745, 1980.
2. Anselmo, V. J., and Zawacki, B. E.: Multispectral photographic analysis: A new quantitative tool to assist in the early diagnosis of thermal burn depth. Ann. Biomed. Eng. 5:179–193, 1977.
3. Barnes, R. W., Shank, G. D., and Slaymaker, E. E.: An index of healing in below-knee amputation: Leg blood pressure by Doppler ultrasound. Surgery 79:13–20, 1976.
4. Berlemont, M., Webber, M. R., and Willot, J. P.: Ten years of experience with immediate application of prosthetic devices to amputations of the legs on the operating table. Prosth. Orthop. Int. 3(8):8–18, 1969.
5. Burgess, E. M.: Immediate postsurgical prosthetic fitting: A system of amputee management. J. Am. Phys. Ther. Assoc. 51:139–143, 1971.
6. Burgess, E. M.: Wound healing after amputation: Effect of controlled environment treatment. J. Bone Joint Surg. 60A:245–246, 1978.
7. Burgess, E. M.: General principles of amputation surgery. In American Academy of Orthopaedic Surgeons, Ed.: *Atlas of Limb Prosthetics; Surgical and Prosthetic Principles,* pp. 14–18. C. V. Mosby, St. Louis, 1981.
8. Burgess, E. M.: Postoperative management. In American Academy of Orthopaedic Surgeons, Ed.: *Atlas of Limb Prosthetics; Surgical and Prosthetic Principles,* pp. 19–23. C. V. Mosby, St. Louis, 1981.
9. Burgess, E. M., and Romano, R. L.: The management of lower extremity amputees using immediate postsurgical prostheses. Clin. Orthop. 57:137–146, 1968.
10. Burgess, E. M., Romano, R. L., and Zettl, J. H.: The management of lower extremity amputations. TR 10-6. U.S. Government Printing Office, Washington, D.C., 1969.

11. Burgess, E. M., and Zettl, J. H.: Immediate postsurgical prosthetics. Orthop. Prosthet. 21:105–112, 1967.

12. Fee, H. J., Friedman, B. H., and Siegel, M. E.: The selection of an amputation level with radioactive microspheres. Surg. Gynecol. Obstet. 144:89–90, 1977.

13. Gulbranson, F.: Immediate postsurgical fitting and early ambulation. Clin. Orthop. 56:119–131, 1968.

14. Holloway, G. A.: Cutaneous blood flow responses to injection trauma measured by laser Doppler volocimetry. J. Invest. Dermatol. 74:1–4, 1980.

15. Holloway, G. A., and Burgess, E. M.: Cutaneous blood flow and its relation to healing of below knee amputation. Surg. Gynecol. Obstet. 146:750–756, 1978.

16. Holloway, G. A., and Watkins, D. W.: Laser Doppler measurement of cutaneous blood flow. J. Invest. Dermatol. 69:306–309, 1977.

17. Kegel, B.: Controlled environment treatment (CET) for patients with below knee amputations. Phys. Ther. 56:1366–1371, 1976.

18. Kerstein, M. D.: Utilization of an air splint after below-knee amputation. Am. J. Phys. Med. 53:119–126, 1974.

19. Kostuik, J. P., Wood, D., Hornby, R., and Mathews, V.: The measurement of skin blood flow in peripheral vascular disease by epicutaneous application of xenon 133. J. Bone Joint Surg. 58A:833–837, 1976.

20. Lassen, N. A., and Holstein, P.: Use of radioisotopes in assessment of distal blood pressure in arterial insufficiency. Surg. Clin. North Am. 54:3–55, 1974.

21. Matsen, F. A., Wyss, C. R., Pedegana, L. R., et al.: Transcutaneous PO_2 measurement in peripheral vascular disease—A preliminary report. Surg. Gynecol. Obstet. 150:525–528, 1980.

22. Moore, W. S.: Determination of amputation level. Measurement of skin blood flow with xenon 133. Arch. Surg. 107:798–802, 1973.

23. Moore, W. S.: Determination of amputation level by measurement of skin blood flow. Arch. Surg. 109:124, 1974 (Letter to Editor).

24. Rabischon, P.: Personal communication, 1974.

25. Sarmiento, A., May, B. J., Sinclair, W., et al.: Lower extremity amputation: The impact of immediate postsurgical prosthetic fitting. Clin. Orthop. 68:22–31, 1970.

26. Sher, M. H.: The air splint. An alternate to immediate postoperative prosthesis. Arch. Surg. 108:746–747, 1974.

27. Wagner, F. W.: The diabetic foot and amputation of the foot. In Mann, R. A., Ed.: *DuVrie's Surgery of the Foot,* 4th ed., pp. 341–380. C. V. Mosby, St. Louis, 1978.

28. Wagner, F. W.: The Syme amputation. In American Academy of Orthopaedic Surgeons, Ed.: *Atlas of Limb Prosthetics; Surgical and Prosthetic Principles,* pp. 326–334. C. V. Mosby, St. Louis, 1981.

29. Weiss, M.: *Myoplastic Amputation, Immediate Prosthesis, and Early Ambulation.* U.S. Department of Health, Education and Welfare, U.S. Government Printing Office, Washington, D.C., 1971.

26

Scoliosis

Gordon L. Engler, M.D.

HISTORY AND PREVALENCE

Spinal column deformities were recognized in ancient Greece. Scoliosis due to trauma or disease processes was defined in the *Corpus Hippocraticum,* a group of Greek textbooks written between the fourth century B.C. and the first century A.D. In addition, kyphosis was identified as a separate entity, although insufficient anatomical knowledge led to some erroneous conclusions. The suggestion of a possible relationship between spinal deformity and pulmonary disease was also made in these early writings.

Today, because of increasing concern for early identification and treatment of spinal deformities, school screening programs have been instituted. Several states, including New Jersey and New York, have legislated mandatory school screening for spinal deformities in children in grades seven through ten. It is extremely important to emphasize the risks and complications associated with untreated scoliosis. In this way, the community health department, parent-teacher associations, and local pediatricians and orthopedists can be expected to cooperate with the proposed plan. Education of the parents and children is required to allay the anxieties and fears often associated with unknown medical problems. School nurses and physical education teachers can be instructed with audiovisual aids, available through the Scoliosis Research Society.

The 30-second examination of a child requires the child to bend forward with the fingertips of both hands held together, while the examiner, usually seated in front of the child, looks down the thoracic and lumbar spine. If any asymmetrical elevation is noted in either area, scoliosis must be suspected. Further examination by a trained orthopedist will then determine whether or not an x-ray is required. This limits the need for x-rays to those children who show a positive clinical abnormality, rather than exposing large numbers of children to radiation. These programs often provide early detection of mild curves that may not progress and that occasionally may spontaneously correct to normal alignment without treatment. Early detection and institution of brace treatment can afford good correction and stabilization of mild progressive curves.

Prevalence

In 1975, Brooks et al.[2] determined that the incidence of scoliosis was 13.6 percent, with a female : male ratio of 1.2 : 1. This study was restricted to students in the seventh and eighth grades. The criteria for establishing the diagnosis of scoliosis included the presence of at least one positive clinical sign, such as elevated shoulder, asymmetrical elevation on forward bend, or pelvic obliquity, as well as a curve measuring at least 5 degrees on an anteroposterior (AP) roentgenogram. The most common type of curve was thoracolumbar. Spontaneous improvement occurred in approximately 22 percent of those patients followed for an average of one year (Figs. 26-1A, B).

In a study of junior/senior high school students, Rogala et al.[10] determind the incidence of idiopathic scoliosis at 4.5 percent, the female : male ratio being 1.25 : 1.0. This ratio varied directly with the severity of the curve. That is, 1 : 1 for cruves of 6–10 degrees, and 5.4 : 1 for curves of more than 20 degrees. This study was conducted with boys and girls from 138 schools during the first year of junior high school (grade seven or eight). The age range was 12–14 years old (average: 13.0). The criteria for diagnosis were a structural deformity noted clinically on forward bending or a curve of 6 degrees or more on a subsequent x-ray of a patient with that clinical finding. Progression was observed in 6.8 percent of the students.

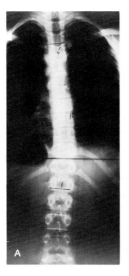 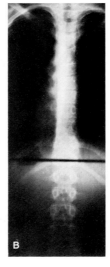

Fig. 26-1. (A) Spontaneous improvement in a right thoracic curve, T4–L1, of 10 degrees. (B) Six months later, erect film shows total resolution with no measurable curve.

In skeletally immature girls with a spinal curve measuring greater than 10 degrees at the initial examination, there was a 15.4 percent incidence of curve progression. No progression was noted in 20 percent of the skeletally immature children with spinal curves measuring more than 20 degrees at the initial examination. Three percent of the cases improved spontaneously, and improvement was seen more frequently in curves measuring less than 11 degrees at the initial examination. Of those examined, treatment was required in 2.75 students per 1000 screened.

Although many prevalence studies have been conducted, a disconcerting variability in results leads one to the conclusion that different diagnostic criteria have led to discrepancies in the statistical analysis. If 10 degrees is used as the "cutting off point" for the diagnosis, the adolescent scoliosis population consists of approximately 25 per 1000.[7]

DEFINITIONS AND NATURAL HISTORY

Scoliosis is defined as a lateral curvature of the spine. In addition to this anatomical variation, the axial skeleton alters in three other major ways. The first is a rotational deformity of the spinal column, the spinous process rotating to the concavity while the body rotates toward the convexity. The greatest rotational deformity occurs at the apex of the curve.

Although it is not known whether it is a precursor or secondary phenomenon of scoliosis, the second alteration is a lateral displacement of the nucleus pulposus within the intervertebral disc space. The displacement of this usually central notochord remnant occurs toward the convexity along the apical segment of the curve, resulting in wedging of the intervertebral disc space as seen on an AP x-ray.

Thirdly, changes in the configuration of the individual vertebral bodies are also noted on an AP x-ray of the spine. Wedging of the vertebral bodies along the apical segment is usually seen in curves of moderate magnitude, that is, those greater than 25 degrees. When wedging of the vertebral body is noted without wedging of the intervertebral disc space, the prognosis is good when early treatment in an appropriate brace is instituted. When, however, intervertebral disc wedging from lateral displacement of the nucleus pulposus is seen, the curve is usually resistant to conservative treatment. Correction or stabilization with an orthotic device is more difficult to accomplish. These curves often require surgery.

Natural History

Neuromuscular Scoliosis. Paralysis accounts for approximately 10 percent of all cases of scoliosis seen. Neuropathic scoliosis includes disorders of lower motor neuron disease, such as poliomyelitis, upper motor neuron disease, such as cerebral palsy, and others, such as syringomyelia. Myopathic diseases would include progressive muscular dystrophy, amyotonia, and Friedreich's ataxia.

Congenital Scoliosis. Children with congenital osseous spinal defects comprise 10 percent of those patients seen with scoliosis. These defects include hemivertebrae, wedged vertebrae, unilateral unsegmented bars, and block vertebrae. In addition, an extravertebral cause, such as fusion of the ribs, can be responsible for scoliosis in this congenital group. Often, several congenital abnormalities occur simultaneously, thus giving rise to the "mixed variety" of congenital scoliosis. In addition, deformities of the spine can be caused by congenital abnormalities of spinal cord development. These include myelodysplasia scoliosis, kyphosis, and lordosis.

Scoliosis due to Associated Diseases. Five percent of scoliosis cases can be ascribed to a variety of associated diseases. These include neurofibromatosis, familial dysautonomia, Marfan's disease, and muscular dystrophy.

Idiopathic Scoliosis. Seventy-five percent of all cases of scoliosis are classified as idiopathic. Investigations[5,12] have shown that there is direct genetic transmission: parents with scoliosis are more likely to have children with curved spines. Yet the transmission is one of incomplete penetrance and variable expressivity, since the disease can vary in incidence and severity within one family. Offspring of families with a prior history of scoliosis should therefore be screened more diligently during their growth phase.

Because most cases of idiopathic scoliosis are genetically transmitted, family planning becomes extremely important. Early detection enables the physician to institute appropriate methods of treatment and prevent the development of serious curves that could otherwise produce severe cosmetic deformity. The fear of transmitting spinal curves genetically should no longer deter parents with scoliosis from having families.

Families who have one or more children affected by scoliosis need psychological support. The physician must explain that proper treatment instituted early can permit the child with scoliosis to lead a normal existence. Modern bracing techniques and dramatic surgical correction can reduce the emotional burden on both the family and the patient.

The physician must emphasize that within a family, some children with scoliosis may not need treatment, while their siblings may require bracing. The physician must allay the anxiety of a mother who feels she has transmitted the disease to her child. The child with a spinal deformity may come from a broken home. The physician must take great care to avoid conflicts within the separated family that would work to the detriment of the patient. Ascribing the cause of the curve to either of the two parents is unimportant. Indeed, all concerned with the treatment program must be made to appreciate that the patient requires continuing pyschological support. It is only with this supportive assistance that any treatment can work; bracing or surgery can only be successful in a child who has the full emotional support of the physician and all concerned relatives.

TREATMENT

Nonsurgical Means

Idiopathic scoliosis is further subdivided according to age of onset. When the curve is identified between the ages of birth and 3 years, the scoliosis is defined as *infantile idiopathic scoliosis*. To be so identified, no osseous abnormality can be present that would otherwise classify it as a congenital scoliosis. When the curve is first identified between the ages of 3 and 10 years, it is classified as a *juvenile idiopathic scoliosis*. This category, for reasons yet undetermined, is more prevalent in England and a few other European countries than it is in the United States.[6,8] The third and largest group of idiopathic scoliosis cases are classified as *adolescent idiopathic scoliosis* and are first identified between the ages of 10 and 17 years.

Treatment in all these groups is essentially related to the magnitude of the curve at the time of the initial examination and the progression as noted on subsequent examination. Many methods of treatment exist. Nevertheless, few modalities have afforded demonstrable stabilization or improvement of the spinal curve.

Exercises. Exercises for strengthening the muscles on the convex side of the curve are often prescribed unaccompanied by other treatment. The efficacy of exercise alone has never been scientifically documented. Indeed, contralateral facilitation of muscular development can be expected in most idiopathic scoliosis patients. Zuk[13] has shown increased spontaneous muscular activity on the convex side of the curve in typical idiopathic scoliosis patients. When therapeutic exercises are combined with a scoliosis brace, however, the result can be significant improvement or stabilization of the curve.

Manipulation. Manipulation has also been attempted for correction of scoliosis. At present, no adequate scientific evidence has been found to substantiate the claim that spinal deformities can be corrected through manipulation. Indeed, delay in obtaining a brace or postponing surgery while undergoing manipulative measures can contribute to significant curve progression.

Traction. Traction alone cannot correct scoliosis. Indeed, stretching muscles and ligaments involved with spinal alignment can hypermobilize the axial skeleton. Gravity can then cause significant progression of an otherwise stabilizing spinal curve. Some attempts have been made to utilize traction at night while maintaining the patient in a spinal brace during the day.[3] This treatment has not proved to afford conclusively better spinal correction than the normal, full-time (day and night) use of a brace.

Electrical Stimulation. Recent research in several centers in the United States and Canada has attempted to correct spinal deformities by electrically stimulating the muscles on the convex side of the curve with implanted or surface electrodes.[1] Although the results of these early projects show promise, conclusive evidence of the efficacy of this treatment in scoliosis has not yet been presented.

Biofeedback. Some research on scoliosis is now being conducted in the field of biofeedback. A signal tone sounds when the patient does not maintain spinal alignment. To turn off the audible stimulus, efforts must be made to correct the spinal alignment. Although still in the experimental stages, and yet to be tested on large series of patients, this device may potentially be efficacious.

Bracing. In general, a curve measuring 18 degrees or less in a growing adolescent can be safely observed for a period of approximately four months. Under normal circumstances, idiopathic scoliosis, if progressive, will advance at the rate of 1 degree per month. If the curve is greater than 18 degrees at the initial examination, or a progression to more than 18 degrees is noted during the observation period, a formal bracing program must be instituted immediately. In a young woman, the onset of osseous maturation usually occurs with the onset of menses at approximately age 12.5 years. Osseous maturation continues over the next four years until the apophyses of the iliac crest and vertebral rings close, or at least are complete in their excursion. Progression is more rapid and dramatic during the first two years, whereas the process slows over the last two years. For this reason, bracing must be considered in the early phase of growth. By accomplishing early stabilization and correction, some flexibility in the brace program can often be permitted in the last two years of growth. If correction and stabilization of the curve have been achieved by age 14, part-time bracing is often possible for the last two years of use.

Once a brace becomes necessary, several difficulties arise. The psychological aspects of enforcing a spinal brace on a growing adolescent cause major social problems. The child may not wish to wear the brace to school or to expose herself during gymnasium classes. Nevertheless, full-time utilization of the brace is mandatory and must be accepted by the patient. This acceptance demands cooperation and emotional support from the family as well as the physician. If other friends or schoolmates already have braces, the task is much easier. A similarity might be drawn between those who wear braces on their teeth, a well-recognized and accepted form of treatment for orthodontic problems.

It is an extremely difficult adjustment for a child to accept wearing a long-term spinal brace. The child has a deformity that requires an orthotic device for an indefinite period of time—until the cessation of growth. Some patients will immediately request surgical correction, preferring the postoperative cast, which is an obvious external device and one readily accepted by the patient's peers. Furthermore, a definite time period is predetermined, at the conclusion of which the cast is removed. This fact makes the cast a much more acceptable condition of treatment. Nevertheless, when the curve measures less than 40 degrees, surgery is usually not required.

A physical education program must be continued while the patient is in the brace. Physical activity allows adequate maintenance of the musculoskeletal system. Activities such as swimming, calisthenics, and other noncontact sports can be performed for short periods of time out of the brace. These should be encouraged. Indeed, if the brace were worn constantly, a certain physiological stiffening and muscular atrophy would ensue. By combining a prescribed amount of physical activity with therapeutic exercises, that weakening can be avoided. In general, the exercise program designed for the patient with a scoliosis brace includes a program of physical conditioning, with emphasis on abdominal muscle tone, hamstring stretching, and pelvic tilt. Upper extremity and shoulder girdle exercises are also of overall benefit.

In recent years, several varieties of braces have appeared. The standard Milwaukee brace is usually now used only for high thoracic curves or thoracic curves of significant magnitude. At present, a low profile or underarm type of brace can be used with effective results for thoracolumbar and lumbar curves. The new braces are plastic and are much lighter than previous heavy metal and leather braces. Caring for the plastic brace is also much easier (Figs. 26-2A, B, C).

Boys sometimes require similar scoliosis braces. Usually a male's muscular development and ligamentous inflexibility permit successful correction to be attained with less than full-time brace utilization. A program of athletics can also be instituted more easily with boys. However, the male with a progressive curve and extensive muscular development often fails to respond to a brace program, and he may require surgery at a later date.

When a brace is required for a child younger than 10 years of age, it is difficult to provide the parent with a definite end point of brace treatment. Some young children will only require a spinal brace full time until the conclusion of osseous maturation. In others a progression of the curve in spite of full-time bracing will demonstrate that the brace is not affording adequate spinal stabilization and that surgical intervention is necessary.

When a dancer or professional or college athlete requires brace treatment for scoliosis, consideration must be given to the normal activities of the patient. In most instances the patient's exercise program is beneficial and can therefore easily be included in the strenghtening exercises designed specifically for scoliosis.

The obese child will not respond favorably to brace treatment because of the interposition of subcutaneous and adipose tissue between the brace and the osseous structures upon which the brace must exert its corrective forces. Indeed, the brace usually does not push on the osseous structures; if it did, decubiti would develop. Rather, the brace affords its correction by encouraging the child to assume an erect posture. The child herself must therefore bring about the correction and muscular realignment of the spinal curve. Office visits are required at three- to five-month intervals. These usually include x-ray examination and orthotic revision of the brace pads. An often-seen initial result of brace treatment

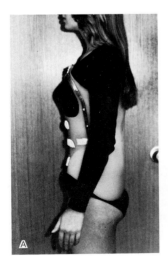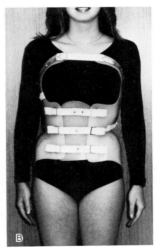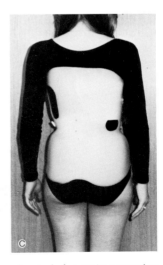

Fig. 26-2A,B,C. A type of low profile or underarm brace presently under study for use in correcting thoracolumbar and lumbar curves. A front closure and the absence of a neck ring make it a more acceptable orthosis to the adolescent.

is a dramatic increase in the child's height. This occurs because of the straightening of the spinal curve and is only in part due to the osseous elongation of the axial skeleton.

It is extremely important to show the child tangible evidence of her curve correction by allowing her to view the x-rays at the periodic examinations. As correction is attained, occasional periods out of the brace may be awarded to the patient for social functions. Visual confirmation that her efforts at correction are succeeding, plus awards of "time off for good behavior," are strong psychological motivations that make compliance with a full-time brace program more palatable.

Some correction and stabilization usually occur after the patient has worn her brace full time for about a year. During this initial period, the brace is worn for 23 hours per day. After the first year, if the curve has been corrected to less than 20 degrees and some stabilization has been identified, some amount of time away from the brace may be permitted. This usually consists of the daytime school hours; the patient continues to wear the brace for sleeping.

When the osseous maturation has run its course, as determined by the vertebral ring and iliac crest apophyses, the curve's stabilization can be tested. This is accomplished by taking an x-ray after the patient has been out of her brace for approximately six to eight hours. If little or no progression has occurred, a weaning program from the brace may be instituted. This weaning usually occurs over a four-month period. When, at the conclusion of osseous maturation, the curve measures 30 degrees or less, little progression can be expected. If at the conclusion of the brace program, however, the curve measures 40 degrees or more, one can usually expect progression, and surgical correction is often indicated. In pregnant women, significant progression can occur in curves measuring more than 40 degrees.

The expectation of the correction afforded by the brace must be explained to the patient and parents. While the brace is being worn, correction can be seen on x-rays. When osseous maturation occurs, and the patient is weaned from the brace, the curve may regress to the original, prebrace magnitude, or slightly worse. For example, a curve of 25 degrees may be corrected to 18 degrees during the brace treatment. After the brace is discontinued, the curve may progress to 25 degrees or 30 degrees between the ages of 18 and 25. Nevertheless, had no brace treatment been instituted and the curve allowed to advance unchecked during the active growth years, a curve measuring 50–60 degrees could be expected at the conclusion of osseous maturation.

Surgery

When a curve greater than 40 degrees is noted in a child of 12 years or older, surgical intervention is usually indicated. Furthermore, in the rare curve that shows progression to greater than 40 degrees in spite of the brace treatment, surgical correction is necessary (Figs. 26-3A, B, C). In addition, some scoliosis patients who present with a significant thoracic lordosis and associated diminished anteroposterior chest diameter respond poorly to brace correction.[9] In fact, the lordosis may be worsened and the scoliosis progress with the use of a brace. In these children, early surgery is usually indicated.

When surgery is the only reasonable choice of therapy, great care must be

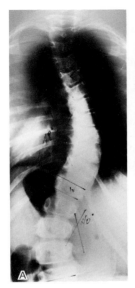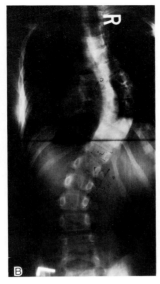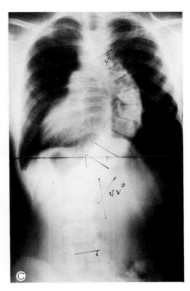

Fig. 26-3. (A) Initial x-rays of a child aged 10 years and 1 month with a right thoracic scoliosis. T5–T12 is 48 degrees; left lumbar T12–L4 is 40 degrees. (B) Five months after institution of a full-time Milwaukee brace worn 23 hours per day, the scoliosis has progressed. Right thoracic T5–T12 is 55 degrees; left lumbar T12–L4 is 38 degrees. (C) Ten months after initial examination and full-time use of Milwaukee brace, the scoliosis has advanced enough to discontinue the brace and recommend an operation. Right thoracic T4–T11 is 64 degrees; left lumbar T11–L4 is 42 degrees.

taken to explain to the parents, as well as to the child, the considerable problems that might ensue if the operation were not performed. The cosmetic deterioration, the onset of severe pain in later years due to osteoarthritis, and the possibility of cardiopulmonary deficiency after the curve progresses to more than 65 degrees are important justifications for surgery. Furthermore, it is much easier to correct and stabilize the spine of an adolescent than that of a mature scoliotic patient. By allowing the curve to progress during the later years of growth, the magnitude of the curve will be greater, and the percentage of attainable correction less.

The risks of the surgical procedure, which involves a spine fusion usually with the insertion of Harrington instrumentation, must also be explained to the parents and child. Three major risks of the operation include paralysis, infection, and the possibility of pseudoarthrosis.

Although its incidence is less than 1 percent, paralysis is the foremost risk in the operative procedure. Paralysis is thought to come from over-stretching the spinal cord and its associated arterial supply, causing an ischemic necrosis of the spinal cord with resultant paralysis. If the Harrington instrumentation is removed immediately after the operation, the paralysis is temporary and full recovery is likely. Preventive measures to avoid paralysis during the procedure include the Stagnara "wake up test"[11] and the monitoring of somatosensory-evoked potentials.[4]

The incidence of infection is usually less than 2 percent. Prophylactic antibiotics have been used in scoliosis operations, but they are often avoided due to the possible promulgation of resistant strains.

The incidence of pseudoarthrosis is usually less than 3 percent. If it does occur, it requires a second operation to reinforce the area of the pseudoarthrosis and alleviate the pain that has ensued.

It is often beneficial to allow the patient and her family to discuss the operation with other patients who have already undergone it. This is best accomplished with the particular physician's own patients, since it is his hospitalization and postoperative regimen that will be followed. Talking with a peer often affords a more realistic understanding of the surgery, the hospitalization, and the cast immobilization.

The physician and the family must have realistic goals and expectations for the outcome of the operation. Certainly the physician is satisfied correcting approximately 60 percent of the curve, although that may allow some rib deformity to persist. The partial nature of the improvement must be carefully explained to the patient and her family so that they realize that a perfect realignment of the spine is not a realistic goal. Emphasis must be placed on the fact that stabilization of the spinal curve will prevent further deterioration and curvature. The fact that the curve can also be corrected with the Harrington instrumentation is a bonus of the newer techniques.

Preoperative preparation of the patient requires a full battery of tests, which include an electrocardiogram, pulmonary function studies, and blood chemistry. In addition, bending x-rays have to be obtained to ascertain the flexibility of the curve and determine if the curve is structural or not; the difference determines the length of the fusion and the position of the instrumentation at the time of surgery. The patient must also be prepared psychologically. Such counseling is best done by the surgeon in his office and in the hospital by a well-trained nursing and house staff with substantial experience in dealing with the problems of scoliosis patients.

Postoperatively, a cast is usually worn from six to nine months. It is common for a patient to go through an initial claustrophobia or depressive state when the cast is initially applied. With assistance from the family and medical staff, the period of adjustment can usually be lessened, and the cast tolerated for the full length of time. Ambulation in the cast is permitted. Restrictions while in the cast include participation in athletics and prolonged periods of standing or walking. Care of the patient's mental as well as physical status must be accomplished, and a program of mild exercises is usually encouraged.

After the cast is removed, the child is usually restricted from contact sports and gymnastics involving the utilization of an apparatus, such as a trampoline or parallel bars. Cross-country skiing, tennis, swimming, and basketball are usually permitted in the regular postoperative program once the cast has been removed.

Although no growth occurs over the area of the fusion, the overall loss in longitudinal height is negligible, because what is lost by fusion is gained by straightening. The loss of flexibility over the fused segment does not seriously affect motion or overall body function. The patient can still bend at the waist and hips and does not assume a ''robot-like'' appearance.

The long-term effects of the fusion are usually beneficial. There will be no development of arthritis, since the joints over the fused segments do not move. Several segments are usually left open below the fusion mass for normal movement. There is no evidence at present to indicate that excessive motion causes deterioration of the lower vertebral segments because of a long, fused segment of thoracolumbar spine.

Although the decision when to operate is determined by a physical examination of the child and a judicious review of x-rays, it is often as important to decide when not to operate. The physician involved in the treatment of scoliosis must appreciate that severe curves may involve more surgery than the patient can tolerate. Furthermore, if no improvement in quality of life for a particular patient can be expected by the operative procedure, surgery should not be recommended. Some patients are not emotionally prepared to undergo the cast immobilization required after surgery. This reluctance is found more often in older adolescents and adults, but it has been seen in some children with previous psychiatric histories.

ADULT SCOLIOSIS

In the adult, surgical correction of severe curves greater than 45 degrees is indicated when pain or progression is noted. The circulation of hormones that become prevalent during the third trimester of pregnancy may cause significant progression of a curve that had previously been stable.

In the postmenopausal woman with untreated scoliosis, osteoporosis may cause further spinal deterioration and vertebral body collapse. The premonition of this fact may also be a reasonable cause for recommending spinal fusion in the 20- to 40-year-old woman.

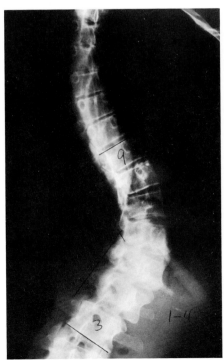

Fig. 26-4. X-rays of a 32-year-old woman. The right lumbar scoliosis from T9–L3 is 67 degrees. In addition, the early lateral spondylolisthesis of L2 on L3 can be seen.

The untreated scoliotic senior citizen often shows a lateral spondylolisthesis, especially in curves of the lumbar spine (Fig. 26-4). The osteoarthritis that ensues because of lateral stress on the displaced vertebral segments can cause great pain in this age group. To avoid osteoarthritis, an operation is prescribed before menopausal osteoporosis and lateral spondylolisthesis have become manifest.

Once a thoracic curve progresses to 65 degrees, an appreciable reduction in pulmonary function can be anticipated. To avoid this condition, surgical correction and stabilization must be accomplished before age 45 or the onset of the menopause.

MANAGEMENT OF SCOLIOSIS FROM OTHER CAUSES

Recommending surgical correction for a scoliosis patient with an associated disease is a complex problem related to the child's overall condition. For example, a patient with meningomyelocele with a motor level of L2 or above usually has a 100 percent chance of developing a spinal deformity. Nevertheless, the extraordinary measures that would have to be undertaken to operate on such a

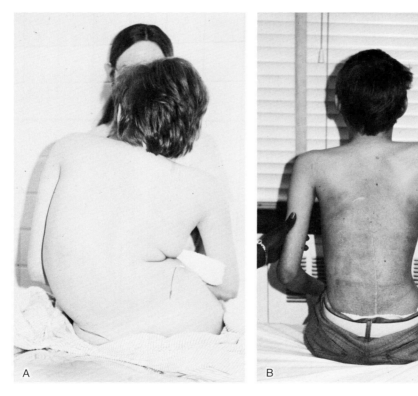

A

B

Fig. 26-5. (A) Before surgery, this patient with muscular dystrophy demonstrated severe scoliosis and pelvic obliquity. (B) After surgery, the thoracic configuration has improved and the upper extremities are more easily used for lapboard activities.

child or adolescent often involve too great a risk to the patient. It is far better to supply the child at an early age with a form of bracing and night splints in an attempt to thwart more severe spinal deformities.

In the young paralytic child, measures must be taken to provide competent bracing early in an attempt to retard the relentless progression of the scoliosis.

In some forms of congenital scoliosis, such as the unilateral unsegmented bar, an early fusion done at age 3 or 4 years may often be necessary. By limiting the fusion to the area of the congenital anomaly, the overall length of the child's spine can be preserved and growth left uninhibited in the remaining segments. No instrumentation is used during the spinal fusion of a congenital scoliosis.

In patients with a significant spinal curve who are confined to a wheelchair, the upper extremities are often used to support the upper body. By correction and stabilization of the spinal deformity, the upper extremities are freed to allow for activities of daily living (Figs. 26-5A, B).

In some patients who use long leg braces and crutches for ambulation, a spine fusion, which often straightens the normal lumbar lordosis, may cause a serious hardship because pelvic motion is required for ambulation. In these instances, it is sometimes necessary to perform a limited anterior interbody fusion with Dwyer instrumentation rather than a long posterior fusion with Harrington instrumentation. In general, a spine fusion is not performed if it could alter or interfere with ambulatory status, and the child or adult is encouraged to continue without the benefits of the operation.

SUMMARY

Untreated idiopathic scoliosis can mean severe disability in life and work. Early institution of adequate bracing can prevent serious cosmetic, emotional, and physical deformities. Surgical procedures to correct scoliosis also play a vital role in the rehabilitation of any patient with a severe spinal deformity.

In the handicapped child with scoliosis, many obvious benefits of surgical correction can be seen in the rehabilitation program. Nevertheless, it is far better to brace early and avoid significant deformities than to attempt extraordinary measures for spinal correction in an already disabled child.

By early detection, application of simple orthotic devices, and appropriate follow-up examination and rehabilitative measures, the need for surgery can be lessened. Nevertheless, when necessary, surgery provides the patient with a solution to a previously little-understood and often inadequately treated orthopedic problem.

REFERENCES

1. Bobechko, W. P.: Scoliosis spinal pacemaker. J. Bone Joint Surg. 56A:442, 1974.
2. Brooks, H. L., Azen, S. P., Gerberg, E., et al.: Scoliosis: A prospective epidemiological study. J. Bone Joint Surg. 57A:968–972, 1975.
3. Cotrel, Y.: Traction in the treatment of vertebral deformity. J. Bone Joint Surg. 57B:260, 1975.

4. Engler, G. L., Spielholz, N. I., Bernhard, W. N., et al.: Somatosensory evoked potentials during Harrington instrumentation for scoliosis. J. Bone Joint Surg. 60A(4):528–532, 1978.

5. Harrington, P. R.: The etiology of idiopathic scoliosis. Clin. Orthop. 126:17–25, 1977.

6. James, J. I. P.: Two curve patterns in idiopathic structural scoliosis. J. Bone Joint Surg. 33B:339–406, 1951.

7. Kane, W. J.: Scoliosis prevalence. Clin. Orthop. 126:43–46, 1977.

8. Lloyd-Roberts, C. G., and Pilcher, M. F.: Structural idiopathic scoliosis in infancy: A study of the natural history of 100 patients. J. Bone Joint Surg. 47B:520–523, 1965.

9. Moe, J. H., Winter, R. B., Bradford, D. S., and Lonstein, J. E.: *Scoliosis and Other Spinal Deformities*. W. B. Saunders, Philadelphia, 1978.

10. Rogala, E. J., Drummond, D. S., and Gurr, J.: Scoliosis: Incidence and natural history. J. Bone Joint Surg. 60A:173–176, 1978.

11. Vauzelle, P. L., Jr., Stagnara, P., Jouvinroux, P.: Functional monitoring of spinal cord activity during spinal surgery. Clin. Orthop. 93:173–178, 1973.

12. Wynne-Davies R.: Familial (idiopathic) scoliosis. J. Bone Joint Surg. 50B:24–30, 1968.

13. Zuk, T.: The role of spinal and abdominal muscles in the pathogenesis of scoliosis. J. Bone Joint Surg. 44B:102–105, 1962.

27

Developmental Neuromuscular Disease

Wilton H. Bunch, M.D., Ph.D.

Neuromuscular diseases are among the most common childhood disorders seen by an orthopedic surgeon. The incidence of these ranges from cerebral palsy, which occurs about 6 times per 1000 live births, to muscular dystrophies, which together account for about 1 per 10,000 live births. The total incidence for the neuromuscular diseases of childhood is somewhere around 8–10 per 1000 births, or nearly 1 percent.

The rehabilitation goals in these diseases are widely variable and depend on the degree of disability. Although the same can be said of adult neuromuscular disabilities, children differ in that they have never previously experienced normal movement and mobility. Thus, children must simultaneously undergo their childhood growth and development and the "rehabilitation" of their neurological disease.

This chapter is organized around two "models" of childhood disabilities. The first, myelomeningocele, is characterized by the child who is born with the defect. The second, muscular dystrophy, is a disability of later onset, and therefore presents a different set of problems. These same considerations hold for other disease entities of childhood, and the application is left to the reader.

THE MYELOMENINGOCELE PATIENT

The goal of rehabilitation is to assist in the recovery of the maximum function possible, consistent with the residual disease process. In the case of a child born with a myelomeningocele, the goal of rehabilitation, or more strictly speaking, habilitation, is to assist in the natural development of the child to the highest level consistent with the neurological defect. The child with a myelomeningocele has many organ systems involved. Problems that arise in any of these organ systems may delay the development of the child, and therefore impede his habilitation. The myelomeningocele child is extremely vulnerable to developmental delay secondary to medical problems, and the prevention of this delay must be the goal of each medical specialist.

The orthopedic surgeon has a great deal to offer in maintaining a normal sequence of development. By assuring that certain milestones of stability and mobility are met, the subsequent cognitive, linguistic, and social development dependent on them can be accomplished. It is imperative therefore that the orthopedic surgeon understand these milestones and provide correct and timely intervention to assist the child in attaining them. This is a different outlook than medical decisions based on the usual orthopedic or rehabilitative stance. It is one of anticipation, prevention, and augmentation rather than repair, replacement, or re-education. The care of most myelomeningocele patients gravitates toward specialized centers instead of being uniformly distributed within the local medical institutions. The result is that most orthopedists and physiatrists are not comfortable with or expert in the care of myelomeningocele children. This is not necessarily bad. What is inexcusable is the orthopedist or physiatrist who feels that all knowledge is contained within his person but who is out of date or otherwise less competent than believed. The bias of the author is that the average neuromusculoskeletal specialist should be able to assess how the child is doing, but probably should not expect to be the only medical contact in that particular discipline.

The discussion proceeds according to the development of the child, rather than on an anatomical basis. Proper treatments for various anatomical deformities are considered in the light of their influence on the overall development of the child. Details of surgical procedures, which are readily available elsewhere, are not provided here.

The Infant

The newborn infant seems so tiny, so helpless, so passive that we sometimes assume that very little is happening. This attitude is wrong. The infant is a competent learner and an active participant in the environment. The newborn child can select what it wishes to see, preferring patterns, faces, and moving objects. When it tires of one pattern, a new pattern will again stimulate its interest. The newborn can discriminate speech and music from noise and demonstrate olfactory discrimination and tactile responsiveness. The newborn is ready to become a part of its world. Yet the newborn infant with a myelomeningocele is separated from the world when placed in an incubator in the intensive care unit. There it is not fondled, it is not handled, it is not picked up, and developmental delay begins at once.

The importance of early interaction between the mother and the child has been extensively studied and is called "bonding." In one study,[12] 28 first-time mothers were given the naked baby for an hour after delivery. During the time the mother's episiotomy was being repaired, she was fondling and cleaning her child. In addition to feedings, the baby was with the mother for five additional hours during each day. A comparison group was shown the baby at birth, and then the child was taken away for bathing and the usual medical care. These children were with their mother for half-hour feedings, but otherwise kept in the nursery. At 5 months, 12 months, and 2 years, the children who had spent more time with their mothers were more advanced cognitively than the normally treated children.

Another study was designed to look at the effect of early contact on the mother.[16] Half of these mothers spent eight hours a day with the child during the postpartum hospitalization. The other half had the child at feeding time only. At two years, there were fewer cases of abandonment, abuse, prolonged neglect, or inadequate care by the mothers who had the additional time with their infants. Whether the effect of this early increased contact is on the child, on the mother, or on both is unclear; nevertheless, the child with a myelomeningocele is denied this contact and is not even with his mother at feeding time. Even when using caution in interpreting these studies, it is safe to say that myelomeningocele children are denied the potential benefit of early contact. In fact, they are frequently denied nearly all contact with the mother for several weeks.

The child who has spent one month in the intensive care unit is measurably delayed. Normally a month-old infant can follow light to the midline, fix both eyes on a light, react positively to comfort, and cry to express demands.[10] The child who has spent the first month in the intensive care unit may not be able to perform any of these activities. Pediatricians are very aware of this information, and they and the neonatal intensive care nurses do their best to minimize the environmental deprivation. However, its impact cannot be denied. The overriding rehabilitative aim is to get the child home with the mother. The orthopedist must be certain that the treatment does not prolong hospitalization at this point.

Initially the orthopedist will be seeing the child with a myelomeningocele because of deformities in the lower limbs. Treatment should not prolong hospitalization. Casting of the knees can usually begin immediately; using serial casts, the knees can be brought into 90 degrees of flexion and stabilized. Since intravenous therapy usually proceeds through the feet, the casts should stop above the malleoli. In this way, they do not interfere with overall treatment but are not being delayed themselves. In contrast, treatment of the feet may have to wait until the "offending" intravenous tubes can be removed. The casts can be changed approximately every three to five days while the child is still in the hospital. Afterward an outpatient schedule should be instituted.

Traditionally, the treatment of congenitally dislocated or dislocatable hips prolongs hospitalization, so care is given to preventing dislocation. Normally the child in intensive care is positioned on its side. If the high hip is dislocatable, the position of adduction and flexion will promote and maintain a dislocation. But if the child is carefully put in a prone position,[17] the hips can be abducted and controlled. This position allows care of the back closure and prevents soiling of the wound as well. If positioned this way in intensive care, many children's hips will stabilize by the time of discharge.

An alternative is the Pavlov harness. Although the device is somewhat clumsy on the newborn, it can be positioned. The hips are held in a position of flexion and slight abduction. Many myelomeningocele centers are combining these two approaches: positioning for intensive care patients and the harness used at the time of discharge.

From 1–6 months of age, the child's development progresses in all spheres. The child learns to smile and, with this gain, the amount of adult interaction markedly increases. The child develops head control and some mobility. This is an opportune time for casting without developmental losses.

If dislocated, the hips should be reduced and immobilized to gain stability. Knee stability and motion should be present. Any treatment of the feet should be nonoperative. If surgery will be required, it should be delayed until about 9 months of age. The rationale for delay is that standing will help to maintain the correction. Accordingly, the period of cast removal should coincide with the projected time the child will begin to stand.

The Sensorimotor Period: Age 6 Months to 4 Years

The concept of a sensorimotor period is derived from psychologists, most notably Piaget. He and subsequent investigators observed that mental development is the result of interaction of the infant and the environment. The child learns by touching, feeling, licking, and dropping things about him. The information gained from the manipulation of things increases mental ability. Any delay in gross motor activity will inhibit this active participation and therefore retard cognitive, linguistic, and social development.[10]

The orthopedist now becomes the most critical person in the child's development. If he is ignorant of these concepts, he may have the child in a heavy bilateral hip spica, which totally prevents all motion. As a result, he may cause frightening developmental delay that he may later attribute to organic brain disease. Yet if the orthopedist uses his devices to augment the motor activity of the child, he may produce rapid increase in cognitive and fine motor skills.

Age 6–12 Months. The first gross motor tasks in this period are the progressive development of head control when upright and the automatic righting reflexes that when developed, lead to independent sitting. Once these are accomplished, hands are then freed for midline activity and play. The major cognitive milestone during this time is the development of the concept of object permanence. No longer is the "out of sight, out of mind" approach of the younger infant adequate. The child of this period is learning that the toy under the blanket is still there and he will search for it. He knows or is learning that the cookie covered by mother's hand is still very worthy of search and discovery. He plays peek-a-boo and knows that covering his eyes will not deprive him of his mother.

Speech at this age is event-specific crying. The mother who persists in shielding a cookie from the prying fingers of a child will hear a loud wail of unhappiness. This is appropriate use of language and communicates a meaning as clearly as does any adult. Similarly, the child of this age who loudly protests the cast saw in orthopedic clinic is not being a "bad child," but is using his language ability to communicate a very real dislike.

These cognitive, fine motor, and speech developments are dependent on sitting. Therefore the child of this age who does not sit will be delayed even if no organic brain lesion exists. Imagine a child with a high neurological level and congenital kyphosis. The child cannot sit because of spinal instability. And when he is propped up, both hands are required to maintain trunk support. Since his arms are his body stabilizers, they cannot participate in motor development, and hand-eye coordination suffers. Because he does not have the hand-eye coordination, the active play with objects and the development of object permanence are delayed. Thus delayed sitting, in effect, retards all other aspects of development.

The orthopedist is able to intervene in this potentially disastrous situation. If an 8-month-old child is not yet sitting, he can be given a light body jacket to hold him upright. With a jacket, the hands are freed to explore and play. Finger feeding becomes possible. The development of concepts about the objects in his environment speeds up, and developmental delay is prevented.

The orthopedist may contribute to developmental delay by having the child in a spica cast and supine during this period. Occasionally there seems to be no alternative, but whenever it is possible a child should be upright. If the sequence of development is needed, most orthopedic treatment still can be undertaken and the child allowed to develop.

Age 1–3 Years. At about the age of 1 year, the normal child begins to stand and walk. With this new mobility, the exploration of his environment expands proportionately. Fine motor control increases, as demonstrated by the ability to stack blocks and feed with a spoon. Most of the child's activities combine gross and fine motor skills, such as moving to reach objects and then manipulating them with ever-improving control.

The development of articulated speech begins during this period, but it is delayed if the child lacks mobility. Why this is so should be easy to understand if one considers the typical 2-year-old child. This is the child who is over, under, around, through, into, and on top of everything in his environment. As a result of this innocently mischievous play, he is constantly being exhorted by his mother to "stop," "get down off that chair," "stop teasing the cat," "go play with your brother," "come to the window and see the birdie," and "get out from under the sink." In contrast, the passively placid, immobile child is not subjected to this constant barrage of language stimulation.

Because upright posture and mobility are so important to a child of this age, they become the predominant orthotic determinants. For the child of 1–2 years, a standing frame can provide the upright position required (Fig. 27-1). Very few children are mobile in these frames, despite the claims of occasional enthusiasts. It is the ease of upright positioning that makes their use well worthwhile.[18] Mobility is more difficult to achieve. Special hand-driven tricycles (Fig. 27-2) and carts are occasionally available or can be devised for the child with a high neurological level.[13] The child with a lower level should begin gait training.

It is important that realistic goals be established for gait training. Numerous studies have shown that only the child with the lower lumbar levels will be a functional ambulator.[9,14] However, it is probably worth an attempt at gait training for higher-level children with the goal of assistance in transfers and the ability to move short distances about the house or school classroom. This goal should be clearly communicated to the parents so that the eventual wheelchair is not

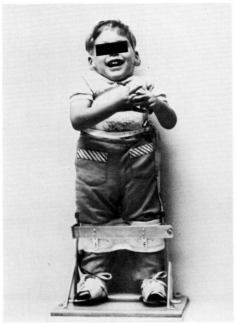
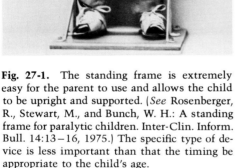

Fig. 27-1. The standing frame is extremely easy for the parent to use and allows the child to be upright and supported. (*See* Rosenberger, R., Stewart, M., and Bunch, W. H.: A standing frame for paralytic children. Inter-Clin. Inform. Bull. 14:13–16, 1975.) The specific type of device is less important than that the timing be appropriate to the child's age.

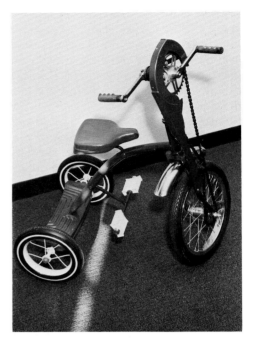

Fig. 27-2. This hand-driven tricycle can be made with standard bicycle parts and a tricycle frame. (*See* Kozole, K., and Bush, M. A.: A hand powered, hand controlled tricycle. Inter-Clin. Inform. Bull. 17:7–12, 1978.) It allows mobility at an economical price.

interpreted as a change of the physician's thinking or as a parental mistake with which guilt is to be associated. Children at higher levels should not be frustrated with excessive demands for distance, which they may lack the strength to accomplish. The obese child may not have the energy to be successful. Those with extremely short attention spans may never master the weight shifts.

Assuming the child is at a lower lumbar level, the question arises whether to start with extensive or minimal orthotics. Each has its advocates. I prefer to start the patient of a lower lumbar level with foot-ankle-knee orthoses, and a trial of gait training once these three areas are stabilized. Occasionally a child will need to have a pelvic belt added for lateral hip stability. After a period of time, most will be able to unlock their knees. Once the knees can be unlocked, the orthoses may be converted to foot-ankle orthoses.

In regard to ambulation and orthotic needs, the twin considerations are mobility and stability. The child must have enough stability during the stance phase to allow movement of crutches or walker. Later, there must be enough stability in stance to allow swing of the other limb. The needs of the child can be asssessed and the orthosis prescribed accordingly.

If foot deformities are a part of the child's problem, they should have been casted through a number of months. Once the child is almost ready to stand, surgical corrections of any remaining deformities should be undertaken. The standing provides a positive force for the maintenance of correction following the surgery. The child can be standing in casts, and little developmental delay will ensue.

If the child is an L3 or L4 level, it is quite probable that progressive hip dysplasia and valgus deformity of the femoral necks will occur during the first three years. If surgery and muscle transfers are undertaken, they should be performed bilaterally to keep the child symmetrical and preferably simultaneously to minimize the period of casting and immobility required. I prefer to transfer the iliopsoas on these patients and combine the transfer with a proximal femoral osteotomy in a single procedure (Figs. 27-3A–C).[5] Others prefer the external oblique to greater trochanter transfer because it adds a motor to the hip.[15] Either procedure should be done in a specialized center so as to ensure competence. A lack of experience on the surgeon's part is an absolute contraindication for surgery.

Spinal surgery may also be needed during these years. Approximately 20 percent of children with myelomeningocele will have congenital anomalies of the spine other than the posterior element defect at the area of myelomeningocele.[4] These anomalies may be manifested as hemivertebrae (incompletely formed vertebrae) or unsegmented areas, and they may occur anywhere on the spine. If these anomalies worsen the spinal deformity, surgery is indicated immediately. They should be treated in the same way that congenital scoliosis is in the child

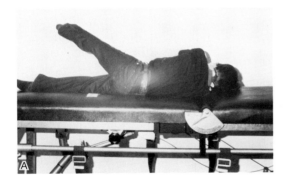
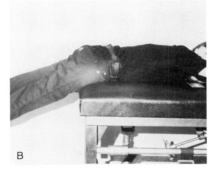
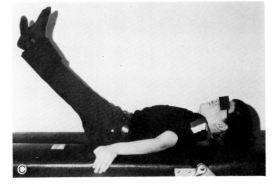

Figs. 27-3A–C. Three years after varus osteotomy and iliopsoas transfer, this boy demonstrates active abduction and extension by the transfer against gravity. He also illustrates that hip flexor power can be maintained despite the transfer of the iliopsoas.

without myelomeningocele. After surgery for an epiphyseal arrest of the vertebral growth place, bracing to prevent additional curvature is usually indicated.[3]

Special considerations exist for spinal surgery in the child with a high level and a congenital kyphosis. Because most of these children will be required to be supine for three to six months after the operation, surgery will contribute to a cognitive and developmental delay. Therefore, from the standpoint of mental and psychological functions, the surgery should be delayed until after the age of 4 years. Yet if the trunk is so unstable that sitting is nearly impossible even with careful use of orthotics, then the child will be retarded because of the kyphosis, and surgery is then indicated. If the curve cannot be controlled with orthotic management and additional bodies are being incorporated into the curve with ever-increasing lordosis in the proximal spine, surgery is indicated, regardless of the age. The physician has to weigh the negative aspects of the postoperative immobilization and the positive aspects of the surgery. For this reason, no rigid guidelines as to timing of surgery can be laid down, but each case must be decided individually on the basis of the progression of the spine and the development of the child.

Age 5 to 10 Years

By the age of 4 or 5 years, the child has learned about his environment and the period of intensive exploration decreases. The child now begins to acquire concepts and the ability to understand and manipulate abstract ideas. The number system, counting, the letters of the alphabet and the way they are put together in words, and the notes on a musical page are all examples of abstract symbols and concepts that the child now explores. Mobility is not as important at this time as previously. If a child has had normal developmental milestones to this point, any operation resulting in decreased mobility will have very little effect on cognitive development. Similarly, if a child with a high level of paraplegia who has achieved mobility at a high price in energy expenditure now becomes less mobile, little is lost from the cognitive and psychosocial aspects.

The second half of the first decade should be relatively quiescent from a musculoskeletal standpoint. The hips should have reached their potential, the feet should be plantigrade, and ambulation is at the highest level of function obtainable. The medical emphasis now is on maintaining the *status quo*. This is more difficult than one might imagine. Three causes of decreasing function must be watched for carefully: development of contractures, dislocation of hips, and changing neurological level.

Contractures. Contractures, particularly about the knee, have a devastating effect on ambulation. Lindseth[14] found that only 3 of 16 patients with knee-extension contractures and 5 of 51 patients with knee-flexion contractures were functional ambulators. Because moderate to severe knee-flexion contractures are usually associated with subluxation, they are particularly difficult to correct. Early recognition and care are mandatory.

It is possible to obtain dynamic control of some knee deformities. If the knee goes into hyperextension in stance phase and has a reasonable amount of flexion, ground-reaction orthoses may be effective. Orthoses make the ankle slightly dorsiflexed and flexion is imposed upon the knee during stance. This condition puts a greater requirement on the quadriceps, which in these patients are usually normal.

If a mild knee-flexion contracture exists, it can be opposed by setting the ankle in a slight amount of plantar flexion. Thus, mid-stance will exert an extension movement at the knee. The forces generated may be large, so the standard band should be replaced with an anterior pretibial shell (Fig. 27-4).

If a contracture exists, the ground-reaction system cannot be used, and above-knee orthoses are required (Fig. 27-5). If the contractures show 30 degrees of flexion or 10 degrees of extension, osteotomies or releases are required. Ideally, many of these could be prevented by early treatment.

Dislocation of the Hips.   The second reason for loss of ambulation is the development of dislocation of the hips in the L4- or L5-level patient. These patients with absent or minimal abduction of the hips slowly develop valgus deformities of the femoral neck, acetabular dysplasia, and dislocation.[5]

The presence or absence of hip dislocation is not thought to influence ambulation. If all levels are considered together, this is probably true. However,

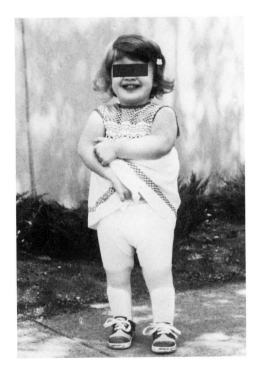

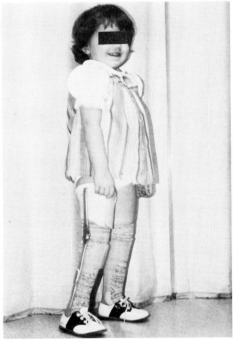

Fig. 27-4.   This anterior stopped orthosis effectively controls knee flexion. The surface layer anteriorly distributes the force over sufficient skin surface to make pressure sores unlikely.

Fig. 27-5.   When above-knee orthoses are required because of excessive force or knee valgus, they should be lightweight. Although not well-shown, this girl has only a lateral upright and joint.

when Lindseth[14] reviewed the ambulatory capacity of his patients of 10–41 years of age, some striking differences were seen. In the patients with L4 and L5 levels whose hips were not dislocated, 23 out of 27 were ambulatory. In contrast, in patients of the same neurological level but with dislocated hips, 8 of 16 were ambulatory. Hips should not be allowed to dislocate under "close observation."

Changing Neurological Level. The third cause of a loss of ambulatory ability is ascending neurological level. As a rule, the neurological level of a myelomeningocele child is stationary and static after his first year. Any deviation from this should be considered pathological until proved otherwise. Ascending neurological function may be due to one of several factors, including diastematomyelia, tethered spinal cord, lipoma of the cord or cauda, and hydromyelia. If a sharp loss of ambulation has been caused by any of these, it is seldom recoverable. Early recognition and immediate diagnosis of progressive neurological defects are the keys to continued ambulatory potential.

If the neurological level or ascending level is markedly asymmetrical or fine motor skill of the hand is diminished, an intraspinal anomaly should be suspected. The least invasive test is the somatosensory evoked potentials (SSEP), which tests the nerve roots sequentially.[19] A single test is not always diagnostic, but deterioration over time is highly indicative of spinal cord pathology.

If there is any question of asymmetry or prolonged latency of the SSEP, many neurosurgeons would recommend immediate myelography, preferably with water-soluble contrast material. This procedure allows visualization of the cord and the path of the nerve root. A low-lying cord or upward path of nerve roots is diagnostic of a tether of the conus and cord. Surgical exploration should be performed only by a neurosurgeon with extensive experience in myelomingocele children.

The child who has escaped the sensorimotor period unscathed by developmental delay is unlikely to experience severe deficits in personality development or mental growth in the next few years. However, continued observation is important to make certain that overt hydrocephalus or hydromyelia does not develop and compromise mental or physical function.

The major vulnerability of the child with myelomeningocele during this period exists in the realm of psychosocial adaptation and self-concepts. For the first time the child is exposed to nursery school and the judgment of children his own age. Heretofore, the feedback the child has received has been entirely from adults. Now it is from peers. It is important that some thought be given to the school setting so that the child will develop a positive self-image in the face of potential negative comments from well-meaning but inquisitive classmates.

The Adolescent With Myelomeningocele

Three separate events—puberty, the ability to think logically, and psychosocial motivation—combine to make up the turbulent period of time referred to as adolescence.[8] Although it is tempting to assume that the adolescent with a myelomeningocele might be less likely to think abstractly than his peers because of his limited childhood experiences, no hard data exist to support such a conclusion. Actually, it is in the area of psychosocial maturation that the teenager with myelomeningocele is at most risk.

Problems During Early Adolescence.   In early adolescence the pre-teen and early teenager begin to expand their horizons beyond the home. They have the ability to visit friends' houses, school, and the neighborhood recreation center with a certain amount of independence. At this stage childhood efforts made to create a functional ambulator can be realistically evaluated. If such efforts were unsuccessful, wheelchair ambulation must be optimized.

Adolescents are preoccupied with their bodies, and narcissistically compare themselves with peers of their own sex. This is potentially a very difficult period for myelomeningocele patients. Not only is the body that they are comparing below normal in terms of strength and agility, but it is further "deformed" by the presence of an ilio-diversion or in-dwelling catheter. The self-image drawn from these painful comparisons can hardly be ideal.

Myelomeningocele teenagers are at a greater disadvantage than a poor body image—their body even seems to be deteriorating, because now the progression of scoliosis is becoming most marked. This event should call for a thorough examination to be certain that a hydromyelia and low pressure hydrocephalus do not exist. Hall et al.[7] have reported that 100 percent of the patients who developed scoliosis in early adolescence had hydromyelia as a contributing or precipitating factor. We have recently treated a pre-teenager with rapidly developing lordosis who had a tethered cord and hydromyelia. At the time of shunt insertion, the intraventricular pressure was in excess of 60 cm of water. After two neurosurgical procedures, the lordosis was markedly improved.

Spinal fusion is required for many myelomeningocele teenagers, usually during early adolescence. The techniques and special indications for anterior and posterior fusion have been reviewed elsewhere.[4,5] Postoperative management is greatly facilitated by the use of total contact plastic body jackets. They permit the control of pressure sores and allow frequent inspection of the skin. With careful attention to the technical details, good stability can be achieved, and patients can be up and attending school during the postoperative period.

In the normal teenager, the early adolescent period is usually a relatively tranquil time. However, for the myelomeningocele child, it may be devastating. During a time when they should be beginning to exert some independence, they are more dependent on not only their parents, but on hospitals, doctors, and other health professionals. When others are developing skills in sports, they are developing sores under their body cast. They may become withdrawn and never develop socially.

Mid-adolescence.   Mid-adolescence is the usual crisis period for normal adolescents and their families. The major conflict is independence, and the struggles may sometimes be ferocious. The myelomeningocele child has not had an opportunity to become more independent during the previous year or so and is now at an ever-increasing disadvantage. In younger children, orthopedists can measure the independence of their patients in terms of independent ambulation. In mid-adolescence, independence now encompasses a great deal more. Decisions involving use of time, where to go, and who to be with may be limited by lack of mobility. However, in the myelomeningocele patient they tend to be limited by the lack of earlier experience and a small number of friends.

Another characteristic of mid-adolescence is the narcissistic exploitation of the ability to attract the opposite sex. Self-worth is frequently measured by the number "chasing" or "being chased" by a given teenager. Clearly, the myelomeningocele teenager may well be eliminated from this activity. It is important that the medical team be aware of this lack and that someone be available for discussion and assistance.

The medical team may well have a chance to be very close to the teenaged patient, because during this period of life a teenager often attempts to identify with extra-parental adults. The adults' acceptance of the adolescent helps to build the self-image and the concept of oneself as an evolving adult. Thus, at exactly the time that the self-image may be most devastated by the peer interactions, it can be most aided by appropriate adult attentions. It is reassuring to know that some myelomeningocele patients can emerge healthy and psychologically intact, given sensitive medical and social support.

Late Adolescence.   For the unimpaired teenager, the turmoil of mid-adolescence finally gives way to late adolescence, in which emancipation is nearly secured. The parent-adolescent relationships are equivalent to those between two adults, and much of the tension is now dissipated. This period centers on the development of mutually caring relationships with those of the opposite sex and the discovery of a functional role in society. Whether the myelomeningocele adolescent will develop these relationships depends on his success in negotiating the previous steps of adolescence.

In summary, during adolescence young people achieve emancipation, and therefore gain independence and control. They also develop an identity and a sense of oneself as an intellectual being, a sexual being, and a functional individual. In each of these areas, teenagers with a myelomeningocele begin with a distinct disadvantage, which may prevent the completion of these tasks. It is imperative that the health care team be sensitive to these problems and give as much assistance as possible.

NEUROPATHIES AND MYOPATHIES

Patients with neuropathies and myopathies are an extremely heterogeneous group. Some children are born weak, whereas others develop their weakness within the first year or so. Others, such as the typical Duchenne's dystrophy patient, seem to be quite normal for the first few years and then become progressively weaker. Obviously the implications of mobility and immobility on normal development will differ according to the degree of disability. If the child is born weak or develops a severe weakness within the first year or two of life, the myelomeningocele model of rehabilitation discussed earlier would apply here, too. If, on the other hand, the child's weakness develops later in life, as with the Duchenne's dystrophy or Kugelberg-Welander form of neuropathy, his early experiences should have been quite normal.

In this section Duchenne's dystrophy is the model for care and rehabilitation. This assumption implies that the child has normal intelligence and neuromuscular function the first few years of life.

Onset of Weakness

Since the onset of noticeable disability is about age 5 years for the average patient, one can assume that a reasonably normal sensorimotor period has been experienced by the child. There should have been no delay in speech or cognitive processes and, in the absence of organic disease, the IQ should be normal. Therefore the child should have started kindergarten as a "normal" child and experienced normal interactions with peers and teachers.

If the child is brought to the physician with complaints of waddling or some weakness, a thorough and definitive diagnosis should be made. The natural history and therefore the information given by the parents is so grossly different for the childhood onset of neuropathies and the congenital myopathies and Duchenne's dystrophy that failure to make this distinction is simply inexcusable. A search for significant family history may provide evidence of some genetic transmission. Enzyme and electromyographic studies should be done prior to biopsy and, in the case of Duchenne's dystrophy, these measures should be adequate for diagnosis. If a biopsy is done, it should be performed in a center with capabilities for histochemistry and electron microscopy. Routine hematoxylin-eosin stains taken in a small community hospital will give no new information and are inadequate standards of practice.

Once the diagnosis is made, the parents' education should begin with genetic counseling and associated emotional support. If the child's disorder is a sex-linked recessive inheritance, as is Duchenne's dystrophy, the mother must be protected from the nearly overwhelming feeling of guilt. It is usually a good idea to have the subject directly introduced and discussed by the clinic's staff.

The child at this age is functioning quite well and specific rehabilitative measures may not seem necessary. Because the eventual development of contractures can play such an important role in the duration of ambulation, a physical therapy program should be instituted and taught to the parents. It should include stretching of the hip flexors, abductors, and heel cords. Patients who have been through such a program almost never require later hip and knee releases. In fact, it is my opinion and experience that the need for these operations is evidence of inadequate early care.

This is a good time to begin to interest the child in hobbies and activities requiring fine motor control rather than strength and gross motor control. Recently we have seen a boy who is quite artistic and this interest was strongly reinforced by the clinic staff. Since his distal musculature will be preserved, he will be provided with interests that will not become impossible to maintain.

Age 10–13 Years

Early in the second decade of a patient's life, the weakness about the hip and knee progresses to the point that independent ambulation is severely threatened. Typically, the child has been walking by alignment stability for several years and now the balance and maintenance of the stability have become increasingly precarious. As the hip extensors weaken, the patient develops compensatory lordosis to move the center of gravity behind the hip. However, this moves the ground-reaction force behind the knee joints, which in turn requires quadriceps strength for knee stability. As the quadriceps become weak, the patient slowly comes up on his toes to move the ground-reaction force ahead of the knee and create knee stability. In the last months of ambulation, the patient is performing a delicate trick of keeping the center of gravity behind the hips and in front of the knees. Finally, this no longer is possible.

The implications of the inability to walk extend beyond the child's physical being. The school experiences become much more difficult, and in many school districts he will be limited in his opportunities. If placed in a wheelchair, certain field trips may be denied him. If architectural barriers are a feature of the school, the library may be off limits. Similarly, the family mobility may become reduced, due to the wheelchair and its increased effort. For these reasons, it seems worth while to prolong walking to the greatest extent possible.

The addition of lower-limb orthotics will usually prolong walking for an average of two years. Orthoses lock the knee, allowing the child to regain the alignment stability at the hips. The mechanical requirements of the orthoses are that they be as light as possible, provide a lock at the knee, and confer stability high on the thigh. A combination of a plastic sheath, such as polypropylene, and metal hinges forms a very strong yet light orthosis.

Surgery allows a child to fit into his orthoses. Usually the heel cords are tight enough to necessitate a lengthening or a tenotomy. If required, hip and knee releases should also be done at this time. Some specialists[20] recommend percutaneous tenotomies, but I prefer a formal, open-heel cord lengthening with transfer of the posterior tibial tendon to the dorsum of the foot. This involves considerably more surgery, but if it is carried out by two experienced teams simultaneously, the anesthetic can be relatively short. The advantage is that the late deformity at the foot and ankle caused by the unopposed posterior tibial muscle is prevented and likely problems of fitting into shoes eliminated. The disadvantage is that occasionally a patient gets postoperative swelling and has difficulty standing on the first postoperative day. Even if swelling occurs, it is important that these patients are out of bed and standing in plaster the day following surgery.

Such devices as crutches or walkers are usually not helpful for children with muscular dystrophy. Because the weakness is symmetrical in the upper and lower trunks, the shoulder stability necessary for crutches is usually lacking. Thus the child who is placed in foot, ankle, and knee orthoses must learn to walk by balancing his weight behind his hips and not attempting to use crutches as the replacement for his hip extensors (Fig. 27-6).

Some involvement with the school is necessary at this point. Once the child is in orthoses, it is necessary that he use them. He should be able to stand for as much time as possible and be allowed to walk. Because he is somewhat slower than other children, the school may complain that it is impossible for him to get from one class to another within the allotted time. All of this may be true. However, most classroom situations can allow a child to leave a minute or two early so as to give him additional time to get to the next class. It is usually necessary for the rehabilitation team to suggest this to the teachers.

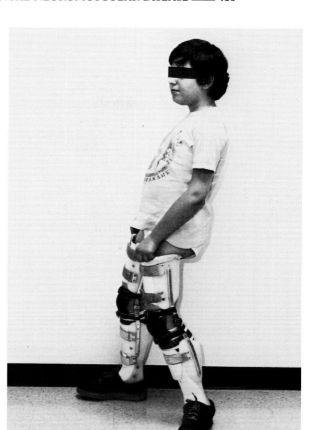

Fig. 27-6. This boy, who has been walking for three years since acquiring orthoses, demonstrates the typical posture of a multiple dystrophy patient. He walks by strongly overshifting his weight from side to side.

The goal of the school is that the patient should be as mobile as other students. This is not unreasonable. However, the school may find an electric wheelchair is the fastest way of moving the child from one class to another and to and from the cafeteria. Therefore it is easy for them to demand that the parents or clinic provide the child with the wheelchair. If this is not medically justified, the rehabilitation team must be prepared to invest the time necessary to educate the school on this point.

Age 13 Years

After two or three years of orthosis-assisted ambulation, the patient's weakness progresses and a wheelchair becomes necessary. The chair should be carefully measured and fitted to the individual.[21] In order to provide independent ambulation, electrical power will be required.

Although a wheelchair provides mobility, it also separates the patient from his peers. Teenagers in wheelchairs have few friends, perceive themselves as extremely isolated, and are uninformed but curious about sex.[11] The lack of sexual information in this group may illustrate the isolation and the dilemma of a wheelchair existence. The boys probably receive no less sexual information from their parents than do their peers, but certainly they receive no more. However, they are denied the locker room conversations and the information that is normally exchanged behind the garage. The early fumbling contacts with the opposite sex are denied them. One boy's total information was the occasional *Playboy* magazine his father brought home. The presence of a physical handicap does not lessen the desires for affection or sexual contact.

The major physical disability of this period is the onset of scoliosis. Of 21 patients followed in their late teens, 12 developed progressive scoliosis severe enough to interfere with their sitting balance. Six of the other nine patients also developed curves of 30–50 degrees by age 20. These curves were never functionally disabling and could be ignored. The presence of lordosis or kyphosis did not influence the progression of scoliosis. In this group of patients, early attempts to brace the spine while in lordosis did not seem to be indicated.

In a retrospective review it became obvious that the patients who walked until the age of 12 but had scoliosis while still ambulatory had progressive curves. Those who were straight at the time they stopped walking did not develop a functionally disabling spinal deformity. It must be repeated that this observation as a predictor applies only to those children who walk until the age of 12.

Over the past seven years, I have fused 15 patients with Duchenne's dystrophy. Out of this group there were no pseudoarthroses, no infections, and only two required intubation overnight. By undergoing surgery within the first year or two after the end of ambulation, these patients' pulmonary functions were still in the 30–50 percent range.[26] It is this reasonable maximum ventilatory capacity that allowed a minimum of pulmonary complications. At the time of this writing, all are still alive and all are still actively sitting. Five of these patients are now at least 20 years old. The experience at Rancho Los Amigos parallels my results.[22] As with the myelomeningocele spinal patients, these children should be operated on in a center where the pediatrician and anesthesiologist are accustomed to patients with neuromuscular defects and skilled in their care.

Older Teenagers

The patient with facio-scapular-humeral or limb-girdle dystrophy does not follow the stereotypical course outlined for the child with the Duchenne's form. Most are functional individuals in the late teenage period and have no ambulatory difficulty. The major functional deficit these patients encounter is weakness about the scapula. When this happens, the scapular stabilizers become progressively weaker and the muscles crossing the glenohumeral joint become ineffective because of the winged scapula. The patient becomes limited in elevation activities, including dressing and personal hygiene.

One approach to treating this problem is to fuse the scapula to the rib cage.[1] In this procedure, a length of about 5 cm of the fifth and sixth ribs posteriorly is incorporated in the bone graft and wired to the scapula. The patient is kept in a shoulder spica for three months to allow for a solid fusion. Following muscle strengthening, after removal of the cast, the patient has increased strength and elevation (Fig. 27-7). Over a period of 10 years, follow-up on this procedure has been gratifying to the patients.

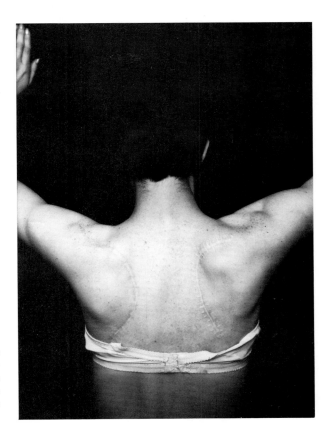

Fig. 27-7. This teenager has limb-girdle muscular dystrophy with the maximum disability in her shoulders. Her left scapula has been fused to ribs 5 and 6. Not only can she elevate her arm higher, but her strength is much greater on the operated side.

SUMMARY

Childhood may be thought of as that period of time in which we accumulate experiences that serve us for the rest of our lives. The neuromuscularly deficient child has a distinct disadvantage in accumulating these experiences; depending on the age at which the disability develops, the sequelae may have impact far beyond the musculoskeletal system.

The process of rehabilitation in the child consists of all medical, social, and educational measures that permit the normal experiences of childhood. The traditional rehabilitation tools—surgery, bracing, and therapy—all have a place in the rehabilitation of the child. However, their effectiveness cannot be measured in the hospital setting, since they are proved only in the school, the playground, and the home.

REFERENCES

1. Bunch, W. H.: Scapulo-thoracic fusion for shoulder stabilization in muscular dystrophy. Minn. Med. 56:391–394, 1973.
2. Bunch, W. H.: Muscular dystrophy. In Hardy, J., Ed.: *Neuromuscular Disease and Scoliosis,* pp. 92–110. C. V. Mosby, St. Louis, 1974.

3. Bunch, W. H.: The Milwaukee brace in paralytic scoliosis. Clin. Orthop. 110:63–68, 1975.

4. Bunch, W. H.: Treatment of myelomeningocele spine. In *Instructional Course Lectures,* pp. 93–95. American Academy of Orthopaedic Surgeons. C. V. Mosby, St. Louis, 1976.

5. Bunch, W. H.: Myelomeningocele. In Winter, R., and Wood, L., Eds.: *Pediatric Orthopedics,* pp. 381–426. J. B. Lippincott, Philadelphia, 1978.

6. Fisk, J. R., and Bunch, W. H.: Scoliosis in neuromuscular disease. Orthop. Clin. North Am. 10(4):863–875, 1979.

7. Hall, P. V., Lindseth, R. E., Campbell, R. L., and Kalsbeck, J. E.: Myelodysplasia and developmental scoliosis. Spine 1:50–58, 1976.

8. Hammar, S. L.: The approach to the adolescent patient. Pediatr. Clin. North Am. 20:782–788, 1973.

9. Hoffer, M. M., Feiweel, E., Perry, R., et al.: Functional ambulation in patients with myelomeningocele. J. Bone Joint Surg. 55A:137–148, 1973.

10. Hostler, S. L.: Development of the infant with myelomeningocele. In *Instructional Course Lectures,* pp. 70–75. American Academy of Orthopaedic Surgeons. C. V. Mosby, St. Louis, 1976.

11. Hostler, S. L.: Personal communication.

12. Klaus, M. H., and Kennell, J. H.: *Maternal-Infant Bonding.* C. V. Mosby, St. Louis, 1976.

13. Kozole, K., and Bush, M. A.: A hand powered, hand controlled tricycle. Inter-Clin. Inform. Bull. 17:7–12, 1978.

14. Lindseth, R. E.: Treatment of the lower extremity in children paralyzed by myelomeningocele. In *Instructional Course Lectures,* pp. 76–81. American Academy of Orthopaedic Surgeons. C. V. Mosby, St. Louis, 1976.

15. Lindseth, R. E.: Personal communication.

16. O'Connor, S.: Quoted in Spezzano, C., and Watermann, J.: The first day of life. Psychol. Today 11:110, 1977.

17. Passo, S. D.: Positioning of infants with myelomeningocele. Am. J. Nurs. 74:1658–1660, 1974.

18. Rosenberger, R., Stewart, M., and Bunch, W. H.: A standing frame for paralytic children. Inter-Clin. Inform. Bull. 14:13–16, 1975.

19. Scarff, T. B., Toleikis, J. R., Bunch, W. H., and Parrish, S.: Dermatomal somatosensory evoked potentials in children with myelomeningocele. Z. Kinderchir 28:384–387, 1979.

20. Siegel, I. M., Miller, J. E., and Ray, R. D.: Subcutaneous lower limb tenotomy in the treatment of pseudohypertrophic muscular dystrophy. J. Bone Joint Surg. 50A:1437–1443, 1968.

21. Stewart, M. M.: *The Wheelchair in Principles of Orthotic Treatment.* C. V. Mosby, St. Louis, 1976.

22. Swank, S., and Brown, J.: Personal communication.

28

Cerebral Palsy

M. Mark Hoffer, M.D.
Martin Koffman, M.D.

HISTORY AND DEFINITIONS

A patient with cerebral palsy has a nonprogressive, nonhereditary disease with many neurological findings. The onset is prenatal and its etiology is ill-understood. Little[13] was the first to describe cerebral palsy. His work was popularized and amplified by Osler and by Freud.[5] Classifications of cerebral palsy have been developed by Balf and Ingram,[1] Minear,[15] Pearlstein,[16] and Phelps.[19] More than 500,000 Americans have cerebral palsy. According to Phelps, one-third of this population has severe involvement and one-sixth has very mild involvement. It is difficult to formulate treatment plans for cerebral palsy patients because of the diffuse manifestations of the disease, but a simple classification scheme has been accepted. This classification is useful in making goals and plans.[10]

There are three general descriptive types of cerebral palsy: spastic, dyskinetic, and mixed. The spastic patient has hyperactive reflexes and clonus. The clonus increases with stretch. The orthopedic surgeon has most to offer this group of patients. Cerebral palsy patients with motion disorders have extremely complicated conditions, and they are more difficult to define and treat. There are precise definitions for spastic motion disorders, such as "athetosis," "chorea," "dyskinesia," and "ataxia." These terms each have different meanings neurologically, but ultimately the differences are not important, because we do not have any specific measures for managing any of these problems. We like to distinguish between those individuals who have problems with control of the limb in the pathway of their motion, and those who have problems in the end point of that motion. Some patients present a mixed picture of spasticity and motion disorder.

The geographic distribution of the disability on the patient's body is another important factor in evaluating cerebral palsy. The hemiplegic suffers mainly from involvement in one side. These people will always walk, and they rarely need any therapy to allow them to speak. Their greatest problem seems to be sensory deprivation in the upper extremity and equinovarus deformity in the lower extremity. It is common for hemiplegic patients to have involvement to a lesser degree in the opposite leg. Single limb involvement also occurs but it is rare.

In patients with diplegia, the lower extremities are more involved than the upper extremities, yet the upper extremities are almost always involved to some extent. Patients with diplegia often have esotropia, too. The involvement for diplegics is usually more severe in the hips and less so in the feet. They tend to have anteverted, adducted hips, valgus, externally rotated knees, and equinovalgus of the feet. The designation of paraplegia is probably not correct for these patients, because that term more clearly defines the individual with spinal cord injury.

The totally involved patient has problems in all four extremities; in addition, speech, swallowing, and cognition are often critically debilitated. Again, we do not use the word "quadriplegia" because we think it is better designated for a patient with a spinal cord injury. It is the totally involved individual, that is, the cerebral palsy patient, who has the most difficulty in ambulating. Ambulation, in fact, is not usually the goal for these individuals. Patients may require surgery and orthoses to aid them in sitting. Scoliosis and dislocated hips do affect the eventual ability of these children to sit and so they may need surgery for the hip and spine.

The reflex levels of these patients are very important to test because they reveal if the patient is developing balance. Children who have not achieved the balance reaction, demonstrated by parachute reflex, and who have persistent obligatory tonic neck reflexes by age three should not be considered candidates for functional ambulation because of their lack of trunk balance. Furthermore, if they do not develop these reactions by the time they are six years old, they will have difficulty with sitting independently.

When studying individual limbs, two general factors must be determined. The sensibility of the limb should be studied by two-point discrimination, graphesthesia, or object identification. The motor control of the limb should be studied for its dependence or independence from patterns of motion involving other limbs. Muscle testing for grades is an excellent way of testing muscles for selective control. However, most cerebral palsied muscles do not have selective control and thus these tests are not valid.

Finally, the most important abilities of human beings involve their cognition and communication. It is difficult to test intelligence unless the person can communicate. Thus these two crucial factors are interrelated. Nonverbal speech programs may aid these patients.

CLASSIFICATIONS OF MOBILITY

We like to think of three types of sitting. A propped sitter is one who has a straight back, loose hips, and can be propped up in a wheelchair. These patients have no balance reactions and often require a loose cerebral palsy bracing as a proper device. Ankle and knee orthoses are not necessary in these sitters, nor are operations on the foot and knee, which are performed for ambulatory patients. Hip releases and surgical stabilization of the spine may be more effective operations. Self-propped sitters may need some support, but they can temporarily maintain themselves at balance. These patients may need modifications of their wheelchairs. Patients who sit independently have balance and support reactions. Attention should be paid to modifying their wheelchair to make sure that they are permitted the ability to transfer. In addition, some of these patients are able to propel the wheelchair backward and it may be necessary to add equipment for foot control.

There are four types of ambulation in disabled individuals. In community ambulation, patients walk both indoors and outdoors during most of their activities and may need orthoses for these activities. These patients require wheelchairs only for long trips out of the community. Household ambulation implies that a patient only walks indoors with the support of some type of apparatus. Household ambulators get in and out of chairs and beds with little, if any, assistance and may need the wheelchair for some indoor activities away from the home only. Physiological or nonfunctional ambulation is more or less a therapy session and individuals in this classification use the wheelchair for their functional needs. Nonambulatory patients may stand and transfer but they are truly sitters because they cannot maintain the balance necessary for forward progression. All hemiplegics can achieve functional ambulation, diplegics who develop balance reactions by age three and have stable hips will walk functionally, and few totally involved patients will achieve functional ambulation.

SURGICAL PLANNING AND OPERATING PROCEDURES

Lower Extremities

It is fortunate that pain happens to be a relatively infrequent indication for surgery in the cerebral palsy patient. Singularly, operations are not often performed for cosmetic purposes alone. By far the most frequent justification for surgical intervention is the expected improvement of function. The deformities and abnormal postures displayed by the cerebral palsy patient from muscle imbalance and imperfect motor control invite a variety of interventions. Unfortunately, surgical correction of a deformity does not always result in improved function. Even so, sometimes it is desirable to advocate prophylactic surgery to prevent progression of a deformity that would otherwise result in loss of function already present. For example, by correcting the progressive subluxation of the hip, loss of ambulation is averted. Nevertheless, there is a suspicious blend of art and science in decision-making when predicting the results of an operation on the peripheral musculoskeletal apparatus in the patient with a central nervous system lesion.

To improve our accuracy in predicting the results of surgery, we rely on classifications, prognostic indicators, empiricism from the experience of others, and information gained by electromyogram (EMG) studies of the timing of "firing" of individual muscles and muscle groups during the performance of certain functional activities.[10,17,18] These tools may be augmented in the future with more kinesiological data and energy cost-of-work studies.

Hemiplegia. All hemiplegics will be independently ambulatory. Equinus deformities can frequently be controlled at an early age by combinations of casting, bracing, and night splints. An Achilles tendon lengthening and split anterior tibial tendon transfer (SPLATT) can be performed for equinovarus attitude of the foot present during the entire gait cycle. Posterior tibialis lengthening may need to accompany the SPLATT procedure if there is fixed varus under anesthesia. The Achilles tendon lengthening must accompany the SPLATT procedure if there is fixed equinus under anesthesia.

If the EMG shows posterior tibialis activity during the swing phase but not during the stance phase, then transfer of the posterior tibialis through the interosseous membrane to the dorsum of the foot may be a more logical procedure than the SPLATT. To transfer the posterior tibialis tendon through the interosseous membrane when it is active through all phases of the gait cycle by EMG is to establish a tenodesis initially resulting in limited ankle motion but which will later stretch out.

Transferring the posterior tibialis to the lateral side of the foot is never indicated.

An equinus foot deformity is rarely solely responsible for a patient failing to walk. The deformity can usually be controlled early with braces and splints until the patient is able to walk; then an operation can be performed. In the previously unoperated-upon foot, a three-level, Hoke-type tenotomy of the Achilles tendon that brings the ankle perpendicular to the tibia with the patient under anesthesia and then casts the ankle in 5 degrees of plantar flexion is the preferred technique. A short leg, weight-bearing cast is postoperatively applied for six weeks.

The technique of advancing the Achilles tendon anteriorly on the os calcis is being evaluated in the treatment of the equinus ankle. Although it is too early to make any definite statements about results, the procedure has its primary application in ankles with adequate motion but in which there is excessive plantar-flexion tone and an equinus gait. We have no experience with os calcis osteotomies in correcting the varus foot in this group of patients.

The hip is rarely a clinical problem in early life for hemiplegics. Occasionally the excessive internal rotation and adduction during gait will require adductor release and a medial hamstring release or a lateral transfer in a child younger than the age of six years who has a passive external rotation range of 20–30 degrees at rest. The medial hamstring (semitendinosus) transfer will be most effective if the gait EMG shows it to be active only during the end of swing phase and into early stance phase, as in the patient without neurological involvement.

More often the adduction and internal rotation attitude during gait will need to be corrected by adductor release. A derotation osteotomy will also be required to correct the anteversion of the femur. Frequently the internal rotation attitude and anteversion is not accompanied by x-ray evidence of hip subluxation, and in these patients the derotation osteotomy can be performed in the distal femur.

The supracondylar approach to the osteotomy has the advantages of permitting early weight-bearing and not leaving hardware in the body for an extended period of time.

Diplegia. Diplegic patients who develop some trunk balance will become ambulatory. Some will be grossly restricted to household ambulation with a pick-up walker, whereas others will be independent community ambulators.

The focus of attention in these patients' lower extremities is at the hips. The hip action brace can be a useful training adjunct to the physical therapy when the patient is learning to walk. But if the hip abduction range begins to shrink, then adductor releases are indicated.[12] Adductor transfer posteriorly to the ischium has not proved to be superior to adductor release alone. The adductor releases must be performed bilaterally in these patients.

If hip subluxation is occurring at any age, then, in addition to adductor releases, derotation-varus osteotomy will be necessary. We tend to use crossed pins to hold the osteotomy in young patients; in the older patients we use a small AO plate or the Coventry screw. In either instance, we have always used a spica cast in the early postoperative period. We release the gracilis, adductor longus, and adductor brevis without performing an obturator neurectomy in these potentially ambulatory children. A crouch gait with excessive lumbar lordosis during gait often calls attention to the presence of hip flexion deformities. If the hip flexion together with the adduction and internal rotation is judged to be contributing to the subluxation of the hip, then other muscles in addition to the adductors will need to be released surgically.

If the patient's ambulation has reached a plateau or is deteriorating over a period of several months while under the supervision of a therapist, and the patient is younger than 10 years old, then surgical correction of the crouch gait associated with excessive lumbar lordosis can be considered. The EMG helps in selecting the iliopsoas or the rectus femoris to release, and it may also aid in analyzing the gracilis or medial hamstring muscles.

Successive or concomitant corrections of the knee flexion deformity by selective distal hamstring lengthenings and tenotomies are indicated in some patients with a crouch gait. A knee flexion deformity should never be approached surgically without proper attention being given to the hip flexion deformity. Attention must also be paid to the possible underactivity of the thigh surae as at least a contributing factor to some of the patient's crouch posture during gait.

Indications for surgery are clinical[3,4,7] and not based on the EMG. Once the decision to operate has been made on clinical grounds, then the gait EMG may aid in selecting the most appropriate muscle among a group to operate upon. The EMG reveals which muscle or muscles are deviating most from their normal phasic pattern of activity during the gait cycle. Surprisingly, several muscles in the lower extremity of diplegics will be firing in a normal manner during walking. Also surprisingly, patients exhibiting the same posture during gait may show different variations from the normal EMG patterns to account for these same postures. For example, the hip flexion attitude may be caused by an abnormal iliopsoas in one patient yet by an abnormal rectus femoris in another. Or, the internal rotation attitude may be due to an abnormal iliopsoas in one patient and to an abnormal medial hamstring in another.

We are less concerned about postures and attitudes, the cosmesis of gait, than we are about the cost of walking, that is, the energy expenditure. Measuring oxygen consumption directly, or indirectly by monitoring heart rates, to determine efficiency of gait and endurance will become more popular in assessing postoperative results.

We are less concerned about the ankles and feet in the diplegics than we previously were.[2] Equinus, although commonly present, is rarely the limiting factor in the patient's ability to walk. Positions at the feet sometimes change in response to hip and knee operations. For that reason, an operation on the feet and ankles is often deferred unless the patient has a significant fixed (not dynamic) deformity, in which case an Achilles tendon lengthening is performed.

Valgus foot deformities are common but are rarely responsible for a patient's failure to progress in ambulation. Orthotic devices are of limited usefulness and peroneal tendon transfers to the medial side of the foot are unpredictable. We find our indications for the Grice procedure to be constricting with time. In many cases we would prefer to wait until the patient is at least 12 years old and then perform a triple arthrodesis if the patient is still a functional ambulator.

However, if the valgus deformities are becoming progressively more fixed and skin changes are taking place at sites of excessive pressure in the shoes, then Grice procedures are required. Proper attention is given to correcting excessive anteversion before the Grice procedures are performed.

Totally Involved Spasticity. The totally involved spastic patient is not and will not be a functional ambulator. Many of these patients have some combination of spasticity and dyskinesia. Those patients with almost pure dyskinesia frequently do walk and the following discussion is not meant to apply to them.

Being able to transfer, assisted or unassisted, is the highest functional level that the total-body-involved spastic patient performs with the use of his lower extremities. These patients will spend most of their waking hours sitting in a chair. This group of patients will include several who appear to resemble diplegics but who have more severe involvement of the upper extremities than usual, or who may resemble hemiplegics with more severe involvement of the unaffected side. Cerebral palsy patients present a continuum of types of severity of geographic involvement.

For the first 8–10 years of their lives, totally involved patients should have aggressive surgical treatment of any subluxation or dislocation of the hip. This treatment encompasses the combinations of soft tissue releases and osteotomies as indicated by static examinations. EMG is of no value in preoperative planning for this group of patients and tendon transfers have never been shown to offer any advantages over releases. Postoperative splinting or bracing for 12 hours a day is often useful. In this age group the hips rarely are painful. We are less aggressive in operating upon deformities about the knees and ankles in these patients, particularly if they are not going to be able to transfer because of the severity of the neurological involvement affecting their balance and use of their upper extremities.

The totally involved patient who has reached adolescence or adulthood needs 90 degrees of painless hip flexion range and balanced spinal curvatures in order to sit propped upright. The adult patient's hip may become painful irrespective of whether it is dislocated. An adult is best managed by paying more attention to the clinical status instead of trying to set up criteria for interventions based solely on the x-ray appearance of the hips.

Proximal hamstring-origin releases from the ischium may be useful to gain hip flexion range for ease of sitting.

A patient who does not have preoperative pain may have it postoperatively. If soft tissue releases alone are not sufficient to gain adequate range of hip motion for sitting, then femoral osteotomy with skeletal shortening would seem to be preferable to the proximal femoral resection in a painless hip.

Once in a while a quadriceps tendon release may be indicated to gain knee flexion range for sitting.

Occasionally spinal stabilization to the sacrum is helpful in controlling the increasing spinal deformity and pelvic obliquity that interferes with sitting. Fusions should include posterior procedures to the sacrum when pelvic obliquity is noted. The addition of anterior thoracolumbar fusions is currently advocated to reduce the pseudoarthrosis rate.

The problem of the painful hip in the cerebral palsied individual has not yet been solved. The results of proximal femoral resection with or without insertion of a constrained implant have been disappointing to date. While initially improved, many of these patients have recurrence of their pain one to two years postoperatively. This disturbance is in frequent association with the presence of excessive amounts of heterotopic bone formation and a decrease in the range of motion that was obtained shortly after surgery.

Upper Extremities

Four factors are to be considered in planning care for the upper limb in cerebral palsy:[11] cognition, sensibility, placement, and control of the muscles of the hand. The problems in assessing cognition and sensibility have already been noted.

Placement of the cerebral palsied hand is a combined problem of body, shoulder, and elbow motion. The range of motion is limited by contracture or spasticity of these parts. The speed of placement is limited by the motion disorders that force the arm to make complicated pathways to an object. The precision of placement is limited by those motion disorders affecting the end point of such placement activity. It is convenient to document the speed and precision of placement of a hand on the opposite knee and on the top of the head.

The muscle control of the upper extremity depends on spasticity. Minor degrees of spasticity may exist in limbs with good function, but severe spasticity leads to fixed contractures of muscle-tendon units and joints. These fixed contractures rarely develop in sophisticated upper limbs and when one sees such deformities, function is surely affected.

The retained perinatal reflexes can influence the posture of the whole upper limb in developing mass flexion-extension patterns. Hands that are obligatory slaves to these primitive mass reflexes also have poor potential for rehabilitation.

Realistic goals for hand use are based on the aforementioned four factors. A patient who has poor cognition, poor sensibility,[24] poor hand placement, and no selective control has four strikes against him. A posture that permits hygiene only is a realistic goal for this child. Yet a patient who has good cognition, sensibility, hand placement, and selective control will have no real need for surgical intervention. Thus, any individual for whom we have a functional goal will have to sacrifice some function, and we would hope that it would be in the motor area where an operation has some effect.

The hygiene and cosmetic operations in patients with four strikes against them consist mainly of correcting wrist flexion, thumb-in-palm, and finger flexion contractures. These patients respond inconsistently to muscle transfers or lengthening procedures. Our general policy is to perform radial to metacarpal wrist fusions with iliac bone grafts and pin fixation. At the same time we lengthen the muscle tendon units by the sublimis to profundis transfer and perform some releases.

Functional procedures are performed in those individuals with good cognition, sensibility, and placement, but who have difficulty with muscle control. The problems in muscle control seem to revolve around three main areas of pinch, grasp, and release. When the thumb-in-palm deformity exists, thumb web releases by Z-plasty and release of the adducted first dorsal interosseous from the thumb metacarpal allow opening of the thumb from the palm.[14] In addition, it may be necessary to augment the thumb extensor by a tendon transfer.[6] Sometimes the thumb metacarpal joint is hyperextended, and for such loose joints, capsulodesis with temporary pin fixation is helpful.

Patients with grasp problems are obliged to use their wrist flexors at the time of finger flexion. This discoordinate action of wrist flexors and finger flexor weakens the effective power of the fingers. Here, a transfer of the wrist flexor to the wrist extensor will allow the patient to flex the fingers in vigorous grasp while the wrist is extended.[9,20,21] Before performing such a procedure, it must be ascertained that when the wrist is held in neutral the fingers can be actively extended. If they cannot, then it is possible that the problem with which the surgeon is faced is one of release.

The patients with problems in releasing find it difficult to open their fingers when the wrist is extended. They are obliged to flex the wrist to open their fingers. In these children there is often synergy between the finger extensors and the wrist flexors. This synergy resembles the tenodesis action seen in paralytics, but in most cerebral palsy patients there is no fixed contracture, the movements being a matter of synergistic activity in release rather than tenodesis. The EMG may help to separate the problems with grasp from those of release and we tend to administer them routinely before an operation. When the flexed wrist release combination is seen, transfer of the wrist flexors to the finger extensors may be helpful.

Numerous other procedures have been introduced for the care of the more sophisticated cerebral palsied hands.[8,22,23] These include sublimis tenodesis for hyperextended proximal interphalangeal joint, the use of the flexor carpi radial muscles, elbow flexor releases, and wrist and finger flexor tendon lengthenings. Flexor slides should not be performed in these more sophisticated hands for fear they will lose significant strength. Wrist fusions are poorly tolerated in functional cerebral palsied hands.

In making surgical plans for the cerebral palsy patient's upper extremity, admittedly each child presents different and unique problems. Current experiments with functional orthoses and needle electromyograms may eventually provide more accurate preoperative judgments in these complex problems.

REFERENCES

1. Balf, C. L., and Ingram, O.: Problems in classification of cerebral palsy in childhood. Br. Med. J. 2:163–164, 1955.

2. Bassett, F. H.: Deformities of the feet due to cerebral palsy. In *Instructional Course Lectures,* vol. 20, pp. 35–41. American Academy of Orthopaedic Surgeons. C. V. Mosby, St. Louis, 1971.

3. Bleck, E. E.: Hip deformities in cerebral palsy. In *Instructional Course Lectures,* vol. 20, pp. 54–82. American Academy of Orthopaedic Surgeons. C. V. Mosby, St. Louis, 1971.

4. Bleck, E. E.: Locomotor prognosis in cerebral palsy. Dev. Med. Child Neurol. 17:18–25, 1975.

5. Freud, S.: *Infantile Cerebral Paralysis,* L. Russin, trans. University of Miami Press, Miami, Fla., 1968.

6. Goldner, J. L.: Reconstructive surgery in the hand in cerebral palsy. J. Bone Joint Surg. 37A:1141–1154, 1955.

7. Goldner, J. L.: General principles in cerebral palsy. In *Instructional Course Lectures,* vol. 20, pp. 20–34. American Academy of Orthopaedic Surgeons. C. V. Mosby, St. Louis, 1971.

8. Goldner, J. L.: The upper extremity in cerebral palsy. In Samilson, R., Ed.: *Orthopedic Aspects of Cerebral Palsy,* pp. 221–257. J. B. Lippincott, Philadelphia, 1975.

9. Green, W. T., and Banks, H.: Flexor carpi ulnaris transplant. J. Bone Joint Surg. 44A:1343–1352, 1962.

10. Hoffer, M. M.: Basic considerations and classifications of cerebral palsy. In *Instructional Course Lectures,* vol. 25, pp. 96–105. American Academy of Orthopaedic Surgeons. C. V. Mosby, St. Louis, 1976.

11. Hoffer, M. M.: The upper extremity in cerebral palsy. In *Symposium on Neurological Aspects of Plastic Surgery,* vol. 17, pp. 133–137. C. V. Mosby, St. Louis, 1978.

12. Hoffer, M. M., Garrett, A., Koffman, M., et al.: New concepts in orthotics for cerebral palsy. Clin. Orthop. 102:100–107, 1974.

13. Little, W. J.: On the influence of abnormal parturition on the child. Trans. Obstet. Soc. London 3:293–296, 1862.

14. Matev, I. B.: Surgical treatment of flexion adduction contractures of the thumbs in cerebral palsy. Acta Orthop. Scand. 41:439–445, 1970.

15. Minear, W. L.: A classification of cerebral palsy. Pediatrics 18:841–852, 1956.

16. Pearlstein, M. A.: Infantile cerebral palsy: Classification and clinical correlation. J.A.M.A. 145:30–34, 1952.

17. Perry, J., Hoffer, M., Antonelli, D., et al.: Dynamic and static electromyography of the triceps surae in children with cerebral palsy. J. Bone Joint Surg. 56A:511–520, 1974.

18. Perry, J., Hoffer, M., Antonelli, D., et al.: Electromyography in the muscles about the hip in cerebral palsy. J. Bone Joint Surg. 58A:201–208, 1976.

19. Phelps, W. M.: Etiology and diagnostic classification in cerebral palsy. In *Proceedings of Cerebral Palsy Meeting.* New York Association to Aid Crippled Children, New York, 1950.

20. Samilson, R. L.: Principles of assessment of upper limbs in cerebral palsy. Clin. Orthop. 45:105–115, 1966.

21. Samilson, R. L., and Morris, J. M.: Surgical improvement of the cerebral palsied upper limbs. J. Bone Joint Surg. 46A:1203–1218, 1964.

22. Swanson, A. B.: Surgery of the hand in cerebral palsy. J. Bone Joint Surg. 42A:951–964, 1960.

23. Swanson, A. B.: Surgery of the hand in cerebral palsy. Surg. Clin. North Am. 48:1129–1137, 1968.

24. Tachdjian, M. O., and Minear, W. L.: Sensory disturbances in the hands of children with cerebral palsy. J. Bone Joint Surg. 40A:85–90, 1958.

29

Poliomyelitis

Alice L. Garrett, M.D.

Poliomyelitis has not been eradicated, although a successful immunization program has made this disease a rarity in the United States. The disease, however, is still epidemic in many parts of the world, and even in this country small outbreaks among the non-immunized attest to the fact that the virus is still present.

A sudden onset of paralysis following a febrile illness accompanied by a stiff neck and pain over the muscle bellies should still arouse a suspicion of polio. Viral studies of the spinal fluid can confirm the diagnosis.

Polio has variable but typical patterns of paralysis. Since polio is a disease of the anterior horn cells in the spinal cord, the distribution of paralysis depends on the portion of the spinal cord affected.[10] Some muscles, such as the opponens pollicis, are often involved; others, such as the short toe flexors, are frequently spared.

The hot packs popularized by Sister Kenny were a great contribution to rehabilitation. With this technique moist heat is applied to the trunk and to each involved segment of the limbs, leaving the joint free for range-of-motion exercises. The heat relieves the muscle pain and permits each joint to be carried passively through a range of motion, thus preventing contractures and stiffness that would otherwise occur during the painful acute stage. It should be kept in mind, however, that some contractures can be beneficial in substituting for residual paralysis in certain areas.[1] This possibility is discussed specifically later.

RESPIRATORY AND TRUNK MUSCULATURE

The threat to life during the acute phase of the disease is paralysis of the respiratory muscles. Frequent testing of vital capacity will enable progressive weakness to be detected and respiratory assistance given early. Paralysis of the shoulder musculature should alert one to probable respiratory difficulty, because the anterior horn cells of these muscles are in close proximity in the spinal cord. Tracheotomy may be necessary if the patient is unable to raise secretions because of respiratory and abdominal muscle weakness. The usual error is to delay instituting these two procedures too long.

Many patients recover enough function to become free of respiratory assistance, but a few will have a continued need. Battery-powered chest and abdominal respirators permit freedom of movement in a wheelchair even for those few who remain completely dependent on mechanical respirators.

Glossopharyngeal breathing[2] can be taught to patients, giving them freedom from respiratory equipment during their waking hours. Patients learn to "swallow" air into the lungs, which allows adequate aeration for quiet activity. Other secondary muscles, such as the neck flexors and abdominals, can also be substituted. However, these muscles are not part of the automatic breathing system; thus they function only when the patient is awake. Respiratory equipment is required during sleep. Only the intercostal muscles and the diaphragm function automatically during sleep.

To obtain an indication of intercostal muscle activity, one must evaluate them in three sections. The upper group can be tested on the supine patient by placing relaxed fingers on the upper third of the anterior chest wall, noting the excursion of the chest and any differences between the two sides. The middle and lower thirds can be assessed by placing the hands laterally on the chest with thumbs touching in the midline. Separation of the thumbs during inspiration reflects excursion of the chest produced by the intercostal muscles.

The diaphragm's action is evaluated by placing the relaxed fingers in the epigastrum. Force from motion of the diaphragm can be palpated.

The abdominal musculature's strength and asymmetry can be estimated by observing the umbilicus during breathing and coughing, noting the movement of the umbilicus toward stronger muscles and the bulging of the abdomen in the weakest quadrants.

Before reconstructive surgery is performed, an assessment of respiratory needs is mandatory.[7] Vital capacity measurements are helpful in judging a patient's need of respiratory equipment during the postoperative period. Measurement of the amount of air exhaled during a maximum effort of expiration following a maximum intake of air provides a guide for determining equipment needs.

Instruments to measure vital capacity are readily available commercially and are a basic part of any respiratory laboratory. Measurements of CO_2 and O_2 levels in the expired air can also be helpful.

For hand or foot surgery, 30 percent of normal vital capacity should be adequate, but for trunk surgery 60 percent should be present. If the vital capacity is less, respiratory assistance should be planned during the postoperative period.

Abdominal muscle paralysis may also affect respiration and can be substituted for by abdominal support. The ability to cough depends not only on adequate inspiration but also on the ability to perform a sudden forced expiration. The abdominal muscles are of paramount importance in this latter maneuver. If abdominal muscles are weak, coughing must be assisted manually to ensure adequate clearing of secretions. In this maneuver, manual pressure is applied to the lower abdomen to provide the force required to bring up secretions.

During the acute phase, proper positioning in bed, accompanied by frequent changes in position, is mandatory to prevent pressure sores. Even in the respirator pressure sores can be avoided by intermittently tilting the patient to the side and supporting the new position by pillows. Special care should be taken to make frequent inspections of the bony prominences of the sacrum, greater trochanters, and heels. Prolonged redness is a danger signal, and pressure in such an area is to be totally avoided. Even in the respirator, range-of-motion exercises for all joints are mandatory.

Spine stability depends upon the strength of the trunk musculature.[3] Without trunk musculature the spine tends to collapse, and the patient becomes unable to maintain the upright position. To some degree, residual stiffness of the paralyzed spinal muscles provides some stability. Therefore these muscles should not be fully stretched; indeed, this helpful contracture should be allowed to remain if paralysis persists.

Fusion of the spine substitutes for lack of musculature and is indicated in any section of the collapsing spine, including the cervical spine,[9] in which severe paralysis exists. Not infrequently, patients with total paralysis of the cervical musculature will have adequate muscles in the lower extremities for ambulation, but not until the neck is stabilized can functional ambulation occur.

Additional problems occur in children with trunk paralysis. Scoliosis* results from asymmetrical paralysis of the trunk muscles or from collapsing of the spine secondary to total paralysis. The extent of spine fusion in these patients not only must include the extent of the curve but also must encompass the collapsing paralyzed segments as well. Otherwise the lever arm produced by the fused segment will result in a grossly handicapping unbalanced spine as the scoliosis progresses in the unsupported areas above and below the fusion.

Many patients with respiratory muscle weakness report an increased breathing capacity following surgery. Although vital capacity is unchanged, the action of the weak muscles on the stabilized spine results in better endurance.

Immobilization of the spine prior to and following spinal fusion has been greatly enhanced by the halo cast. The halo attaches directly to the skull, and the cast is molded to give a firm purchase on the pelvis, lessening the need for thoracic pressure. Immobilization is then assured for patients with respiratory limitations, with high spinal curvatures, or with collapsing spines. Internal fixation devices also aid in correction and immobilization for these patients.

Abdominal fascial transplants can support weak abdominal muscles. Strips of fascia lata are placed between the lowest stable rib and the opposite anterior pelvic crest. The two crossed strips substitute for the oblique abdominal muscles. If the potential is there, some increase in strength can occur when constant overstretching is controlled by the fascial grafts.

_____

* See Chapter 26.

UPPER EXTREMITY MUSCULATURE

The arm must be able to lift an object against gravity in order to be useful. Therefore the shoulder muscles must be better than fair in order to be functional. Wheelchair patients with poor shoulder muscles may be fitted with mobile arm supports attached to the wheelchair.[11] With the arm thus supported against gravity even poor muscles can functionally move the arm, allowing the patient to get his or her hand to the mouth and cover a lapboard, desk, or table area. These mobile arm supports must be individually fitted and balanced for each patient to substitute for the weakest muscles and to allow the stronger ones to manipulate the device. Therapists experienced in adjusting these devices are critical to their effective use.

For ambulatory patients no such effective device exists. It is better to think of a shoulder fusion to allow scapular muscles to control shoulder motion. Shoulder position in a fusion is determined by a number of factors. It is better to lose the ability to elevate the arm fully than to be unable to adduct to the side fully. The "salute" position is too high. The position of rotation is also critical, since the extremes of rotation are lost. It is better to be able to reach the face and front of the chest–desk area than to rotate externally to reach the back of the head. The most significant loss is in the degree of internal rotation necessary to attend to bathroom needs. Therefore both shoulders should not be fused. Fusion of a totally paralyzed arm has some benefits, such as ease in dressing. This fusion definitely should not be in much abduction and not in an excess of internal rotation. Interscapular fascial transplants can substitute for paralyzed scapular adductors.

The elbow flexors must be of sufficient strength to lift not only the arm but also the object it carries. Again, mobile arm support can be a substitute aid for the wheelchair patient, but again, for the ambulatory patient there is no effective device. A slight elbow flexion contracture can be very beneficial in a patient with weak flexors. The strength necessary to initiate flexion from a fully extended position is much greater than from a flexed position. Therefore, some flexion contracture is useful and should not be stretched out in a patient with partial paralysis.

Opponens paralysis is typical of polio. Its lack results in a 50 percent loss of hand function—with paralysis the web space between the thumb and index finger tends to shorten. This contracture grossly limits grasp and is very difficult to stretch out. However, an opponens hand splint applied early will prevent this contracture. To be functional the thumb pad should meet the finger pads of the index and middle fingers when their metacarpophalangeal joints are almost fully flexed. If the opponens is an isolated paralysis, an opponensplasty is an excellent procedure to restore the other half of the hand. The ring finger sublimus is the ideal motor if the muscle is present in good strength. Hand splints, besides preventing contractures, can effectively substitute for certain paralysis. A lumbrical bar allows the long finger extensors to extend the fingers, thus making it possible to open the hand. If the hand is flail, hand function is still possible through the use of the flexor hinge splint if the wrist extensors are present.[8] With this splint, extension of the wrist forces the metacarpophalangeal joints to flex, thus providing grasp. Surgery can substitute for this splint by fusing the thumb and interphalangeal finger joints and tenodesing the long extensors and flexors. The operation will supply force to the normal automatic opening and closing of the hand that occurs with wrist motion. Contracture of the long finger flexors and extensors provides a functional automatic grasp powered by wrist musculature when finger flexors and extensors are paralyzed.

Between these two extremes of a flail hand and an isolated opponens paralysis lie many possibilities of splinting and tendon transplants, depending upon the degree of paralysis. The most important concept to apply is to stabilize joints that do not have motor control. One cannot expect muscles of short excursion to provide power over long excursions, nor can tendon transplants be counted on to control too many flail joints. It is better to have precise control of a few key motions in both directions. Always judge the potential function against that obtained by a flexor hinge and splint. To justify surgery, the expected function must exceed the automatic grasp.

Before any surgery of the upper extremity is considered, the weight-bearing functions of the arms with crutches must be considered. A shoulder fusion does not prevent crutch walking, but a metacarpal block would. An opponensplasty, as well as elbow and other hand transplants, must be protected from heavy-duty weight bearing.

LOWER EXTREMITY FUNCTION

A full range of motion of both hips and knees is important for full function. There is usually a tendency for hips to become contracted in flexion, external rotation, and adduction, and the knees tend toward flexion contractures. Proper positioning in bed and passive range of motion are mandatory during the acute stage. Hip flexion contractures are to be avoided in all patients, including those in wheelchairs. Although mild flexion contractures do not interfere with sitting, in the supine position they exert a lordotic pull on the spine. This pull can compromise the abdominal and even the thoracic cavities. A preventive prone positioning program for nonambulatory patients should be begun early and continued indefinitely to combat the prolonged flexion position necessitated by wheelchair use.

For ambulation the antigravity muscles must be functioning or substituted for. If the hips have a full range of motion, standing is possible with both legs flail by using two long-leg braces fixed at the knee and ankle. The patient stands in hyperextension at the hip, resting against the anterior capsule of the hip, which is reinforced by the "y" ligament. Obviously, hip flexion contractures prevent this locking action. A swing-through or a four-point gait is possible if upper extremity function permits the use of a crutch and if hip hikers are present to move the legs forward. The presence of gluteals of good strength and the ability to advance the leg forward are enough to eliminate the need for crutches.

Advancement of the leg can be accomplished by hip flexors of poor strength. Knee flexors of at least fair strength will also provide adequate hip flexion. During stance, knee flexion results in the knee falling ahead of the hip. Knee extension then advances the leg.

A patient with two flail legs requires good strength in the trunk and upper extremities to ambulate functionally. Muscle imbalance about the hip is a potential cause of contractures, with motion limited in the direction of the weakness. Unopposed flexors in particular are a problem. Imbalance between abduction and adduction in the growing child may result in subluxation and even dislocation of the hip. If such an imbalance is present, x-rays of the hip should be taken at regular intervals to pinpoint this avoidable complication before secondary acetabular dysplegia develops. Early muscle transplants, such as adductors to the ischium and gluteus medius to the greater trochanter,[6] should be considered before acetabular dysplasia occurs and bone surgery is required to correct this secondary deformity. A varus osteotomy of the femur may also be necessary to correct excessive anteversion. Bone surgery without correction of muscle imbalance will not prevent recurring deformity.

Transfer of the gluteus medius to the greater trochanter will not prevent Trendelenburg's symptom, since it takes near-normal muscle strength to stabilize the hip laterally. This transplant then needs crutch protection to maintain its strength and prevent dislocation of the hip.

Long-leg braces for flail legs should have the ankle joint fixed in slight dorsiflexion to compensate for the hyperextended hip position, and the knees should be locked in extension.

An absent quadriceps can be replaced by strong gluteus maximus action or strong plantar flexion of the ankle. Of all the losses of antigravity muscles, absence of the quadriceps is the least handicapping. If the plantar flexors are also weak, a short-leg brace with an up stop can substitute for them, thus obviating the need for a long-leg brace. If the gluteals are strong enough, even climbing stairs is possible. Full knee extension is necessary, and a knee flexion contracture of even a few degrees will make a long-leg brace necessary for knee stability. In the foot a fixed-ankle, short-leg brace will provide foot and ankle stability. Fixing the ankle in plantar flexion is not necessary to make the knee stable. Plantar flexion makes rolling over the foot during walking difficult and may produce a progressive genu recurvatum. In fact, in a growing child an absent quadriceps replaced by gluteus maximus and plantar flexion may induce a progressive genu recurvatum and require a long-leg brace with a free knee to limit hyperextension. If possible, however, hyperextension should be controlled by a short-leg brace limiting plantar flexion. Another indication for a long-leg brace in a growing child may be an increasing medial instability of the knee secondary to a valgus force at the knee when the flail leg is externally rotated at the hip during gait.

Not infrequently in the flail foot the short toe flexors may still be functioning. In such cases there is a tendency to produce a varus foot. Since these flexors serve no useful purpose in this foot, surgery to stop their deforming action should be considered. However, the most common cause of a varus deformity in a flail leg is a long-leg brace in which external tibial torsion was not built in. With the knee joint of the brace centered at the knee's axis of motion, the foot is forced into a varus position to get into the shoe. The shoe can be placed at a maximum of 15 degrees external rotation, but any greater torsion must be put into the uprights of the brace.

Muscle imbalance in the foot can result in deformity. Function can be compensated for with a brace with up or down stops or a fixed ankle position, but a brace cannot stop muscle imbalance from acting as a deforming force on the growing bones in the foot. Therefore, surgery to correct the muscle imbalance may be indicated, irrespective of whether or not bracing can be eliminated.[12] Bone stabilization may be necessary to correct bone deformity and furnish stability to joints uncontrolled by muscle action.

The energy requirements for walking with severe paralysis may be handled by teenagers and even young adults. However, for older patients the sitting position becomes more and more desirable. Changing levels of physical activity with increasing age must be kept in mind whenever such procedures as hip fusion are considered.

Long-leg braces attached to a back brace or even a pelvic band provide an exercise program, as do parallel bars, but not true ambulation. Functional ambulation includes the abilities to move between sitting and standing, to lock and unlock braces, and to put on and take off braces. This is not to say that taking a few steps with help does not give some advantages; for example, the ability to get into public bathrooms and theater seats may make many more activities possible, activities that do not allow wheelchair access. However, wheelchair transportation may leave a person much more energy to devote to more intellectual pursuits instead of having to expend it in the physical labor of getting from place to place. The same philosophy applies to powered wheelchairs. Better to have mobility with mechanical aids rather than arrive at the destination too fatigued to function or be unable to navigate independent of other people.

INEQUALITY OF LEG LENGTH

Bone growth is stimulated by weight bearing and by muscle action. Paralysis occurring in a growing child will have an adverse effect on the rate of growth of the long bones associated with the paralyzed muscles. Obviously, the younger child with the most growth potential will be at greatest risk of a significant problem. In a flail leg the lack of muscle action on the bone results in less growth potential than in the other muscled leg. The physician should follow the differential rate of growth by scanographs and bone-age films of the wrist.[5] Through serial studies the rate of growth and the resultant leg-length discrepancy expected at the end of growth can be estimated.[4] The upper tibial epiphysis or lower femoral epiphysis on the longer leg can then be surgically obliterated at a certain age in order to keep the discrepancy in leg lengths to a minimum. Tables have been constructed to show the expected growth from both these epiphyses; their development contributes most to total leg length. These tables relate to bone age, not chronological age. Therefore, concomitant films of the wrist are just as important to follow as the actual lengths of both legs. A small discrepancy in the paralyzed leg is an advantage in easing the clearance of that leg during gait. Therefore, the legs should not be equalized; rather the shortening should be kept to the optimal level. The short leg can also be lengthened to obtain the desired result.

The worst leg-length discrepancies result in contractures severe enough to prevent weight bearing. Prevention of contractures, or correction of them if they are present, is especially important in the growing child. Since nothing can be done about the lack of muscle stimulation in the flail leg, the prevention or correction of contractures, together with use of appropriate orthoses, will ensure that at least the weight-bearing stresses will continue to stimulate bone growth.

EDUCATIONAL AND VOCATIONAL GOALS

Education must not be compromised in these patients. Intellectual capacity is not impaired, and these patients can compete with their normal peers if they are not deprived of the educational and vocational training opportunities. Manual labor will not be possible for those with any degree of paralysis, meaning that educational opportunities become of even greater importance. Accordingly, therefore, after the acute illness efforts must be directed at obtaining full mobility and maximum use of hand function with the least interference to educational pursuits. Timing of surgery should be arranged to keep the loss of school or work days to a minimum.

The sudden loss of function that this illness brings to a child or adult may mean a gross shift in living patterns and future plans for both the patient and the family. Social workers and psychologists knowledgeable about the special problems faced by these families and the medical care necessary to attain maximum function for the patients can be of utmost value. Many families without such help may not survive or may adopt coping behaviors that are not in the best interests of all concerned. Grief, depression, and anger are all emotions expected, and it is the unusual patient and family that could not benefit from professional help in meeting these emotional crises.

Vocational and educational training in itself is not enough. Transportation to and from work and facilities for independent living may be necessary adjuncts to successful rehabilitation. The closer a patient can come to using public transportation and conventional living facilities, the easier it will be to return to the mainstream of life. However, some patients may require special vans that accommodate a wheelchair, and some may need special living arrangements. Whatever is required that can be made available will enhance independence and come closer to keeping the individual within society. It is important to realize that control over events and making one's own decisions about the future are paramount. As soon as the acute crisis is over, the concern should be to shift decision-making away from health personnel to the patient.

REFERENCES

1. Adkins, H. V., Robins, V., Eckland, F., et al.: Selective stretching for the paralytic patient. Phys. Ther. Rev. 40:644–648, 1960.
2. Dail, C. W., Affeldt, J. E., and Collier, C. R.: Clinical aspects of glossopharyngeal breathing. Report of use by one hundred postpoliomyelitic patients. JAMA 158:445–449, 1955.
3. Garrett, A. L., Perry, J., and Nickel, V. L.: Stabilization of the collapsing spine. J. Bone Joint Surg. 43A:474–484, 1961.
4. Green, W. T., and Anderson, M.: Skeletal age and the control of bone growth. In *Instructional Course Lectures,* vol. 17, pp. 199–217. American Academy of Orthopaedic Surgeons. C. V. Mosby, St. Louis, 1960.
5. Greulick, W. W., and Pyle, S. I.: *Radiographic Atlas of Skeletal Development of the Hand and Wrist,* 2nd ed. Stanford University Press, Stanford, 1959.
6. London, J. T., and Nichols, O.: Paralytic dislocation of the hip in myelodysplasia. J. Bone Joint Surg. 57A:501–506, 1975.

7. Nickel, V. L., Perry, J., Affeldt, J. E., and Dail, C. W.: Elective surgery on patients with respiratory paralysis. J. Bone Joint Surg. 39A:989–1001, 1957.

8. Nickel, V. L., Perry, J., and Garrett, A. L.: Development of useful function in the severely paralyzed hand. J. Bone Joint Surg. 45A:933–952, 1963.

9. Perry, J., and Nickel, V. L.: Total cervical-spine fusion for neck paralysis. J. Bone Joint Surg. 41A:37–60, 1959.

10. Sharrard, W. J. W.: Distribution of permanent paralysis in the lower limb in poliomyelitis; clinical and pathological study. J. Bone Joint Surg. 37B:540–558, 1955.

11. Smith, E. M., and Juvinall, R. C.: Design refinement of the linkage feeder. Arch. Phys. Med. Rehab. 44:609–615, 1963.

12. Westin, G. W.: Tendon transfers about the foot, ankle, and hip in the paralyzed lower extremity. J. Bone Joint Surg. 47A:1430–1443, 1965.

30

Skeletal Tuberculosis

Donald R. Gunn, M.B., Ch.B., M.Ch.Orth., F.R.C.S. (Ed.), D.Sc.Hon.

The great majority of cases of skeletal tuberculosis involve joints. A tuberculous infection of bone or tuberculous osteomyelitis is a relatively rare form of the infection. In the spine, the joints that are most often involved are the intervertebral disc and the adjacent vertebral bodies. It is rare for less than two bodies and one intervening disc to be involved and common for four or five vertebral bodies and the related intervertebral discs to be included in the area of disease. Involvement of the posterior joints and the posterior elements of the spinous processes, laminae, and transverse processes is rare and is almost always a backward extension from disease starting in the vertebral bodies.

In the extremities the large joints are most often involved and the large joints of the lower extremities are more often attacked than those of the upper extremities. Thus, tuberculosis of the hip and knee is the most common form of tuberculosis of the skeleton except for spinal tuberculosis. Tuberculosis does occur in the large joints in the upper extremity, shoulder, elbow, and wrist but is not as common as it is in the hip and knee. Tuberculous osteomyelitis, when it is seen, usually occurs in the short long bones of the hands and feet. Occasionally tuberculous osteomyelitis of the ribs has been identified.

PREVALENCE AND CAUSES

Tuberculosis remains a widespread disease in the Middle East, Africa, and the Far East. In 1976, Seddon[6] estimated that in all of its forms it may involve as many as 20 million infectious cases worldwide. Even in the technically advanced countries that now consider the disease to be somewhat unusual, tuberculosis may cause more deaths than any other notifiable infectious disease. Whereas in the past an appreciable number of cases were due to infection by the bovine bacillus, most patients today are infected by the human strains of the bacillus. This is particularly so in the Middle and Far East, where cow or buffalo milk is seldom a part of the diet. Even when it is used, milk is always boiled.

Only a relatively small portion of the total number of cases involves bones and joints, which is thought to be 5 percent of the total. However, 5 percent of 20 million is still a large number of cases. This number may be subdivided into two approximately equal groups, those who show infections of the spine and those having involvement of joints other than the spine.[6]

HISTORICAL NOTES ON TREATING TUBERCULOSIS

Prior to the introduction of effective antituberculous drugs, the basis of treatment was rest. Both local rest to the involved part and rest to the patient as a whole were prescribed. Additional supportive measures included a good diet, fresh air, and excellent nursing. Complete rest was aimed for, and it was felt that this rest needed to be prolonged, uninterrupted, and even enforced. This was the era of long stays in the hospital and sanitorium, the patient spending months and even years in bed, immobilized with suitable splints or frames.

Long periods of hospitalization as demanded by this regimen also required extensive educational facilities supported by occupational therapy and physical therapy whenever possible. Although there is no doubt that rest plays an important part in the healing of lesions for some patients, it must also be remembered that complete rest on this scale had detrimental effects. Osteoporosis from disuse and renal calculi were relatively common and all the problems and sequelae that arose therefrom. Over the years there were many attempts to ablate or abbreviate tuberculous infection of bone, but they were all almost universally unsuccessful for the reason that primary wound healing was seldom achieved. The end result was a draining sinus with mixed infection. Those patients with a significant tuberculous infection plus a superimposed secondary infection became likely candidates for the development of amyloidosis, a disease process that killed a great many of these patients.

Effective drug therapy became available after 1945 and consisted of the administration of streptomycin by injection and para-aminosalicyclic acid (PAS) and isoniazid by mouth. Various combinations of these three drugs were used for lengthy periods of time, but the important thing was that they were effective in almost any combination. It has recently been demonstrated that the streptomycin supplement to PAS and isoniazid was of no demonstrable benefit and would appear to have been unnecessary.[5]

A second positive aspect of drug therapy is that it allows for successful operations. Tuberculous joints and the abscesses that often result from them can be opened, drained, and closed with a high expectation of satisfactory primary wound healing. In addition, it has proved to be possible to debride a tuberculous lesion of the bone or joint and perform primary bone grafting with a good chance of success because of the effectiveness of these drugs.

The combination of effective drugs and surgery has reduced the hospital time to relatively brief periods of days or weeks as opposed to months or years. In the pre-drug era, splints and frames to immobilize limbs and spines were fabricated with skill and ingenuity by bracemakers and orthotists in order to achieve the maximum immobilization of the unfortunate patient. To review these devices against the background of modern treatment produces the feeling of wonderment that patients could tolerate and survive those medieval-appearing devices.

DIAGNOSIS AND DIAGNOSTIC TOOLS

A carefully taken history and an accurately recorded and detailed clinical examination remain the bases of the diagnosis of skeletal tuberculosis. One other factor, however, is important: an awareness that the disease still exists and can turn up in surprising situations. Skeletal tuberculosis *is* a sleeper disease, usually unsuspected and consequently undiagnosed.

Any examination of the spine should include measurement of height and correlation with the patient's age. Inspection of the spine will reveal deformities, the most common of which are kyphotic deformities in the dorsal and dorsolumbar region. Gross limitation in movement of the neck is common and reversal of the normal lordotic curve plus limitation of movement in the lumbar spine are also often seen. Neurological function distal to any suspected spinal lesion must be carefully assessed, and because tuberculosis of the spine usually involves the vertebral bodies, the first function of the spinal cord to be involved is motor function. Sensory loss is a comparatively late aspect of neurological damage in this disease. Skeletal tuberculosis is often associated with pulmonary tuberculosis or infections of the genitourinary tract and a careful evaluation of these systems must also be part of the routine evaluation.

The examination of the extremities will be directed toward pain or limitation of function of joints. When identified, these disabilities will be associated with muscle wasting, swelling, tenderness, limitation of movement, or fixed deformity of the joints. Premature epiphyseal arrest, a relatively common feature of this disease, often leads to significant shortening in addition to the reduction in length produced by the destruction of the joint itself.

Laboratory investigations have not been of significant and specific help. The sedimentation rate has proved to be a useful indicator and should be repeated at monthly intervals once the diagnosis has been established. A high sedimentation rate at one time indicated that the patient should not have surgery, but now it is accepted that a high sedimentation rate is in fact an indication for surgery. Once the lesion has been surgically debrided, a rapid drop in sedimentation rate over the next one to two months can be expected. This decrease can be an indicator of success of the surgical procedure plus, of course, the effect of the antituberculous drugs.

In skeletal tuberculosis, the main diagnostic tool has been the use and interpretation of x-rays. Although a complete skeletal survey is preferable, it is often not practical, whereas good x-rays of the involved area of the skeleton plus good chest x-rays are essential. X-rays, however, are by no means an accurate predictor of tuberculosis; the rate of diagnostic error based on x-rays alone has proved to be in the region of 25 percent.[5] Computerized axial tomographic scanning of the spine has not been used to an appreciable degree in detecting tuberculosis, but it is already evident that it produces useful diagnostic information in other infectious processes in the spine and will no doubt prove valuable for tuberculosis as well.

BASIC PRINCIPLES AND TECHNIQUES

As the full effectiveness of antituberculous drugs has become increasingly appreciated, it is evident that the rigid forms of immobilization once used over long periods of time are no longer necessary. In the 1950s, when operations for skeletal tuberculosis became much more feasible, it was strongly felt that operative clearance of the infected lesion would not only abbreviate the period of treatment needed but would also enhance the final results.

In tuberculosis of the spine, the clear advantages of operating have not really proved to exist and comparative studies conducted in Korea, Africa, and Hong Kong have produced some interesting findings. Five different mechanical treatment regimens were studied, one common factor being that all patients received antituberculous drug therapy (Fig. 30-1). The five different regimens were: no restraint or immobilization; a plaster of Paris jacket supporting the spine but allowing the patient to be ambulatory and even leave the hospital; rest in bed for six months; minimal eradication of disease by an operation; and radical excision of the tuberculous focus with bridging of the resulting defect in the spine by autogenous bone graft (Fig. 30-2). Results of these studies have been published in the British Medical Research Council bulletins and they show that more than 80 percent of the patients in each group achieved satisfactory results.[1-4] The best results of all were produced by the radical surgical approach, but the percentage of satisfactory results was less than 10 percent better than those treated by the simpler efforts (Fig. 30-3). The results of these controlled studies, monitored by the Medical Research Council of Great Britain, indicate that spinal tuberculosis can be treated adequately by good drug therapy and immobilization. Yet the study also seems to indicate that the immobilization can be quite minimal in the form of a plaster body jacket, that ambulation is allowable, and that the regimen does not require prolonged rest in bed or in the hospital.

However, certain cases of spinal tuberculosis do require operation, and these patients form two groups. First is a small group that does not respond well to drug therapy, as exemplified by the child who remains unwell, whose appetite perhaps remains poor and sedimentation rate remains high, and who on serial x-rays shows evidence of increasing destruction.

A small clinical test of some importance in some parts of the world is that the child who does not suntan easily is sick. Children under treatment for tuberculosis who on exposure to the sun turn pink and then pale again are not doing well, which perhaps may be another indication for a surgical approach.

The second group of patients in whom surgery is required are those with spinal tuberculosis and evidence of spinal cord or cauda equina compression. Any

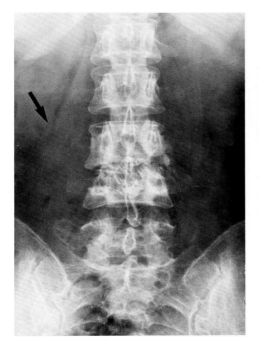

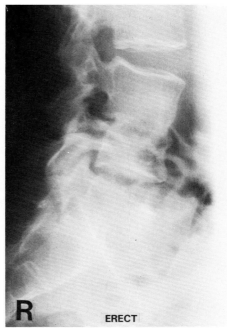

Fig. 30-1. Tuberculosis involving the third and fourth lumbar vertebrae. Note the significant destruction, particularly of the fourth lumbar vertebra, and the formation of a large abscess.

Fig. 30-2. Tuberculosis of the lumbar spine, showing some bony union after debridement and drug treatment.

deterioration in neurological function should, if possible, be dealt with surgically. There is no question that patients with partial or complete paraplegia have improved after a drug regimen alone, but equally there is no question that the nervous tissue can be decompressed more quickly through an operation.

The treatment of tuberculosis of the large joints of the extremities has also changed significantly over the last decade or two and will continue to change. Some years ago it was felt that the only satisfactory result from a tuberculous infection of a joint of the lower extremity was a bony ankylosis (Fig. 30-4). The emphasis has changed gradually, with the trend toward attempting to maintain some mobility in the joint. In this area considerable judgment is required. A child with an early infection of hip or knee should be immobilized. After a reasonably short period of time and with the cover of antituberculous drugs, an attempt should be made to mobilize the joint. This step can be taken only in patients whose x-rays show no bony destruction or minimal bony destruction. If the attempt at immobilization is successful, then gradual progression to weight bearing may be attempted over a period of several weeks or months (Figs. 30-5 and 30-6). In those patients who originally had significant destruction of articular surfaces, arthrodesis may still prove to be the most satisfactory long-term answer. However, attempts to regain or maintain movement in some of these joints are probably justifiable, but disappointments will inevitably be encountered.

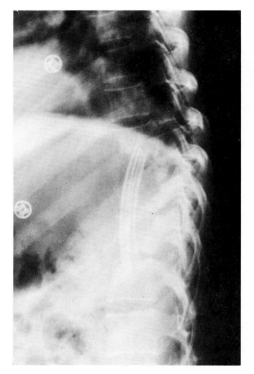

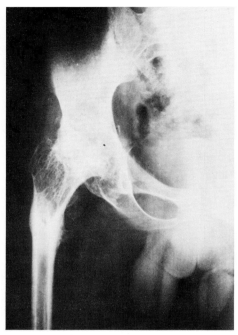

Fig. 30-3. Extensive tuberculosis involving five vertebral bodies treated by excision and rib grafting.

Fig. 30-4. Arthrodesis of a hip severely damaged by tuberculosis.

Finally, those patients who because of extensive joint disease have had an arthrodesis may in due course become candidates for total joint replacement and remobilization of an arthrodesed joint. At present, the only joint to which this procedure would certainly apply would be the hip joint. Perhaps the shoulder joint could be considered as well. In our present state of knowledge, it would be unwise to attempt to immobilize an arthrodesis of the knee by total joint replacement.

Mobilizing tuberculous joints, whether they have tuberculous synovitis or have received interposition arthroplasties, is a procedure requiring skill and prolonged physical therapy. The physical therapist and occupational therapist are very important parts of the team treatment approach to healing tuberculous joints.

TREATMENT OF CHOICE

There is no question that the basis of treatment of tuberculous lesions of the skeleton is well-maintained and well-supervised antituberculous drug therapy. Further treatment of tuberculous lesions of the spine will depend to a great extent on the facilities available. Although good and even excellent results can be obtained by the use of external splints and by having the patient ambulate, the best results are still obtained surgically. However, this constitutes major surgery

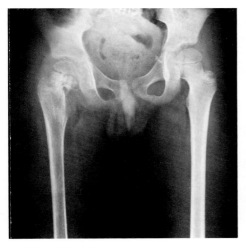

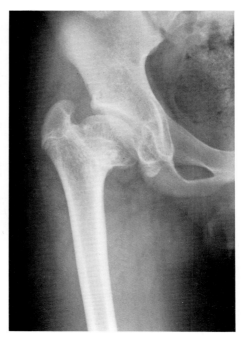

Fig. 30-5. Tuberculosis destroying the neck of the femur involving the hip joint.

Fig. 30-6. The same case shown in Figure 30-5, but five years after conservative management with rest, traction, and drug therapy.

and requires excellent facilities. In those patients demonstrating neurological involvement of the spinal cord or cauda equina, surgical treatment is the approach of choice.

ALTERNATIVES TO THE TREATMENT OF CHOICE

No satisfactory alternative really exists to the use of adequate antituberculous drugs. As noted, there has been a considerable move away from institutional treatment of tuberculous patients, and more and more the outpatient approach or brief hospital stay is acceptable. Surgery for tuberculosis of the spine is less necessary than it was thought to be some years ago, but the stage where it plays no part has not been reached.

FUTURE AVENUES IN REHABILITATING SKELETAL TUBERCULOSIS

In cases of tuberculosis of the spine there will be further efforts to minimize the development of the spinal deformity, which in the case of tuberculosis is a kyphotic deformity. With this in view, the use of internal devices, such as posteriorly placed springs, may finally prove to play a part.

In tuberculosis of the weight-bearing joints, the guiding principle used to be to produce a joint that was painless and stable, and, if possible, would move. The priorities of treatment were in that order. Thus, an arthrodesis of a joint that led to a painless and stable joint fully met the first two criteria. To produce a joint that was painful, stable, and mobile was of no satisfaction to the patient. However, our aim must be to attain all three of those priorities, which should become more and more possible as further experience is gained in various forms of arthoplasty for infected joints.

ACKNOWLEDGMENT

The illustrations have been made available by Professor P. Chacha of the University of Singapore.

REFERENCES

1. Medical Research Council Working Party on tuberculosis of the spine. J. Bone Joint Surg. 55B:678–697, 1973.
2. Medical Research Council Working Party on tuberculosis of the spine. A study in Pusan, Korea. Tubercle 54:261–282, 1973.
3. Medical Research Council Working Party on tuberculosis of the spine. J. Trop. Med. Hyg. 77:72–92, 1974.
4. Medical Research Council Working Party on tuberculosis of the spine. A study in Hong Kong. Br. J. Surg. 61:853–866, 1974.
5. Pillay, V. K.: Personal communication.
6. Seddon, H. J.: Editorial. J. Bone Joint Surg. 58B:395–397, 1976.

31

Neck Pain

Henry H. Bohlman, M.D.

Neck pain is one of the most common complaints confronting the physician and therapist. A general understanding of the various causes of neck pain is an important asset in planning an orderly regimen of diagnosis and treatment.

For many years there has been a general misconception that all neck pain originates from neural compression. Any pain-producing disease that affects the peripheral joints and musculoskeletal system may also involve the cervical spine and cause pain.[11,13] That is, trauma, tumors, and inflammatory diseases, as well as degenerative processes, may result in a painful neck syndrome.

The pathophysiological mechanisms by which neck pain is produced are: direct external neural compression of the cervical roots or spinal cord; central, or intrinsic, neural cord pressure; degenerative disc or joint disease; intrinsic osseous or ligamentous lesions; and abnormal motion or instability. Cervical spine pain may radiate to distal sites because of direct neural compression or by stimulation of deep somatic nerve endings found in the joints, bone, and outer layers of the disc itself.[4]

Depending upon the cause, the pain will travel down the arm in different patterns. If the cause of pain is by direct nerve root compression, the pain pattern will follow a dermatomic distribution to the shoulder in the case of the fifth cervical root, or into the arm, forearm, and fingers if the lower cervical roots are involved. Generally, pain originating from deep somatic nerve endings of the joints or bone will produce inner scapular pain with aching of the arm or forearm. This shoulder pain is associated with generalized paresthesias of the hand.

PAIN FROM DIRECT NEURAL COMPRESSION

A laterally herniated intervertebral disc most commonly occurs without a history of trauma. It may produce external, anterior compression of a nerve root with specific sensory and motor abnormalities plus the loss of sensation in a particular dermatome pattern as well as weakness of specific muscle groups innervated by that particular nerve. The resulting pain of a laterally herniated cervical disc is radicular in distribution and unilateral but referred pain to the pectoral, inner scapular, or occipital regions may occur (Figs. 31-1A, B).

A centrally herniated disc, however, may produce anterior spinal cord compression with myelopathy and radiculopathy because of anterior horn cell impairment. The size of the osseous spinal canal is very important in predisposing the patient to significant neural compression. A congenitally narrow cervical canal (less than 16 mm) is often associated with spinal cord compromise following a herniated disc. Pain of a central disc herniation may be in the neck, back, or even in the legs (Figs. 31-2A–C and 31-3A–C).

Formation of chondro-osseous spurs in the cervical spine may result in compression of the nerve roots if it is posterolateral at the joints of Luschka or in

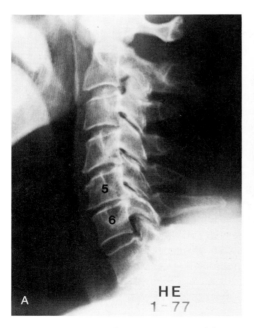
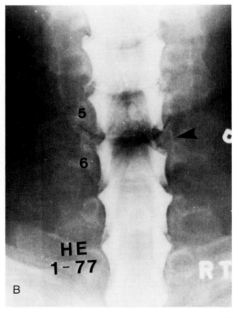

Fig. 31-1. (A) Lateral roentgenogram of the cervical spine of a 50-year-old man, without antecedent trauma, who presented with severe neck pain radiating to the right inner scapular region, shoulder, arm, and forearm. Physical examination revealed marked limitation of extension of the neck (20 degrees). Reproduction of pain and paresthesias of the right arm, forearm, thumb, and index fingers occurred with neck extension and right lateral rotation. There was weakness of the right biceps muscle and loss of sensation to pin prick in the right volar thumb area. Cervical spondylosis affects the fourth, fifth, and sixth levels. (B) Anteroposterior view of the cervical myelogram revealed a central as well as right lateral filling defect. It indicated soft disc herniation with nerve root compression in the sixth cervical vertebrae of the right side.

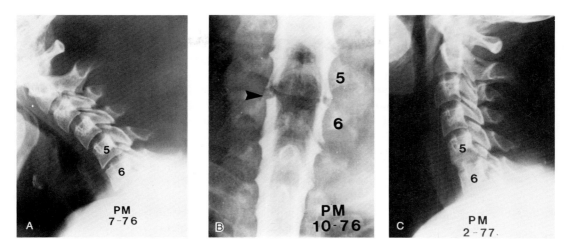

Fig. 31-2. (A) This 30-year-old woman was struck from behind while driving her car three years ago. She sustained a flexion-extension neck injury with immediate neck and right arm pain. Physical examination revealed severe limitation of extension of the cervical spine (20 degrees) with pain. She had no neurological deficit. Chronic neck and arm pain persisted for three years after nonoperative treatment. This figure demonstrates the lateral flexion roentgenogram of the cervical spine with slight narrowing of the disc space between the fifth and sixth cervical levels, but it is otherwise normal. (B) Anteroposterior view of the patient's cervical myelogram reveals a predominantly central disc herniation with filling defect between the fifth and sixth cervical levels. Pain was produced by spinal cord compression without neurological signs. (C) Lateral roentgenogram five months after Robinson anterior cervical discectomy and fusion. The patient's pain was entirely relieved and she was able to return to work in a factory.

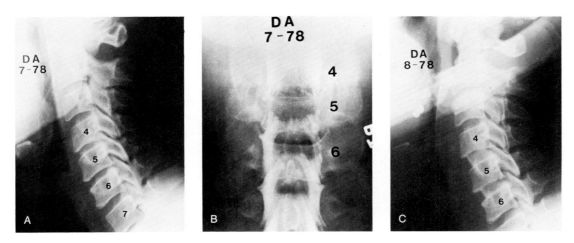

Fig. 31-3. (A) Lateral roentgenogram of the cervical spine of a 35-year-old man who had been injured in a vehicular accident nine months before. The patient struck his head and had immediate neck pain followed by bilateral shoulder and upper arm pains with paresthesias of the arms and legs. Neck pain persisted after nonoperative treatment. Physical examination revealed bilateral biceps and triceps weakness, as well as leg paresthesias on hyperextension of the cervical spine. There is mild narrowing of the C4–C5 and C5–C6 disc spaces. Signs of myelopathy were present and included bilateral Hoffmann's reflexes as well as clonus. (B) Anteroposterior view of the cervical myelogram. The large central filling defects at C4–C5 and C5–C6 indicate compression of the spinal cord. (C) Anterior discectomy and fusion were performed, confirming large extruded discs at C4–C5 and C5–C6. The patient's paresthesias and weakness were relieved. The bone grafts have been in place for one month.

spinal cord compression if the spur is more centrally located at the posterior aspect of the vertebral body.

One of the earliest signs of neural compression is pain, believed to be ischemic in origin because the intrinsic blood supply to the nerve roots and cord is blocked before the axoplasmic flow and physiological neural function cease. The result of that cessation is paralysis. In addition, there are somatic nerve endings in the dura and root sheaths. The pain of neural compression may be intermittent and related to the position of the neck and cervical spine. Hyperextension of the neck produces increased bulging of a herniated disc and further compresses the neural structures against the inwardly buckled posterior ligamentum flavum. Pain reproduced by hyperextension of the neck is often the first sign of a centrally herniated disc; the patient may actually refuse to allow extension of the neck. Extension of the neck with lateral rotation may reproduce lateral nerve root compression and radicular pain radiating to the shoulder, arm, and fingers. Paresthesias may be associated with any of these maneuvers, specifically, in the arms with root compression and in radiation to the torso and legs with spinal cord compression. The concepts of mechanisms of increased neural compression with various motions of the cervical spine are obviously important when considering treatment of any cervical disorder, whether by physical therapy, immobilization, or surgical intervention.

A meticulous physical examination should include range of motion of the cervical spine recorded in degrees of extension, flexion, and rotation as well as the patient's response to those maneuvers. Frequently, the patient will be tender to palpation over the spinous process of the offending vertebral segment. Accurate neurological examination, including motor, sensory and reflex changes, aids the examiner in classifying the particular pain disorder, such as nonradicular or somatic, radicular, and myopathic with long tract signs.[3]

Electromyography may be helpful in determining specific nerve root levels of pathology, yet the technique can be totally negative with early nerve root compression. Electromyogram examination and nerve conduction studies may, however, differentiate peripheral nerve compression in the extremity from proximal root compression when pain is referred to the shoulder, arm, and hand.

For purposes of documentation as well as diagnosis, physical therapists, nurses, and other allied health professionals can record a detailed neurological examination prior to attempts at treatment.

Historically, it is well known that herniated cervical as well as lumbar discs with nerve root compression can usually be treated successfully by nonoperative measures. It is certainly my experience that even those patients with significant cervical nerve root compression and resultant muscle weakness will, in the majority of cases, resolve the paralysis and pain syndrome without surgery. The soft herniated cervical disc usually occurs during the early stage of disc degeneration in the third, fourth, or fifth decade of life without antecedent trauma. Patients with neck pain in their sixth or seventh decade should be suspected of having tumors of bone or other lesions producing the radiculopathy.

Nonoperative measures that have stood the test of time in successful treatment of herniated cervical discs include soft collar or rigid cervical orthosis immobilization, intermittent cervical traction, and administration of such drugs as the nonsteroidal anti-inflammatory agents, muscle relaxants, and pain medications. Both the patient and therapist should be instructed in the use of immobilization and traction devices so that the head and neck are not in an extended position, aggravating the situation. The soft collar should be worn with the narrow position anteriorly. For the same reason head-halter traction in the lying or sitting position must be utilized with the neck in slight flexion or neutral position so that further aggravation of the condition does not occur by extending the spine. The response of the patient to these treatment modalities often determines the progression of the treatment plan. In most cases the patient is instructed to wear the soft collar all waking hours during the day and at night if the pain is awakening the patient. Cervical traction is carried out daily. Moist or dry heat is applied during the traction session to relieve muscle spasm. If the patient is hospitalized, traction can be carried out intermittently during the day.

The usual favorable early response to treatment will be a decrease in the intensity and duration of the patient's pain. When the patient notes a marked decrease in pain, then the next sign of improvement ordinarily will be increased motor strength in the involved arm. With further improvement, the pin prick sensory loss will return, accompanied by relief of paresthesias, but the latter sign may take months. I do not believe there is a place for manipulation of the cervical spine in cervical disc disease. Compressed nerve roots are already swollen and inflamed. Therefore further motion of the neck by manipulation or forced exercises serves only to exacerbate the condition. In addition, ultrasound is of questionable benefit and is not necessary. Many physicians practice with injections of "trigger points" with steroids and local anesthetics to relieve pain. These treatments do not seem to be beneficial. The cervical spine and nerve roots have an amazing capacity to heal if they are rested by cervical orthoses and recumbency.

In a small percentage of cases, the herniated cervical disc is so large that the root compression is not resolved by nonoperative management. Depending upon the severity of pain and neural deficit the patient is experiencing, if in six to eight weeks the situation is not improved, then operative excision of the disc may be indicated. Before operating, cervical myelography is carried out to localize the specific pathological disc level. The safest and most reliable technique of cervical disc excision was first described by Robinson and Smith in 1955.[14] This technique involves an anterior approach to the cervical spine. The entire offending disc and ruptured fragment are removed, followed by a fusion with bone graft. Modern surgical technique involves the use of a high-intensity headlight as well as magnification by ocular loops. The bone graft is used to open or distract the disc space and foramina to more normal size and to stabilize the offending segment by preventing further progression of osteochondral spurs. Frequently, the patient will awaken from anesthesia without the radicular pain that was present preoperatively, and over the following days and weeks the muscle paralysis resolves. Usually, the last modality to recover is the sensory deficit. A rigid brace is worn following surgery for six to eight weeks or until the bone graft is healed radiographically.

The patient with a herniated cervical disc producing myelopathy and long tract signs has a more serious and potentially disabling problem. Cervical myelopathy is frequently associated with radiculopathy, so that the patient may have ataxia and hyperreflexia as well as weakness or atrophy of the upper extremities. Extreme caution is necessary in order not to extend the cervical spine in a cervical orthosis or traction devices when treating a patient with recognized myelopathy. Often these individuals have a very narrow cervical spinal canal, plus spondylosis with spur formation at the posterior vertebral body margin. Extension of the neck may produce increased pain and neurological deficit. Again, rigid immobilization of the cervical spine is a most important early treatment. Historically, cervical myelopathy has been treated by conservative means. But it is my belief that the spinal cord is in jeopardy and even in the presence of neurological improvement, operative intervention is usually necessary to prevent ultimate progression of the disease or spinal cord damage from minor trauma, such as a fall in this ataxic person. Once again, the safest means of treating the herniated cervical disc associated with myelopathy is by anterior cervical discectomy and fusion, preferably by the Robinson technique.[2]

As always, when contemplating surgery, a cervical myelogram is made to determine which level or levels of the cervical spine need attention. The prospects for patients with cervical myelopathy, even if severe, are very good as far as neurological recovery is concerned unless the patient has had severe paralysis with bladder and posterior column (position and vibratory sense) dysfunction for a long period of time. Historically, laminectomy carries a significant risk of further neural damage (greater than 20 percent) as well as deterioration years after surgery. Anterior cervical discectomy and fusion remove the offending disc, stabilize the pathological segment, and prevent further progression of chondro-osseous spur formation and spinal cord irritation. Postoperative immobilization in a rigid cervical orthosis is mandatory until the bone graft is healed.

PAIN FROM CENTRAL OR INTRINSIC CORD PRESSURE

Uncommonly, a patient may present with neck pain as a chief complaint and the underlying pathology is a central cervical cord cavitation or syringomyelia. This central cyst affects the fibers of the lateral spinothalamic tract where they cross over in the central part of the cord. The patient loses the sensations of pain and temperature in dermatomes on both sides of the body. The pyramidal tract and anterior horn cells are affected, causing motor paralysis in the legs and arms. This lesion is not to be treated by physical therapy and usually requires operative drainage by a posterior cervical approach or laminectomy. The central cord signs may be spontaneous in origin, or rarely occur after spinal cord injury, but both are present with neck pain and progressive neurological loss.

Tumors of the spinal cord may be extramedullary (external) or intramedullary (internal) and produce pain as the first symptom. Pain may be distributed over specific root dermatomes or more centrally in the torso and legs. Documentation of a neurological deficit with motor paralysis and sensory loss, usually dissociated, on the opposite side of the body confirms the tentative diagnosis. Pain in this situation may occur at night, is frequently constant, and is unrelieved by lying down or immobilization. A cervical myelogram or computerized axial tomography scan is indicated if a tumor is suspected.

PAIN FROM DEGENERATIVE DISC AND JOINT DISEASE

The origin and pathophysiology of degenerative disc disease are not totally understood but may be related to previous trauma, congenital anomalies, and the aging process.[1,3,6] The cervical spine is quite mobile and subjected to more stress than the more rigid thoracic spine. With aging the disc loses its water content and becomes friable; the disc space narrows, producing abnormal motion at that particular segment. It is likely that the combination of abnormal mechanics and disc degeneration causes chondro-osseous spur formation at the margins of the vertebra and zygoapophyseal joints, leading to the clinical and radiological picture of osteoarthrosis of the spine. The joints of the cervical spine are not really different than any other peripheral joints that can become inflamed and result in a syndrome in which pain is radiated to more distal sites of the extremity. The evidence of degenerative disc disease is high in the general population, occurring in 40 percent of adults by the fourth decade and in 70 percent of adults by the sixth decade.[7] Therefore neck pain with distal radiation is quite common and can occur without signs of neural compression. However, the peak incidence of discomfort seems to be between 40 and 49 years of age.[11,13]

The etiology of pain in degenerative cervical disc and joint disease is more obscure than with obvious neural compression syndromes. However, certain factors can be identified that are related to the production of the pain. Anatomically, the facet joint capsules, the outer layers of the annulus fibrosis, and the anterior and posterior longitudinal ligaments have all been shown to be innervated by γ- or C-nerve fibers with simple terminations in these structures.[4,5,8] Also, bone itself has innervations that travel with the vascular supply. Therefore it can be postulated that with abnormal motion or distortion of such soft tissue as the annulus, longitudinal ligaments, and joint capsules, stimulation of the C-nerve fibers occurs and a pain syndrome is created. This pain, although it may be referred to other sites, is not in the radicular pattern of pain from nerve root compression.

The diagnosis of the etiology of neck pain without neural compression becomes more difficult. A complete physical examination is essential. It may reveal limited cervical spine motion, especially extension, if osteoarthrosis is present, and pain on palpation of the posterior cervical spine may identify which segment is pathological. Pain from degenerative disc disease may radiate to the occiput, shoulder, inner scapular area, and arm. Generally, the higher level of cervical spine pathology causes pain radiation into the upper scapular area, whereas lower cervical disc disease is likelier to cause pain radiation more distally into the arm or lower scapular area. The patient may complain of subjective paresthesia without an absolute radicular pattern. Frequently, the patient will volunteer that lying down or immobilization of the head and neck relieves the pain, which is a diagnostic clue to methods of treatment.

Before 1954, the treatment of symptomatic degenerative disc disease was totally conservative. However, in 1955 Robinson and Smith published the first report of successful treatment of this entity by anterior discectomy and fusion, the purpose of which was to remove the offending disc and stabilize the abnormal motion segment. This operation has been universally successful in selected patients who are first unrelieved with conservative treatment.[9,10,12]

Initially nonoperative measures are similar to those described for treatment of the herniated cervical disc. Immobilization with a cervical orthosis is important during daytime activities. Anti-inflammatory agents and mild pain medication are taken. Cervical traction is useful but not as successful as in the acutely herniated soft disc. Traction may be utilized to relieve painful muscle spasm, but it is of doubtful value in distracting the disc affected by osteoarthrosis. Heat may be very helpful. Moist packs or radiant heat with an infrared lamp can be applied.

Immobilization and physical therapy will not arrest the basic process of disc degeneration and chondro-osseous spur formation, but for most patients it may stop the pain syndrome. If, however, the pain becomes chronic and disabling, that is, if the patient is unable to resume normal activities, and the pathological cervical level can be identified, then an anterior cervical discectomy with fusion will usually relieve the pain. A cervical myelogram is always made before operation to identify pathological levels. The ideal situation is the patient with a single level of disc disease, since statistics show that the greater the number of levels fused, the poorer the results will be (Figs. 31-4A–G).

Another major indication for operative intervention is cervical spondylosis with myelopathy. Ordinarily, the spondylitic patient who develops signs of cord compression has a pre-existing, congenitally narrow canal that becomes further compromised by the ingrowth of chondro-osseous spurs. Although this patient needs immediate immobilization and rest of the cervical spine, the response of improvement in neurological function may be only temporary. Traction is not indicated in these patients and may actually be dangerous if hyperextension of the spine occurs to produce further spinal canal compromise. Cervical spondylosis with myelopathy usually presents with gait difficulties and is most frequently not painful. If surgery is indicated, only then is a cervical myelogram performed. All levels causing spinal cord compression require anterior discectomy and fusion, which may be as many as three or four. The results of the Robinson technique of anterior fusion in this entity are excellent.[14] No attempt is made to remove posterior osteophytes because of the threat of iatrogenic spinal cord injury. Once fusion is complete at the affected osteoarthritic levels, the previously formed reactive spurs will be absorbed by the normal process of bone remodeling, since motion is alleviated at these levels. In addition, the spinal cord irritation is relieved once the segment is stabilized with the bone graft.

Following surgery and healing of the bone grafts, physical therapy is essential to patients with myelopathy. They need gait training and muscle strengthening. Occasionally they will experience loss of position sense and not be aware of where their feet are being placed during ambulation. This condition necessitates the use of temporary walking aids, such as a parallel bar, a cane, or a walker. In most cases functional recovery can be expected.

One of the more difficult problems facing the physician and therapist is the patient with neck pain secondary to disc disruption, but without disc protrusion. This patient usually has a history of trauma (a flexion-extension injury), develops neck, inner scapular, and shoulder pain, subjective paresthesias, and shows no positive neurological findings on examination. In addition, the roentgenograms fail to reveal any evidence of spondylosis or a level that would show the cause of the problem. Pathologically, cervical spine injuries may cause disruption of a disc not visible to routine roentgenograms, and although the patient may be treated with all

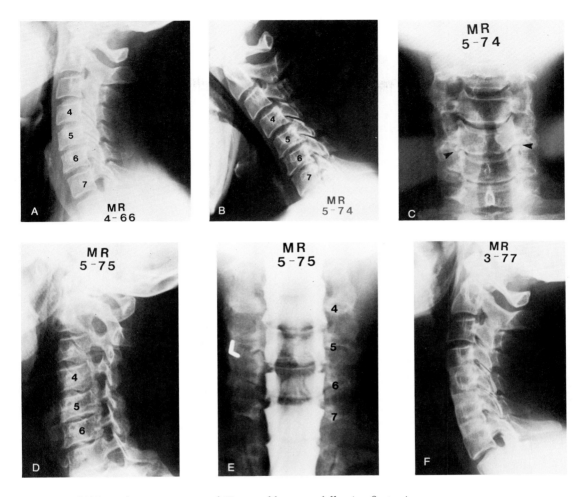

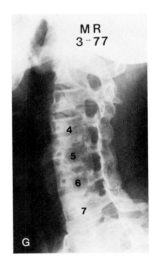

Fig. 31-4. (A) Lateral roentgenogram of 40-year-old woman following first episode of cervical and arm pains in 1966. Physical therapy and soft collar immobilization relieved the patient's pain. There is only minimal narrowing of the C5–C6 disc, indicating early disc degeneration, and very little chondro-osseous spur formation. (B) Eight years later, the patient had repeat roentgenogram taken because of another bout of severe neck and arm pains and bilateral paresthesias of the forearms, thumb, and index fingers. Physical examination revealed limitation of extension of the cervical spine (30 degrees) with pain. However, there was no neurological deficit. Physical therapy and collar immobilization failed to relieve the patient's symptoms. Note the lateral view of the cervical spine, which indicates progression of the cervical spondylosis with narrowing of the discs and chondro-osseous spur formation at the C4–C5, C5–C6, and C6–C7 levels. (C) Anteroposterior roentgenogram of the cervical spine in 1974 reveals the large spurs laterally at the joints of Luschka between the C4–C5, C5–C6, and C6–C7 vertebrae. (D) Oblique view of the cervical spine demonstrates moderately sized spurs protruding into the foraminae at C4–C5, C5–C6, and C6–C7 levels. (E) Anteroposterior view of the cervical myelogram illustrates predominately central defects at the C4–C5, C5–C6, and C6–C7 levels. (F) Anterior discectomy and fusion by the Robinson technique were carried out at the C4–C5, C5–C6, and C6–C7 levels without any attempt to remove osteophytes. Two years after surgery, the patient's pain and symptoms have been relieved and the osteophytes have resorbed by the process of normal bone remodeling. (G) Oblique view demonstrating enlargement of the foraminae at the C4–C5, C5–C6, and C6–C7 vertebrae following spontaneous resorption of the chondro-osseous spurs.

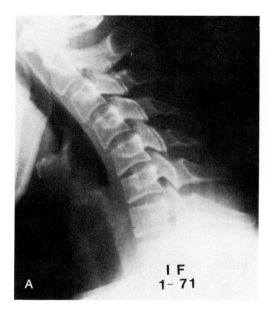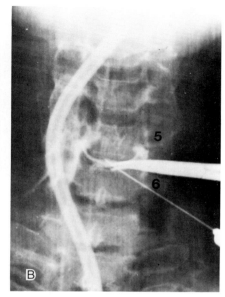

Fig. 31-5. (A) Lateral cervical roentgenogram of a 35-year-old woman who had injured her neck skiing in 1965, six years before. Neck pain and right shoulder and inner scapular pain persisted until 1971. The physical examination demonstrated subjective paresthesias of the right forearm and hand, but not weakness or sensory loss. The flexion roentgenogram did not identify any apparent abnormality of the cervical spine. (B) Operative discograms were carried out, revealing cervical disc disruption of the C5–C6 level. Note how the dye outlines a cleft in the disc as well as extravasating out along the nerve root sleeves. The Robinson technique of anterior cervical discectomy and fusion immediately and permanently relieved the patient's pain and paresthesias.

forms of nonoperative therapy, the pain will not resolve.[1] If after one or two years the pain is still disabling, special radiological studies may be indicated, including dynamic flexion and extension views and operative discography.[4] Disc disruption and rents in the annulus may be identified in this situation by instilling saline and contrast material into the central portion of the disc. If the discogram is positive, greater than 3 mm of dye will be accepted and outline a horizontal cleft in the disc. The dye will then be discharged through the posterolateral rent in the annulus along the nerve root sleeves. Excision of the offending disc and fusion in this situation will relieve the pain (Figs. 31-5A, B).

PAIN AS A RESULT OF ABNORMAL MOTION OR INSTABILITY

Abnormal motion of the cervical spine may be the result of trauma, rheumatoid arthritis, or osteoarthritis.[2] Instability between the second and seventh cervical levels as defined by White and Panjabi[15] is subluxation greater than 3.5 mm anteriorly or translatory displacement of the vertebral bodies as well as an angula-

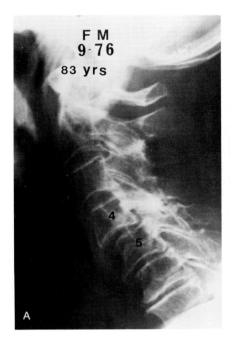 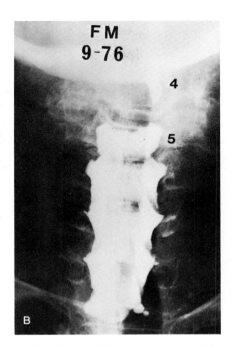

Fig. 31-6. (A) This lateral roentgenogram was taken of an 83-year-old man presenting with neck pain, shoulder pain, bilateral deltoid weakness, and myelopathy manifested by difficulty walking and hyperreflexia. There was no history of preceding trauma. There is marked cervical spondylosis with spontaneous anterior subluxation of the fourth and the fifth cervical vertebrae. (B) Anteroposterior view of the cervical myelogram revealed almost complete block of the dye column at the C4–C5 level, a sign of severe compromise of the spinal canal and cervical cord compression. Anterior discectomy and fusion at the C4–C5 level was performed without reduction of the subluxation. Five months following operation, the patient's symptoms were relieved, and the spine was stabilized.

tion between two vertebrae of greater than 11 degrees compared to either adjacent interspace. The findings indicate ligamentous laxity of a pathological extent. Trauma tears the ligament complex and rheumatoid arthritis causes general ligament laxity. The osteoarthritis results in zygoapophyseal joint erosion with facet capsular laxity, but it can also produce compensatory subluxation above very stiff lower cervical segments (Figs. 31-6A, B). Atlantoaxial dislocations may produce neck and occipital pains (Fig. 31-7). Regardless of the etiology of ligament instability, abnormal motion may result in neural compression pain or deep somatic pain. Even the dura and nerve root sheaths have deep somatic innervation and compression of these structures prior to the onset of paralysis may produce a referred pain of somatic nature.[13]

When roentgenographic examination demonstrates instability of the cervical spine in conjunction with neck pain or radicular pain, immobilization by external means is necessary. Usually a rigid orthosis should be used. Gross instability following traumatic subluxation or dislocation may require halo cast or brace fixation, especially when it is associated with an incomplete neurological deficit. Chronic pain syndromes resulting from spinal instability will only temporarily be

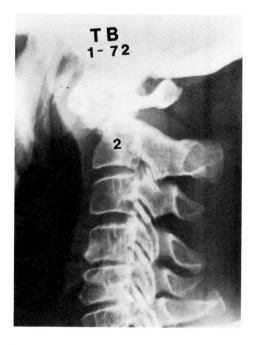

Fig. 31-7. This lateral roentgenogram was taken of a 56-year-old man with known rheumatoid arthritis who was struck on the back of the head by a wing of a plane following his giving flight instructions to another pilot. He developed severe neck and occipital pains with myelopathy. He has atlantoaxial dislocation with marked forward shift of the posterior arch of the atlas toward the odontoid process. Stabilization by posterior atlantoaxial arthrodesis was performed to relieve his symptoms.

improved by external immobilization. Therefore they usually require internal fixation with an anterior or posterior arthrodesis (Fig. 31-8). If most of the laxity is in the posterior ligament complex, then posterior fusion is indicated. But if the laxity is associated with disc disruption and anterior compression of the nerve roots or spinal cord, then anterior decompression and fusion should be performed. Even when levels 2 and 3 of the lower cervical spine are fused, there is very little loss of functional neck motion, since approximately 45 percent of motion occurs at the upper levels of the cervical spine and occiput. Once union of the arthrodesis

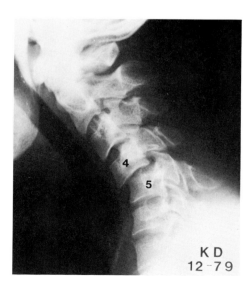

Fig. 31-8. This lateral roentgenogram was taken of a 30-year-old man following a vehicular injury. After rigid immobilization, neck and shoulder pain persisted for three months. No sensory loss or weakness was demonstrable on examination. The posterior ligament complex did not heal enough to prevent chronic subluxation, which is associated with disc disruption and pain. Posterior arthrodesis was performed with wire fixation and iliac grafting from the fourth to fifth cervical levels, and it relieved the patient's symptoms.

has occurred, usually at three months, a vigorous exercise program is carried out to regain motion without pain. Most patients can return to fairly normal activities after arthrodesis of the spine.

SUMMARY

Rehabilitation of the patient with neck pain should be directed at the basic pathological process or cause of the pain. Not all neck, shoulder, and arm pains stem from neural compression. Osteoarthritis, rheumatoid arthritis, abnormal cervical motion, and intrinsic spinal canal problems may all produce neck pain as a result of stimulation of the C-fiber system, which is perceived as pain in more distal structures, such as the shoulder, interscapular region, and arm.

Nonoperative treatment of neck pain is directed toward the basic problem. Immobilization by external support prevents irritation of deep somatic nerve endings and compressed neural structures. Cervical traction in the neutral position is appropriate for the younger patient with a soft herniated disc, but not for the older spondylitic patient. Application of heat to the musculature of the cervical region is beneficial in relieving muscle spasm and the symptoms of arthrosis of the spine. No indication exists for manipulation of the cervical spine in the treatment of painful neck disorders.

Anti-inflammatory agents may be prescribed in cases of arthrosis of joints or of inflammation of the nerve roots secondary to compression by herniated discs. Narcotics and tranquilizers for painful cervical spine disorders should be used with caution and for short periods of time.

When nonoperative treatment fails to relieve cervical pain and the basic pathological process has been delineated, operative decompression and fusion by the anterior approach may be most beneficial in obliterating the syndrome. Occasionally, posterior fusion is indicated. Once the arthrodesis has healed and the cervical spine is stable, the rehabilitation process may be completed to return the patient to useful activities.

REFERENCES

1. Bohlman, H. H.: Pathology and current treatment concepts of cervical spine injuries. In *Instructional Course Lectures*, vol. 21, pp. 108–115. American Academy of Orthopaedic Surgeons. C. V. Mosby, St. Louis, 1972.
2. Bohlman, H. H.: Cervical spondylosis with moderate to severe myelopathy. A report of seventeen cases treated by Robinson anterior cervical discectomy and fusion. Spine 2:151–162, 1977.
3. Bohlman, H. H.: The neck. In D'Ambrosia, R. D., Ed.: *Musculoskeletal Disorders, Regional Examination, and Differential Diagnosis,* pp. 178–224. J. B. Lippincott, Philadelphia, 1977.
4. Cloward, R. B.: Cervical discography. Ann. Surg. 150:1052–1053, 1959.
5. Cloward, R. B.: The clinical significance of the sinu-vertebral nerve of the cervical spine in relation to the cervical disk syndrome. J. Neurol. Neurosurg. Psychiatry 23:321–326, 1960.
6. Compere, E. L.: Origin, anatomy, physiology and pathology of the intervertebral disc. In *Instructional Course Lectures,* vol. 18, pp. 15–20. American Academy of Orthopaedic Surgeons. C. V. Mosby, St. Louis, 1961.

7. Kellgren, J. H., and Lawrence, J. S.: Osteoarthritis and disk degeneration in an urban population. Ann. Rheum. Dis. 17:388–397, 1958.

8. Mulligan, J. H.: The innervation of the ligaments attached to the bodies of the vertebrae. J. Anat. 91:455–465, 1957.

9. Riley, L. H.: Cervical disc surgery: Its role and indications. Orthop. Clin. North Am. 2:443–452, 1971.

10. Riley, L. H., Robinson, R. A., Johnson, K. A., and Walker, A. E.: The results of anterior interbody fusion of the cervical spine: Review of 93 consecutive cases. J. Neurosurg. 30:127–133, 1969.

11. Robinson, R. A.: The problem of neck pain. J. Med. Assoc. State Ala. 33:1–14, 1963.

12. Robinson, R. A.: Cervical spine. In Milch, R. A., Ed.: *Surgery of Arthritis,* pp. 24–47. Williams & Wilkins, Baltimore, 1964.

13. Robinson, R. A.: Anterior cervical fusion in cervical spine degenerative disease. In Gurdjian, E. S., and Thomas, L. M., Eds.: *Neckache and Backache,* pp. 176–198. Charles C Thomas, Springfield, Ill., 1970.

14. Robinson, R. A., and Smith, G. W.: Anterolateral cervical disc removal and interbody fusion for cervical disc syndrome. Bull. Johns Hopkins Hosp. 96:223–224, 1955.

15. White, H. A., and Panjabi, M. M.: *Clinical Biomechanics of the Spine.* J. B. Lippincott, Philadelphia, 1978.

32

Low Back Disability

Vert Mooney, M.D.

THE PROBLEM

Back pain is an extremely common human phenomenon; perhaps 80 percent of all persons in modern industrial society will experience back pain at some time during their active life.[20] Fortunately, most of the time the problem is self-limiting in that overall recovery of 70 percent within a month can be expected, and within two or three months, perhaps 90 percent of individuals will be free of pain.[14] Unfortunately, recurrences are frequent, and three or more episodes of back disability can occur in up to 70 percent of afflicted patients.[15]

For the employed population, back pain constitutes a particularly significant disability. Those individuals who have back pain for longer than six months to such a degree that they are incapacitated from work have only a 50 percent chance of ever returning to work.[18] Back-pain patients who have experienced more than six months' incapacity to work are roughly in the same numbers as those having heart trouble as a source of unemployability.[8] Various investigators have tried to evaluate the impact of this common disability. In one study of English workers, back pain was found to be the source of 70 weeks' annual absence for 100 men employed.[1] One percent of all work days lost is believed to be due to back pain.[11]

Despite the appreciable economic and human impact evidenced by these statistics, the medical world is still not clear about the specific etiology of most back pain. A herniated disc is thought to account for relatively few back complaints.[12] The rather specific causes, such as tumors, fractures, osteoporosis, intra-abdominal or intrapelvic disease, and metabolic bone disease, account for a very small percentage of the overall numbers of backache sufferers who appear in the physician's office.

In an effort to separate that which we know from that which we do not know, we at the Southwestern Medical School Spinal Pain Center have developed a working diagram for diagnoses, as shown in Table 32-1. These diagnoses are established on clinical (via a history and a physical examination) and radiographic grounds. As will be noted, the first two diagnoses merely separate pain complaints that are essentially mechanical, category 2, from those that involve nerve root irritation, category 1. The great majority, of course, fall into category 2, which may be identified as segmental instability. The third category is in a class by itself in that the degree to which persistent complaints are based on intraspinal scarring rather than pre-existent and recurrent disease cannot be clearly assessed by the clinician. The fourth category becomes self-evident with x-rays. The fifth category implies the specific phenomenon known as pseudoclaudication. The diagnosis is based largely on a history of symptoms due to a narrowing of the caliber of the spinal canal. A myelogram is required to establish the diagnosis. Categories 6 and 7 are extremely vague and, after category 2, they are the most commonly identified. Soft tissue strain implies an acute onset coupled with some sort of trauma, and thus some mechanical cause is responsible for the process. The condition is assumed to underlie any chronic back pain problem without

Table 32-1. Categories of Clinical Syndromes for Diagnosing Back Pain*

1. _____Nerve Root Involvement = Leg/Arm Sign/Symptoms	
_____Sensory loss	_____Sitting straight-leg raising
_____Motor loss	_____Reflexes ↓
_____LeSeague	_____↑ Leg pain with walking
_____Cross LeSeague	_____Valsalva leg pain
2° to Disc_____ Skeletal_____ Both_____ Other_____	
2. _____Degenerate/Post-Injury Segment(s) = Back/Neck Pain	
_____Instability symptoms	_____Postural relief
_____Muscle tenderness/spasm	_____Episodic
_____Range restriction	_____Traumatic event
3. _____Post-Surgery Syndrome = History_____	
_____Nerve root signs	_____Root symptoms
_____Instability symptoms	_____Bizarre pain pattern
4. _____Fracture_____	
5. _____Spinal canal stenosis_____	
6. _____Soft tissue strain_____	
7. _____Deconditioned_____	
8. _____Congenital/developmental skeletal_____	
9. _____Metabolic arthritis_____	
10. _____Metabolic bone_____	
11. _____Malignancy_____	
12. _____Other_____	

* Courtesy of the Southwestern Medical School Spinal Pain Center.

significant or believable findings. The other diagnostic categories are relatively rare and specific laboratory tests are required to establish them.

In contrast with cardiac problems, one of the more unfortunate characteristics of chronic back disability is the lack of a definitive test to establish the diagnosis. There is no electrocardiogram for chronic back pain and even radiographic findings are of extremely questionable significance. Certainly skeletal variations at the lumbosacral junction, mild scoliosis, spondylolysis, and moderate degenerative changes do not correlate with incidence of back disability in pre-employment radiographic assessments.[16] Clinicians are aware that incidential findings of major degenerative lumbar disease may occur in individuals with no back complaints at all. Indeed, when tested, 25 percent of adults who have no back complaints at all will have an abnormal myelogram.[13] Other specific diagnostic tools, such as diskography, must separate a naturally occuring degenerative phenomenon from what appears to be the same type of degenerating phenomenon in another individual who is symptomatic.

Although physicians once thought that most chronic back disability came primarily from the degenerating disc, experience has shown that other innervated structures appreciatively contribute to pain as well. The use of the radiographically controlled facet injection[19] has confirmed that the facet joints themselves are major contributors to chronic back pain. In fact, relief for varying periods of time can be achieved by injecting anesthetic and steroid agents into the lumbar facets. Unfortunately, radiographic findings infrequently offer clues to the symptomatic source of pain complaints in the facet joints. Moreover, the location of pain complaints are not specific to the skeletal-segmental level. Pain referred to the buttock and down the leg can occur in exactly the same location from noxious stimuli emanating at any of the lower three lumbar segments.[19]

Thus, not only is it the commonness of this disability, but the lack of specific objective findings that make treatment a confusing matter. Because of the reigning uncertainty, a wide variety of treatments may be advocated and "confirmed" as being effective. For example, in a study in Busselton, Australia, in 1975, surgical care and spinal manipulation were both found to be 79 percent effective in relieving chronic back disability.[10] In this study, in which an orthopedic consultant polled the entire working community, about 40 percent of the adult population indicated that they had experienced back problems within the past three years. Only 1.6 percent of the total number of back pain sufferers had undergone operations for their back problems, the same success record as was observed for manipulation. Traction helped only 41 percent of the cases, exercises helped 55 percent, and medication, about 75 percent. This study revealed that medical practice has not established any clearly effective format for treating this ubiquitous and essentially incurable disease process.

THE COST

The problem of back rehabilitation would not be of as great an importance if it were not for the cost. It is a disease process that tends to affect individuals in their most productive years. Although it is by no means life-threatening, back pain can effectively remove sufferers from the work force and, thus, place additional demands upon society. One of the most thorough analyses of the cost problem was made by Leavitt et al.[17] In their study, 100 consecutive low-back pain cases leading to disability claims were reviewed. These cases constituted 22 percent of all disability claims received by the insurance carrier in the period being examined.

The study was undertaken to identify what cases might be expected to be most costly, and the results were as follows: 75 percent of the individuals with workmen's compensation claims went back to work without incurring significant costs, 25 percent accounted for nearly all the costs incurred, and 20 percent claimed persistent disability three years following the onset of the condition.

From this study, certain variables were found not to be predictors of a return to work. These included the physician's prognosis for return to work, date of injury to date of notification, employment history, and accident or injury codes. Factors that were predictive for a costly settlement were an extended time lag between date of injury and the first referral to a second physician, the time lag between the date of injury and the last day worked, hospitalization, and mention of surgery. And of course, the initiation of litigation was consistently predictive of costly settlement. The initial diagnosis of pathology could not separate those who were going to be most costly to the insurance company from those who would return to work. However, in the costly cases, the majority showed, in retrospect, inconsistency of the objective findings, changes in pain patterns, and inconsistent relationship of pain to physical activity. Psychological impairment was commonly documented. The most consistent medical findings in the costly group were delay in specific medical care and delay in hospitalization if required. This group accounted for 87 percent of the insurance dollar paid. Less than 50 percent of all costs to the insurance company went toward medical treatment or support during the treatment. Thus, it was the recommendation of Leavitt et al. that more intensive early medical care be instituted and that the insurance carriers attempt to monitor the effectiveness of care more closely in an effort to reduce costs. In a study of medical costs across the nation, Pheasant[21] demonstrated that hospital-related costs for backache in 1974 came to about $1.4 billion, about 1.5 percent of the entire health care dollar for that year. Of the 28 percent of those hospitalized for back pain and treated by surgery, the operation accounted for 60 percent of the total hospitalization costs.[21]

Although the implication of such statistics is that surgical care is both costly and without guarantee of success, other factors must be considered. From a study of 116 patients operated on for lumbar disc disease, Surin[25] analyzed the number of days patients took for sick leave for 10 years before surgery and compared these records to those for 10 years after surgery. From the beginning of the observation period, a steadily increasing incidence of number of days on sick leave was documented. The event of surgery seemed to have little more than a transitory effect on reducing the incidence of days off because of back disability. The one factor that seemed to correlate with shorter postoperative disability and decreased postoperative sick leave was a short interval from onset of complaint to surgical care.[25] This study, along with others,[9,23] indicates that a protracted delay between complaint and an operation correlates with less favorable results. Here again, the implication is that significant positive findings in the form of signs and symptoms should be rapidly followed by an operation say, within six months. In

Surin's study,[25] those patients who did less well had certain traits common in their preoperative history. They were more often sick in general, more often on sick leave for low-back troubles, and were usually doing heavy work. Finally, their signs and symptoms of sciatica were not usually severe and consequently surgery was delayed.

Thus, delay in diagnosis and treatment correlates with greater expense and less favorable results. Yet specific diagnoses are extremely difficult to achieve without significant signs and symptoms. The underlying theme of this whole discussion, however, reinforces the view that in that small minority of patients who will continue with chronic pain disability, very vigorous diagnostic and treatment programs must be undertaken.

THE WORK-UP

It is usual to separate acute from chronic disability. It is also useful to establish a work-up format allowing comparisons of one patient to another. For this purpose, pain drawings, patient questionnaires, and specific physical check-off sheets are useful.

The patient's pain drawing, shown as Figure 32-1, is extremely useful in evaluating complaints and assessing the progress of treatment. In our own unit, the patient fills out an orange form when first seen, and at the follow-up visits, fills out the same type of pain drawing, only on a different-colored page, which

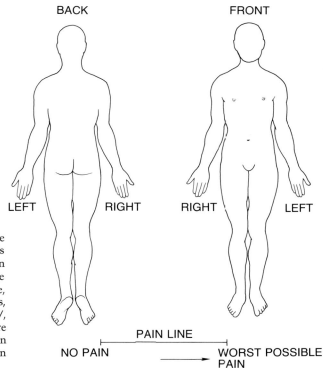

Fig. 32-1. A blank for a pain drawing. The patient is instructed to show where his pain is on the body and mark how strong the pain in on the line below the bodies. Pain is marked on the body according to the following key: ache, ∧∧∧∧, burning, = = = = = = =, numbness, 0000, pins and needles, ..., stabbing, //////, other, XXXXX. Patient is also asked to compare arm pain to neck pain and to compare leg pain to back pain. (Courtesy of the Southwestern Medical School Spinal Pain Center.)

Table 32-2. History Form for Patients with Chronic Back Pain*

DATE:_____

Name_____ Age_____

Present job_____ How long_____ Last job_____

1. What date (roughly at least) did your present pain start?_____
2. How long have you had any problems with back, neck, legs or arms_____(circle affected part or parts)
3. How long have you been unable to work or do normal housework?_____
4. Did your pain start gradually_____suddenly_____injury_____where_____
5. Do you get short of breath or a tight feeling in your chest with your back or neck pain?_____
6. Do you notice your pain after you exercise or exert yourself?_____
7. Does your pain ever radiate down your left arm or elsewhere?_____ Please describe_____
8. If sudden onset, please describe what happened_____

9. My pain is: check the appropriate box.	Better	Worse	No different
With cough or sneeze	___	___	___
Sitting in straight chair	___	___	___
Sitting in soft easy chair	___	___	___
Bending forward to brush teeth	___	___	___
When I wake in the morning	___	___	___
Middle of night	___	___	___
Mid-day	___	___	___
Lying flat on back	___	___	___
Lying flat on stomach	___	___	___
On side with knees bent	___	___	___
Riding in a car	___	___	___
When looking up	___	___	___
When I am tense	___	___	___

	Yes	No
10. My back sometimes gets stuck when I bend forward.	___	___
After walking, bending forward relieves my pain.	___	___
My back feels like giving way when I bend forward.	___	___
My pain stops me when I walk a certain distance.	___	___
I have trouble with urine and bowel control.	___	___
11. Have you been in a hospital for back, leg, neck or arm pain?	___	___

Number of times_____ Give dates_____
12. Have you had myelograms (x-rays of spine with dye injection)? Number of times_____
13. Have you had neck or back surgery? Number of times_____ Please give type and dates_____
14. Have you been in the hospital with other medical problems? Number of times_____ Describe_____

* Courtesy of the Southwestern Medical School Spinal Pain Center.

Table 32-2. History Form for Patients with Chronic Back Pain (*continued*)

15. What treatments have made your pain better?
    What treatments have made your pain worse?
16. What brought you to this office?
17. Do you have an attorney helping you?
18. Do other members of your family have significant back or neck
    trouble?_____(relationship) Who?
19. Do you have to change jobs?_____To what?_____
20. Are you under any pressure at home? _____ at work? _____
    mild _____ moderate _____ severe _____
21. What is the most aggravating thing about your pain?
22. What was the date of your last physical examination and name of doctor who
    did it?
    Pelvic done?   Rectal done?

PHYSICAL EXAMINATION:

    Lumbar spine: No   Yes

	No	Yes	
Scoliosis:	( )	( )	Mark with S's on drawing
Muscle spasm:	( )	( )	
Ecchymosis:	( )	( )	Mark with E's on drawing
Point of tenderness:	( )	( )	Mark with T's on drawing

        Range of motion: Flexion_____°'s
                              Right bending_____°'s
                              Left bending_____°'s
                              Extension_____°'s

    Neurological examination:

Straight-leg raising:		Right_____	Left_____
Deep tendon reflexes:	K.J.	Right_____	Left_____
Normal (√)	A.J.	Right_____	Left_____
Depressed (↓)	Ant. Tib.	Right_____	Left_____
Absent (⁰)	E.H.L.	Right_____	Left_____
Increased (↑)	F.H.L.	Right_____	Left_____

    X-rays: Normal_____
            Fracture_____Skeletal variation_____Degenerative changes_____
            Location_____

Diagnosis category # _____(Other diagnosis)_____
DICTATED _____ A.M. ( )   P.M. ( ) DATE_____
                      SIGNATURE: _____

MAILED DATE: _____
INITIAL: _____

becomes a permanent part of the file. The main purpose of these drawings is to establish a clear-cut understanding among patient, physician, and physical therapist as to the nature of complaints. Explaining the pain in words is often difficult to do in a specific or instructive manner, yet patients can be surprisingly discrete and concrete in identifying their pain complaints if they can point them out on a structural and physical basis. These localizations of pain are consistent and reliable in assessing a patient's progress. Moreover, especially in chronic cases for whom various behavioral aspects are interwoven with the structural causes of pain, this aspect of the subjective disability can be well demonstrated by the sometimes bizarrely sketched pain drawings. These bizarre pain drawings do correlate with abnormal psychological testing and thus give some insight into personality traits.[22] Although the patient's history for acute onset can be relatively short and descriptive, a chronic pain complaint on initial evaluation requires a much more specific work-up. We use a questionnaire form, reproduced as Table 32-2, to have patients identify, in concrete terms, the most important aspects of their current and past history. Specifically, the various postures that affect their pain are significant if the pain complaint is structural. For instance, it is unlikely that somebody with a degenerative disc, herniated disc, or facet arthropathy could tolerate lying prone. Most often, lying on the side with the knees bent is a position of relief. Review of these questions at follow-up time often offers an opportunity to evaluate the consistency of a patient's complaints. As will be recalled from Leavitt et al.'s study, the aspect of patient work-up correlating most significantly with prolonged and unsuccessfully treated back disability was inconsistency of complaints.

Finally, a specific statement of physical findings is important. The sensory examination on this form is quite limited. The drawing itself often reflects abnormalities in sensory examination and can be confirmed by the physical examination. For the patient with specific deficits of neurological function, additional commentary can be made. Various examinations, such as cross-legged referral of pain and Cram's test (acute buttock pain resulting from lateral popliteal pressure in the flexed knee of an individual with positive, straight-leg raising)[5] are rare but considered pathognomonic for nerve root involvement. In a busy practice or clinic, the initial work-up, including the history and physical examination, can be administered by an allied health professional. A more demanding physical examination, according to the experience and training of the physician, can be made in light of these preliminary findings.

At follow-up, variations can be identified when compared to the concrete findings on the questionnaire, the patient's pain drawing, and the physical examination sheet. This procedure avoids excessive verbalization in patient charts and is, in general, far more accurate in evaluating progress.

Despite any attempts to provide a solid data base for initial evaluation and prognosis, in most instances the physician is usually left with a vague diagnosis that in a medical-legal sense can best be identified as a lumbar syndrome. In this situation, no prognosis or treatment is suggested by the examiner. Unhappily, this escape from a decision frequently allows the clinician to avoid forcing upon himself some conceptual framework of pathology to which he can apply a rational treatment plan. Thus, for his own record, it is useful to have some sort of diagnostic category, each with an implication for a treatment plan.

TREATMENT FOR ACUTE BACK DISABILITY

The discussion so far suggests that a vigorous treatment plan is wasted on most patients because within three months, more than 80 percent of them have resolved their problem spontaneously. Nonetheless, some effective form of therapy should be prescribed that is honest with the medical facts as we understand them today and that is as economical as possible. For most sufferers of low-back pain without overwhelming complaints, the "back school" approach is most useful.

By "back school" we mean a kind of patient education. The concept of back school was initiated in 1970 by the Swedish therapist Mary Ann Zachrisson-Forssell. Since then it has been tried with considerable variation in America and Europe. The instruction begins with description of pertinent anatomy in terms understandable by even the less well-educated. Various audiovisual aids, of course, are useful. The initial discussion leads into a presentation of those postures and positions most beneficial to the back. Thus, straightening of lumbar lordosis is advocated and the use of the semi-Fowler resting position is presented. From the postural aspect, dynamic control of these postures is advocated. Various exercises aimed at strengthening the abdominal and gluteal muscles are presented. Usually the course is taught in groups so that exercises can be attempted. There are wide variations in opinion as to what exercises are most favored or beneficial; at present, no clear-cut advantage of one type over another seems available. Muscle strengthening, however, would seem to have a great advantage no matter what disease process was being treated. Next the patient is led into discussions about work postures and health habits, followed by a more general consideration of the disadvantages of protracted pain, from the physical and especially emotional standpoints. Various methods are used to establish some enthusiasm for healthy behavior. In general, back school is run by a physical therapist, although in various programs physicians, psychiatrists, psychologists, and other clinicians also participate. The aim of back school, however, is patient education about the disease process and, most of all, making the patients themselves responsible for returning to healthy behavior.

Although the approach may seem simplistic, it cannot be considered destructive, it certainly is not costly, and, in fact, it has been demonstrated to work as effectively, if not more so, than any other method. Bergquist-Ullman and Larsson[3] conducted an excellent prospective blind study in which this method was compared to placebos and more vigorous physical therapy using exercises and mobilization techniques (manipulations). The method was as helpful as the more vigorous physical therapy program and significantly better than the placebo (short-wave diathermy). The patients in the back-school group returned to work sooner and had fewer recurrences of disability than those in an average industrial population. This study also indicated that various vocational factors correlated with more prolonged off-time or frequency of pain complaints. Frequent bending and twisting, fixed postures, repetitive work, no need of concentration, and discontentment about work were all factors that hindered rapid resolution of pain. Although the incidence of acute back problems among office workers and manual workers was about the same as their overall percentage of employment, the manual workers returned to work more slowly and had more frequent relapses. This situation seems to support the view that, among other things, physical capacity to perform is related to success of treatment and defense against recurrences. Accordingly, the back-school method emphasizes that back disability is often part of the human condition, that everyone bears responsibilities for his own health, and one cannot place all blame at the door of other individuals, especially the employer. Back school also removes much of the mystique about back disability. Because patients are endowed with more responsibility for their care, they are more unlikely to fall prey to various "magic cures" unless their specific validity is demonstrated.

For many patients with acute, severe, disabling pain, a lecture series and training program would certainly not be satisfactory. Those who can tolerate it financially are best handled by bed rest. A recent study among military personnel has demonstrated that bed rest speeds the patients back to full duty faster than relegating them to light duty.[26] Moreover, anti-inflammatory medication did not seem to enhance the rate of return to full duty. However, it is seldom possible in modern society to rest in bed for several weeks. Other methods of pain resolution are necessary. The traditional analgesics are certainly reasonable, but prolonged narcotic intake does not comprise appropriate management. An alternative is the use of various injection maneuvers to achieve more rapid relief of symptoms and return to a physical activity program.

Here the validity of categorical diagnosis is important. If the problem is mainly considered to be segmental instability, injection of the facet joints under fluoroscopy is appropriate. These complaints tend to involve back pain without a considerable degree of sciatica. If the problem is lumbar radiculitis (category 1 with nerve root involvement), epidural injection by the caudal or lumbar route often can give sufficient temporary relief to allow the patient to mobilize and return to nearly normal activity. It must be recognized that no study has demonstrated that the injection forms of treatment are definitive and offer a potential for cure in excess of natural and spontaneous recovery rates. In fact, in a well-controlled study wherein disc hernias proved by myelogram to be associated with crisp neurological signs were treated by steroid versus saline epidural injections, the results were about the same in that approximately the same percentage of patients got well or required surgical care.[24] Nonetheless, these treatments by injection can provide relief from acute pain, avoid habituation to disability and prolonged time off from work, and allow more normal physical function.

CHRONIC BACK PAIN

It is in this aspect of care that back rehabilitation becomes an economic and clinical necessity. The chronic problem, one that has become so disabling that work activity is no longer available and that has failed to improve by the traditional therapies of surgery, medication, or bracing, requires a more comprehensive approach.

Failures in treatment confound the clinician regardless of his specialty or place in the treatment chain. The clinician-scientist is constantly faced with the problem of insufficient diagnostic work-up for crystallizing the problem properly, as well as insufficient treatment approaches for the specific diagnosis. The failed first operation on an industrial worker's back has only a 10 percent potential to be successful on the second occasion.[2] Assuming the technical achievement of the first surgery was the best possible, the patient was worked up in the usual way, and the diagnosis was secure, why was there failure to respond to treatment? The answer may involve the relationship between emotional disability and successful treatment, given the same treatment for the same signs and symptoms. In patients treated with chymopapain, those with marked deviations in their psychological test had a very poor success rate, contrasted to those with fairly standard results on psychological tests who were doing extremely well.[27] Obviously behavioral aspects of chronic pain disability take their toll on some affected individuals.

Some aspects of chronic disability are probably enhanced by medical care. For example, it is quite common to keep supplying analgesics to an individual suffering from chronic benign pain. The analgesics seldom seem to be successful, and they become progressively less so as time passes. With the discovery of endogenous, narcotic-like analgesics known as enkephalins, it is quite reasonable to expect that the production of these pain-controlling agents would be suppressed by exogenous material.[7] Delays in instituting effective therapies, prolonged, medically reinforced habituation to disability, and litigation suggesting that healthy behavior will reduce the ultimate amount of financial settlement are all factors the medical profession helps to reinforce in the prolongation of disability. When prolonged pain behavior has occurred and the objective findings have been insufficient or corrected, the only possible approach to problem resolution is one using multiple therapies.

The underlying approach to back rehabilitation is the focus on healthy behavior in increasing levels of function and performance. There are numerous ways to approach these goals, all largely based upon empirical competence and personnel available. In our own experience, three factors are critical in the comprehensive care and rehabilitation of chronically disabled patients from back pain:

1. Knowledgeable consultation and guidance are necessary from a physician astute in the disease process of degenerative back disability. Nothing can be more embarrassing than efforts to rehabilitate chronic back pain that is, in reality, metatastic cancer. Medical authority is essential to assure that the patient is being ethically and correctly treated.

2. Successful back rehabilitation also depends on the presence of a health professional comfortable with various aspects of physical training. Usually a physical therapist is involved, but a trained physician's assistant, occupational therapist, or nurse can perform this function just as well.

3. The emotional component of chronic pain must be understood and communicated to the patient. This task is best filled by a psychologist, but it may be accomplished by another individual knowledgeable and experienced in this area of human behavior. Or, several members of the rehabilitation team may approach a patient from different points of view and contribute to a successful rehabilitation process.

In a fully organized program, the patient should expect to be involved in a rehabilitation milieu lasting all day. Various group activities should be interspersed with a session on training and education. In an ideal inpatient program, patients live in a dormitory setting and take their meals together. More than a few patients are necessary to achieve the most successful group therapy. At least six seem to be required, but approximately 10 or 12 work together best. Larger groups tend to get unwieldy and lose focus. The program certainly should have various exercise projects as a major treatment. Walking and bicycle riding are included in the exercise program. If a pool is available, aquatic exercises known as swimnastics are very useful. Various other regimens, such as biofeedback, muscle relaxation tapes, electrical stimulation, group counseling sessions, vocational evaluation, and lectures on healthy behavior all can be incorporated into this type of comprehensive program. It is difficult to identify exactly what phase of the program is the most beneficial; in fact, it probably varies from one patient to another. Certainly an enthusiastic staff who sincerely believe in the effectiveness of their work is a necessary ingredient to the success of such a program.

From a comprehensive program in back rehabilitation, what results can be expected? First, what are the criteria of success? Certainly return to work is the most definite. However, given the social and economic situation of America today, this goal may not be realistic. Someone already receiving Social Security disability certainly has no motivation to return to a job that was distasteful in years past. Other improvements to note would be the reduction in medication, decreased use of health care facilities, and probably the most realistic commentary on healthy behavior—increased activity. Unfortunately, comprehensive rehabilitation facilities tend to be seen as last resorts by both the medical community and patient population. Thus, a patient's arrival at such a facility occurs many months and even years after an onset of disability. Accordingly, high levels of success are not possible. Cairns et al.[4] compared the success rate of a comprehensive inpatient facility (Rancho Los Amigos Spinal Pain Center) with an outpatient facility at Downey Community Hospital. Both centers used the classic multidisciplinary approach already described,[4] and the patients at both settings

Table 32-3. Comparative Success Rates in Rehabilitation at Inpatient and Outpatient Facilities*

	INPATIENTS, %†	OUTPATIENTS, %†
Initial decrease in pain	75	54
Decrease maintained	55	92
Initial increase in activity	80	67
Increase maintained	68	95
Decrease in medications	50	71
No more treatment	57	66
Unable to work	45	27
Ready for vocational rehabilitation	3	5
In vocational rehabilitation	11	5
Working	15	52

* From Cairns, D. P., Mooney, V., and Crane, P.: Spinal pain rehabilitation: A comparison of inpatient and outpatient treatment results and development of predictors for outcome. Presented at International Lumbar Spine Society Meeting, Göteborg, Sweden, May 1980.
† One hundred patients followed for a year.

Table 32-4. Time Off from Work as an Influence on Success of Rehabilitation for Inpatients and Outpatients*

VARIABLES INVOLVED IN RETURNING TO WORK	UNABLE DUE TO PAIN	VOCATIONAL REHABILITATION		WORKING
		Ready for	In	
Outpatients				
Age, years, p = 0.004	45.7	38.4	39.2	40.8
Problem time, months, p = 0.004	31	25.6	14.8	33.7
Time off work, months, p = 0.000	19.4	12.4	14.4	4.8
Number of operations, p = 0.007	0.7	0.4	0.4	0.3
Inpatients				
Age, years, p = 0.08	46	42	42	39
Problem time, months, p = 0.14	97.4	76	111.3	41.3
Time off work, months, p = 0.06	40.3	5	36	17.3
Number of operations, p = 0.06	1.4	0.7	1.9	0.6
MMPI—Hs, raw score, p = 0.01	24.6	22.0	27.2	21.3
MMPI—Hy, raw score, p = 0.01	32.3	31.0	36.5	28.9

* From Cairns, D. P., Mooney, V., and Crane, P.: Spinal pain rehabilitation: A comparison of inpatient and outpatient treatment results and development of predictors for outcome. Presented at International Lumbar Spine Society Meeting, Göteborg, Sweden, May 1980.

were all in their mid-40s. However, the time off from work at the inpatient facility averaged three years, whereas those in the outpatient facility averaged only 14 months. Table 32-3 summarizes the results from both the programs.

In reviewing these results, it is not surprising to find that one of the most important factors influencing the results of treatment was time. Time off from work was found to be the major consideration in predicting treatment outcome, as shown in Table 32-4. The longer a person reacts to his pain by being disabled, the more likely environmental factors in addition to tissue pathology begin to control his disability.* This view is expressed again and again by experts and experienced individuals working in the area of chronic pain control.[6] In the behavioral approach to rehabilitating disability from chronic pain, the patient's environment must somehow be controlled in order to reduce the level of disability. Correspondingly, verbal remarks about increasing pain are not necessarily associated with decreased activity. A patient may indeed return to work and increase his activity to such a point that although continued verbalizations of pain are heard, the statements no longer affect his basic functioning.

* See also Chapter 11.

SUMMARY

In order to achieve significant success caring for patients with chronic and acute back disability, it is still necessary to rely on basic principles of scientific medicine. Every effort in identifying a structural diagnosis must be undertaken. The physician must be prepared to challenge the effectiveness of various modalities of treatment and discount those that cannot demonstrate effectiveness. There is no place for witchcraft and wishful thinking in this area of care any more than there is in total hip surgery. Reliance on such modalities as ultrasound and diathermy has never been demonstrated to offer any alleviation of pain. Education, reassurance, and especially emphasis on the patient's own responsibilities are the hallmarks of excellent rehabilitation.

In this area of patient care, as in rehabilitation of other disorders, reliance on allied health professionals is the key to effective and economical treatment programs. The use of trained individuals as educators and therapists removes surgeons from a role for which they are poorly trained and usually poorly motivated to tolerate. The physician controlling the rehabilitation program must be prepared to accept differing opinions and even other frameworks of care if they can be demonstrated to be effective and without risk to the patient. Here, as in rehabilitation of other diseases, the physician must be prepared to be the coach of the team and an authority figure and be willing to take responsibility for the effectiveness of the whole program. To say that the pain problem is in the patient's head offers no help to the patient for relief or understanding. If the physician has insufficient time or background to counsel and guide the patient, he must associate himself with persons capable of doing so. For effective rehabilitation, function must be emphasized. Alleviation of pain by multifaceted approaches using the emerging knowledge of behavioral medicine certainly has demonstrated its effectiveness. Appreciation of the sociological as well as legal aspects of the current disability is important. Anger or reaction to the system will not solve problems, nor will delay. Back rehabilitation involves resolving problems as soon as is feasible. The patients' participation in their own recovery is necessary. Every effort should be made to reduce the secondary gain from chronic disability. The role of the specialist in musculoskeletal disability is vital in order that definitive treatment can be accomplished emphatically. Operations must be advocated when necessary, although postoperative care must also be placed in the context of the person. If the patient is one with a lifestyle or personality that may potentiate his pain, rapid progression into a rehabilitation environment of function and vocational expectation is necessary. The orthopedist, with his appreciation of function and finite goals, is ideal in directing a rehabilitation program for the individual disabled from back pain.

REFERENCES

1. Anderson, J. A. D.: The back pain in industry. In Jayson, M., Ed.: *The Lumbar Spine and Back Pain,* pp. 45–50. Pitman Medical Publishing, London, 1976.
2. Beals, R. K., and Hickman, N. W.: Industrial injuries of the back and extremities. J. Bone Joint Surg. 54A:1593–1611, 1972.

3. Bergquist-Ullman, M., and Larsson, U.: Acute low back pain in industry, a controlled prospective study with special reference to therapy and confounding factors. Acta Orthop. Scand. Suppl. 170, 1977.

4. Cairns, D. P., Mooney, V., and Crane, P.: Spinal pain rehabilitation: A comparison of inpatient and outpatient treatment results and development of predictors for outcome. Presented at International Lumbar Spine Society Meeting, Göteborg, Sweden, May 1980.

5. Cram, R. H.: A sign of sciatic nerve root pressure. J. Bone Joint Surg. 35B:192–195, 1953.

6. Fordyce, W.: *Behavioral Methods for Chronic Pain and Illness.* C. V. Mosby, St. Louis, 1978.

7. Goldstein, A.: Opioid peptides (endorphins) in pituitary and brain. Science 193:1081–1086, 1976.

8. Haber, L. D.: Disabling effects of chronic disease and impairment. J. Chronic Dis. 24:469–487, 1971.

9. Hakelius, A.: Prognosis in sciatica. A clinical follow-up of surgical and non-surgical treatment. Acta Orthop. Scand. Suppl. 129, 1970.

10. Hay, M. C.: Prevalence of some orthopedic problems in a community survey. In *Seminar on Medical Rehabilitation of Musculoskeletal Disorders,* pp. 131–134. Royal Perth Hospital, Perth, Australia, 1975.

11. Helander, E.: Incidence of industrial off time. J. Soc. Med. T. 50:398–404, 1973.

12. Hirsch, C.: Etiology and pathogenesis of back pain. Isr. J. Med. Sci. 2 (3):362–370, 1966.

13. Hitselberger, W. E., and Witten, R. M.: Abnormal myelograms in asymptomatic patients. J. Neurosurg. 28:204–206, 1968.

14. Horal, J.: The clinical appearance of low back disorders in the city of Göteborg, Sweden. Comparison of incapacitated probonds with matched controls. Acta Orthop. Scand. Suppl. 118, 1969.

15. Hult, L.: The Munkfors investigation. Acta Orthop. Scand. Suppl. 16, 1954.

16. LaRocca, A., and McNabb, I.: Value of pre-employment radiographic assessment of the lumbar spine. Can. Med. Assoc. J. 101:49–54, 1969.

17. Leavitt, S. S., Johnston, T. L., and Beyer, R. O.: The process of recovery: Patterns in industrial back injury. Part II. Predicting outcomes from early case data. Indust. Med. Surg. 40:7–15, 1971.

18. McGill, C. M.: Industrial back problems—a control problem. J. Occup. Med. 10 (4):174–178, 1968.

19. Mooney, V., and Robertson, J.: The facet syndrome. Clin. Orthop. 115:149–156, 1976.

20. Nachemson, A. L.: The lumbar spine: An orthopedic challenge. Spine 1 (1):59–71, 1976.

21. Pheasant, H. C.: Backache—its nature, incidence and cost. West. J. Med. 126:330–332, 1977.

22. Ransford, A. O., Cairns, D., and Mooney, V.: The pain drawing as an aid to psychologic evaluation of patients with low back pain. Spine 1 (2):127–134, 1976.

23. Roslund, J.: Indications for lumbar disc surgery. Unpublished thesis, Karolinska Institute, Stockholm, 1974.

24. Snoek, W., Weber, H., and Jorgensen, B.: Double blind evaluation of extradural methylprednisolone for herniated lumbar discs. Acta. Orthop. Scand. 48:635–641, 1977.

25. Surin, V. V.: Duration of disability following lumbar disc surgery. Acta Orthop. Scand. 48:466–471, 1977.

26. Wiesel, S. W., and Rothman, R. H.: Acute low back pain—an objective analysis of conservative therapy. Spine (in press).

27. Wiltse, L. L., and Rocchio, P. D.: Pre-operative psychological tests as predictors of success of chemonucleolysis in the treatment of low back syndrome. J. Bone Joint Surg. 57A:478–483, 1975.

33

Rheumatoid Arthritis

J. Pierce Conaty, M.D.

Rheumatic diseases are those conditions in which musculoskeletal pain and stiffness, with its associated varying disabilities, are prominent. Arthritis is the general term used when joints are involved.[21] This chapter will consider the three main entities of polyarthritis of unknown etiology: rheumatoid arthritis, juvenile rheumatoid arthritis (JRA), and ankylosing spondylitis. All three can produce profound musculoskeletal changes and offer rehabilitation challenges.

Approximately 20 million persons have arthritis in one form or another; about 5 million are afflicted by rheumatoid arthritis. The National Center for Health Statistics of the Department of Health, Education, and Welfare collected data on the prevalence of rheumatoid diseases.[15] Evidence of rheumatoid arthritis was found in 3.2 percent of the population examined and was considered "classical" or "definite" in 30 percent of those persons.

Rheumatic complaints are the second greatest cause of incapacity and are responsible for the largest share of chronic disability in this country, contributing to millions of workdays lost. There is no other group of diseases that "rarely kills" yet causes so much suffering in so many for so long. As Katz has stated, "rheumatic diseases do not impose a death sentence, but imprison the patient for life."[15]

Physicians and members of the allied health professions treating rheumatoid arthritis appreciate the complex, protean, and usually progressive nature of the disease. An understanding of the disease process and course it is likely to follow is mandatory. Results of treatment inspected in the light of multiple disabilities can only be meaningful if the patient's total functional activity is considered. In this way guidelines for rehabilitation, that is, lessening the sequelae of permanent disability,[20] are established.

The problem of a short listing of representative activities from which an initial classification of functional ability can be developed is well-known. Estimates of function do not distinguish between incapacity as a result of disease activity and incapacity secondary to deformity. However, the functional classification of the American Rheumatism Association provides a suitable basis for repeat assessments of this ongoing disease process (Table 33-1). In their classic study, Duthie and associates[8] used this classification system to evaluate functional capacity at the time of hospital admission, at the time of discharge (objective documentation as to the benefits of hospitalization), and at follow-up nine years later (assessing the course of the disease). At the nine-year assessment, 21 percent of the patients had no disability (Grade I), 41 percent were moderately incapacitated (Grade II), 27 percent were more severely crippled (Grade III), and 11 percent were totally dependent (Grade IV), as shown in Figure 33-1.

Conaty and Nickel[6] have documented that patients do improve with hospitalization, yet they experience a post-discharge functional regression or a gradual functional loss as the disease progresses. An update to this study would be useful to see if our current sophisticated diagnostic measures, newer drug therapy, and more advanced surgical techniques would alter the prognosis and course of the disease process.

The exact prevalence of JRA is unknown but it is thought to be 0.06 percent of the school population. Ansell and Bywaters[2] estimate that between 6 and 8 children per 100,000 under the age of 15 years have rheumatoid arthritis. Their criteria are that JRA is arthritis occurring before the age of 16 and manifested by two of the following signs: pain, swelling, and limitation of motion in four or more joints reliably observed over three months, or in one joint for a similar period with biopsy confirmation.

Table 33-1. Functional Classifications of American Rheumatism Association

Class I	Complete. Able to carry on all usual duties without handicap
Class II	Adequate for normal activities, despite handicap of discomfort or limited motion at one or more joints
Class III	Limited. Can perform little or none of duties of usual occupation or self-care
Class IV	Largely or wholly incapacitated. Bedridden or confined to wheelchair; little or no self-care

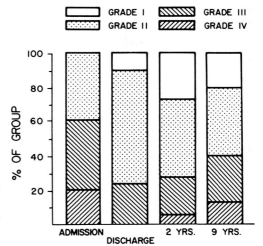

Fig. 33-1. Evaluation of the functional capacity of rheumatoid arthritis patients by using the classification system of the American Rheumatism Association. Reproduced by permission of Duthie, J. J. R., Brown, P. E., Truelove, L. H., et al.: Course and prognosis in rheumatoid arthritis. A further report. Ann. Rheum. Dis. 23:193–204, 1964.

JRA can generally be separated into three clinically distinct patterns, each with a different course and prognosis. These varieties are the acute systemic form, the monoarticular or nonsystemic form, and the polyarticular form. The acute systemic form can sustain disease activity for years, resulting in considerable disability. The monoarticular form responds readily to medical and surgical treatment, does not progress to the polyarticular type, and therefore rarely affords rehabilitation challenges. The polyarticular type closely resembles the adult disease, with active joint disease leading to increasing contractures.

Ankylosing spondylitis is also less common than rheumatoid arthritis, with reported incidents in the population at large at 1 in 2000 (0.05 percent).[18]

The clinical course and associated prognosis are extremely variable in ankylosing spondylitis. For most patients, the disease offers no social or economic problems, particularly if the patient is well-controlled. Approximately 90 percent of the patients with ankylosing spondylitis work full time and support their families. Only about 5 percent reach total incapacitation. Erosive hip disease, not spinal involvement, occasionally will produce the major disability requiring an extensive rehabilitation program.

HISTORICAL NOTES

Over the last half century, rheumatologists and surgeons have continually searched for an expedient solution to relieve arthritic disabilities.

Early attempts at surgical removal of the diseased synovial tissue enjoyed a modest vogue for 10–15 years in the late 1920s and 1930s, only to fall into disfavor because of reports expressing disparate results.[19] After 1960, interest in synovectomy was revived, with a marked increase in surgery performed early in the course of the disease. The word "prophylactic" became popular, and it was even suggested that removal of synovial tissue in one joint had a beneficial effect on the overall disease process. Subsequent observation of recurrences after synovectomy has now made it clear that the operation is not always successful and it certainly does not alter the course of the disease.[16] A more detailed discussion of synovectomy is presented later in this chapter.

In 1949 the original and impressive observations on the effect of corticosteroids on rheumatoid arthritic patients were made by Hench et al.[13] What followed was more than a decade of use and, in many cases misuse, of what we now know to be a hazardous medication. Taken in large doses for a long period of time, corticosteroids produce predictable and serious side effects. Its use is now discouraged despite its spectacular capacity to reduce joint inflammation and pain.

In the last 15 years the major advance that could be termed a breakthrough in the treatment of rheumatoid arthritis has occurred in the field of orthopedic surgery. Associated with this progress has been a marked improvement in the rheumatologist-surgeon liaison, for now most of the younger rheumatologists have an excellent understanding of surgical indications. Yet the soundness of Duthie and associates'[7,8] basic hospital regimen, outlined nearly 30 years ago and consisting of bed rest, plaster splints to affected joints, aspirin to tolerance, and physical therapy, cannot be overemphasized. Contemporary treatment has developed from this foundation.

DIAGNOSTIC TOOLS USED IN SELECTING THE MODE OF REHABILITATION

Early and proper diagnosis of an arthritic entity forms the basis of all treatment and subsequent formulation of a suitable rehabilitation program. This is particularly true in the general community, where the patient is initially seen by the primary physician who may be a family practitioner, a rheumatologist, or an orthopedic surgeon. The diagnostic tools of a good history and a careful physical examination are time honored. Laboratory tests are helpful in determining the extent of the disease activity and may help in offering some clue as to the prognosis. The diagnostic criteria for rheumatoid arthritis have been outlined by the American Rheumatism Association and are listed as Table 33-2. The diagnosis of rheumatoid arthritis requires seven of the criteria. In the first five criteria, the joint signs or symptoms must be continuous for at least six weeks.

Significant laboratory abnormalities in rheumatoid arthritis include elevated sedimentation rate, anemia, elevated rheumatoid factor titers (RA), and synovial analysis showing inflammatory Group II fluid with a low complement. Although it is never an unfailing diagnostic indication, the higher the titer factor the more likely is rheumatoid arthritis, particularly with titers higher than 1:1280. Higher factors are likely in the more severe forms of the disease and in those patients with extra-articular manifestations of rheumatoid arthritis.

Laboratory tests in the JRA patients are not as specific as in the adult. In the polyarticular form of the disease, the routine laboratory tests are similar to those noted in the adult population. However, the rheumatoid factor tests are positive in only 10–20 percent of patients. Positive tests for antinuclear antibodies (ANA) average 20 percent.

Table 33-2. American Rheumatism Association Criteria for Rheumatoid Arthritis*

Conditions

1. Morning stiffness
2. Arthritis in at least one joint
3. Swelling of at least one joint
4. Swelling of at least one other joint
5. Symmetrical simultaneous swelling of two joints
6. Subcutaneous nodules
7. Typical roentgenographic changes
8. Positive agglutination test
9. Poor mucin clot test
10. Characteristic synovial biopsy
11. Characteristic nodule histology

Ranking

Classical:	7 criteria (criteria 1–5 must be present for at least six weeks)
Definite:	5 criteria (criteria 1–5 must be present for at least six weeks)
Probable:	3 criteria (criteria 1–5 must be present for at least six weeks)
Possible:	at least two of the following: morning stiffness, persistent or recurrent arthritis for at least three weeks, history or observation of joint swelling, subcutaneous nodules, elevated erythrocyte sedimentation rate or C-reactive protein, iritis (in JRA)

* Original data from American Rheumatism Association; modified for use at Rancho Los Amigos Hospital.

The unusually high incidence of the antigen HLA-B27 in patients with ankylosing spondylitis has allowed the correct diagnosis in cases otherwise difficult to recognize. More than 90 percent of patients with ankylosing spondylitis are B27-positive, thereby making the differentiation from mechanical or noninflammatory back disease rather easy.

BASIC PRINCIPLES OF REHABILITATION

The process of rehabilitation is a multidisciplinary therapeutic program to recover maximum function in patients with permanent or protracted impairment. Rehabilitation in rheumatoid arthritis, adult or juvenile, encompasses six major factors: assessment, education, physical therapies, medical management, surgical treatment, and psychosocial counseling.

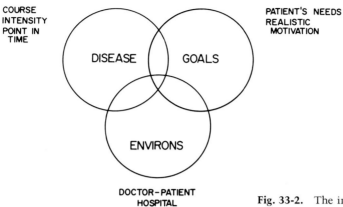

COURSE
INTENSITY
POINT IN
 TIME

PATIENT'S NEEDS
REALISTIC
 MOTIVATION

DISEASE   GOALS

ENVIRONS

DOCTOR-PATIENT
HOSPITAL
FAMILY
POST-DISCHARGE LOCATION

Fig. 33-2. The interlocking elements necessary for making assessments. Courtesy of J. P. Conaty.

Assessment

Assessment implies an appreciation, understanding, and interpretation of the disease, the patient's needs (goals), the environs, and the overlap created by all three. These elements are diagrammed in Figure 33-2.

Assessment of the disease must consider its pattern and the intensity of its ongoing process in the evaluation. Knowledge of the natural course of rheumatoid arthritis and the value of appropriate treatment provides two inescapable facts: a small but significant percentage of patients eventually do become incapacitated, yet this incapacitation, in whole or in part, may be reversible. The physician may have difficulty in foreseeing the future in patients with rheumatoid arthritis because of the varied course of the disease, but much can be learned from the pattern of the process. If incapacity occurs late and functional loss is due to pain and weakness, the response to treatment should be favorable. If, however, incapacity occurs early, indicating a more aggressive form of the disease, then improvement, although initially possible, may prove to be short lived. A contractural deformity, particularly if severe and associated with gross weakness, indicates neglect.

Assessment of functional goals must consider the patient's needs, not the doctor's. It infers realism, not theory, and recognizes motivation. The patient may frequently express the desire to ambulate with less pain but may, at the same time, disregard serious upper extremity functional loss unless pain in this area is a major factor. The treating physician, particularly if a surgeon, may find such an assignment of priorities difficult to accept. Substitutional motor patterns frequently minimize overall functional loss in the upper extremity, but the loss of the ability to ambulate because of pain provides no alternatives.

Goals should be set before a patient is admitted to the hospital, but if they have not, they should be quickly established after the admission work-up by the various disciplines. Functional goals need not always be equated with potential.

On rare occasions, wheelchair dependence may be more sensible for both the function and safety of the patient. Alteration of goals, occasionally upward but usually downward, may be indicated during the hospital stay. However, the initial functional goal, respecting the patient's needs and those established by a seasoned observer, usually stands.

Assessment of the environs considers a number of factors. A warm relationship with the doctor must exist, be it in the community or in the framework of a special arthritis unit. In such a unit, the allied health professionals should be supportive of the physician, who must exercise leadership and show respect for all fellow professionals. Delegation of various aspects of patient care by the physician is desirable but surrendering medical responsibilities to members of the allied health team is unacceptable.

The initial and ongoing changing assessment of upper and lower extremity function is one of the two primary responsibilities of the physical and occupational therapists; the second is the application of the basic therapy modalities. The data provided to the surgeon by the therapist should provide basic information necessary in determining appropriate surgical treatment. The surgeon should be wise enough to require such helpful guidance but the decision is his as to the timing of a specific procedure in any given patient. Barring complications, postoperative management ideally is shared by the surgeon and the therapist. However, management of such complications again becomes the sole responsibility of the operating surgeon.

The charge nurse must provide day-to-day overall in-house evaluation as it pertains to response to medications and various therapies, physical and psychosocial. The liaison nurse prepares the rehabilitated patient for discharge and re-entry into the community and follows the course of this patient in the home setting, reporting back any subsequent adversities. The total inpatient care, discharge planning, and subsequent outpatient follow-up are directed by the physician. Avoiding this responsibility is tantamount to ultimate failure of the categorical unit.

The special unit hospital milieu provides a subtle benefit; the milieu should allay patients' apprehensions and fears. However, sometimes a patient with strong denial or depressive patterns will derive no benefit from the milieu and will be threatened by and respond poorly to all aspects of the hospital environs.

The patient's family should be concerned and supportive of all phases of the treatment. They should be able to communicate with all members of the allied health team. Patients coming from and returning to an overindulgent home setting will usually relapse to their pre-admission functional level. Occasionally a readmission at a later date is sought when an overindulgent family unit is about to collapse because of age or physical debility of the key member, that is, the wife, husband, or parent. By this time the patient is usually too far relapsed, physically and mentally, to be helped by a rehabilitation program. An extended care facility is the preferred alternative. The most promising situation is therefore one in which a well-motivated patient presents himself to the rehabilitation unit and asks for help in increasing his abilities to function. He should have plans to return to a supportive family and community and expect to enjoy the benefits of his functional gains.

Education

In the community setting, all aspects of outpatient disease education are the responsibility of the physician treating the rheumatic disease entity, unless he has knowledgeable allied health support in the office or clinic.

The need for education is not necessarily related to the degree of involvement. It should begin with early disease and, if necessary, continue on through the period of late disease complicated by varying degrees of disability. Educating hospital patients about all aspects of their disease is a tremendous contribution of the nursing, occupational and physical therapy, clinical psychology, medical social service, and vocational rehabilitation professions. Regardless of all this talent, the physician enjoying the full resources of a special unit is still responsible for providing his share of the patient's education on a one-to-one basis.

Physical Therapies

Basic physical therapies for patients with rheumatoid arthritis encompass prevention of deformity, instruction in use and abuse of the joints involved, instruction in the use of self-help devices, and exercise programs.

Prevention of deformity includes proper positioning with rest, proper posture when upright, and the use of appropriate resting splints. The latter includes splints for the wrists, knees, and ankles, and they can be made of plaster or polypropylene. The polypropylene shell splint developed at the University of California Biomechanics Laboratory has shown a measure of success in controlling valgus deformity of the hindfoot and ankle. Functional splinting of the hand is ineffective in preventing deformity, particularly at the metacarpophalangeal (MCP) level.

Education in the area of physical measures relates principally to the overuse and abuse of the involved joints. These violations should be explained to the patient by the physician, nurse, and therapist. Many of a patient's everyday endeavors, such as abuse in transferring (loading the flexed MCP joints), overuse in knitting, and strain because of obesity, do fall under the category of misuse. The degree of improvement possible in the range and strength of joint motion should be explored through an appropriate exercise program.

Increased function with self-help devices should be determined primarily by the knowledgeable occupational or physical therapist. Aids include the wide range of devices to offset lost upper extremity function, wheelchair adjustments, and alterations in the home setting to accommodate the needs of the disabled patient and his equipment.

Exercises designed to avoid fatigue are instituted when the patient has full range. Exercise should be minimized during any "joint flare" accompanied by increased pain and swelling. Active assistance exercises are preferred when the patient lacks full range of motion of the involved joint. Resistive exercises are performed with caution, they should be well supervised, avoided in a "disease flare," and worked through a limited range. Resistive exercises are generally required after surgical arthroplasty.

Medical Management

Drug therapy plays a key role in the management of any inflammatory joint disease but it should never be abused. A great variety of medications are available and discussed in detail in all textbooks on the rheumatoid diseases. Only a synopsis is included here.

Anti-inflammatory Agents. Salicylates administered in full dosage offer the most effective relief of pain and stiffness. Given 8–14 of the 5-grain tablets daily in divided doses, the serum salicylate level reaches an acceptable 20–30 percent.

Corticosteroids should be used only in those patients who fail to respond to other anti-inflammatory agents, intra-articular steroids, and remittive drugs (gold salts). Five mg of prednisone daily is usually tolerated well. Steroids reduce inflammation but do not alter the course of the disease.

Remittive Agents. Long-term administration of gold salts stands the best chance of bringing the disease into remission. Details of administration are outlined in all texts on arthritis. A total of 1 g is given in divided doses. A response can be expected after receiving 400–500 mg. Reactions to gold salts are common. Penicillamine, still considered somewhat experimental, can also produce a remission but there is a considerable delay (two to three months) from beginning of therapy to clinical improvement.

Cytotoxic Immunosuppressive Agents. These hazardous agents should be used only by those familiar with their use and toxic effects. They should be reserved for those patients who have failed to respond to other forms of treatment and demonstrate rapid progression in joint destruction and extra-articular complications, such as severe vasculitis.

Intra-articular corticosteroids are of great value, particularly if used after joint aspiration of a large effusion. Intra-articular cytotoxic agents are still under investigation.[9] Strong analgesics are discouraged, and narcotics are absolutely avoided except under extreme circumstances.

A well-planned drug therapy program can control the majority of the ambulatory outpatient rheumatoid population. However, the long-term prognosis for the hospitalized patient is guarded. The ultimate course of rheumatoid arthritis depends largely on the way it begins. Although results do vary, the course of the disease is unfavorable in the presence of the conditions listed in Table 33-3.

Surgical Treatment

Historically, the orthopedic surgeon has dealt with chronic musculoskeletal deformities, such as poliomyelitis and osseous tuberculosis, and has understood the development of deformity, the loss of function, and the methods for overcoming chronic disability. The surgeon has the unique ability to direct both the nonoperative and the surgical rehabilitation, and his presence can create an environment that ameliorates the negative attitude of patients toward reconstructive surgery.

Table 33-3. Poor Prognostic Indicators of
Rheumatoid Arthritis*

1. Females usually have a worse prognosis
2. Insidious onset
3. Symmetrical disease
4. Initial marked activity that persists
5. Early multiple joint effusions
6. Early constitutional symptoms
7. Early appearance of nodules
8. Extra-articular manifestations, notably vasculitis
9. Early appearance of roentgenographic erosions
10. Early elevations of rheumatoid factor
11. Prolonged interval between onset of the disease and
    first medical evaluation

* Adapted from Katz, W. A.: Rheumatology. In Katz,
W. A., Ed.: *Rheumatic Diseases,* 1st ed., pp. 3–4. J. B. Lippincott, Philadelphia, 1977.

The era of orthopedic surgical intervention in the treatment of rheumatoid arthritis has come of age, producing documented functional improvement.[6] Reconstructive procedures relieve pain, increase function, and thereby decrease disability. Yet they do not cure the disease and they may not totally eradicate the local disease process in the joint operated upon.

The success of any surgical procedure depends primarily on the proper selection of the patient for surgery and the correct operative procedure. The surgeon's involvement encompasses an understanding of the disease process, understanding of appropriate surgical goals, and surgical know-how, as well as the patient motivation and allied health support previously discussed.

The surgeon must realize that he is intervening in an ongoing disease process that ultimately might erase the functional benefits of any given procedure. He should also recognize that he can literally make a career out of operating on a single, severely involved rheumatoid patient. "Most reconstructive procedures help to a degree, but the true surgical excellence depends on the recognition of the genuine needs of the patient and a true appreciation of the potential gain from each procedure and its proper timing."[6] The accuracy of the preoperative profile of the patient's potential is the benchmark of success.

The rheumatoid patient is chronically ill and more often than not is chronically depressed. Both entities are treatable and should be sorted out prior to any surgical intervention. Chronic depression is an enormous deterrent to the success of any treatment regimen. A disease flare does not preclude surgical intervention as long as the patient is under maximum medical control.

High competence in surgery is mandatory when operating on the rheumatoid patient, but the preoperative evaluation is the most important. Rheumatoid arthritis, particularly as it relates to joint replacement, can offer some degree of technical forgiveness. Polyarticular involvement eases the long-term mechanical stresses on the operative joint and is contrary to the single osteoarthritic joint undergoing total replacement. The recurrence of local disease or overall disease progression is the mortal enemy of long-term surgical success.

The following orthopedic procedures are indicated for treating rheumatoid arthritis, JRA, and ankylosing spondylitis.

Synovectomy. Popular a decade ago, this procedure now has limited application to adults and children. Earlier retrospective studies from various centers[5,10-12,14,19] would seem to indicate that synovectomy was beneficial in the knee joint, the elbow, the MCP joints, and the proximal interphalangeal (PIP) joints. McEwen,[17] who conducted a controlled evaluation of synovectomy in the treatment of rheumatoid arthritis in the knee, the MCP and the PIP joints, recently reported his results at the end of three years. His conclusions were:

> The synovectomized joints were better than the controls, in a number of aspects at the end of one year.
>
> By the end of three years the differences had essentially disappeared in hand cases, but soft tissue swelling remained less in the synovectomized knees than in the control knees.
>
> There were no statistically significant differences between the synovectomized and the control joints after three years with regard to bony erosions on radiographic examinations.[17]

McEwen will report his findings again after five years of follow-up observation. A similar controlled evaluation has been carried out in the United Kingdom with almost identical results.[3]

Synovectomy is indicated only in the non-erosive knee joint of a young wage-earning patient, for whom "buying time" is important. The possibility of success is enhanced in the patient with seronegative disease or monoarticular involvement. Anti-inflammatory or remittive agents, not synovectomy, should be used to control the synovitis in finger joints.

Dorsal wrist clearance of synovial tissue is required if extensor tendon rupture occurs, a development usually combined with some form of wrist stabilization. Volar clearance is indicated with carpal tunnel complaints and should be carried into the palm and fingers when "triggering" happens.

Joint synovectomy should be performed as part of any arthroplasty procedure, despite the current acceptance that synovectomy in itself does little to prevent recurrent articular damage.

Soft Tissue Releases. These are frequently indicated in the JRA patient with polyarticular-type disease and who is prone to contractural deformity. Releases may be performed in the hip, knee, hindfoot, and wrist. Operations on the hindfoot or wrist may need to be accompanied by appropriate tendon transfers.

In the adult, soft tissue release may be required in the posterior knee joint, either as a primary procedure or as a preliminary to arthroplasty. Candidates for knee replacement with 50 degrees or more of flexion contracture, depending upon the type of prosthesis and the functional goals of the patient, may first require posterior release.

The efficacy of soft tissue releases in relieving nerve entrapment syndrome is unquestioned.

Osteotomy. Long bone realignment, indicated in trauma residuals and degenerative knee disease (tibial osteotomy of the Coventry type), is rarely performed in any form of inflammatory arthritis. The total effectiveness of joint replacement in the involved joint has negated any true indication for osteotomy in rheumatoid arthritis.

Cervical or lumbar spinal osteotomy is occasionally indicated for ankylosing spondylitis in order to correct an unacceptable flexion deformity. The level contributing to the major flexion deformity can be cervical, thoracic, or lumbar. This must be determined preoperatively. Cervical extension osteotomy involves great danger, but the results of the procedure, described by Simmons,[22] can be spectacular in correcting a chin-on-chest deformity.

Lumbar osteotomy, first described by Smith-Peterson et al.[24] 35 years ago, has proved to be a time-honored successful procedure in correcting thoracolumbar flexion deformity. Harrington compression rods can be used to ensure maintenance of correction while the fusion matures.

Arthroplasty. The various types of arthroplasties have played a major role in surgical management of the rheumatoid arthritic patient for half a century. They include resection arthroplasty, interpositional arthroplasty, surface replacement, and total joint arthroplasty. The basic requirement of a successful arthroplasty continues to be painless, stable motion.

Resection arthroplasty is now usually confined to metatarsal head and proximal phalanx resection (Hoffman- and Clayton-type procedures), and the various resection techniques about the great toe, which are considered part of the total forefoot reconstructive procedures.[4]

Interpositional arthroplasty, popularized by the innovative cup arthroplasty of Smith-Peterson et al., has been replaced by the newer surface arthroplasty or total replacement.

The surface replacement arthroplasty currently enjoying popularity is the procedure in which the acetabular and femoral head surfaces are replaced with high-density plastic and metal surfaces, both cemented in place. Although technically somewhat difficult, excellent initial results have been reported by Amstutz et al.[1] Some of the unconstrained total knee replacements resecting minimal bone (Marmor-type) can be considered as a form of surface replacement. Intact ligaments and a firm capsular sleeve are required for stability.

The success of total joint replacement in the hip and knee is now legend. The selection of the type of prosthesis used in the knee, for total or minimal constraint, depends upon the degree of knee stability that develops once the deformity is corrected.

Silastic MCP arthroplasty has enjoyed a widespread acceptance. Postoperative therapy and hand splinting to maintain proper positioning while the realigned soft tissues undergo repair contribute greatly to the operation's success.

Arthrodesis. Arthrodesis remains a frequently performed procedure despite improved arthroplasty techniques. Fusion can provide total pain relief and stability when mobility is of lesser or no concern. Arthrodesis is useful in alleviating the following disabilities:

Erosion of the unstable cervical spine, particularly when there are neurological findings of cord compromise.

Painful varus (in children) or valgus (in adults) high-foot deformity, in which subtalar fusion or triple arthrodesis is performed. The procedure should be carried out before the ankle joint is destroyed.

Deformities of the MCP joint of the thumb, the interphalangeal joint of the thumb, or both.

Fusion of the PIP joints in a functional position.

The unstable wrist. In addition, the so-called pseudoarthrodesis (relying on firm scar tissue for adequate stability) still may be preferred to total wrist replacement, particularly in the young or in those patients with inadequate wrist extensors.

In the severely involved patient, the staging of multiple procedures may be required. In a patient with equally involved hips, knees, and forefeet, the best plan seems to be bilateral forefoot procedures, followed by hip replacement, one at a time (two operations), followed by knee replacements, perhaps both knees at the same time.

In the upper extremity, operations are always performed unilaterally. With wrist, thumb, MCP and PIP joint involvement, the following routine has proved efficacious: simultaneous wrist and PIP stabilization followed eventually by simultaneous MCP arthroplasty and thumb fusion.

Psychosocial Counseling

The presence of psychosocial problems in chronically disabled patients should be apparent to all observant clinicians. In the community, the detection of and solution to these problems may fall upon the treating physician, who may well seek the help of a practicing clinical psychologist or psychiatrist.

In the special-unit hospital setting, a large portion of the psychologist's and medical social worker's time is spent in collecting data to evaluate these complex psychosocial histories. In this way their approach differs somewhat from the community need of short-term concept of crisis intervention. The medical social worker is frequently dealing with an older, traditionally oriented population in need of financial counseling. These patients may need to hear that their severe disability entitles them to receive some form of public assistance, which may be very difficult to accept. Some people can never come to terms with this fact, affording some problems in establishing a rehabilitation program.

The clinical psychologist deals with the frequently observed major problems of anxiety, which responds well to therapy. Prolonged anxiety will lead to depression. Depression in its severest form leads to suicide. Depression is also medically treatable. Denial is a defense against depression and frequently results in the patient not securing adequate medical treatment. Denial may serve a purpose but is eventually self-defeating. Depression may ensue when denial breaks down.

Other commonly observed factors requiring counseling, education, and psychotherapy include marital problems, low self-esteem or poor body image, expectations that the operation will result in a total cure, and subjective pain in excess of objectively observed pain.

The psychotherapist appreciates that surgical intervention is an anxiety-provoking experience, particularly with today's need for informed consent. Each disease flare-up may also precipitate an anxiety reaction of another loss or a regression to earlier functional levels necessitating a stage of adjustment. The primary goal of counseling is to help the patient become more self-accepting, to live with the disease, to be open to changes that can be made, and to exercise those options.

REHABILITATING JRA PATIENTS

Assessing cases of JRA is more difficult than for adult forms. The case history as provided by the parent may be guarded, because the parent is protecting the child. Objective evaluations must relate to function, which require knowledgeable personnel. Interpretation, too, is troublesome. Unlike most adults, children have difficulty in defining their problem. A child's true physical status must be inferred from behavior, then interpreted for the family and used to formulate therapeutic goals properly. These goals are:

> Relief of joint pain via the proper use of anti-inflammatory medications, splinting, and an occasional surgical procedure.
> Improvement of function, especially the prevention of deformity as it relates to growth.
> Educating the family to cope with the child's disease. Relief of pain and functional improvement may be totally frustrated in the presence of genuine psychosocial difficulties. The home is the key to successful treatment.
> Appreciating the complexities of the disease's activity. All members of the various disciplines involved in treatment should realize that disease activity fluctuations alter function and that such fluctuations require physical and psychological support and a modification of the home program.

Singsen and associates,[23] reporting on total hip replacement in children with arthritis, noted that the success of the surgery depended to a great degree upon the motivation of the patient:

> Young patients, and to a lesser degree, their parents, may quickly grasp at this procedure as the solution to many difficulties. This is particularly true if children are desperate to be like their peers. However, the children frequently do not comprehend the limited benefits that may be gained from total hip replacement and the need for at least a full year of intensive postoperative physical therapy. Many children with arthritis have a very limited view of the long-term consequences of their disease process. At this age, lack of maturity may obstruct the realization that total hip replacement is only one small part of the total process of rehabilitation.[23]

The surgeon should realize that this is true of any operative procedure performed on the juvenile rheumatoid patient. Upper extremity reconstruction may prove less straightforward than lower extremity reconstruction. In older children, their need for functional improvement may depend upon IQ, aptitude, and occupational considerations.

The treatment program should be consistent and provide a realistic perspective. Consistent medical management should avoid the "ups and downs" in function that produce parental resistance. If variations in the program develop, the goals of the family and the treating medical team may diverge. The family is not willing to cause their child pain, and their goal becomes one of a comfortable existence for the child. Parents usually side with the less aggressive treatment program and may join any member of the treatment team who advocates "doing the easiest thing first." All efforts should be directed toward having these children reach adulthood emotionally and physically independent.

REHABILITATING PATIENTS WITH ANKYLOSING SPONDYLITIS

Fewer than 5 percent of patients with ankylosing spondylitis become totally dependent. An erosive hip disease associated with marked limitation of motion of the hip and accompanied by a rigid lumbar spine may result in a major disability. Bilateral total hip replacements are frequently indicated. The results of this operation are not as gratifying as those in rheumatoid arthritis, but relief of pain is predictable. Postoperative heterotopic bone formation, commonly seen in the days of cup arthroplasty, is not as frequently observed with total hip replacement. The reason for this is unknown. However, the postoperative range may be limited as a result of long-standing extrinsic soft tissue tightness.

Lumbar and cervical osteotomy can be performed to correct the severe flexion deformity that produces visual compromise and poor body image. Spinal deformity can be prevented with early education, anti-inflammatory medication, and posture and exercise regimens.

ALTERNATIVES TO TREATMENT OF CHOICE FOR ALL ENTITIES

On occasion, the treatment team must accept the fact that some patients and some patients' families may elect not to accept, in whole or in part, the advised treatment program. This decision may be based on a denial of the extent of the disability or on a genuine acceptance of the *status quo.*

Perceptive allied health members must also appreciate that, at times, certain aspects of the patient's emotional behavior must not be invaded. To do so may prove unrewarding or destructive. Physical disability may form a sound basis of mutual self-support in a compatible home situation with each member's role, the helper and the helpless, necessary for balance. To disrupt this creates problems.

THE FUTURE

There are three promising future directions in the rehabilitation of rheumatoid arthritis and its allied conditions. One avenue involves the identification of the etiology of rheumatoid arthritis, negating any need for rehabilitation. Another promising direction is the continuing increase in medical-surgical liaisons. This liaison has taken us to newer levels of successful patient care. The future should offer further improvement. Also expected is the growth of objective documentation about functional gains after treatment. Many centers now perform lower extremity kinesiology studies pre- and postoperatively, and these tests provide a true measure of objectivity as it relates to time, distance, and velocity. Upper extremity functional testing has always been more difficult to evaluate objectively. Functional hand assessment is straightforward in the post-trauma patient, but the multiple joint involvement of the rheumatoid arthritic patient with substitutional patterns and opposite hand assist makes objective documentation of functional gains and losses extremely difficult. Practical hand-assessment tests must be based on functional activities recording ability or inability to perform certain basic single-handed tasks within a certain amount of time.

REFERENCES

1. Amstutz, H., Graff-Radford, A., Gruen, T., and Clark, I.: Tharies surface replacements: A review of first one hundred cases. J. Bone Joint Surg. 2A:211, 1978. (Abstr.)
2. Ansell, B., and Bywaters, E. G. L.: Juvenile chronic polyarthritis. In Scott, J. T., Ed.: *Copeman's Textbook of Rheumatic Diseases,* 5th ed., pp. 365–388. Churchill Livingstone, Edinburgh, 1978.
3. Arthritis and Rheumatism Council and British Orthopaedic Association: A controlled trial of synovectomy of the knee and metacarpophalangeal joints in rheumatoid arthritis. Ann. Rheum. Dis. 35:437–442, 1976.
4. Clayton, M. L.: Surgery of the forefoot in rheumatoid arthritis. Clin. Orthop. 16:136–140, 1960.
5. Conaty, J. P.: Surgery of the hip and knee in patients with rheumatoid arthritis. J. Bone Joint Surg. 55A:301–314, 1973.
6. Conaty, J. P., and Nickel, V. L.: Functional incapacitation in rheumatoid arthritis: A rehabilitation challenge. J. Bone Joint Surg. 53A:624–637, 1971.
7. Duthie, J. J. R., Brown, P. E., Knox, J. D. E., and Thompson, M.: Course and prognosis in rheumatoid arthritis. Ann. Rheum. Dis. 16:411–424, 1957.
8. Duthie, J. J. R., Brown, P. E., Truelove, L. H., et al.: Course and prognosis in rheumatoid arthritis. A further report. Ann. Rheum. Dis. 23:193–204, 1964.
9. Ellison, M. R., and Flatt, A. E.: Intra-articular thiotepa in rheumatoid disease. Arthritis Rheum. 14:212–222, 1971.
10. Ellison, M. R., Kelly, K. J., and Flatt, A. E.: The results of surgical synovectomy of the digital joints in rheumatoid arthritis. J. Bone Joint Surg. 53A:1041, 1971.
11. Eyring, E. J., Longert, A., and Bass, J. C.: Synovectomy in juvenile rheumatoid arthritis. J. Bone Joint Surg. 53A:638–651, 1971.
12. Geens, S., Clayton, M. L., Leidholt, J. D., et al.: Synovectomy and debridement of the knee in rheumatoid arthritis: II. Clinical and roentgenographic study of thirty-one cases. J. Bone Joint Surg. 51A:626–642, 1969.
13. Hench, P. S., Kendall, E. C., Slocumb, C. H., and Polley, H. F.: Effects of cortisone acetate and pituitary ACTH on R. A., rheumatic fever and certain other conditions; study in clinical physiology. Arch. Intern. Med. 85:545–666, 1950.

14. Inglis, A. E., Ranawat, C. S., and Straub, L. R.: Synovectomy and debridement of the elbow in rheumatoid arthritis. J. Bone Joint Surg. 53A:652–662, 1971.

15. Katz, W. A.: Rheumatology. In Katz, W. A., Ed.: *Rheumatic Diseases,* 1st ed., pp. 3–4. J. B. Lippincott, Philadelphia, 1977.

16. McEwen, C.: Early synovectomy in the treatment of rheumatoid arthritis. N. Engl. J. Med. 279:420–422, 1968.

17. McEwen, C.: Multicenter evaluation of synovectomy in the treatment of rheumatoid arthritis. Arthritis Rheum. 20:765–771, 1977.

18. Ogryzlo, M. A.: Ankylosing spondylitis. In Hollander, J. L., Ed.: *Arthritis and Allied Conditions,* 8th ed., pp. 669–723. Lea & Febiger, Philadelphia, 1972.

19. Pardee, M. L.: Synovectomy of the knee joint. A review of the literature and presentation of cases. J. Bone Joint Surg. 30A:908–914, 1948.

20. Perry, J.: Personal communication.

21. Rodnana, G. P., Ed.: Primer on rheumatic diseases, 7th ed. J.A.M.A. Suppl. 224:April 30, 1973.

22. Simmons, E. H.: The surgical correction of flexion deformity of the cervical spine in ankylosing spondylitis. Clin. Orthop. 86:132–143, 1972.

23. Singsen, B. H., Isaacson, A. J., Bernstein, B. H., et al.: Total hip replacement in children with arthritis. Arthritis Rheum. 21:401–406, 1978.

24. Smith-Petersen, M. N., Larson, C. B., and Aufranc, O. E.: Osteotomy of the spine for correction of flexion deformity in rheumatoid arthritis. J. Bone Joint Surg. 27A:1–11, 1945.

34

Degenerative Arthritis

Randall J. Lewis, M.D.

Degenerative arthritis is a progressive, noninflammatory disorder affecting both the axial skeleton and the extremities. It is characterized by progressive loss of articular cartilage, bone proliferation, and varying degrees of stiffness or instability, leading to loss of function. The most common presentation of degenerative joint disease (DJD) is pain, and it is for pain or stiffness that most patients seek medical attention.

Osteoarthritis is by far the most common disease affecting the musculoskeletal system, afflicting more people than all other arthritides combined. The incidence of symptomatic osteoarthritis increases with age. Although significant DJD is unusual before the fourth decade, Gordon[1] estimates that 20 percent of the population older than age 60 years of age suffers from symptomatic degenerative joint disease. With the increasing number of elderly individuals in the population, interest in degenerative joint disease as both a medical and social problem has become greater. Fortunately, medical and surgical advances over the past decade have given the physician a broader range of effective therapy for symptomatic osteoarthritis.

Osteoarthritis often is divided into primary (idiopathic) and secondary types. With the latter, there is a recognizable mechanical abnormality that leads to deterioration of the joint, often at a relatively early age. Congenital hip dysplasia, Legg-Calvé-Perthes disease, intra-articular fractures, and instability due to loss of ligamentous support are a few of the well-known causes of secondary osteoarthritis. Aging of the articular cartilage and abnormal mechanical stress on the joint are the two most plausible theories for the etiology of primary osteoarthritis, although genetic factors have been implicated as well.[5] The early morphological changes in both cartilage and bone have been extensively categorized.[2] The end result of the disease is always a net loss of articular cartilage, with marginal bone proliferation and subchondral sclerosis.

TREATMENT MODALITIES

The treatment of osteoarthritis is rehabilitation in the truest sense: returning the patient to a satisfactory functional level. Degenerative arthritis, no matter how advanced, is not treated if it is not symptomatic. Although the patient may have osteoarthritis in multiple joints, treatment should be geared to those areas that are functionally incapacitating or persistently painful. The modalities used should be appropriate to the severity of functional impairment: total joint arthroplasty is inappropriate treatment for a stiff but functional hip in a patient who requires only occasional aspirin for discomfort, whereas continued aspiration, long-term administration of anti-inflammatory agents, and severe curtailment of physical activity are equally unsuitable approaches for the middle-aged patient with disabling osteoarthritis of the medial compartment of the knee.

Although osteoarthritis is not a systemic disease, oral anti-inflammatory agents and mild analgesics are effective in relieving symptoms, and they should be used for treatment initially. Aspirin is the drug that best combines analgesic and anti-inflammatory properties.[3] It is safe, effective, inexpensive, and tolerated well by most patients. It can be used in plain or buffered form. If aspirin is ineffective in relieving symptoms, any of the newer nonsteroidal agents (ibuprofen, tenoprofen, tolmetin, or napsylate) can be tried and used as a maintenance regimen. Patients may fail to respond to one agent and achieve excellent results with another of similar potency. A brief course of phenylbutazone or indomethacin may quiet acute inflammatory symptoms but is inappropriate for long-term maintenance because of potential gastrointestinal and bone marrow toxicity. There is no place for systemic steroids in the treatment of osteoarthritis.

Intermittent administration of intra-articular steroid injections for osteoarthritis is controversial. Although steroid injections may dramatically relieve acute inflammatory symptoms, repeated dosage carries the risks of interfering with cartilage nutrition, skin atrophy, and infection of the joint. The necessity for repeated injections suggests an untreated mechanical basis for recurrent symptoms; joints involved in such a pattern should be evaluated as candidates for surgery.

Heat, cold, biofeedback, acupuncture, and a whole host of external modalities have been used to treat degenerative arthritis, and each has its adherents. Patients often report that heat is the most effective agent in relieving stiffness and aching, and they often will work out their own regimen for using it. The beneficial effects of heat may be as much systemic as local. Ten to 15 minutes in a warm shower or tub, morning and evening, is inexpensive, convenient for the patient, and often remarkably effective. Whirlpool baths, ultrasound, and hospital heat treatments seem to offer little more than a good soak in the tub at home and are more costly, less convenient, and less readily available.

Mechnical support, traction, and exercise all play important roles in the treatment of degenerative joint disease. Because their value and use vary with the region involved, they will be discussed in relation to individual joint symptoms in the next section.

Surgery is often the definitive treatment for osteoarthritis, especially if it is accompanied by significant mechanical abnormalities. The advent of total joint replacement, particularly for the hip and knee, has provided an effective and often dramatic way to treat advanced degenerative joint disease. The greatest benefits of surgical treatment have been in the area of pain relief and the increase in activity level that such relief permits. As the effectiveness and predictability of reconstructive surgery have increased, the indications for operative treatment have broadened. Reconstruction of the arthritic joint should be considered a part of the therapeutic armamentarium to be used at an appropriate stage of the disease, rather than as a last resort when all possible physical and pharmacological manipulations have been exhausted. Medical, surgical, and mechanical modalities are complementary and should be used in a well-conceived program for the functional rehabilitation of a diseased joint.

THE AXIAL SKELETON

Nowhere do the twin etiologies of aging and abnormal mechanical stress come together more neatly than in osteoarthritis of the back and neck. The spine may be regarded as two segmental columns, anterior and posterior, enclosing the spinal cord (see Fig. 34-1). As aging proceeds, the annulus of the disc loses its elasticity and bulges outward with consequent loss of the normal disc height. Loss of the normal relationships in the anterior column leads to abnormal stresses on the facet joints of the posterior column (Fig. 34-2). The response of the posterior structures to these stresses is narrowing of the joint space, marginal bony proliferation, or

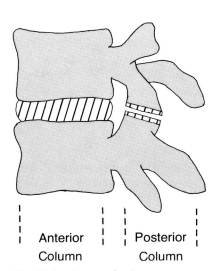

Fig. 34-1. A normal spine.

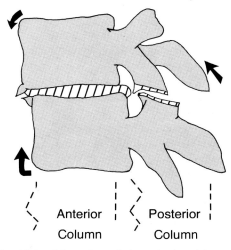

Fig. 34-2. Disruption of the spinal architecture with disc degeneration and collapse. Note osteophytes encroaching on neural foramen.

formation of osteophytes. Osteophytes also form anteriorly at the joints of Luschka in the cervical region and at the posterior and anterior margins of the vertebral body throughout the spine. The net result is narrowing of the neural foramina and encroachment on the spinal canal. Any disc protrusion anteriorly or hypertrophy of the ligamentum flavum posteriorly further compromises the canal. The net result is nerve root compression, with pain, abnormal neurological findings, and disability.

The Neck

Osteoarthritis in the cervical spine may present with neck pain or with pain radiating to the shoulder or interscapular area. Pain may be spontaneous or evoked by certain motions and activities involving extension of the neck or rotation of the head, such as backing up a car. Radiation of pain in the distribution of a specific dermatome, muscle weakness, and reflex and sensory changes all serve to localize the level of the root impingement. Because the disease is commonly present at multiple levels, repeated careful physical examination is important to discern where the disease is significant. Electromyographic and nerve conduction studies are helpful in determining anatomical levels and differentiating peripheral entrapment, such as carpal tunnel syndrome and thoracic outlet pathology from cervical spine disease. They are not, however, a substitute for careful, repeated, neurological evaluation.

In the absence of neurological deficit, initial treatment should be conservative. Heat applied in any of a variety of ways, support in the form of a cervical collar, and anti-inflammatory medication should be instituted. An acute attack of symptoms may be relieved by a brief course of potent nonsteroidal anti-inflammatory medication, such as phenylbutazone or indomethacin, always given in conjunction with physical modalities. For less acute symptoms, salicylates or other nonsteroidal medication may be more appropriate. Careful explanation of the nature of the disease process and of the importance of mechanical support and heat help to alleviate the patient's anxiety and ensure compliance with the treatment regimen. Forewarning of the potentially chronic nature of the problem and dispelling expectations of a quick recovery may be important in avoiding discouragement if symptoms persist beyond a few weeks. Cervical traction (2.25–4.50 kg) applied at home may help to relieve symptoms and is both inexpensive and convenient. It may also be applied in conjunction with a firm cervical collar. The collar has the advantage of portability and may be used throughout the day without restricting a patient's activity. Traction may sometimes be effective when a collar alone will not suffice. Intermittent cervical traction is useful but must be applied in a supervised setting. Desk workers, especially secretaries and typists, often exacerbate their symptoms by working. They may require reduced duty schedules and prolonged use of a collar for support as well as maintenance of good cervical posture. The patient must avoid heavy lifting. Because of the potential chronicity of symptoms, it is desirable to avoid narcotic analgesics. In the absence of neurological deficit, it is wise to persist with a conservative, well-supervised regimen for 6–12 months before considering surgical intervention. The presence of objective neurological impairment, however, should prompt consideration of surgery. With the acute onset of neurological abnormality or the progression of a deficit, myelography should be performed without delay, and any remediable lesion should be treated surgically.

The Lumbosacral Spine

The etiology of degenerative disease in the lumbosacral spine is identical to that in the neck. Schmorl and Junghanns[4] observed that 90 percent of the population demonstrated disc changes beyond the seventh decade. Radiographic changes of degenerative disease are generally present beyond the third decade. Because of the universality of lumbar spine changes, careful evaluation of the clinical situation is mandatory, and a functional approach to the problem should be adopted. Disc space narrowing, osteophytes, hypertrophic facets, and even degenerative spondylolisthesis do not require treatment, but pain, restricted motion, and weakness do.

The patient may present with acute pain or a gradual increase in symptoms. Pain may be localized to the low back region or may radiate to the buttock or posterior thigh and calf. Pain radiating to the foot may indicate an L5 or S1 root lesion but is of no greater significance. The patient may demonstrate a marked list to one side. Pain is often exacerbated by sitting or by rising from a chair.

The primary aim of treatment is to relieve pain. First, the patient must be placed on a program of strict bed rest for mechanical unloading of the spine. He is instructed to remain in bed, lying supine or on the side, sometimes using a pillow under the knees. Bed rest should be interrupted only for toilet activities until the acute pain has eased. To save money, this program is generally begun at home. Additional modalities, such as heat and massage, may help relieve the discomfort. When the pain decreases, the patient is permitted several brief periods out of bed, during which he may stand or walk but not sit; sitting is permitted only for meals.

Muscle relaxants and narcotic analgesics are useful in treating acute symptoms. They should be used judiciously, however, for fear of developing dependence. Anti-inflammatory medication or a defined regimen of salicylates are often preferable. It is essential, however, to stress the primary importance of mechanical rest.

Once the acute symptoms have subsided, the patient is allowed progressively more activity, with careful avoidance of heavy lifting and prolonged sitting. A program of flexion and stretching exercises is begun to improve posture and abdominal muscle tone. A lumbosacral corset or light back brace may be of help. For obese patients, weight reduction is mandatory. High-heeled shoes should be discouraged because they require the wearer to flex the knee and hip for balance, involving secondary hyperextension of the lumbar spine to maintain an erect posture. Encouragement and a positive attitude on the part of the physician are essential to the success of the rehabilitation program. At George Washington University Medical Center, we have instituted group exercise and posture instruction classes directed by a physical therapist. Patient education in proper lifting techniques, avoidance of prolonged sitting, and faithful adherence to a moderate regimen of flexion and stretching exercises are stressed. Although a back support may help in mobilization and may be useful for vigorous activity over the long term, we prefer to have the patient develop his own musculature to support the back. In obese patients a support is of little use because it cannot gain adequate purchase to immobilize or support the spine.

If a supervised regimen of bed rest at home, exercises, support, and medication is not effective, a trial of traction in the hospital may be warranted. A careful search for intraspinal pathology should be made. Myelography or axial tomography may be necessary to demonstrate anterior pathology or spinal stenosis. Appropriate decompression should be performed for canal impingement. (A psychosocial evaluation is also important, because underlying problems may adversely influence a patient's symptoms and response to treatment.) Spinal fusion may be indicated if instability is present and other pathology has been ruled out. Because of the unpredictability of spinal fusion, we often use a trial of either a plaster or molded plastic jacket for six weeks in questionable cases. If the symptoms are relieved by external immobilization, spinal fusion may be offered to the patient. If the symptoms are not relieved by immobilization, fusion is unlikely to help.

THE UPPER EXTREMITY

The Shoulder

Primary osteoarthritis of the shoulder is rare. Before making the diagnosis, a careful search for a rotator cuff tear, tendinitis, or impingement syndromes must be performed. These soft tissue problems are more often the cause of shoulder pain than the actual joint degeneration. In the true osteoarthritic shoulder, a regimen of heat, exercises to maintain mobility, nonsteroidal anti-inflammatory agents, mild analgesics, and intermittent steroid injection often achieves symptomatic control. When these are insufficient, joint replacement may be indicated. Diagnosis and management of shoulder joint replacement are discussed in greater detail in Chapter 35.

The Elbow

Osteoarthritis of the elbow is usually post-traumatic. Pain and stiffness in varying proportions are the presenting complaints. Heat and systemic medication should be used to relieve symptoms and active range of motion exercises instituted to maintain mobility. Generally, passive stretching should not be done, because the irritation caused by the passive stretch often increases the symptoms and results in unimproved or even greater stiffness.

When symptoms predominantly involve the radiocapitellar joint (generally following an old fracture of the radial head or capitellum), radial head excision may be beneficial. Humeroulnar arthritis or panarthritis is more difficult to treat. Stiffness, the hallmark of elbow arthritis, tends to recur after the operation. Arthroplasty may be effective in relieving pain but rarely results in an appreciable increase in the range of motion. It is therefore the painful osteoarthritic elbow with acceptable motion that is best treated by arthroplasty. A painless, stiff elbow will not be markedly improved by surgery. Further advances in the treatment of elbow osteoarthritis will have to address the problem of stiffness.

THE LOWER EXTREMITY

The Hip

The advent of dependable, effective arthroplasty has revolutionized treatment of the osteoarthritic hip (Fig. 34-3). Total hip replacement is now the accepted treatment for degenerative hip disease in patients past middle age, providing they have sufficient pain or functional impairment to warrant surgical intervention. Along with dependable, rapid relief of pain, the procedure allows a rapid return to weight-bearing and requires only a modest rehabilitation program, making it applicable to even elderly patients. The details of postoperative rehabilitation for total hip replacement are described in Chapter 36.

Before considering total hip arthroplasty, the physician can prescribe various nonsurgical modalities that may provide substantial symptomatic relief and allow the patient to maintain a reasonable level of activity. These measures may forestall, or on occasion obviate, the need for reconstructive surgery. Salicylates or other nonsteroidal anti-inflammatory agents may be used as a maintenance regimen. A program of active exercises once or twice daily will also help to preserve range of motion. Assisted flexion of the hip to the chest and internal and external rotation are performed in the supine position. The patient is instructed to lie prone at least 30 minutes per day and perform active extension exercises of the hip, raising the leg off the bed, 20 times per day. This exercise will help retard the development of flexion contracture. Similarly, the patient is specifically instructed never to sleep with a pillow beneath the leg, since that will tend to worsen contractures.

By far the most effective physical modality, however, is a cane used in the hand opposite the symptomatic hip. Forces over three times the body weight are applied across the hip joint during normal walking. A cane used in the opposite hand drastically decreases the moment arm of the applied force against which the abductors must pull, reducing the forces across the hip joint by about 50 percent. Proper use of a cane often achieves dramatic results and allows many patients to resume a moderate activity level without severe discomfort.

When the foregoing measures fail to provide adequate pain relief or allow reasonable function, surgical rehabilitation is indicated. We do not use potent anti-inflammatory agents over a long period, nor do we suggest regular use of two external supports before recommending total hip arthroplasty. Because of long-

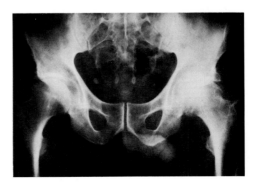

Fig. 34-3. An osteoarthritic left hip. Note joint space narrowing and sclerosis.

term concerns about loosening of the cement-bone bond and metal fatigue involving the femoral component, many centers are using surface replacement arthroplasty and porous coated components, implanted without cement, for selected patients. The role of these procedures *vis à vis* standard replacement arthroplasty is yet to be determined.

The Knee

The knee is comprised of three functioning compartments: the medial, the lateral, and the patellofemoral. Degenerative arthritis of the knee tends to involve one or two compartments selectively, most often the medial or patellofemoral. The pattern of arthritic involvement and the severity of symptoms determine the rehabilitation regimen.

Early osteoarthritis without significant angular deformity, contracture, or joint space narrowing is best treated by anti-inflammatory agents and exercises. The exercise program is of primary importance to maintain strength and stability; this importance must be explained to the patient. The patient is instructed to perform 100 straight-leg raises on the affected side two or three times per day. Quadriceps setting may be added. Progressive-resistance exercises or anything else that involves resisted extension of the knee are specifically prohibited. Although successful in rehabilitating acute injuries and following ligament reconstruction, such exercises exert large forces across the patellofemoral joint. Because some degree of patellofemoral arthritis is generally present, the symp-

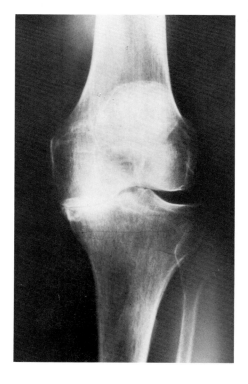

Fig. 34-4. Medial compartment arthritis of the knee. Note loss of normal valgus alignment.

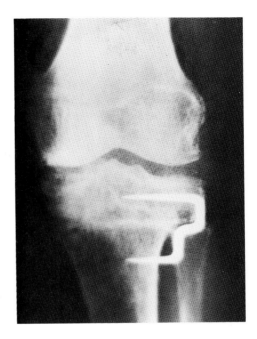

Fig. 34-5. The same patient after high tibial osteotomy to realign the leg. The patient experienced great relief from pain.

toms will be made worse by application of large forces across the arthritic joint surfaces, thus defeating the entire rehabilitation regimen. Conversely, the simple straight-leg raising usually alleviates patellofemoral symptoms if followed explicitly. One should also caution the patient against sitting or sleeping with a pillow beneath the knee because it will lead to progressive flexion contracture.

When moderately advanced disease is present, with joint space narrowing, instability, and angular deformity, the regimen of exercises and anti-inflammatory agents should again be started. If symptoms persist, however, prompt consideration should be given to surgery. Most often the varus or bowleg deformity will be present with medial compartment symptoms (Fig. 34-4). High tibial osteotomy effectively restores normal alignment and provides symptomatic relief. If it is performed before severe deformity is present, an excellent long-term result can be expected. Because it conserves normal tissue, this procedure does not preclude, and indeed may forestall, subsequent replacement arthroplasty (Fig. 34-5). For this reason, it is especially useful in the younger and middle-aged patient with long life expectancy and significant functional demands. Because the symptoms and deformity are progressive, undue delay in performing surgery may be harmful; the deformity may progress to the point that osteotomy is no longer reliable. Meniscectomy removes a significant weight-bearing structure in the involved compartment and should not be performed. We have not found debridement or "housecleaning" procedures useful.

Severe deformity, multiple compartment disease, and elderly patients who are prone to postoperative stiffness are best treated by total knee arthroplasty. The details of rehabilitation following knee replacement are presented in Chapter 36.

The Ankle

Degenerative arthritis of the ankle is almost always post-traumatic. Some relief may be obtained from analgesics and anti-inflammatory medications. Exercises are generally not helpful. Immobilization often lessens the symptoms and may be achieved by a high-top boot, a plastic ankle-foot orthosis, or a molded or laced ankle boot. If bracing fails to relieve symptoms, surgery is indicated. Arthrodesis is the established treatment. The role of replacement arthroplasty is yet to be determined.

FUTURE DIRECTIONS

Further progress in the treatment of osteoarthritis will undoubtedly occur as better prostheses are developed for end-stage disease. Of equal importance will be the diagnosis of degeneration at an early stage when aggressive therapy may halt progression and avert the eventual need for joint replacement. Further research into the etiology of primary osteoarthritis may also provide clues to prevention, the ultimate therapy.

REFERENCES

1. Gordon, T.: Osteoarthrosis in U.S. adults. In *Population Studies of the Rheumatic Diseases, Proceedings of the Third International Symposium,* pp. 391–397. Excerpta Medica Foundation, New York, 1966.
2. Mankin, H. L.: The reaction of articular cartilage to injury and osteoarthritis. N. Engl. J. Med. 291:1335–1340, 1974.
3. Riordan, F. H., III: Pharmacologic treatment in osteoarthritis. In *American Academy of Orthopaedic Surgeons' Symposium on Osteoarthritis,* pp. 80–85. C. V. Mosby, St. Louis, 1976.
4. Schmorl, G., and Junghanns, H.: *Die Gesund und die Kranke Wirbelsaule in Rontgenbild und Klinik,* 3rd ed. George Thieme Verlag, Stuttgart, 1933.
5. Sokoloff, L.: *The Biology of Degenerative Joint Disease.* University of Chicago Press, Chicago, 1969.

35

Upper Limb Joint Replacement

Alfred B. Swanson, M.D., F.A.C.S.
Genevieve deGroot Swanson, M.D.
Judy Leonard, O.T.R.
Barbara Ziemba, O.T.R.

Articular pathology caused by trauma, rheumatoid arthritis, osteoarthritis, or infection is as old as mankind. Restoring function to unstable, stiff, or dislocated joints continues to be a complex challenge of reconstructive surgery. A successful arthroplasty should be stable, mobile, durable, retrievable, and free from pain. The postoperative care and rehabilitation program are of great significance to the final result of the arthroplasty. Individual variations presented by patients demand a great knowledge of the many factors involved as well as the ability to select the best-suited surgical and rehabilitation plan.

BASIC CONCEPTS OF ARTHROPLASTY

In order to bring the subject of rehabilitation after joint implant procedures in the upper extremity into perspective, it is first necessary to classify the various possible materials and methods used and understand the basic differences among them.

Classification of Implant Materials

Implant materials that can be used in reconstructive surgery of the extremities can be classified according to their physical characteristics: rigid (metals), semi-rigid (high-density polymers), and flexible (elastic polymers or elastomers).

There are different applications for each type of implant material. The rigid and semi-rigid materials have been most commonly used in total joint replacement prostheses. The flexible materials (silicone elastomers) have been used as an adjunct to resection arthroplasty. The two methods of arthroplasty differ appreciably.

Classification of Implant Fixation

Stabilizing the implant in the desired position for function is an important consideration for total joint replacement procedures and for flexible implant arthroplasty. Stabilization may be obtained by using:

> Fasteners, such as pins, screws, bolts, nails, and sutures.
>
> Mechanical interlocking, as with a stem, collar, sleevelike cap, or grooving on the implant.
>
> Physical bonding at the interface between the material and host with methyl methacrylate.
>
> Direct chemical bonding, that is, organic fixation of synthetic material to host tissues may be possible with some of the new ceramic materials, although the permanence of this bond is questionable.
>
> Ingrowth of tissue into the implant's fibers of loosely woven textiles or metallic fiber materials. The properties of such material must be seriously considered when used inside a synovial cavity, which will reject these relatively inert materials if they have rough surfaces and therefore an increased surface area. The time of immobilization necessary for tissue ingrowth results in joint stiffness and delays rehabilitation.
>
> Encapsulation around a smooth surface silicone implant with the use of capsuloligamentous reconstruction. All implants become encapsulated.

Classification of Arthroplasty Types

The possible combination of various types of implant materials and basic designs could be infinite. However, the basic designs for implants can be classified as follows: interposition arthroplasty, condylar replacement implant, ball and socket implant, the interlocking hinge with or without a transfixion pin, and the flexible hinge.

Classification of Arthroplasty Methods

Three different concepts of arthroplasty have emerged: resection arthroplasty, articulated joint replacement, and implant resection arthroplasty. These methods differ markedly in their concepts, designs, applications, material characteristics, and postoperative management.

Surgical Resection. Resecting bone in a stiffened, contracted joint can improve motion by shortening skeletal structures, lengthening soft parts, providing new gliding surfaces, and allowing nature to develop a new joint space with a supportive fibrous joint capsule. However, the results of this method are unpredictable because the prolonged postoperative fixation can compromise the expected range of motion. Furthermore, the joint space can gradually narrow and stiffness and subluxation may result. Bone absorption and remodeling at the amputated bone end are frequent occurrences, producing further shortening and joint instability. The unpredictable results of simple resection arthroplasty have been a challenge to continued research.

Articulated Joint Replacement. In this method, a mechanical model takes over the function of the joint. These so-called total joint or articulated joint replacements include three basic types of implants: unconstrained, semiconstrained, and constrained (fixed axis). The articulated implant usually requires fixation to the bone with cement. This approach certainly has attractive possibilities from the engineering standpoint and has found success mainly in the weight-bearing knee and hip joints. A problem remains, however, with the total dependency on insubstantial synthetic materials at the boundary between it and the human tissues. As a result, any implanted device is only as successful as its biomechanical and biological tolerance by human host tissues. The method used to replace small joints of the extremities with mechanical hinges or partial implants has met with mixed success and limited acceptance;[3] in many cases the bone has not tolerated the hard material. Bone absorption and material breakdown have negated many of the early good results obtained. Articulated implants made of rigid materials designed to replace the small joints of the hand have proved technically difficult for the operator and biomechanically unforgiving. Furthermore, it is extremely difficult to cement implants into small bones without injuring the bone or failing to get an adequate permanent fixation. Again, the results are biomechanically unforgiving. At the level of the wrist, articulated implants are popular but they have presented problems related to excessive removal of bone stock and loosening of the devices. At the level of the elbow and the shoulder joints, articulated implants are the subject of continuous research and development;[8] some have shown a moderate success. Yet loosening or fracture of the devices due to the severe torque forces present at these joints continue to present difficulties.

Implant Resection Arthroplasty. In our earlier observations of the simple resection arthroplasty technique, it appeared to us that is we could in some way provide internal support to guide the healing process, the ideal joint substitute could perhaps be found. From this hypothesis, the senior author originated in 1962 a research project to design and develop flexible (silicone) implants to be used as an adjunct to resection arthroplasty.[8] This is an easier and safer alternative because it helps nature build her own joint system through the resection arthroplasty concept. The method provides an excellent functional restoration, although not an anatomical one. By minimizing the demands of the synthetic materials and simulating the biomechanics of the human joint system, it is much more likely that the improved resection arthroplasty will be long lived and free of disastrous complications.

From the rehabilitation standpoint, articulated implants require less postoperative immobilization and guided mobilization than in resection arthroplasty, with or without a flexible implant, because they are less dependent on the encapsulation healing process. However, in order to obtain an optimal range of motion and strength, an equally intensive rehabilitation effort will be required.

GENERAL PRINCIPLES OF REHABILITATION

Wounding of any part of the body produces a vascular reaction and edema. This reaction can result in scar formation that in turn can cause stiffness. From the early stages of treatment, every measure should be taken to decrease, if not prevent, unnecessary residual stiffness. Knowledge and strict application of certain basic principles of care are therefore essential to obtain the optimal result. They include proper operative dressing, immobilization in a functional position, and postoperative elevation, motion, and exercises. A brief review of these principles as they apply to implant arthroplasty procedures in the hand, wrist, and elbow, and to total joint replacement of the elbow and shoulder will be discussed.

The patient must be an active participant in the rehabilitation process. The best method to obtain the patient's full cooperation is to provide him with detailed information about the surgical plan, the specific course of postoperative management, and a realistic evaluation of future goals and forseeable limitations.

Constrictive operative dressings and early passive movements should be avoided. Proper elevation of the hand and the extremity will enhance venous return, decrease the escape of fluids into interstitial spaces of the injured parts, and reduce edema. Early motion of the operated joints, when indicated, is important to maintain muscle length, reduce edema, prevent ligament contracture and adhesions of tendons and other gliding surfaces, and maintain the hand's architecture. Motion should be encouraged at the level of the joints not operated upon to avoid sympathetic dystrophy. The rheumatoid patient has usually experienced some loss of motion and functional impairment already. He should be frequently examined for any loss of mobility of the elbow and shoulder, for even a few degrees of loss of abduction and external rotation may signal an impending shoulder-hand syndrome. If instituted early and continued throughout the treatment program, circumduction exercises of the shoulder and active movements of the digit, especially with the hand elevated, will avoid many of the disastrous effects seen in improperly treated patients.

Specific exercises for the reconstructed part must follow an organized and supervised regimen. Exercise programs should be gradually progressive and carried out with a minimum of pain. Passive movements should be avoided in the very early stages. The patient should learn how to relax the muscles as well as contract isolated muscle groups. It is advisable for the patient to use the extremity protectively during the early postoperative phase. The postoperative rehabilitation program must be continued for at least three months after surgery because of the tendency of these previously stiffened joints to tighten up. It is best to be gradual rather than abrupt in discontinuing the exercises and wise to recommend a weekly self-evaluation of the range of motion to maintain the desired results. Following this, the patient can safely use the extremity for the activities of daily living and working. However, the patient should continue to exercise and splint as necessary for up to a year after surgery. Rough usage of the hand is not recommended.

Rehabilitation techniques are highly individualized, varying with each reconstructive surgeon and each joint treated. A physical therapist, occupational therapist, or other trained personnel can be of assistance in carrying out postoperative therapy programs. However, they require close supervision by the physician for proper adherence to the prescribed program.

POSTOPERATIVE REHABILITATION FOR FLEXIBLE IMPLANT ARTHROPLASTY OF THE DIGITS

The postoperative care and rehabilitation program are critical for the quality of the outcome of finger joint implant arthroplasty. In the flexible implant arthroplasty method, the implant acts as a dynamic spacer that separates the bone ends while maintaining alignment of the joint, as an internal mold to support the development of the new joint capsule, and as a flexible hinge. This concept can be expressed as follows:

$$Bone\ resection\ +\ implant\ +\ encapsulation\ =\ new\ joint$$

One of the most important functions of a flexible implant is to maintain internal alignment and spacing of the reconstructed joint while early motion is started, with the implant acting as a dynamic spacer. Early guided motion is essential in promoting the development of a new, functionally adapted fibrous capsule. That collagen formation and development can be guided is a basic concept to be understood by surgeons who undertake arthroplasty procedures.[5] As with simple resection arthroplasty, if motion is restricted during the healing phase, there will be poor mobility of the joint. Therefore the host tissue or collagen reaction must be used advantageously. The fact that the collagen capsule can be reinforced at surgery and trained postoperatively is used prospectively in the formation of the new joint.

If arthroplasty is to be considered, the patient must be cooperative and in good general condition. The skin and neurovascular status must be adequate and the elements necessary to produce a functional musculotendinous system must be available, along with adequate bone stock to receive and support the implant. Adequate facilities must also be available for the operative and postoperative therapy.

Variations of the arthritic involvement presented by many patients demand great mastery of the factors implicated. Reconstructive procedures of weight-bearing joints of the lower extremity that will require walking with crutches should precede upper extremity reconstruction. Excessive manual labor and awkward hand weight-bearing, such as seen in some crutch walkers, should be avoided after surgery. If crutch walking cannot be avoided, special platform-type crutches should be used. Multiple reconstructive procedures must be staged appropriately. Tendon repair and synovectomy of tendon sheaths should be done six to eight weeks before joint reconstruction in the rheumatoid hand. However, if the extensor tendons are ruptured and the metacarpophalangeal (MCP) joints dislocated, arthroplasty of the MCP joints is done before the finger joints. In swanneck deformity, arthroplasties of the MCP and proximal interphalangeal (PIP) joints are performed at the same stage. However, in boutonniere deformity, it is preferable to reconstruct the PIP joint before the MCP joint. Any tendon imbalance or bone and joint malalignment must be corrected; otherwise it will affect the long-term result of joint replacement. Precise anatomical dissection, adequate soft tissue release, respect for gliding surfaces, prevention of edema, and early guided movement in functional planes are essential for good results in arthroplasty procedures.

The postoperative dressing should support the arches of the hand, control its alignment, and provide adequate compression without constriction. It is fashioned with Dacron batting applied longitudinally, and it includes a small palmar plaster splint to maintain the wrist in neutral position. Pressure on the radial side of the hand should be avoided; proper alignment of the digits can be supported by applying Webril gauze strips to the ulnar side of the digits. Proper elevation of the hand and extremity will enhance venous return and reduce edema. The use of a special arm sling that can be attached to an intravenous infusion stand has been very helpful. Slings should not routinely be worn when the patient is in the upright position, as they may prevent use of the extremity.

The greatest challenge in postoperative rehabilitation of finger joint arthroplasty is maintaining a proper balance between good healing of the surrounding scar tissue while applying proper amounts of tension across the scar to obtain the desired range of motion. Controlled motion during this period will train the new capsule to have sufficient looseness for flexion and extension and sufficient tightness in the medial-lateral plane for rotation and angular stability. An adjustable and dynamic brace is necessary to guide the motion of the joint across desired planes and prevent recurrent deformity during the early postoperative course. Scar formation will vary according to the joint involved, the type of surgery performed, and the differences in collagen reaction of each patient. The associated tendon deficiencies also vary. It is therefore the responsibility of the operating surgeon to control the process by providing a well-organized rehabilitation program. The patients receive specific instructions and are regularly followed in the early postoperative period. They are instructed to sit comfortably to stabilize the proximal joints, including those of the shoulder, elbow, and wrist, and to concentrate their movement at the reconstructed joints. Once the sutures are removed, the patients can precede their exercises with an oil or lotion massage. The follow-up should be meticulous and include objective measurements of the patient's progress, because it is as important to the patient's prognosis as the surgical procedure. To fail to understand this is to miss the opportunity of a complete success.

THE DYNAMIC BRACE

We have designed a brace to facilitate early postoperative motion in our patients who undergo finger joint implant resection arthroplasties. Its use has greatly improved the anatomical and functional results. The brace prevents undue stretching of associated reconstructed tendons and ligaments, and it assists the digital extensors and flexors, which are frequently weak from long-standing deformity, accompanying tenosynovitis, and fibrosis. The dynamic brace has three major functions: to provide complete and adjustable correction of residual deformity, control motion in the desired plane and range, and assist flexor and extensor power.

The basic brace for finger joint arthroplasty consists of a dorsal splint that provides a stable base for outriggers and supports the wrist. The brace is available in three basic sizes. Three transverse straps attached to the dorsal splint are made of malleable metal for easy adjustment to the shape and size of the forearm. Adjustable Velcro straps are attached to these transverse straps to hold the brace in position. Two Velcro straps are placed around the forearm and one across the palm; the latter has a palmar pad to help maintain the arches of the hand and prevent rotation of the brace. A transverse bar to which finger slings are attached is fitted onto a dorsal arm. The position of the transverse bar can be adjusted in all three planes. The finger slings are made of soft plastic with multiple perforations and are connected to the transverse bar with rubber bands. Small radially placed outriggers may be added for correction of pronation deformity often present in the index and middle fingers of rheumatoid hands. A longer bar can be used for thumb abduction. All of these outriggers are attached with thumb screws. A flexion cuff is used to help correct flexor weakness. This sheepskin cuff is attached to the dorsal splint, passes around the digits, and draws them into flexion by the pull of a Velcro strap attached through a loop on the proximal portion of the brace. With this cuff, the finger joints can be passively brought into flexion for prescribed periods of time during the day. A figure-eight elbow strap is used to prevent distal migration of the brace when the cuff is used.

POSTOPERATIVE REHABILITATION FOR ARTHROPLASTIES OF THE METACARPOPHALANGEAL JOINTS

Goals and Special Considerations

In our experience, the results of an organized postoperative program for these patients are so much better than those of any other method that every attempt should be made by the surgeon to provide this type of care.[8,9]

The ideal motion to be obtained following implant resection arthroplasty at the MCP joints is adequate flexion of the ulnar digits, allowing the surface of their pulps to touch the palm at the distal palmar crease for adequate grasp of smaller objects. Full flexion of the index and middle fingers is less critical for grasping, since these digits are mainly used for pinch activities. A degree of spreading of the fingers into abduction, especially of the index finger, is important. Full extension at these joints is also important for performing normal hand activities and maintaining the balance of the distal joints. Chronic flexion deformity of the MCP joints can further aggravate hyperextension tendencies at the PIP joints. Pronation deformity of the index finger and occasionally the middle finger can be a problem in the rheumatoid hand and can, to some degree, be corrected in the postoperative program.

Patients who have normal PIP joints frequently will not gain the full expected motion at the MCP joint following arthroplasty because they tend to flex the PIP joint during their exercise program and thus immobilize their MCP joints. To gain active motion of the MCP joints in these patients, we occasionally will tape small padded aluminum splints on the dorsum of the PIP joints for the first three or four weeks after surgery to encourage the patient to localize all flexion force at the MCP joint. This seems to improve the range of motion obtained. Occasionally, temporary Kirschner wire fixation of the PIP joints can also be used for the same purpose.

Brace Fitting and Treatment

The voluminous, conforming, operative hand dressing is left on until the postoperative swelling has decreased, usually in three to five days. The dynamic brace is applied over a lightly padded dressing after removal of the postoperative dressing. If the brace is not available, guided early motion may still be obtained by applying a lightweight, short arm cast fitted with outriggers and similar rubber-band slings.

The dorsal wrist splint, with a 0.62 cm felt pad placed between the forearm and the brace, should be applied loosely enough so that it is not constrictive, yet tightly enough so that it does not rotate on the forearm and hand. If there is a tendency toward continued swelling, the limb may be elevated with the wrist supported in extension against an intravenous infusion stand. Active exercises in the elevated position may then be carried out.

The rubber-band slings are placed on the proximal phalanges to guide the alignment of the digits into the desired position. The pull of the slings should be adjusted in a slight radial deviation to prevent recurrent ulnar drift. The tension of the rubber bands should be tight enough to support the digits and yet loose enough to allow 70 degrees of active flexion; this is especially true of the little finger, which may have weak flexion power. The brace may require adjustment once or twice a day in the early postoperative course. The thumb outrigger is usually applied because of the patient's tendency to bring the thumb over the fingers on flexion. Formation of this habit should be avoided because the lateral pressure of the thumb on the index finger could result in recurrent ulnar drift deformity.

If there is a tendency toward rotation (pronation) in the index or middle fingers, additional outrigger bars are applied to provide a rotation force at the MCP joint based on the concept of a force couple. A force couple is defined as two equal and opposite forces that act along parallel lines. It is obtained by applying the loops to the digit that shows a tendency for pronation, as shown in Figure 35-1. A rubber-band sling is fitted from an additional outrigger to the distal phalanx of the digit tending to pronation. The combined pull of two slings provides a torque force in the direction of supination on the digit without interfering with flexion and extension movements.

The extension portion of the brace is worn continuously day and night for the first three weeks. Meanwhile, specific flexion measures are prescribed. The flexion exercises in the brace with the extension slings in position are carried out,

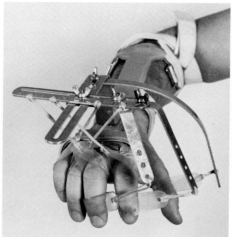

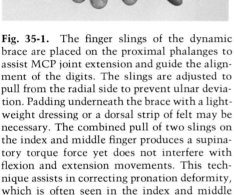

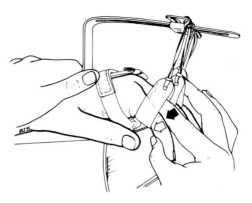

Fig. 35-1. The finger slings of the dynamic brace are placed on the proximal phalanges to assist MCP joint extension and guide the alignment of the digits. The slings are adjusted to pull from the radial side to prevent ulnar deviation. Padding underneath the brace with a lightweight dressing or a dorsal strip of felt may be necessary. The combined pull of two slings on the index and middle finger produces a supinatory torque force yet does not interfere with flexion and extension movements. This technique assists in correcting pronation deformity, which is often seen in the index and middle fingers of rheumatoid hands. Note the thumb outrigger to control abduction and the slings for the little and ring fingers.

Fig. 35-2. Active and passive flexion exercises are carried out in the brace starting on the third postoperative day. No more than 0.9 kg of force should be applied when assisting passive flexion, as shown here. The arm is positioned over a book to help stabilize the proximal joints yet allow the digits movement. Proper adjustment of the tension of the rubber bands is essential for full range of motion. The extension portion of the brace is worn continually for the first three weeks.

starting at three days postoperatively, both actively and passively (with no more than 0.90 kg of force) on an hourly basis (Fig. 35-2). The ideal goal of zero degrees extension to 70 degrees flexion is constantly stressed. The patient is seen at least three times by the physician or the therapist during the first week, and the brace is carefully readjusted as necessary. Only exceptionally, that is, if the little finger exhibits marked flexor weakness with adequate extensor stability, can the extension sling be removed from this digit during the exercise periods.

During the second and third weeks, the extension portion of the brace is also worn continuously day and night. If there is severe flexor weakness and good extension, the extensor sling can be removed one to two hours a day to achieve greater active flexion of the MCP joints. If the patient appears not to be obtaining 70 degrees of flexion, several measures can be taken. Should most of the motion be occurring at the PIP joints, they can be immobilized with small, dorsal, taped-on, and padded aluminum splints to help localize the flexion force at the MCP joints. The rubber bands may be lengthened to decrease the extension force applied. Occasionally, temporary Kirschner wire fixation of the PIP joints can also be applied for the same functional purpose.

At three weeks any residual lack of flexion should be treated energetically. The flexion cuff may be worn one to two hours twice a day to flex the MCP joints passively. As this cuff is used, the figure-eight elbow strap should be applied to prevent distal migration of the brace (Fig. 35-3A). The patient may use the flexion cuff to obtain further flexion during active flexion exercises. Other devices for improving flexion in the presence of adequate extension are those for traction. Finger slings on the proximal phalanges can be attached volarly to the loop of a special Velcro wrist strap or to the wrist strap of the dynamic brace (Fig. 35-3B). If the distal interphalangeal (DIP) and PIP joints are stable, dressmaker hooks can be glued to the fingernails with a cyanoacrylate adhesive. Individual rubber bands are then attached from the loop of the special wrist strap to the nail hooks. Initially this is done over a 5.62 cm wooden dowel to encourage flexion (Fig. 35-3C). As the flexion increases, the size of the dowel is progressively reduced to obtain even more flexion. A finger crutch can also be substituted for the dowel. Eventually this traction device is used without any grasping device. A small Band-aid is applied over the hooks to avoid snagging them between exercise periods. Traction methods allow better alignment and more control over the desired amount of flexion pull for each individual finger. With an adequate extensor mechanism, they can be started during the early postoperative course in certain cases presenting severe preoperative stiffness or flexion weakness. In these difficult cases a functional compromise can be reached by sacrificing a few degrees of extension.

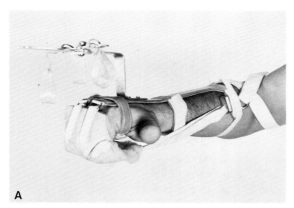

A

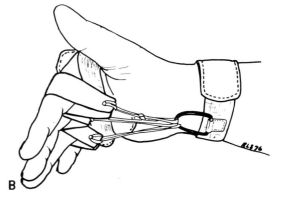

B

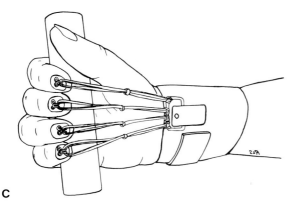

C

Fig. 35-3A–C. Passive flexion devices that can be used by the third postoperative week. (A) The flexion cuff is placed in a position for passively assisting flexion of the joints. The Velcro strap pulls to the radial side and may be used by the patient to increase the stretching effort gradually. The figure-eight elbow strap should be used to prevent distal migration of the brace. (B) Finger slings placed on the proximal phalanges are attached to the loop of a special Velcro wrist strap or to the strap of the dynamic brace to provide flexion traction. (C) If the interphalangeal joints are stable, this is an extremely efficient method of obtaining passive flexion of the MCP joints after arthroplasty.

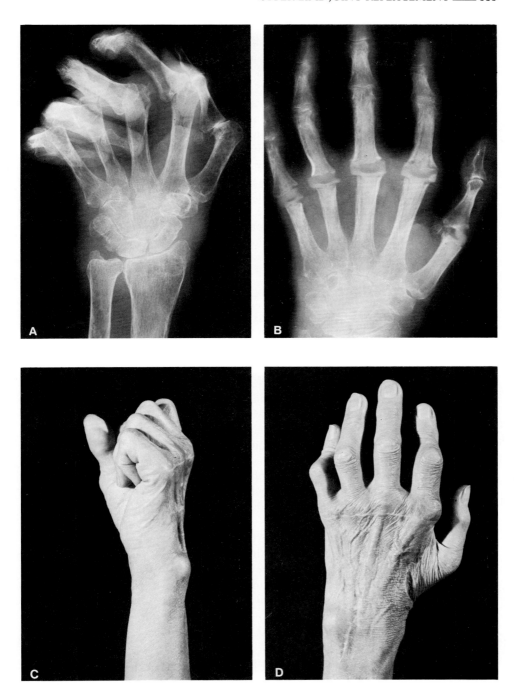

Fig. 35-4A–D. Preoperative radiogram and the results (two years later) of flexible-implant resection arthroplasty of all five MCP joints. Note the improved appearance of the hand: the correction of deformities is good, as is the tolerance of the implants on the radiogram. The patient remains free of pain and has a functional range of flexion and extension.

The extension portion of the brace is usually worn solely at night, starting at the fourth postoperative week and continuing for another three weeks. In cases in which there is a persistent extensor lag, a tendency for flexion contracture, or a deviation of the digits, continued part-time support with the brace must be prescribed for several more weeks or even months. The patient should follow a continued exercise and stretching program for three months postoperatively to maintain the movement obtained in the early phase. After this time, the final range of motion will have been established (Figs. 35-4A–D).

Collagen maturity and scar contracture vary from patient to patient. The associated tendon deficiencies also vary. Therefore the use of the brace in the postoperative period requires tailoring and careful follow-up by the operating surgeon. The patient's progress is evaluated by measuring the range of motion with accurate goniometer readings; the movements of the digits are observed without the brace to be sure that the patient is getting the desired result. The reconstructed joints start tightening up during the second postoperative week and will be quite tight by the end of three weeks. If the desired range of motion has not been obtained by three weeks, it will be difficult to gain further improvement in motion.

POSTOPERATIVE REHABILITATION FOR THUMB METACARPOPHALANGEAL JOINT ARTHROPLASTIES

Flexible-hinge implant arthroplasty of the thumb MCP joint may be indicated for reconstruction of the painful rheumatoid, degenerative, and post-traumatic disabilities with severe destruction of the MCP joint, and for associated stiffness of distal joint or basal joints, or boutonniere deformity when the MCP joint is destroyed and the distal joint needs fusion. This procedure has provided adequate stability and the increased flexion permitted is especially important for fine coordinated movements. Following implant insertion and repair of the extensor mechanism, the DIP joints is temporarily fixed in extension with a small Kirschner wire passed longitudinally through the finger pulp into the flexor tendon sheath. This is removed in two to three days.

The conforming surgical dressing is removed after three to five days. Because stability rather than mobility is desired, the thumb MCP joint is maintained in zero degrees of extension for three to four weeks with a padded aluminum splint. The splint extends to the distal end of the thumb and runs proximally to the wrist. It is taped in position around the thumb and wrist. No special exercises are prescribed after splint removal except for normal functional adaptations. Forceful activities should be avoided for six to eight weeks postoperatively.

POSTOPERATIVE REHABILITATION FOR PROXIMAL INTERPHALANGEAL JOINT ARTHROPLASTIES

Postoperative care for the PIP joint depends upon several factors. There are three basic situations: reconstruction of a stiff PIP joint, reconstruction of a swan-neck deformity, and reconstruction of a boutonniere deformity.

When the implant arthroplasty has been performed without a tendon reconstruction for a stiff PIP joint, active movements of flexion and extension should be started within three to five days after surgery. The ideal range of motion following this surgery is of zero degrees of extension to 70 degrees of flexion. Small, taped-on, padded aluminum splints to hold the digit in extension are worn mainly as night splints and may be used for several weeks postoperatively, depending upon the degree of extensor lag present. A few degrees of extensor lag can usually be expected in this type of surgery. The same splint may also be applied slightly to the ulnar or radial side of the dorsum of the digit to correct any associated angulatory deformity. Active flexion-extension exercises can be performed with a variety of exercise devices. If necessary, the DIP joint may be temporarily pinned with a Kirschner wire to concentrate the action of the flexor profundus at the PIP joint. These pins can be removed after about three weeks.

If the implant resection arthroplasty of the PIP joint has been performed for a swan-neck deformity in association with a tendon reconstruction procedure, a padded, taped-on aluminum splint is usually placed on the digit after the postoperative edema has subsided. The joint is immobilized in 10–20 degrees of flexion, and the splint is left on for ten days until the exercises are begun. It is important to obtain at least 10 degrees of flexion contracture of these joints in order to prevent recurrent hyperextension tendencies. Unless the central slip has been released, there may be an imbalance of the joint in favor of extension. During the healing phase, the digit should be held in the flexed position with the aluminum splints at least on a part-time basis. The DIP joint must not remain in severe flexion—it may be temporarily pinned in a neutral position. Pinning will localize the flexion forces at the PIP joint and help the recovery of movement. The MCP joint should be supported in extension with the rubber-band slings of the brace or with the reverse lumbrical bar. After the second week, gentle passive flexion exercises of the PIP joint can be started if necessary.

If the implant resection arthroplasty procedure has been done to correct a boutonniere deformity, it is important to maintain the extension of the PIP joint and allow flexion of the DIP joint. The DIP joint, if in severe hyperextension, should be released by sectioning the lateral tendons over the middle phalanx or by lengthening the lateral tendons. The reconstruction of the extensor mechanism should be protected for approximately ten days with an extension splint applied after the postoperative swelling has decreased. In this situation, the aluminum splint should immobilize only the PIP joint in extension for three to six weeks, depending on the degree of extension lag present. The distal joint should be allowed to flex freely. Active flexion and extension exercises are usually started 10–14 days after surgery in alternation with the extension splint. The splint is worn at night to hold the PIP joint in extension until the position of the joint is stable, which may require ten weeks.

A Kirschner wire passed into the flexor sheath through the fingertip can be used as a temporary internal splint for immobilization of the DIP or PIP joints. A 0.087 cm wire is carefully passed through the fingertip from the distal to proximal joints; the wire should end up touching the palmar aspect of the proximal end of the proximal phalanx. It is left in place for several days or until the postoperative swelling has decreased sufficiently to permit the application of splints with circumferential bandaging.

The exercises for the PIP joint can be carried out actively and passively,

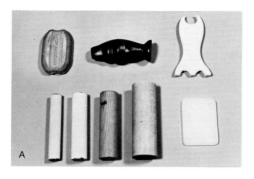

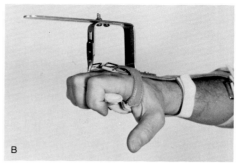

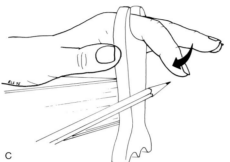

Fig. 35-5. (A) A variety of exercise devices are needed to increase joint motion and strength. (B) The reverse lumbrical bar can be used to support the proximal phalanges and eliminate motion of the MCP joints during flexion exercises. Note the palmar pad for maintaining the transverse arches of the hand preventing rotation of the brace. The flexion cuff can be applied to force flexion gently if necessary. (C) We designed a "finger crutch" to help support the proximal phalanx in extension during flexion exercises.

always taking care to support the MCP joint in extension. This can be done with the opposite hand, either over the edge of a book or with a variety of orthotic devices, as shown in Figure 35-5A. Extension of the MCP joints can also be supported with the reverse lumbrical bar attached to the dynamic brace or to a special wrist splint (Fig. 35-5B). Passive flexion can then be obtained with the flexor cuff or with rubber-band traction to fingernail hooks. A dowel can also be used to support the MCP joints. We have developed a small "finger crutch" that we have used in a similar fashion to the Bunnell wood block to support the proximal phalanx during the exercises. It is made of a 0.62 cm plywood or hard rubber material (Fig. 35-5C). We have also developed another exercise device, shown in the upper middle of Figure 35-5A. The shape of the device supports the proper anatomical position of the digits and the arches of the hand. It is made in progressive sizes to obtain an improved range of motion. Passive stretching of flexion contractures of the PIP joint can be carried out by blocking hyperextension of the MCP joint with the standard lumbrical bar and by applying extension force to the middle phalanx with the extension rubber-band slings of the dynamic brace (Fig. 35-6).

POSTOPERATIVE REHABILITATION FOR DISTAL INTERPHALANGEAL JOINT ARTHROPLASTIES

A double-hinged implant can be an adjunct to resection arthroplasty of the DIP joint. It may be indicated for correction of degenerative or post-traumatic disabilities when preservation of joint motion is desired and the following

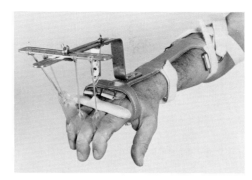

Fig. 35-6. Passive stretching of a joint requires the use of the three-point principle of pressure application. The brace can be adjusted to stretch the PIP joints in extension with the lumbrical bar in normal position for cases of flexion deformities. This adaptation of the brace should not be used after MCP joint arthroplasty because it may produce a subluxation of the base of the proximal phalanx toward the palm.

conditions are present: destroyed and painful joints; stiffened joints in which soft tissue release alone would be inadequate; and presence of adequate bone, ligamentous integrity, a potential tendon system, and an adequate skin and neurovascular system.

The postoperative care is similar to that of a mallet finger. The DIP and PIP joints are splinted in full extension for the first two weeks. Then only the distal joint is immobilized in extension for another four weeks—the PIP joint is allowed to flex freely. After this time, use of the digit is resumed. Active extension and flexion exercises are prescribed. As in any finger joint arthroplasty, rough activity is not recommended.

POSTOPERATIVE REHABILITATION FOR IMPLANT ARTHROPLASTIES OF THE CARPAL BONES

Silicone carpal bone implants can be used as spacers following resection of diseased carpal bones (trapezium, scaphoid, or lunate). These implants can satisfactorily maintain joint space and alignment following bone resection.[8] Adequate capsuloligamentous support and continuity around these implants are essential for early and late stability, and they must be obtained at surgery. The role of the palmar ligament structures in maintaining stability of carpal implants is critical. Carpal bones are completely surrounded by a capsuloligamentous structure; any disruption in these supporting structures following trauma or total resection of a carpal bone will result in instability of the implant replacement. Therefore when resecting carpal bones a thin shelf of bone is left at the base of the excision to preserve the ligamentous integrity. If a defect in these structures is present, it should be repaired with a tendon graft or a tendon slip from an adjacent tendon. When intercarpal stability is good or a firm capsuloligamentous system can be reconstructed, good long-term results can be expected. The implant must be kept in anatomical position during the healing period so that the encapsulation will become secure. Ideally the implant should not be permanently fixed to the surrounding bones, because that would result in localization of forces at the fixation point that can cause bone absorption, tissue necrosis, and implant failure. Consequently, temporary fixation of the carpal implants to an adjacent carpal bone is recommended. This type of fixation can be achieved with a suture or a pinning technique. Such temporary measures have become feasible now that implants are manufactured of a more tear-resistant silicone material.

IMPLANT ARTHROPLASTY OF THE THUMB BASAL JOINTS

The problems presented at the thumb basal joints must be correctly evaluated, and they are different in osteoarthritis and rheumatoid arthritis. Therefore, based on the senior author's long-term experience, two distinct methods of implant arthroplasty have been designed: the standard trapezium implant replacement[8] and the trapeziometacarpal joint implant arthroplasty.[8] The use of an implant in resection arthroplasty of the thumb basal joints has definite advantages over simple resection arthroplasty or fusion procedures. By acting as a space filler, it helps to preserve the anatomical relationships of the basal joints of the thumb after resection arthroplasty. The implant aids stability and prevents the tendency toward subluxation that may occur after simple resection arthroplasty. It also obviates the disadvantages of rigidity and poor positioning of the thumb that frequently present after fusion procedures. The important motion at the base of the thumb is maintained without loss of stability; there is good pain relief and improved strength. Meticulous capsuloligamentous reconstruction around these implants and correction of any associated deformity of the thumb are essential for good results.

The trapezium implant is a flexible, one-piece, intramedullary stemmed implant designed to help preserve the anatomical relationships of the thumb basal joints after resection arthroplasty of the trapezium. It is maintained in proper alignment by a triangular intramedullary stem that fits into the first metacarpal and by capsuloligamentous reconstruction around the implant. The head of the implant has a slightly concave surface to provide a more stable fit on the rounded articular surface of the scaphoid. In osteoarthritis, the trapezium is usually the center of a generalized or pantrapezial arthritic process. Fusion or interpositional arthroplasty of the trapeziometacarpal joint does not remove the diseased tissue in the other three joints. Therefore a total trapeziectomy will be necessary in most of these cases to eliminate all arthritic pain. In the presence of good bone stock, a trapezium implant can be used as an adjunct to this resection arthroplasty. This procedure is also indicated in post-traumatic arthritis, such as following an old Bennett's fracture, or in rheumatoid arthritis with localized bony changes when the following conditions are present: localized pain and palpable crepitation during circumduction movements, with axial compression of the thumb ("grind test"); loss of motion, with decrease of normal pinch and grip strength; radiological evidence of arthritic changes of the trapeziometacarpal, trapezioscaphoid, trapeziotrapezoid, and trapezium-second metacarpal joints, singly or in combination; or unstable, stiff, or painful distal joints of the thumb or swan-neck collapse deformity.

Many patients, especially those with rheumatoid arthritis, present disabilities of the thumb basal joints with severe displacement, absorption, or fusion of the contiguous carpal bones, all of which make trapezium arthroplasty difficult. Instead of carrying out a trapeziectomy, a limited resection of the base of the metacarpal and distal surface of the trapezium is done. A specially designed convex condylar implant is then used as an adjunct to the trapeziometacarpal resection arthroplasty. Because of the narrowness of the joint space, the usual range of motion obtained with the standard trapezium implant cannot be expected. A stable, pain-free, functioning thumb joint is obtained if the recommended technique has been followed.

The postoperative care and rehabilitation program are similar for both the trapezium and trapeziometacarpal implant arthroplasty methods. The wound is closed and drained and a secure dressing, including anterior and posterior plaster splints, is applied. It is also possible to apply a plaster cast at the end of the operative procedure; the cast should be bivalved and the extremity elevated because of the potential postoperative swelling. After four to five days the dressing is changed and the drains removed; a short arm-thumb spica cast is then applied. If a Kirschner wire is used, a small window is made over the area of exit of the pin to prevent wobbling of the wire by the cast. In two to three weeks the wire is extracted. After six weeks, the cast is removed and the patient is instructed to start a guarded range of motion, to include pinch and grasp activities. A small 2.5–5 cm diameter dowel can be grasped in the first web space to improve abduction and build strength in the hand and forearm.

POSTOPERATIVE REHABILITATION FOR SCAPHOID AND LUNATE IMPLANT ARTHROPLASTIES

Use of a silicone scaphoid implant may be considered upon diagnosis of the following clinical conditions: acute fractures, comminuted or grossly displaced; pseudarthrosis, especially with small proximal fragments; Preiser's disease; avascular necrosis of a fragment; or failures of previous surgery. Use of a silicone carpal lunate implant may be considered upon diagnosis of the following clinical conditions: Kienböck's disease; long-standing dislocations; localized osteoarthritic changes; or resistance to nonoperative measures. These procedures are contraindicated when there is a possibility for nonoperative treatment; generalized arthritis of the wrist; severe carpal instability with inadequate or irretrievable ligament or bone support to stabilize the implant; or greatly decreased bone space.

Once the operative procedure is completed, the incision is closed and drained. A secure dressing that includes an anterior plaster splint is applied. In scaphoid implant arthroplasty a long arm-thumb spica scaphoid cast is applied after three to five days, with the wrist in 20–30 degrees extension and slight radial deviation. In lunate implant arthroplasty, a short arm cast with the wrist in slight extension is applied. The cast is worn for six to eight weeks. If a pin is used, a window is made over its exit site and is removed after four weeks. The cast can also be applied at the end of the operative procedure providing it is bivalved and the extremity is kept elevated. Full use of the wrist is resumed at 12 weeks.

Postoperative roentgenograms should be made to evaluate the position of the implant. Serial roentgenograms should be made over the long-term postoperative course to evaluate the maintenance of the position of the wrist bones and the implant.

POSTOPERATIVE REHABILITATION FOR ULNAR HEAD IMPLANT ARTHROPLASTIES

An ulnar head replacement arthroplasty may be considered for disabilities of the distal radioulnar joint in rheumatoid, degenerative, and post-traumatic dysfunctions of this joint. Specific indications include presence of pain and weakness of the wrist joint unimproved by nonoperative procedures and instability of the ulnar head that shows radiographic evidence of dorsal subluxation and erosive changes. The procedure can also be used to correct sequelae of a simple ulnar head resection that failed.

At the end of the procedure, a voluminous, conforming hand dressing that includes a plaster palmar splint is applied, with the patient's hand in slight dorsiflexion. On the third postoperative day, the drain is removed and, if there is no swelling, a short arm cast or splint is applied in the same position to protect the wrist from excessive activity for three to four weeks. The best immobilization is obtained by using a long arm cast with the forearm in supination. However, most rheumatoid patients are quite inactive so that a lesser degree of immobilization is adequate. After cast removal, exercises similar to those described for radiocarpal joint implant arthroplasty are prescribed.

POSTOPERATIVE REHABILITATION FOR WRIST IMPLANT ARTHROPLASTIES

A wrist implant arthroplasty is indicated in case of arthritic or traumatic disability resulting in instability of the wrist from subluxation or dislocation of the radiocarpal joint; in severe deviation of the wrist that causes musculotendinous imbalance of the digits; in stiffness or fusion of the wrist in a nonfunctional position; or in stiffness of a wrist when movement is a requirement for hand function. The wrist reconstruction should usually be performed before surgery of the finger joints. Some feel the method is contraindicated in workers performing heavy manual labor, but others have reported using it successfully in such patients.[8] If the implant arthroplasty does not meet functional requirements, wrist fusion can be done later.

Once the procedure is completed, a voluminous, conforming hand dressing is applied that includes a plaster splint with the wrist in neutral position. The extremity is elevated for three to five days. A short arm cast keeping the wrist in neutral position is applied and fitted with outriggers to hold rubber-band slings for supporting finger extension if digital tendons have been repaired. The cast is worn for two to four weeks. During the period of plaster immobilization, the patient is encouraged to carry out active exercises for the MCP and interphalangeal joints. Isometric gripping exercises of the forearm muscles are started two to three weeks after surgery. Following cast removal, wrist exercises are progressively instituted. Flexion-extension exercises are carried out while the forearm is supported on a firm surface. The wrist is over an edge of, say, a table. Ulnar and radial deviation exercises are performed while the arm is held firmly and the hand is moved from side to side. Pronation-supination exercises for the forearm are done with the arm firmly against the body. If the patient shows a tendency to tightness, some active and passive stretching exercises are prescribed. A good ratio of stability to mobility is sought, because a joint that is too loose may be unstable. About 50–60 percent of normal flexion-extension movements is ideal. Three months after surgery, the active range of motion should be approximately from 45 degrees dorsiflexion to 45 degrees palmar flexion and 10 degrees of radial and ulnar deviation. The patient is cautioned against any activity, such as heavy labor or certain sports, that could produce repetitive stresses at the level of the wrist joint.

ELBOW JOINT IMPLANT REPLACEMENTS

The elbow is the intermediate joint of the upper extremity, forming the mechanical link between the first segment—the arm—and the second segment—the forearm. It has great importance in placing the hand in a functional zone. The problems of implant replacement at the level of the elbow joint are complex, since they are based on the specific anatomical and biomechanical requirements of this joint. Anatomically, the elbow constitutes only one joint with only one joint cavity. Biomechanically, it has two distinct functions: rotation involving the proximal radioulnar joint and flexion and extension involving the true elbow joint.

Implant replacement may be required at two different sites in the elbow joint: the capitellar-radioulnar joint and the ulnohumeral joint. Treatment of disabilities of the capitellar-radioulnar joint can be carried out by radial head resection arthroplasty with or without the use of a radial head implant.[8] Disabilities of the ulnohumeral joint can be treated in several ways, depending on the patient's age, activity requirements, and the level and severity of the disease process. Various therapies of choice consist of resection arthroplasty with or without interposition of biological materials, as for example, fascia lata or dermis; arthrodesis; hemiarthroplasty to replace the distal humerus, proximal ulna, or radial head; flexible (silicone) implant resection arthroplasty with reconstruction of the elbow ligaments; and articulated implant replacement with or without the use of a radial head component. These implants can be unconstrained, semiconstrained, or constrained.

RADIAL HEAD IMPLANT ARTHROPLASTY

Replacement of the radial head with a silicone implant can be indicated for rheumatoid, degenerative, or post-traumatic disabilities presenting pain, crepitation, and decreased motion at the radiohumeral or proximal radioulnar joint with joint destruction or subluxation visible on radiograms. Other indications include resistance to nonoperative treatment, primary replacement after fracture of the radial head, and symptomatic sequelae after radial head resection. Evidence of joint narrowing secondary to radiohumeral joint synovitis is not a contraindication to radial head implant replacement combined with elbow synovectomy. Inadequate bone stock or dislocation of the radius from the ulna are contraindications for radial head implant arthroplasty.

The operative dressing includes a posterior plaster splint applied when the elbow joint is in 90 degrees flexion. The splint is removed after three days and a light dressing is applied. Active flexion-extension and pronation-supination exercises are allowed and their frequency is increased progressively. The patient must avoid heavy lifting or stressful use of the elbow during the healing period. Full activity of the joint is resumed at six weeks. If necessary, gentle stretching exercises can be started at four to six weeks to increase the active range of motion. Early postoperative movements facilitate rehabilitation and increase the range of motion.

ULNOHUMERAL JOINT IMPLANT REPLACEMENT

A successful implant replacement of the elbow joint will be one that can restore a destroyed elbow to a pain-free, mobile, stable, and durable joint. It will have to tolerate compression and shearing stresses applied in flexion and extension in the sagittal plane as well as the torque stresses added when the elbow is used in the horizontal plane. However, full dependency on any synthetic device should never be expected.

The main difficulties in developing a total elbow joint prosthesis have centered on the fixation of the device, bone absorption at the bone-implant interface, and durability of the material. The physician and biological engineer have made great progress in the treatment of the destroyed elbow.[1,2] However, implant replacement of the elbow joint is still at an experimental and developmental stage. Postoperative management depends on the surgical techniques used. A secure repair of the triceps tendons incised in the operative exposure of the elbow is necessary. Protection of this repair must be considered during the rehabilitation phase for six weeks. Failure to obtain adequate extension of the elbow may be due to problems of the operation or failure in the postoperative rehabilitation program. Since active extension must be delayed, passive movements are emphasized. Guarded active extension may be started at three weeks, avoiding heavy resistance until the sixth or eighth week. When the ligament repair at the elbow is insecure, external bracing or bracing incorporating elbow hinges may be prescribed.

A rehabilitation program following a total elbow replacement may be indicated to improve the final range of motion and strength. If the soft tissue repair is considered to be secure, active, and gentle, assisted elbow flexion-extension and forearm pronation-supination are started between the fourth and sixth postoperative day. The arm is kept in a resting position so as to counteract gravitational forces. Motion at the shoulder, wrist, and hand is also encouraged. In some cases the use of static and dynamic elbow splints can be useful. The range of elbow flexion is slowly increased to 100 degrees, taking care to avoid stretching, pain, or resistance to the triceps muscle for at least two weeks or longer. After three weeks, light activities of daily living are possible, as is gentle prolonged stretching if indicated. Regular follow-up visits are mandatory to check progress in range of motion and strengthening.

SHOULDER IMPLANT REPLACEMENT

Implant replacement for the shoulder joint is at a developmental stage. Adequate results have been reported for pain relief and partial return of function.[1,4] However, a variety of problems have been met, including faulty implant design, difficult surgery due to complex anatomy of the area, difficulty in restoring the biomechanical requirements for shoulder joint function, and less than adequate durability of implant fixation. Two basic implant categories have been proposed: the first is a hemiarthroplasty in which the head of the humerus is replaced with an intramedullary stemmed implant. This operation has been reasonably successful in patients with sequelae of a fracture dislocation of the upper end of humerus. The second procedure encompasses a so-called total joint category in which four basic implant types are represented: an unconstrained type in which the humeral head and glenoid are resurfaced (Neer type);[6] a bipolar or bicentric implant type in which the humeral and glenoid components are joined, yet the glenoid component is not fixed (Swanson type);[8] a semiconstrained implant with a conforming component for the glenoid (McNab and English type); and a constrained implant in which the humeral and glenoid components are connected to each other and are also fixed to the bone (Lettin-Stanmore, Post, Gestina types).[7]

TOTAL SHOULDER ARTHROPLASTY

The immediate postoperative care for the shoulder replacement procedure requires protection of the anterior incision and the reattached shoulder cuff or deltoid muscles. Surgical variables may alter the postoperative plan and require use of a Velpeau dressing, a shoulder spica cast, or abduction brace. In typical cases, the extremity is positioned to avoid humeral abduction, maintain some humeral flexion, and restrict the extremity with a sling-swathe dressing. When supine, the humerus should rest on a foam wedge pillow placed under the arm to provide 20 degrees of forward flexion of the shoulder. This position has been found satisfactory for patient comfort and for protecting the usual surgical repair. The patient is not usually expected to exercise the extremity until four to five days after surgery. Until that time he or she is expected to accept the responsibility for maintaining the position described and to learn to relax the muscles, avoiding tension in the neck, upper back, and shoulder.

On the fourth or fifth postoperative day, an exercise program of passive forward flexion is started and carried out for five-minute periods, eight to ten times daily. These are done in a supine position (Fig. 35-7A). During this period, the patient may ambulate with the arm placed in a sling to maintain the described position. Support of the arm is continued with the positioning pillow, and the elbow is now extended with the palm up. During the first six weeks, it is imperative that the patient avoid active flexion or abduction or leaning on the

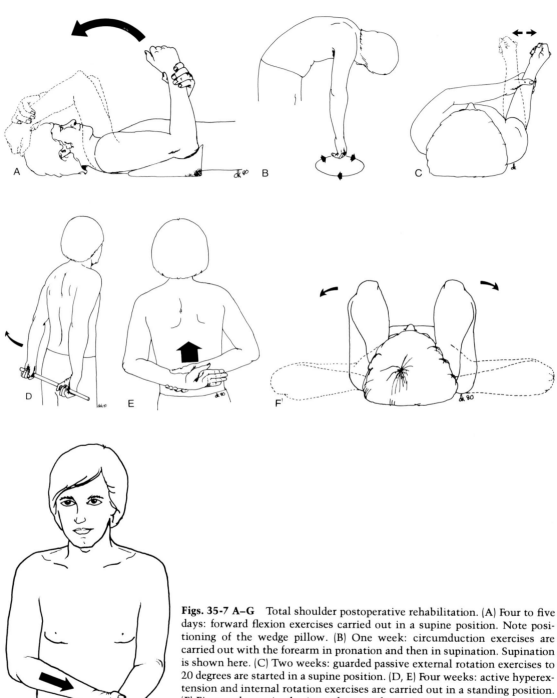

Figs. 35-7 A–G Total shoulder postoperative rehabilitation. (A) Four to five days: forward flexion exercises carried out in a supine position. Note positioning of the wedge pillow. (B) One week: circumduction exercises are carried out with the forearm in pronation and then in supination. Supination is shown here. (C) Two weeks: guarded passive external rotation exercises to 20 degrees are started in a supine position. (D, E) Four weeks: active hyperextension and internal rotation exercises are carried out in a standing position. (F) Five weeks: active horizontal external rotation exercises are shown here. Passive pulley exercises are started as well. (G) Six weeks: progressive resistive isometric exercises in forward flexion and internal and external rotation are instituted. Internal rotation is shown here.

operated extremity during activities of daily living. Excessive external rotation may disrupt the operative repair of the anterior shoulder.

At the first postoperative week, the circumduction exercises shown in Figure 35-7B are added. The sling may be removed at mealtime to permit limited hand activity. A week later the sling may be discarded. The patient may allow the arm to hang naturally at the side. Circumduction exercises are continued, enlarging the circles. Flexion exercises are now done in a standing position and are guided through a passive range of motion with the healthy hand. Guarded passive external rotation to 20 degrees is started (Fig. 35-7C). At the fourth postoperative week, active exercises of hyperextension and internal rotation are started from a standing position (Figs. 35-7D, E). During the fifth week, horizontal external rotation is added to the patient's tolerance (Fig. 35-7F). Passive pulley exercises are introduced in addition to the passive exercises. A rope with handles attached is passed around a pulley installed at a suitable height on a wall. The patient sits down, firmly grasping both handles, thus using the active pull of the healthy extremity to passively mobilize the operated one. During the sixth week, progressive resistive isometric exercises are initiated for forward flexion and for internal and external rotation. The opposite hand may be used to provide resistance, as demonstrated in Figure 35-7G.

Moist or dry heat may be beneficial prior to the exercise program. They are followed by pendulum and pulley exercises for relaxation, in which gradual progress is made to the more difficult motions. If a greater range of motion is desired, the active exercises of forward flexion, external rotation, and flexion with abduction can be done more vigorously. At 12 weeks postoperatively, active abduction of the shoulder is encouraged. At this time, the patient is expected to achieve 70 percent of the normal range of motion in shoulder flexion and external rotation. Patients are encouraged to continue daily exercises up to a year after surgery in order to maintain the range of motion and develop additional strength.

REFERENCES

1. Cofield, R. H., Morrey, B. F., and Bryan, R. S.: Total shoulder and total elbow arthroplasties: The current state of development, part II. J. Contin. Ed. Orthop. 7:17–25, 1979.

2. Dee, R.: Personal communication, 1980.

3. Flatt, A. E.: *The Care of the Rheumatoid Hand,* 3rd ed. C. V. Mosby, St. Louis, 1977.

4. Lettin, A. W. F., and Scales, J. T.: Total replacement of the shoulder joint (two cases). Proc. Roy. Soc. Med. 65:373–374, 1972.

5. Madden, J. W., and Peacock, E. E., Jr.: Studies on the biology of collagen during wound healing: Dynamic metabolism of scar collagen and remodeling of dermal wounds. Ann. Surg. 174:511–520, 1971.

6. Neer, C. S.: Replacement arthroplasty for glenohumeral osteoarthritis. J. Bone Joint Surg. 56A:1–13, 1974.

7. Post, M., Haskell, S., and Finder, J.: Total shoulder replacement. J. Bone Joint Surg. 57A:1171, 1975.

8. Swanson, A. B.: *Flexible Implant Resection Arthroplasty in the Hand and Extremities.* C. V. Mosby, St. Louis, 1973.

9. Swanson, A. B., Swanson, G. deG., and Leonard, J.: Post-operative rehabilitation program in flexible implant arthroplasty of the digits. In Hunter, J. M., Schneider, L. H., Mackin, E. J., and Bell, J. A., Eds.: *Rehabilitation of the Hand,* pp. 477–495. C. V. Mosby, St. Louis, 1978.

36

Lower Limb Joint Replacement

William P. Fortune, M.D.

The evolution of joint replacement surgery took shape as a result of the attempts by a number of investigators to solve the problem of the arthritic hip. Gluck[7] in 1891 in Berlin implanted an ivory ball and socket joint and attempted to achieve fixation with a luting agent. He is regarded as the original pioneer in total hip replacement as we currently understand the procedure. In 1923, Smith-Peterson of Boston adopted mold cup arthroplasty as the method by which the arthritic hip could promote growth of new layers of cartilage and thereby assist the natural repair process. The main disadvantages were the comparatively long period of hospitalization, the duration of rehabilitation, and the need for walking aids extending often to 12 months.

Since the early 1950s, the English surgeons Charnley and McKee, through their research and clinical applications, must be given credit for the major breakthrough that has taken place in total hip replacement. Charnley[2] regarded the coefficient of friction as the primary factor affecting the design of the hip joint and subsequently other major joints, and he also introduced the use of acrylic cement as the luting substance. The overall benefit to patients suffering from severe arthritic problems of the major joints of the lower limb is undoubtedly greater as a result of the developments of newer materials, improved designs of prosthetic systems, refinement of the surgical team's skills, and the close relationship that the rehabilitation team of therapists, nurses, engineers, and materials scientists brings to the care and management of the patient undergoing total joint replacement for the lower limb.

TOTAL HIP REPLACEMENT

Reconstruction of the adult hip by replacement has met with success and is now accepted as a relatively safe operative procedure. When we talk about total hip replacement, however, we must define whether we are referring to the conventional stemmed femoral systems or to the recent addition of the double cup resurfacing systems.[4] The concepts of each system are markedly different, the patient population requirements vary considerably from one to the other, the operative techniques and skills required for the resurfacing are more demanding, and the postoperative rehabilitation is appreciably different with regard to weight-bearing protection and joint control development.

In the space of the 19 years (1962–1981) since Charnley adopted acetabular components made of high-density polyethylene, we have systematically gone through three generations of conventional total hip systems. As our knowledge and experience increased, so too have significant modifications in prosthetic design and improvement in materials and operative techniques taken place. Paralleling these advances, excellence in operative rehabilitation has kept pace.

In my experience, the success or failure of any joint replacement is directly related to the close and orderly integration of three areas of the patient's odyssey. These are the preoperative rehabilitation period, the surgical rehabilitation period, and the postoperative rehabilitation period.

The Preoperative Rehabilitation Period

Patient Selection. The foremost reason that a patient seeks the care of an orthopedic surgeon for consideration of total hip replacement is pain. The severity of the accompanying deformity (limited motion and contractures), inability to walk with or without aids, and inability to work or to enjoy a quality of life consistent with the patient's ability are directly related to the severity of pain. The decision to operate often depends on many factors, including age, type of work, medical status, quality of bone, and the patient's anxiety and goals.

The conventional total hip with modifications as we know it today has given literally hundreds of thousands of patients a new and wonderful life with improved function and freedom from pain. However, the problems of mechanical failure emphasize the absolute importance of proper patient selection and patient preparation.

Patient Preparation. The preparation of the patient is, to my mind, the key to the subsequent rapport that has to be developed between the patient, family, surgeon, and the rehabilitation experts. Realistic goals must be outlined by the surgeon so that the patient has a clear understanding of what should be anticipated. The patient and family must understand that all running and jumping activities after surgery are absolutely and unequivocally inimical to the long-term survival of the arthroplasty. Many times it is helpful for the new patient to be given a list of patients who have had the intended procedure. This allows the new patient to have a more direct access to the answers of questions that he or she is asking from someone who has experienced all of the preparation anxiety, operative pain, and the frustrations and joys of the postoperative period.

The preoperative physical therapy program has to be consistent in degree and intensity with the patient's pain. Specific exercise programs are unrealistic and only serve to burden the patient with more discomfort. However, swimming is an excellent method for preoperative stretching and muscle toning. This period also allows the patient to be instructed in the proper use of walking aids for ease of postoperative ambulation activities. Our patients are admitted two days before surgery, and this period of time is sufficient to allow for adequate medical, social, and physical preparation.

The basic diagnostic method other than physical examination is the interpretation of x-rays: weight bearing, obliques, and crosstable laterals. The bone scan is quite helpful in determining candidates for resurfacing total hip arthroplasty.[4] Routine laboratory tests are obtained with specific emphasis on preoperative clean-catch urine cultures to screen out patients with potential urinary problems, which might systematically seed the arthroplasty.

The patient who has unilateral hip disease differs considerably from the patient with bilateral hip problems and certainly from the individual with upper as well as lower multiple joint involvement.[16] Staging of multiple procedures must be thought out and planned with care. As a general principle, patients with bilateral hip disease are best managed if the operations are performed during the same hospitalization and as close together as safety allows.

Two-stage bilateral total hip replacement one week apart has been this author's usual approach. However, in some selected problem cases, a single one-stage bilateral total hip replacement has been advantageous, allowing for a faster rehabilitative recovery period.[11] The close staging of the procedure is particularly indicated for those patients who have marked deformities and contractures.[15] The patients in these two groups are selected if there are no medical or surgical contraindications and if there is unanimous agreement among the patient's attending physician, anesthesiologist, and surgeon.

The patient with bilateral hip and knee deformities presents another problem, one that is essentially a direct extension of the preceding. To ensure patient safety, the basic principle in surgical rehabilitation is to perform the operations temporally as close together as possible. In general, my approach has been to perform the hip operation first as outlined earlier, wait 10–14 days for recovery and intervening rehabilitation, and then perform a single-stage bilateral total knee replacement operation. Such phasing allows a more rapid surgical correction of deformities, contractures, and limb malalignment. The postoperative rehabilitation program can be initiated sooner, the number of hospital admissions and anesthetics is reduced, and the patient is able to enter the postoperative period of rehabilitation unconstrained by pain, deformity, and contractures in another synergistic joint.

The Surgical Rehabilitation Period

All things being equal, the quality, utility, and ultimate function of the arthroplasty are determined at the time of its implantation. The rehabilitative surgical team must understand the normal kinematics of the hip, for such knowledge is fundamental to the outcome of the operation. The principle of having the moment arms about the hip in ratio of 2:1 (Fig. 36-1) is the essence of hip

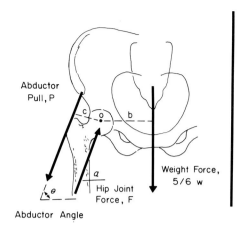

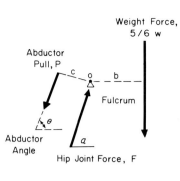

Fig. 36-1. The moment arms $b:c$ are in a ratio of $2:1$. The re-establishment of this ratio places the point 0 (which is the sum of all the moments about the hip and must be equal to zero) in a normal location.

reconstruction.[2] When this is fulfilled, the patient's postoperative course is smooth, and optimal motion and balance are achieved. The surgeon accomplishes this primarily by the technique of medialization of the acetabular prosthesis. It insures that the abductor muscles will be placed in the best position to carry out their role as primary hip (pelvic-femoral) stabilizers. This also helps reduce the forces about the hip as a result of pathomechanics and allows the acetabular component to be seated under good pelvic bone stock. A second and equally important principle of hip reconstruction is developing proper tension in the soft tissues about the hip; this is accomplished by selecting the correct prosthetic neck length. Therefore medialization and correct neck length allow the surgeon to re-establish essentially normal hip kinematics.

Stability is important to function. It is directly influenced by the previous two points, and to a major extent by the orientation of the acetabular and femoral components. The surgeon attempts to facilitate range of motion and enhance stability by placing the acetabular component in an abducted position of 30–35 degrees from the horizontal and opening the mouth of the prosthesis 15–20 degrees from the vertical plane. By placing the femoral component in a neutral version position, maximum stability and range of motion are achieved. When these principles are adhered to, the complications from subluxation and dislocation are substantially diminished.

Trochanteric osteotomy is frequently necessary for the optimal performance of the operation. However, it does modify and extend the postoperative rehabilitation period. Currently, most hip surgeons prefer to leave the abductor-trochanteric complex intact whenever possible.[9] The complications of infection and thromboembolism are a constant source of concern to the surgeon. Prophylactic antibiotics, antibiotic irrigating solutions used to lavage the wound during the operation, improved surgical team techniques, and environmental modifications in the operating rooms have combined to decrease the infection rate to less than 2 percent in many centers and to less than 1 percent in others.

Thromboembolism is constantly a life-threatening complication and is in terms of frequency the number one complication in total hip replacement. Pulmonary emboli occur in approximately 10 percent of cases and fatal emboli in about 2 percent. The author's preferred program for prevention is early movement, early ambulation, elastic thigh length hose, warfarin for women, and either aspirin or warfarin for men.

The Postoperative Rehabilitation Period

Immediate Program.   As soon as the dressings are applied, an Ace bandage hip spica is wrapped in place and elastic hose donned. The patient is then carefully transferred to a bed in the operating room once the anesthesiologist has awakened the patient. In the event of spinal anesthesia, the patient is not moved until the lower limbs are cautiously controlled so as to guard against subluxation or dislocation in the face of poor or absent muscle tone.

Immediate anteroposterior and crossbed lateral x-rays are taken to assure that the arthroplasty is in its reduced position; if it has dislocated, then it can be reduced immediately. If it is found to be reduced, then both lower limbs are placed in bilateral balanced slings, a wide one under the thigh and the other under the calf (Fig. 36-2). Both legs are then positioned in a wide, abducted position and the patient is taken to the post-anesthetic recovery room. The postoperative rehabilitation process begins at this point.

Once he is fully awake the patient sees the respiratory therapist, who begins the postoperative deep breathing and coughing routine that was explained during the immediate preoperative hospitalization. When stabilized, the patient is transferred to the orthopedic floor, where the orthopedic nurses adjust the bed position if necessary and encourage the patient to begin active calf and ankle exercises to prevent venous stasis. When the patient is fully alert and awake, he is encouraged to do these simple exercises ten times per hour.

During postoperative rounds, the orthopedic team, which includes the house staff, orthopedic nurses, and surgeon, attempts to have the patient actively flex and extend the hip with the leg supported. This is an invaluable aid in allowing the most apprehensive patient an opportunity to realize that moving the limb will not produce injury. Many patients are afraid that if they move the hip or limb they will damage the arthroplasty, and they thus maintain a very rigid extremity. This self-induced muscle spasm and guarding only intensify the postoperative pain by increasing to some degree the relative muscle hypoxia induced by the spasm. By gently flexing and extending the hip a few times with the limb supported, the vast majority of patients are able to relax these large muscles and are thereby made more comfortable during the first 24 hours after the operation.

The first day after the operation, all patients who have intact trochanters are

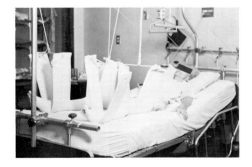

Fig. 36-2. Both lower limbs are supported in balanced slings in wide abduction. This position is helpful in balancing the pelvic-femoral relationships of both hips.

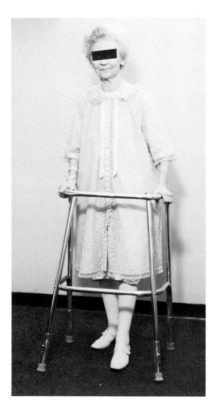

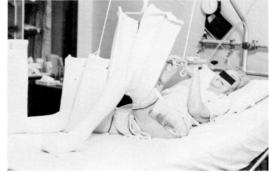

Fig. 36-3. The foot of the operative extremity (left) is placed on the floor so as to reduce the forces across the hip during ambulation. Note: _No toe touching._

Fig. 36-4. A knee-sling system allows for an active-assistive hip flexion and extension exercise program that permits more rapid joint control. Note fishnet in place of tape for dressing.

allowed to sit at the edge of the bed for a few moments and then permitted to ambulate with a walker for a few steps. During this time, the bed linen is changed—the patient may sit no longer than 5 minutes. Preoperatively the patient has been instructed in the use of the walker and in the three-point partial weight-bearing gait. All patients are instructed in the importance of placing the entire plantar aspect of the foot (sole and heel)—_not toe touch_—on the floor (Fig. 36-3). With the entire foot resting on the floor, the muscles about the hip can be made relatively inactive and the resulting forces across the operated hip reduced, thereby making ambulation easier and more comfortable. The patient is allowed out of bed once on this day but may ambulate again in the evening if he so desires.

The second postoperative day begins with the removal of the Hemovac-Aernovac tubes; the intravenous lines are discontinued, and the patient is switched to oral antibiotics. The antibiotics are continued until the final intra-operative cultures are reported. The patient begins a program of active-assistive hip and knee flexion and extension exercises with the help of a knee sling and pulley system incorporated into the balanced abduction slings (Fig. 36-4). The patient is encouraged to perform this program three times per day for ten repetitions each. Most patients are able to do this with minimal difficulty and a more rapid control of the joint appears to develop. The patient is encouraged to ambulate twice this day for a distance of the patient's choosing.

The patient may sit for not longer than 15 minutes, once again to avoid venous

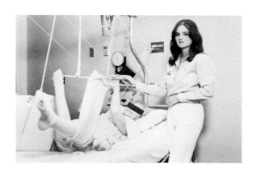

Fig. 36-5. An active abduction program under supervision by the seventh postoperative day.

stasis. Calf and ankle exercises continue to be encouraged by all members of the rehabilitation team. Patients with unilateral total hip replacement are helped out of and into bed from the operated side; this is to protect against adduction, which might lead to subluxation or dislocation. The patients with bilateral total hip replacement are protected in abduction during the process of getting out of and into bed.

The third through sixth postoperative days include essentially the same program of bed exercises, with a gradual increase in the number of times up for ambulation. On day seven the patient is usually transferred to conventional or forearm crutches, depending on the patient's preference, and stair activities are begun. The bed sling program is modified to include gluteal settings, ten times, three times a day, and an abduction component is added to the knee sling routine (Fig. 36-5). The skin staples or sutures are removed at this time.

The majority of unilateral hip replacement patients are able to get in and out of bed independently after seven days, can negotiate stairs comfortably by day eight or nine, and are ready for discharge by the tenth day. By the time of discharge, the patient without trochanteric osteotomy can negotiate essentially full weight-bearing comfortably with crutches.

The patient is discharged on an active hip flexion program three times a day for ten repetitions sitting on a table top. The abduction program is performed by lying in bed and actively abducting the legs simultaneously for the same frequency, as with the hip flexion program. Use of a smooth wooden or plastic surface approximately 120 cm in length and 30 cm wide is helpful in accomplishing this exercise.

Long-Term Programs. The patient is seen in follow-up one week after discharge for a wound and joint control check. At this time an assessment is made with regard to abductor control and lurch. If the patient has control, an active abduction program against gravity is outlined, and the patient is given a cane for use in restricted areas (Fig. 36-6). If the patient is obese, not well-motivated, or has poor joint control, no change is made in the exercise format or ambulation aids. Swimming is encouraged as soon as the wound will allow.

The vast majority of total hip patients are able to follow and carry out their own home rehabilitation program without the assistance of a physical therapist. However, in those instances in which the patient for whatever reason cannot progress on course, then the therapist becomes actively involved in the patient's

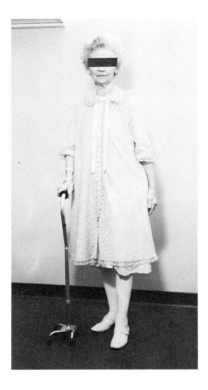

Fig. 36-6. Most patients can ambulate with a cane 14–21 days after their operation. This patient could do so on the sixth day following conversion of a prosthesis to a conventional total hip replacement.

care. It is imperative that normal abductor control be established. Until such time as it is, the patient is protected by using a cane in the opposite hand. Most patients with conventional total hip replacements are free of crutches in four to six weeks, and many have developed excellent hip kinematics by six to eight weeks, making them completely free of a cane.

The patient is next seen at six weeks and modifications are made in the program. At this point most patients are able to tolerate an active hip extension program against gravity and this is added to the other exercises. As mentioned throughout this section, elimination of the abductor weakness and abductor lurch is primary to the long-term survival of the arthroplasty. The prolonged weakness and lurch cause abnormal strains in the upper femur that directly increase the bending moment on the femoral component. These abnormal forces over a period of time deform and loosen the components. A resurfacing system will tend to magnify the abnormal strains and stresses at the femoral cup-bone junction so that stress fracturing will occur, leading to failure of the arthroplasty.[4]

Trochanteric osteotomy is often essential in the surgical management of a particular problem; it also means that the postoperative rehabilitation program must be modified. Often these patients may require more blood replacement and are therefore not ready for an early mobilization routine.

However, in uncomplicated cases in which the trochanter is removed, the patient is allowed out of bed by the second or third postoperative day. Here it is essential that the rehabilitation team recognize the need for a protected non-weight-bearing program that includes a gait pattern that will allow the hip musculatures to inhibit themselves from generating their full force of contraction. However, the general knee-sling exercises are the same. It is essential to maintain a relatively abducted attitude of the limb for the first few weeks during ambulation. Stair activities are begun at the same time but the limb is protected from weight bearing. The patient is usually discharged between the 10th and 14th postoperative day on the same program as for the patient with the intact trochanter.

Weight bearing must be protected with crutches for at least 12 weeks. Active antigravity abduction and hip extension exercises must not begin until there is adequate radiological evidence of osseous healing at the osteotomy site; this usually is not seen for at least 8–12 weeks after the operation. Once there is good evidence, then the graduated program of abductor and extensor strengthening can be initiated. Again, the goal is to develop and maintain a gait without abductor weakness and lurch. Often this patient will require some type of walking aid as late as six months after total hip replacement. However, once the trochanter has healed and good abductor strength and control have developed, the function and control of the arthroplasty are equal to those of the intact trochanter patient.

Resurfacing total hip replacement is comparatively new and is still considered to be by many clinical investigators a relatively experimental approach to the problem of the arthritic hip. It offers to young and middle-aged patients a procedure that is a reasonable alternative to conventional total hip replacement.[4] It does require more demanding skill on the part of the surgeon, plus a modification in the postoperative management with regard to weight bearing that is reminiscent of the mold cup arthroplasty program. Because the femoral head must be reamed and sculpted, the cancellous trabecular bone must be allowed to repair itself. Therefore weight bearing must be scrupulously controlled for approximately 12 weeks after the operation. During this time, however, the postoperative exercise program proceeds as outlined for the patient with an intact greater trochanter. The vast majority of these operations are accomplished without trochanteric osteotomy.

Of all the groups of total hip recipients, the patient having a resurfacing arthroplasty must be protected by using a cane until the lurch is converted; if this is impossible for any reason, the patient should remain married to the cane to try to avert femoral neck-cup failure. Periodic bone scanning is helpful in assessing the quality of the femoral head beneath the metal cup.[4]

Dislocation is an unwelcome interruption in the smooth progression of the postoperative rehabilitation process. Yet it occurs even when the components have been properly selected, positioned, and oriented. When the dislocation occurs immediately following surgery, it should be reduced at once so that the process of rehabilitation may proceed. However, when the dislocation occurs weeks after the operation, then the hip must be reduced immediately and the patient placed in balanced sling suspension with the hips in wide abduction for six weeks. The period in the sling is necessary to allow the stretched tissues to heal and the abductors to accommodate to a new position. Knee sling exercises in abduction may be instituted after two to three weeks in the slings. Once the six weeks have passed, careful mobilization can be started again, being sure to maintain wide abduction of the limb accompanied by active abduction, extension, and hip flexion exercises. Protected weight bearing will be continued until normal hip kinematics have been re-established.

There is nothing more gratifying than to see a patient who has had severe pain and associated deformities rehabilitated through the efforts of orthopedic nurses and physical and occupational therapists. The occupational therapist often is able to instruct the patient in the use of certain extension aids that are of help in donning socks, hose, and footwear. The combined efforts and expertise of these members, along with the skill of the surgical and engineering members, assure the continuance of improvement in the quality of life for patients with arthritis of the hip.

TOTAL KNEE REPLACEMENT

The basic concepts that Charnley developed for total hip replacement have been refined and modified by himself and other investigators. By 1968 Gunston,[8] working in Charnley's laboratory, developed the first condylar resurfacing system for the knee and thereby opened the "era of unlinked knee arthroplasty." These changes, like the hip systems before them, have revolutionized the operative treatment of knee arthritis.

The knee is anatomically and functionally a more complicated articulating machine than the hip joint. The hip depends primarily for its inherent stability upon the osseous male-female relationship. Knee stability, however, is a function of the soft tissue constraints: specifically, the major ligaments, capsule, the menisci that help deepen the joint surfaces, and the muscle-tendon groups that span and power the joint.[6]

The femorotibial alignment (valgus-varus) is fundamental to knee anatomy because it directly affects the patellofemoral articulation. The patellar mechanism is intimately concerned with normal knee function, and when malalignment is present for whatever reason, it may be a direct causative factor in arthritic problems that ultimately bring the patient to the surgical rehabilitation team.

The complexities of knee kinematics are proportionally related to these anatomical relationships. The knee is not a hinge joint, but rather a machine that changes its fulcrum of motion through the entire flexion-extension arc and thereby defines a centroid of instant centers. The knee therefore exhibits varying modes of motion in the sagittal plane, exhibiting characteristics of rolling, rocking, sliding, and gliding. Rotation in the femorotibial articulation is an essential part of normal knee kinematics, and this factor is a basic consideration in prosthetic design. The translational movements of fore and aft shear as well as mediolateral shear are similarly important aspects of motion.

The posterior cruciate ligament, of all the major knee ligaments, is considered to be the primary determinant of knee kinematics. This structure directly controls the magnitude of forward translation of the femur on the tibia during the critical phase of gait when the knee is in the flexion phase and under load. When it is absent or attenuated, the femur will tend to sublux or dislocate anteriorly off the tibia. Therefore a greater effort is required from those muscle groups, namely, the hip extensors and the gastrocnemius complex, that dynamically control the flexion moment about the knee. The appreciation of this most important kinematic data is essential to choosing an arthroplasty design.[3]

What Is A Total Knee?

After Walldius[14] first replaced the femorotibial joint with a hinged prosthesis in 1951, the concept of knee prosthetic replacement for this entire articulation revolved around a hinge. This was the generally accepted procedure for the severely involved arthritic knee until 1968. Gunston[8] designed an unlinked condylar prosthesis held to bone with acrylic cement, and he thereby changed the course of major knee replacement surgery.

During the last 12 years, a number of significant design modifications have been implemented. In addition, surgeons have made fundamental improvements in their knowledge and understanding of normal kinematics and pathomechanics.[5,6,10] We now appreciate the soft tissue envelope or sleeve of the knee joint and the role it plays in fostering as well as correcting deformities. Our understanding of fixed versus unfixed deformities has also deepened.

Angular, flexion, rotatory parameters, and bone substance loss have become understood in an overall view. Leading surgeons and engineers have been able to develop concepts of unlinking the articulating surfaces and have created prosthetic systems with varying degrees of constrainment inherently designed into the bearing surfaces. As a result of increased knowledge and improved operative techniques, the majority of patients who come for total knee replacement today can be offered a relatively unconstrained prosthesis.[10] The patient can be assured of significant correction of the deformities, relief of pain, and improvement in function and quality of day-to-day life from systems resembling the normal bearing surfaces of the knee and requiring less implanted hardware. The rehabilitation team offers the patient a major improvement in the final outcome as compared to 20 years ago.

The Preoperative Rehabilitation Period

Patient Selection.   Pain, again, is the primary reason that the patient seeks consideration for operative correction. However, the complexities of the knee joint directly influence the decision that the experienced and skilled knee arthroplasty surgeon makes in the selection of the appropriate total knee system.

This decision is based upon the degree of angular deformity, flexion deformity, rotatory deformity, and bone substance loss. It also is based upon whether or not there is a fixed or correctable deformity at the time. All these data are basic to the final decision as to what will be the best system for correcting the problem. The fundamental principle of total knee surgery at this point is that the most unconstrained system should always be used.[3] This principle will assure a longer period of time free from the problems of failure, particularly those related to the bone-cement bond.

Patient Preparation.   Many patients who come for total knee replacement have severe, almost incapacitating pain, and one might expect that the postoperative course would fade by comparison. However, a small percentage of patients in this group will have a rocky postoperative course because of their inability to tolerate the postoperative pain. No matter how disabled the patient is before surgery, it is, in my experience, virtually impossible to identify these individuals preoperatively. It has been my policy to make sure that any patient in whom there might be the slightest suspicion of possible postoperative problems with regard to mobilization talks with other total knee patients. This has been an invaluable aid in preventing postoperative complications.

Again, as with the total hip patient, preoperative exercises must be carefully tailored to the patient's clinical problem. In most instances, a program of quadriceps setting or isometric exercises can be tolerated by the patient preoperatively, and we encourage a program of daily repetitions for quadriceps muscles, ten times, four to six times a day. It is particularly unrealistic for many of these patients to do anything more because of the pain and disability present. When the patient is admitted to the hospital, the postoperative program is outlined and ambulation training instituted.

The Surgical Rehabilitation Period

The knee, probably more than any other major joint, requires the strict adherence of the surgical rehabilitation team to basic kinematic knowledge and the principle that directs the selection of the most unconstrained system capable of correcting deformities and achieving stability with a good range of motion.[3] To achieve optimal results for the total knee patient, normal mechanical alignment (Fig. 36-7) of the knee relative to the weight-bearing axis intersecting the hip, knee, and ankle must be re-established. The concept of condylar replacement allows for duplication of anatomical knee relationships and the establishment of more normal polycentric motion. To obtain full motion with stability, the surgeon balances the ligaments and supporting soft tissue structures so as to ensure their proper length-tension relationships.

When there are no significant deformities and when passive correction to neutral can be achieved, the surgeon can then proceed in an orderly fashion.

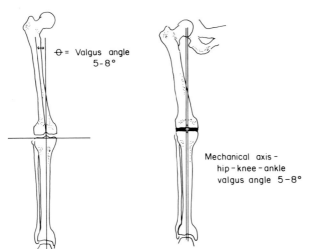

θ = Valgus angle
5-8°

Mechanical axis –
hip – knee – ankle
valgus angle 5-8°

Fig. 36-7. The mechanical axis falling in a straight line intersecting the hip, knee, and ankle will subtend the valgus angle θ of 5–8 degrees.

Appropriate jigs are used to prepare the bone surface. The proper thickness of the tibial component has to be selected to ensure re-establishment of the normal mechanical alignment and the length-tension relationships of the supporting soft tissues of the knee. However, when the deformities are fixed because of adaptive changes in the soft tissue supports, the surgical rule of release and balancing of these contractures is invoked before any bone preparation is carried out. The surgeon releases these tissues in a systematic, meticulous, and orderly fashion until the deformity can be corrected to neutral. When that has been accomplished, the surgical team proceeds as outlined before, always cognizant of the fact that the least constrained prosthesis is to be implanted. When this surgical approach has been undertaken, the postoperative course and management will vary greatly from that of the less complicated case. In the case of bilateral involvement, it is appropriate to undertake a bilateral one-stage replacement when safety can be assured, based upon the skill and support of the surgical team as much as the intra-operative status of the patient after the first procedure.

The Postoperative Rehabilitation Period

Immediate Program. The postoperative course and rehabilitation program are markedly different from that of the patient who has had total hip arthroplasty. Initially, pain is the most important factor separating the total knee patient from the total hip patient. The pain that these patients experience is real and much more intense. Therefore they require more frequent medication for the first 36–48 hours after surgery. As a result, the surgical team may not want to mobilize this patient until three or four days after the operation. The patients are placed in a very large, bulky, cotton compression dressing with anterior and posterior plaster splints; these constraints make movement in bed awkward and difficult, especially if a bilateral procedure has to be undertaken.

However, the rehabilitation team begins its program on the operation day. The respiratory threrapist sees the patient initially, regardless of the anesthesia used. Active ankle motion is encouraged as soon as the patient returns to the orthopedic floor and repetitions ten times per hour are encouraged so as to prevent venous stasis. I prefer that the foot of the bed be elevated to 45 degrees for adequate venous drainage as long as there is no inherent arterial insufficiency and the heel is kept free of the bed by placing soft rolled bumpers under the ankles. The patients are also placed on prophylactic antibiotic and antithromboembolic medication.

One operative complication frequently seen following total knee surgery is peroneal nerve problems. In the main they are related to some type of neurapraxia that occurs either as a result of correcting a valgus external rotation contracture or, more commonly, from improperly applied postoperative dressings and splints. When the complication is recognized soon after the operation (within the first few hours), releasing the dressing and reapplying it loosely are often sufficient to correct and prevent permanent nerve damage. Every member of the rehabilitation surgical team should be aware of this problem and strive for its recognition and elimination.[5]

On the second postoperative day, the drainage tubes and the bulky compression dressing are removed. A new dressing is applied and held in place with a fine mesh tubular sleeve, the elastic hose are donned, and a knee immobilizer brace with a Velcro strap is applied. An active program of quadriceps exercises is instituted, ten repetitions, three times a day. Active straight-leg control is begun with assistance, and the patient may be allowed out of bed one time for a brief period of ambulation. If the patient experiences significant pain, then the program is begun on the third day. The sooner the patient gains active joint control, especially of the knee, the smoother will be the postoperative course and the greater the eventual range of motion and function attained.

In our initial groups of total knee patients nine years ago, the postoperative management included rest without motion for the first five to seven days because of our concern about wound healing.[5] We found that our incidence for postoperative manipulation was much higher, by almost 30 percent, than it is now with the program of active-assistive exercises instituted earlier. We utilize a midline incision and have not had any wound healing problems.[10]

On the third or fourth day, a knee-sling exercise program is added to the straight-leg raising and ambulation activities. The patient supports the thigh with the sling and pulley arrangement and actively draws the heel along the sheet. The patient is then encouraged to extend the knee actively as much as possible against the force of gravity; this is done three times a day for ten repetitions.

On the fifth day the patient begins to add an active-assistive, flexion-extension program while seated at bedside. The orthopedic nurses assist with this exercise program three times a day every day. The frequency and continuity of such an intimate approach are invaluable for attaining rapid and early joint range and control and for the long-term benefit of having an excellent range of motion with full extension and flexion.[5] At George Washington University Medical Center, the surgeon and the surgical house staff team actively participate with the nurses in the program.

At no time is any forcing, pushing, or stretching carried out; in fact, they are prohibited. Instead the knowledge of the basic reciprocal reflex arc of Sherrington is invoked. With the patient comfortably seated at bedside and the rehabilitation therapist (be it nurse, therapist, or surgeon) seated comfortably opposite the patient, the therapist actively encourages the patient to flex the knee, at the same time resisting that effort by gently positioning his or her hand against the back of the leg. In this way the hamstring muscles are firing under resistance to produce a shortening contraction while the quadriceps mechanism concurrently undergoes a relaxation or lengthening contraction. What results is an increase in the flexion arc through a relatively painless process. As the flexion-extension progresses, the patient gains easier kinematic sense and control of the joint. The patient substitutes less and less with extraneous hip and back movements, and a more normal, fluid, reciprocal rhythm is developed.

Over the fifth through seventh days, the patient is allowed to ambulate free of the knee immobilizer as soon as good active quadriceps control is developed. The patient may sit with the knee flexed to comfort, but while in bed, the immobilizer is used. The immobilizer is used for a period of six to eight weeks postoperatively at night to ensure that no loss in the extension range occurs.

Over the years I have noted in some cases a loss of extension upon return for the first postoperative visit as compared to that upon discharge. This happens frequently in patients who have had significant flexion contractures prior to arthroplasty. Many of these patients feel more comfortable with the knee partially flexed in bed, and it does not take very long to lose the extension gained by surgery. Our team is diligent in its attempt to prevent this complication.

In general, most patients can comfortably flex the knee to between 75–90 degrees by the ninth or tenth postoperative day. They may have full extension or lack only 5 or 10 degrees. However, in those infrequent instances when the patient cannot proceed with the program and is only at about 50 degrees by the ninth or tenth day, it is best to manipulate the patient (Fig. 36-8). Otherwise the longer one waits the poorer the results will be. The manipulation is done with the help of the anesthesiologist. It is performed in the patient's room under careful and safe control and using Pentothal sodium as the anesthetic agent. The patient is allowed to rest that day; the exercise program is reinstituted the following day. Often a short course of anti-inflammatory medication is helpful in supporting the program after the manipulation. All patients who have low pain thresholds are medicated prior to their bedside exercises.

Ambulation activities continue with walker aid until the ninth or tenth day, when most patients are able to be switched to crutches and usually discharged 14 days after surgery. Stair-climbing activities are begun at the same time crutch walking is instituted.

When the patient is discharged he or she should be ambulating independently with crutches and have an active range of motion arc from 0–5 degrees of extension and 85–90 degrees of flexion. The sutures or staples are usually removed between days 10 and 12, and the wound held with adhesive paper strips. The patient and family are instructed in the home program prior to discharge and, as with the total hip patient, a postoperative brochure is given to the knee patient.

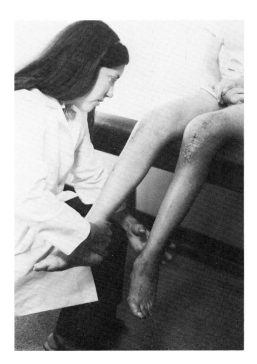

Fig. 36-8. A patient 12 days following a single-stage, bilateral, total knee replacement that required manipulation under anesthesia because of limited motion. Manipulation should not be postponed, in the author's view.

The Long-Term Program. The patient returns for the first postoperative visit a week after discharge for wound, venous stasis, and joint control evaluation. Again, if any great problems arise in maintaining the exercise program, then the physical therapist is actively included in the regimen. If there are no problems, the patient begins progressive, isometric, and resistive exercises for the quadriceps and an active knee flexion program in the prone position for maximizing knee flexion. At this time approximately 50–60 percent of patients may be switched to a cane and the crutch can be discontinued gradually.

The second visit occurs at the sixth week after the operation. By this time, at least 80 percent of unilateral total knee patients are using a cane or free of walking aids. At this point the average arc of motion in the patients with either a Kinematic or Duopatellar posterior cruciate ligament (Figs. 36-9A, B) retaining prosthesis is 95–100 degrees from 0 degrees of extension.

During visits three and six months later, the surgeon monitors the patient's progress. Most patients gain their optimal range of motion arc some 6–12 months after their operation. In most patients who have had a condylar prosthesis, such as the Kinematic or the Duopatellar systems, the team can realistically expect an overall flexion arc in the range of 110–120 degrees with full extension.

The postoperative rehabilitation regimen of the patient who requires realignment by extensive soft tissue release so that the fixed deformity can be converted to a correctable one is predicated upon the postoperative program for ligamentous and soft tissue injury repairs. Since the experienced knee replacement surgeon is attempting to implant the least amount of prosthetic hardware and use the least amount of bearing constraint, which directly affects the longevity of the prosthetic-cement-bone bond, these supporting soft tissues must be allowed to

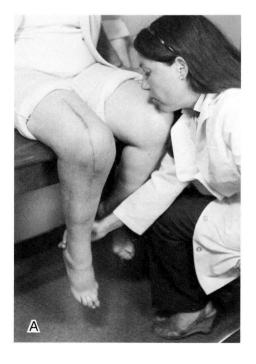

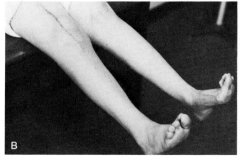

Fig. 36.9. (A) Twelve weeks after a kinematic total knee replacement, this patient is actively flexing to 95 degrees sitting. Note the therapist resisting active hamstring contraction for maximum quadriceps relaxation. (B) The same patient is exhibiting complete, full, active extension and ambulating without walking aids at 12 weeks postoperatively.

heal and re-establish joint stability. Therefore after surgery this patient's course is modified as follows.

Once the wound has healed and the postoperative swelling has subsided, during which period the patient is protected in plaster splints, a carefully applied cast brace is fitted that will protect from any varus-valgus stress, yet allow 20–60 degrees of flexion and extension. By so doing, it is hoped that a new band of scar tissue will be formed to supplement the supporting structures. The cast brace is kept on for a minimum of eight weeks and a maximum of 16 weeks. When it is removed, the patient is placed in a traditional knee metal brace for further protection and the knee mobilization and progressive resistance exercises are instituted. Weight bearing progresses in a normal fashion according to the individual patient's progress.

Some patients may periodically experience pain related to the incision area, the medial and lateral quadriceps retinacular regions, or to the pes anserinus complex. The sensitivity is often transitory, caused as it is by pulling and stretching of those tissues, and it is invariably relieved by a short course of anti-inflammatory medication. The advent of condylar replacement that is unlinked in form, made of metal and plastic, and that is based on the principles of proper soft tissue length-tension relationships has allowed the rehabilitation surgical team to offer to patients with advanced arthritis of the knee incalculable relief from pain, correction of contractures and deformities, and an improvement in the degree and quality of life unknown by their predecessors.

TOTAL ANKLE REPLACEMENT

The ankle is the most inherently stable major weight-bearing joint. Kinematically it performs simple planar motion of one degree of freedom in the sagittal plane.[1,12,15] It has a large load-bearing surface area through which tremendous compressive forces are exerted: they approximate five times body weight at certain points in the gait cycle. The average total range of motion in health is between 75 and 80 degrees. In walking, only 25–35 degrees of motion are required; however, in ascending and descending stairs, 50–60 degrees are needed for normal ankle-foot function.

Primary degenerative arthrosis of the ankle is largely unknown because this joint is so finely machined. It is exquisitely stable, has simple planar motion and a relatively thick articular cartilage, and possesses a large surface area by which these high compressive loads are dissipated.

The commonest causes of ankle arthrosis are rheumatoid arthritis, post-traumatic problems, and talar injuries. Gait studies reveal that during level walking only 10 degrees of extension (plantar flexion) and 14 degrees of flexion (dorsiflexion) are required and the centroid of motion is located in the body of the talus.[13]

Kinematically a cylindrical design appears to offer optimum clinical results, allowing a range of motion from 15 degrees of extension to 15 degrees of flexion.[13] An articulating surface area of at least 9 cm², which exhibits a compressive yield strength six times that which it will be called upon to withstand, appears to offer the patient a reasonable substitute to the inherent ankle problem.

The Preoperative Rehabilitation Period

Patient Selection. Total ankle replacement at best is an operation offered infrequently and then only to a very small percentage of patients suffering from arthritis of the ankle. Whereas the ratio of total hip to total knee replacement is approximately 2:1, the ratio of total hip to total ankle replacement is at least 30:1. Because of the high forces generated across this joint and the increased likelihood of prosthetic failure, only two groups are generally considered to be proper candidates for this type of ankle arthroplasty. The first is the patient with rheumatoid arthritis, who comprises the largest group by a ratio of 10:1 compared to the next type of patient, who is a non-obese individual older than 60 years of age suffering from post-traumatic arthritis and who already has some subtalar joint involvement.

Patient Preparation. This aspect of patient management does not constitute a prolonged period other than to outline the hazards of overuse of the prosthesis and explain that there is a significant probability of failure. Some of the general principles of postoperative management are reviewed. No specific exercises are given preoperatively but ambulation training is instituted.

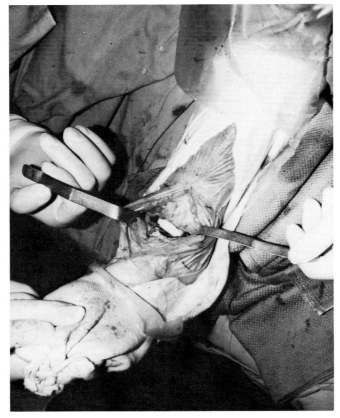

Fig. 36-10. Careful retraction of skin and subcutaneous soft tissue to prevent necrosis.

The Surgical Rehabilitation Period

Three areas are of concern to the surgical team. The first is wound care during the operation, because one of the common complications as a result of this procedure is delayed wound healing. A straight longitudinal incision is utilized and meticulous care is given the skin during retraction (Fig. 36-10).[15]

The second area of concern is to avoid intra-operative fracturing of the malleoli; often this occurs because of the osteoporotic nature of the bone and the very restricted operative field for surgical exposure. If this complication arises, the fractures can be treated with appropriate internal screw fixation and the postoperative course modified very little (Figs. 36-11A, B).[1]

The third area of surgical concern is that of impingement.[13] Since present total ankle surgery does not actually resurface the talofibular weight-bearing articulation, the patient will frequently experience pain in that specific area during weight bearing. The surgeon attempts to prevent this problem from occurring by carefully resecting a part of the fibular articular area.[13]

The Postoperative Rehabilitation Period

The general medical and orthopedic nursing management follows for this patient as for recipients of total hip and knee replacements. Initially the wound is protected in a large bulky dressing with anterior and posterior splints, the bed and leg elevated to control wound edema, and active ankle motion is encouraged even in the plaster splints. Pulmonary therapy is instituted as usual.

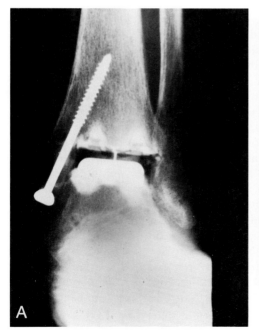 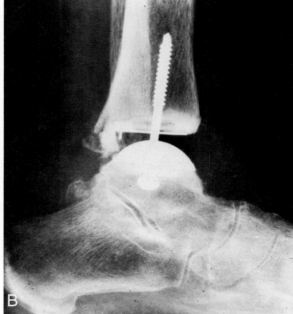

Fig. 36-11. (A) Anteroposterior and (B) lateral weight-bearing views of total ankle arthroplasty.

Because wound healing can be a serious problem at times and edema a major factor in this process, the patient remains at bed rest with the leg elevated and the original surgical dressing in place for the first three to five postoperative days, the surgical drain tube having been removed at 48 hours. The dressing is removed and a gelo-type, semicompression rigid dressing applied from toes to midcalf. The patient is then begun on an active program of dorsal and plantar motions for ten repetitions four times a day. Partial weight bearing using the walker or crutches is allowed by the fifth day after the operation. If malleolar internal fixation is necessary, then the patient is placed in a well-fitting short leg walking cast five to seven days later, when partial ambulation is allowed.

As long as there are no complications, the total ankle patient is usually discharged sometime between the 8th to 12th day after surgery and seen in the office a week later. The active program of ankle flexion and extension is encouraged for periods of six times a day. An elastic knee-length hose is substituted for the dressing or cast when appropriate, and walking aids are usually completely discontinued by 6–12 weeks after surgery.

The majority of patients can expect an improvement in overall ankle motion of 20–30 degrees and nearly total relief of pain. A carefully performed total ankle replacement can be a very gratifying operation, for it does effect significant improvement in the patient's ability to function in day-to-day walking activities. However, it is still an area in which continued basic and clinical research is necessary for design modifications and improved fixation methods so that untimely failures can be prevented.

FUTURE RESEARCH

There are two avenues of current and future research that hold promise for reducing the percentage of prosthetic failure. One has to do with newer techniques in forging metal components that enhance the strength characteristics of these components and thereby significantly decrease the likelihood of failure by fracture. The problem of failure as it relates to loosening has been addressed recently by improved techniques in the use of the polymethyl methacrylate at the time of implantation. Secondly, a clever area of advancing research has to do with porous-surfaced implants. By using porous surfaces, one can reduce the stresses on the implant itself and thereby do away with the need for a grouting substance. These studies have been underway in North America for the past three years. We at the George Washington University Medical Center are trying to solve the problem of fixation in the laboratory by utilizing a biodegradable material that gives immediate prosthetic fixation. This is then coupled with a porous material allowing long-term ingrowth for fixation. If this type of approach proves to be valid, it will allow the patient to load the implanted joint more rapidly. A number of prosthetic implant systems now offer a wide selection of sizes and shapes so that the prosthesis can be adapted to the patient and not the patient to the components. The horizon appears promising for future patients requiring implant surgery.

REFERENCES

1. Buchholz, H. W., Engelbrecht, E., and Siegl, A.: Totale Sprunggelenksendoprothese Modell "St. Georg." Chirurg. 44:241–247, 1973.
2. Charnley, J.: Total hip replacement by low friction arthroplasty. Clin. Orthop. 72:7–21, 1970.
3. Fortune, W. P.: A general overview of various total knee prostheses—their relative indications. In National Academy of Sciences Report, V 101 (134), SRS-500-75-001 and DHEW No. 105-76-4103:215–224, pp. 350–359. National Academy of Sciences, Washington, D.C., September, 1974.
4. Fortune, W. P.: The Indiana conservative total hip; a review of 50 cases with a three year experience. Paper presented before the American Academy of Orthopaedic Surgeons, Atlanta, Georgia, February, 1980.
5. Fortune, W. P., and Adams, J. P.: Geometric total knee arthroplasties: A report of fifty cases. In *The Knee Joint,* pp. 251–260. International Congress Series, Excerpta Medica, Amsterdam, 1974.
6. Freeman, M. A. R.: Total replacement of the knee. Orthop. Rev. 3:2–25, 1974.
7. Gluck, T.: Referat uber die Durach das moderne Chirugische Experiment. Arch. Klin. Chir. 41:186–193, 1891.
8. Gunston, F. H.: Polycentric knee arthroplasty. J. Bone Joint Surg. 53B:272–277, 1971.
9. Harris, W. H.: A new approach to total hip replacement without osteotomy of the greater trochanter. Clin. Orthop. 106:19–26, 1975.
10. Ranawat, C. S., and Shine, J. J.: Duocondylar total knee arthroplasty. Clin. Orthop. 94:185–191, 1973.
11. Salvati, E. A.: One-stage bilateral total hip replacement. Orthop. Rev. 9(5):143–147, 1980.
12. Samuelson, K. M., Tuke, M. A., and Freeman, M. A. R.: A replacement arthroplasty for the three articular surfaces of the ankle utilising a posterior approach. J. Bone Joint Surg. 59B:376–377, 1977.
13. Stauffer, R.: Personal communication.
14. Walldius, B.: Arthroplasty of the knee using an endoprosthesis. Acta Orthop. Scand. 24:43–51, 1957.
15. Waugh, T. R., Evanski, P. M., and McMaster, W. C.: Irvine ankle arthroplasty: Design, operative technique and preliminary results. J. Bone Joint Surg. 58A:729, 1976.
16. Welch, R. B., and Charnley, J.: Low friction arthroplasty of the hip in rheumatoid arthritis and ankylosing spondylitis. Clin. Orthop. 72:22–32, 1970.

37

Benign and Malignant Musculoskeletal Tumors

Dempsey S. Springfield, M.D.
William F. Enneking, M.D.

REHABILITATION AND TREATMENT

Rehabilitation of the patient with a musculoskeletal tumor begins as soon as the physician suspects the diagnosis. Usually the patient is yet to be disabled, and the degree of disability will be determined by the treatment of the tumor. Through a well-planned evaluation and treatment program, the patient's disability may be kept at a minimum without compromising accepted tumor surgery techniques. A well-thought out approach to the patient, the patient's family, the evaluation and diagnosis of the tumor, and the final treatment program can mean the difference between a productive individual and a debilitated one. Mismanagement of any aspect of the patient's treatment may lead to an unnecessary handicap. This chapter describes methods of evaluating and treating patients with musculoskeletal tumors that attempt to maximize the patient's function yet not compromise necessary tumor therapy. Following the necessary treatment and the incumbent loss of function, standard specific rehabilitative programs should be instituted, as discussed in other chapters of this volume.

Until the last ten years, patients with cancer, including musculoskeletal malignancies, had been largely categorized as totally disabled. The poor prognosis and commonly performed amputative surgery created an aura that precluded these patients from being returned to the productive society. This trend is changing. The public is beginning to accept patients with cancer, even those who are incurable, back into society. The physician is recognizing the importance of making the most of the life these patients have remaining, and many patients whose diagnosis was once associated with almost certain death can now expect a better than even chance for survival. Most rehabilitative efforts for the patient with musculoskeletal malignancy have concentrated on the post-treatment period. However, the most effective rehabilitation begins before treating the tumor. Waiting until treatment has been instituted may markedly reduce the eventual functional capabilities of the patient.

The team approach to rehabilitating patients with musculoskeletal tumors is required. Recent advances in chemotherapy provide the physician an added therapeutic modality. Radiation therapy techniques have improved and must be considered in the treatment plan of each patient. An aggressive surgical approach to pulmonary metastases has significantly prolonged life and should not be overlooked in the overall management of the patient. The psychiatrist, psychologist, and social worker should be included, as well as the occupational and physical therapists. All of these individuals can assist the primary physician in planning for and treating the patient. When each member of the team has an opportunity to offer recommendations, the success of rehabilitation is greatly increased.

Early Referrals to Centers

Patients with suspected or proved musculoskeletal tumors should be treated in a center specializing in this area. Musculoskeletal tumors are uncommon, and the practicing physician who sees only an occasional musculoskeletal tumor should not be expected to treat these patients. Usually the history, physical examination, and x-rays provide sufficient information to justify a referral to a center for treating musculoskeletal tumors. Patients with suspected tumors, benign or malignant, should be referred prior to biopsy. More often than not, the surgical plan is affected by the initial biopsy as much as by the histological diagnosis, and often the biopsy precludes surgical excision without ablation. A biopsy should not be performed prior to a thorough evaluation; indeed, it should be the final diagnostic test before definitive therapy, since there is evidence to suggest that a delay between biopsy and definitive surgery reduces the patient's chance of survival. For these reasons, all patients with suspected musculoskeletal tumors should be referred before biopsy.

Psychosocial Aspects of Care

The physician caring for the patient with a tumor is faced with two relationships and two, often opposing, demands. The physician develops a personal relationship with the patient and must gain the patient's trust. He must also develop a relationship with the patient's tumor. These two relationships often provide conflicting situations because adequate treatment of the tumor often requires ablative surgical resection in an otherwise active, healthy person. It is only with careful integration of these two relationships that optimal rehabilitation is achieved. Proper treatment of the patient demands adequate treatment of the tumor. The challenge is to assist the patient before the operation in accepting the necessary treatment, planning the least disabling adequate treatment program, and providing a postoperative program that will allow the patient to retain maximum function.

Developing the proper relationship with the patient and the patient's family is crucial to the success of the treatment program. The physician must understand the patient's perspective and desires and the patient must trust the physician and accept his advice. Honesty is the best means of gaining the patient's trust. Keep the family and patient informed of the results of tests and the status of the evaluation to provide peace of mind to the patient. Keep the treatment options open until the diagnostic evaluation is complete, and finally discuss fully the situation and therapy options with the patient and family. Allow the patient to take part in the decision-making process. Some patients prefer amputation and early prosthetic replacement to the prolonged healing process of limb-saving procedures, whereas others are willing to endure a long period of convalescence to preserve an extremity or joint function. Inclusion of the patient in the treatment program is the best method of assuring full cooperation in the post-therapy rehabilitative program. The physician should not expect the patient to be an active participant only after treatment has been accomplished.

Evaluating the Tumor

Thorough evaluation of the tumor is required before formulating a treatment plan. The physician should systematically examine the tumor and its relationship to the patient prior to surgical manipulation. A biopsy done prior to diagnostic tests may alter the results and undermine an accurate reading. A complete history, physical examination, screening x-rays of the tumor, chest x-ray, and routine laboratory work are the minimal prebiopsy requirements. The additions of [99]technetium bone scanning, arteriography, computerized axial tomography, and routine tomography of the tumor or chest are necessary to characterize and localize the tumor accurately.[2,8] Once the tumor has been thoroughly evaluated, a differential diagnosis is established; then treatment alternatives are discussed.

The biopsy should be performed following this evaluation, and, whenever practical, definitive surgical therapy completed under the same anesthetic. This reduces the potential for contaminating the wound with tumor cells and eliminates the patient's agonizing period of waiting between confirmation of the diagnosis and the operation.

Planning the biopsy is crucial to the treatment of the patient. Examples of poorly positioned incisions, inadequate tissue, and other complications of biopsy procedures justify the adage, "the attending physician should perform the biopsy, and the resident the definitive surgery." Poorly placed biopsy incisions may preclude limb-saving surgery or appreciably increase the risk of a postoperative error. All tissue contaminated at the time of biopsy must be removed en bloc with the tumor. If the biopsy is made without regard to the subsequent definitive surgery, a great deal of tissue can be unnecessarily compromised. An *incisional* biopsy should be performed when the physician suspects a malignant tumor, or when he is not sure of the diagnosis. An *excisional* biopsy should be performed when the physician is confident the tumor is benign and excision is indicated.

Although inclusion of the patient in the decision-making process is of primary importance, the postoperative functional status of the patient should not compromise the treatment of the tumor. When amputation is indicated, the physician should have developed the patient's trust to the point that amputation can be accepted. The physician should not let his sympathy with the patient interfere with adequate tumor surgery. Adequate removal of the tumor is the first priority—reconstructing the defect resulting from the excision is the second. The excision should not be compromised to improve function. In many instances, prosthetic replacement of a limb offers better function than would a limb-salvaging procedure that carries a greater risk of recurrence.

Surgery

Up to the day of surgery, the rehabilitative program for the patient with a musculoskeletal tumor, benign or malignant, is similar. Once surgery has been performed, patients are separated into categories depending on the type of reconstruction rather than upon their diagnosis. The categories of tumor removal are: incisional biopsy, marginal excision, wide excision, and radical resection.[10] The reconstruction after one of these operations varies according to the exact anatomical location of the tumor. The postoperative rehabilitation is a function of both the type of surgical excision and type of reconstruction.

Incisional biopsy is the removal of a portion of the tumor, with some of the tumor left in the wound. It may be either a preliminary diagnostic maneuver leading to the definitive surgical procedure or the only surgical procedure for tumors treated by nonsurgical means. Examples of the latter are Ewing's sarcoma, reticulum cell sarcoma, and metastatic carcinoma. Careful planning of the skin incision placement and the tissue to be removed includes consideration of the consequences of biopsy. Incisional biopsy of soft tissue tumors rarely produces significant functional impairment and does not require formal postoperative rehabilitation. The removal of bone for biopsy, on the other hand, leads to significant reduction in strength.[1] The reduction should be carefully assessed and steps taken to protect the bone from fracture. Whenever possible, biopsies should be done on the soft tissue component of the tumor. When cortical bone must be removed, it should be obtained from the surface with the least compressive or tensile forces. The upper extremity usually requires only immobilization via a sling, but protection of the lower extremity may require non-weight-bearing on crutches, plaster protection, brace protection, internal fixation, or a combination of these. The appropriate protection is easily provided if considered prior to fracture. Active exercise for the biopsied limb should begin in the postoperative period.

Marginal excision is the en bloc removal of the tumor by dissection about the pseudocapsule. Microscopic disease is left in the wound if the tumor is malignant or locally invasive, but excision is adequate if the tumor is benign. Benign tumors are better treated by marginal excision rather than intracapsular excision or curettage if they require removal. Marginal excision of a benign soft tissue tumor rarely, if ever, produces a significant functional deficit, and patients can be expected to return to their preoperative status. Marginal excision of bone tumors may require surgical reconstruction and physical rehabilitation. The reconstruction following marginal excision is usually a graft of the bone defect. Small cortical defects may be grafted with iliac bone graft, the bone protected for two to four months, and the patient should be able to return to his preoperative state. Large cortical defects and defects in anatomical sites exposed to large stresses require more mechanical strength than that furnished by an iliac bone graft. Cortical grafts of the tibia fibula provide excellent mechanical strength after they are internally repaired.[4]

Additional support may be provided by metallic devices or methyl methacrylate. Postoperative protection is required for varying lengths of time, depending on the nature and extent of the defect. A cortical graft weakens as it undergoes creeping substitution, and the bone should be protected for two years.[3] Fatigue fractures of long grafts are common, but they heal spontaneously.[3] In the lower extremity, a long leg, ischial weight-bearing, drop-lock brace will protect grafts. When marginal excision removes part or all of a joint, arthrodesis and hemiarthroplasty are the treatment alternatives, and standard rehabilitative procedures are followed.

Wide excision is the en bloc removal of the tumor along with a surrounding cuff of normal tissue. It is the treatment of choice for locally aggressive benign tumors (recurrent giant cell tumor or fibromatosis) or low-grade malignancies (parosteal osteosarcoma, low-grade chondrosarcoma, or grade 1 fibrosarcoma). Reconstruction following wide excision may vary from minimal for small, soft tissue tumors located within a muscle, to amputation, for a tumor involving major vessels and nerve. Planning a wide excision and reconstruction usually requires thorough preoperative staging and consideration of many types of reconstruction.

Radical resection is the en bloc removal of the tumor and the entire anatomical compartment in which the tumor is confined. High-grade malignant tumors that require radical removal usually need amputation, but occasionally in well-selected cases a limb-saving procedure can be performed. Because the reconstructive procedures following wide excision and radical resection are similar, they will be discussed together.

The initial aspect to consider in selecting from various methods of reconstruction following wide or radical tumor removal is the patient's overall status. Young patients with "curable" disease are willing and should be encouraged to invest the postoperative time required in realizing the benefits of a limb-saving procedure. Older patients with limited life spans or patients with metastatic disease who are receiving palliative surgery may be better served by amputation and prosthetic replacement. Patients with upper extremity lesions should be encouraged along the lines of excision or resection and reconstruction rather than amputation because of the usual superior function compared to prosthesis. Even those patients with a flail shoulder, flail elbow, or a neurologically compromised extremity function better than do current upper extremity prostheses. Each patient presents a unique challenge, but some principles have been formed through the years.

Excision or resection of tumors about the shoulder girdle is often accomplished without ablation of the extremity. As long as the brachial plexus is not within the resection plane, function of the upper extremity can usually be maintained. Tumors of the scapula can be successfully managed with a scapulectomy.

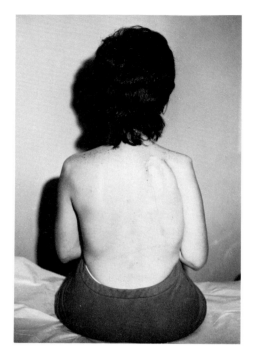

Fig. 37-1. A 31-year-old woman after a scapulectomy for a low-grade fibrosarcoma. The cosmesis is not excellent, but the patient has about half the normal active shoulder flexion, extension, and abduction.

In Figure 37-1, the patient has an unstable shoulder and the cosmesis is not excellent, but abduction to 60 degrees, forward flexion to 45 degrees, and full rotation of the humerus with a normally functioning hand are appreciably better than would be possible with a prosthesis. Resection of the shoulder joint is best reconstructed by using fibular grafts to obtain an arthrodesis to the remaining scapula (Fig. 37-2). Patients with an arthrodesis have significantly better function than those who develop a pseudoarthrosis. Arthrodeses of the elbow or wrist are superior to amputation or pseudoarthroses.

Pelvic tumors are often resectable without ablation. A classification of the types of resection with options for reconstruction has been published.[5] Function is best when arthrodesis is accomplished between the proximal femur and remaining pelvis (Fig. 37-3). Reconstruction following wide segmental excision of diaphyseal

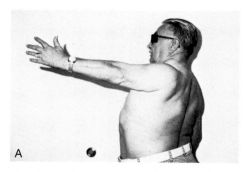
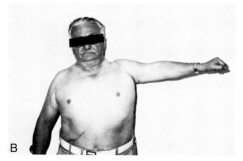

Figs. 37-2A,B. A 56-year-old patient after resection of acromion, glenoid, humeral head, and adjacent soft tissue for a chondrosarcoma. Reconstruction consisted of arthrodesis of remaining humerus to scapula. Function is excellent.

tumors is possible without amputation (Fig. 37-4). The grafted extremity must be protected for at least two years, and to achieve successful rehabilitation the patient must be willing to invest this time. Tumors about the knee may be successfully managed by resection and arthrodesis[6] (Fig. 37-5), a commonly performed procedure because of the propensity of musculoskeletal tumors to be located in the distal femur or proximal tibia. The patients are usually fully weight bearing in a long leg brace by six months and free of the brace by two years. Once the cortical bone grafts are internally repaired, the patient is completely functional within the limits of a knee fusion. Patients with tumors below the proximal tibia that require wide or radical removal are usually best reconstructed with standard below-knee prostheses.

Soft tissue tumors offer a special challenge.[10] Motor deficits produced by nerve resection can be compensated for through tendon transfers. The principles established through the experience gained in reconstructions of patients with poliomyelitis are directly applicable to postoperative reconstructions of patients after soft tissue tumor excision or resection. Function lost following the resection of the radial and ulnar nerves in the upper extremity and the common peroneal nerve in the lower extremity may be replaced through the use of standard bracing

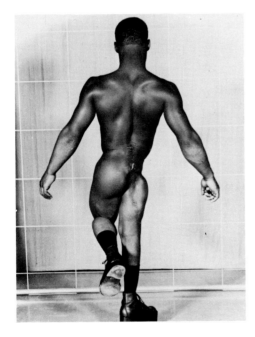

Fig. 37-3. This 17-year-old male underwent a pelvic resection for a low-grade fibrosarcoma. Despite a shortened lower extremity, function is excellent, with an arthrodesis of pubis to femoral shaft. Reprinted with permission from Enneking, W. F., and Dunham, W. K.: Resection and reconstruction for primary neoplasms involving the innominate bone. J. Bone Joint Surg. 60A(6):745, 1978.

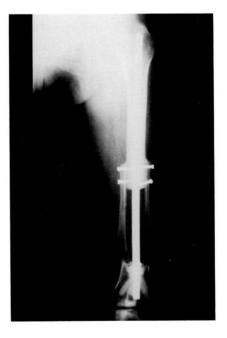

Fig. 37-4. The x-ray of a 37-year-old woman's femur after a resection of the distal diaphysis for an intraosseous chondrosarcoma. Dual cortical grafts with intramedullary fixation constitute a satisfactory method of reconstructing segmental shaft resections.

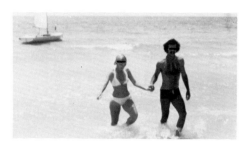

Fig. 37-5. This 25-year-old woman is standing on the leg reconstructed with a resection arthrodesis of the knee after wide excision of a recurrent giant cell tumor.

or surgery. The need for inclusion of the sciatic nerve in the resection of a tumor does not automatically indicate the need for amputation. In selected patients, a flail, partially anesthetic, and braced lower extremity functions better than does a hip disarticulation prosthesis. The rehabilitative challenge in orthopedic oncology is in planning and performing adequate tumor surgery while maintaining maximal functional potential.

Patients with musculoskeletal tumors treated by radiation and/or chemotherapy require the rehabilitative services of the orthopedist. Through physical therapy programs, patients receiving radiation therapy can maintain excellent function

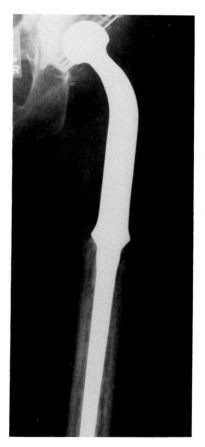

Fig. 37-6. This x-ray is of a custom-made acetabular and proximal femur replacement. At present, this prosthetic reconstruction is most effective in the hip. Future developments should make either allograft or prosthetic replacement of other major joints clinically practical and reliable.

of their irradiated part. Patients with pathological fractures are best managed with immediate internal fixation to prevent the complications of inactivity and morbidity of non-union.[7] The orthopedic surgeon should strive to keep the tumor patient, even one with metastatic disease, mobile.

The tumor amputee should be treated just like the amputee whose cause was not malignant. A better prognosis has been found among patients whose amputations were the result of tumor surgery compared to those whose amputations were due to the complications of atherosclerosis.[9] Usually, the tumor amputee is young and robust. Although adjuvant chemotherapy produces weight and mood fluctuations, well-motivated patients can benefit by early fitting of standard prostheses.

FUTURE DIRECTIONS

Future directions in rehabilitating patients with malignant musculoskeletal tumors fall into three categories. Currently, surgery remains the primary treatment. The improved survival rates are based on adequate surgical removal of the primary tumor combined with adjuvant chemotherapy that suppresses the micrometastasis so often present at the time of surgery. Advances in adjuvant therapy should someday reduce the need for radical surgery. Certainly, with respect to soft tissue tumors, this hope is being realized.[11] The second category is in the development of improved implantable devices to replace surgically excised tissue. These implants may be metal, ceramic, plastic, or allograft, and we hope that the surgeon will be able to replace increasingly large defects and complex joints with a high degree of success in the future (Fig. 37-6). Thirdly, prosthetic replacements for both the upper and lower extremities require improvements. Functional myoelectric prostheses that provide sensory feedback will be available soon. Of special concern is the hip disarticulation prosthesis, which is currently unacceptable, yet commonly required by the tumor amputee.

CONCLUSIONS

Rehabilitation of the patient after musculoskeletal tumor surgery is unique in that the physician has the opportunity to plan prospectively for reconstruction of the deficit and to favorably influence the ultimate functional capabilities of the patient. Through thorough preoperative evaluation and carefully planned tumor surgery, patients can be rehabilitated effectively. Every effort should be made to include these patients in integrated postoperative rehabilitative programs so as not to segregate them from other patients requiring rehabilitation.

REFERENCES

1. Burstein, A. H., Curvey, J., Frankel, V. H., et al.: Bone strength. The effect of screw holes. J. Bone Joint Surg. 54A:1143–1156, 1972.
2. Chew, F., Hudson, T. M., and Springfield, D. S.: Unpublished data.
3. Eady, J.: Unpublished data.

4. Enneking, W. F., Burchardt, H., Puhl, J. J., and Piotrowski, G.: Physical and biological aspects of repair in dog cortical bone transplants. J. Bone Joint Surg. 57A:237–252, 1975.

5. Enneking, W. F., and Dunham, W. K.: Resection and reconstruction for primary neoplasms involving the innominate bone. J. Bone Joint Surg. 60A:731–746, 1978.

6. Enneking, W. F., and Shirley, P. D.: Resection arthrodesis for malignant and potentially malignant lesions about the knee using an intramedullary rod and local bone grafts. J. Bone Joint Surg. 59A:223–236, 1977.

7. Harrington, K. D., Sim, F. H., Enis, J. E., et al.: Methylmethacrylate as an adjunct in internal fixation of pathological fractures. J. Bone Joint Surg. 58A:1047–1055, 1976.

8. Hudson, T. M., Haas, G., Enneking, W. F., and Hawkins, I. F., Jr.: Angiography in the management of musculoskeletal tumors. Surg. Gynecol. Obstet. 141:11–21, 1975.

9. Pritchard, D.: Personal communication.

10. Simon, M. A., and Enneking, W. F.: The management of soft tissues sarcomas of the extremities. J. Bone Joint Surg. 58A:317–327, 1976.

11. Suit, H. D., Russell, W. O., and Martin, R. G.: Management of patients with sarcoma of soft tissue in an extremity. Cancer 31:1247–1255, 1973.

Index

Page numbers followed by f represent figures; page numbers followed by t represent tables.